The Native American Herbalist's Bible

7-in-1 Companion to Herbal Medicine

The Only Gardener and Forager Guide to Native Herbs and Wildflowers You'll Ever Need to Craft Traditional Herbal Remedies

Linda Osceola Naranjo

Disclaimer

The publisher and the author are providing this book and its contents on an "as is" basis and make no representations or warranties of any kind with respect to this book or its contents. The publisher and the author disclaim all such representations and warranties, including but not limited to warranties of healthcare for a particular purpose. In addition, the publisher and the author assume no responsibility for errors, inaccuracies, omissions, or any other inconsistencies herein.

The content of this book is for informational purposes only and is not intended to diagnose, treat, cure, or prevent any condition or disease. You understand that this book is not intended as a substitute for consultation with a licensed practitioner. Please consult with your own physician or healthcare specialist regarding the suggestions and recommendations made in this book. The use of this book implies your acceptance of this disclaimer.

The publisher and the author make no guarantees concerning the level of success you may experience by following the advice and strategies contained in this book, and you accept the risk that results will differ for each individual. The testimonials and examples provided in this book show exceptional results, which may not apply to the average reader, and are not intended to represent or guarantee that you will achieve the same or similar results.

First Printing Edition, 2021

Printed in the United States of America
Available from Amazon.com and other retail outlets

Table of Contents

The Native American Herbalist's Bible 1

The Forgotten Art of The Ancestors of Medicine

Traditional Herbalism, Modern Methods, and Spiritual Practice for the Medicine Man of the 21st Century

Linda Osceola Naranjo

Introduction

"Everything on the earth has a purpose, every disease an herb to cure it, and every person a mission. This is the Indian theory of existence."
Mourning Dove [Christine Quintasket] (1888-1936) Salish

W e live in a country where the cure for virtually any disease and ailment is within our grasp. In our forests, meadows, plains, and gardens grow small, seemingly insignificant flowers and herbs, plants that we don't look twice at, and trees of which we don't even bother to learn the name. Yet, they are the key to a better, healthier, and more sustainable way of life.

Our forefathers, more attuned with nature than we could ever imagine to be, understood that, and took carefully and sparingly the gifts that Nature offered to heal themselves and grow stronger.

We have lost that knowledge.

Only starting from the 1970s, a renewed interest in botanic medicine has uncovered the depth of the Native American knowledge of plants and their healing powers. The research has not only helped herbalists, but physicians and scientist as well that re-discovered substances that the Native Americans people knew about for hundreds of years.

This book is the extended edition of the best-selling *The Native American Herbalist's Bible: 3-in-1 Companion to Herbal* Medicine, offering four more volumes on gardening techniques, growing healing plants and wildflowers, and pediatric healthcare.

This is the unabridged companion to Native American herbs, their traditional and modern use, complete with appropriate doses and usage, gardening tips and techniques for both medicinal plants and wildflowers. The book is completed by a list of simple and effective recipes for the most common ailments for both adults and children.

You don't need to put at risk the delicate natural balance of your body and that of your loved ones by taking drugs and medications, if an easily available natural solution is just outside your door. Harvest carefully or grow your own herbs, learn to know your body and what works best for you, communicate with the nature surrounding you, and you will in a small way bring back a culture that for too long has been treated as inferior.

This book will teach how to find and treat the herbs the way the native American tribes did: from the forest to your herbalist table, but you will have to find your way to listen to your body and the plants around you.
To aid you in your holistic journey, we have decided to divide the book in seven handy volumes.

This first volume will give you a full theoretical approach to Native American medicine and the herbal medicines methods and preparations.

The second volume is a complete encyclopedia of all the most relevant herbs used in traditional Native American medicine, complete with modern examples, doses, and where to find them, making it a very effective field guide.

The third volume is a "recipe book" of sorts: it offers easy herbal solutions to the most common diseases a budding naturopath can encounter. It is meant as a jumping point to find your own way to treat yourself and your fellow man and will come in handy even to the most experienced herbalist.

The fourth volume provides a complete theoretical and practical approach to Native American traditional planting techniques and how they can be implemented in modern gardens.

The fifth volume is the native gardener's almanac for medicinal herbs. Foraging is not always an option and a lot of herbs are handy to have in your garden: this volume will guide you through the herbs that you can and (should) have in your garden.

The sixth volume continues the guide to the plants you can plant in your gardens focusing on healing wildflowers, which are not only good for your health, but for the planet as well, and they are not bad on the eyes either!

The seventh volume focuses on native pediatric healthcare. Treating children is a very delicate undertaking, their physiology is more sensitive to external agents, especially drugs. Natural herbalist treatments are effective and gentle in treating common, less severe, pathologies and they won't needlessly weaken your child's immune system. The herbs listed in this last volume have been carefully researched to specifically treat children and their ailments, avoiding any allergic reaction and boosting their immune system.

I am happy to guide through a life-changing journey in search of lost knowledge, amazing healing plants, and carefully crafted herbal remedies and I hope it will help you nurture a stronger relationship with the nature surrounding us and the many gifts it bestows upon us.

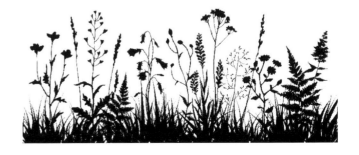

Native American Medicine and Modern Uses

S ince the 1970s and ever more so today, there is a growing interest in the medicinal uses of herbs and plants for complementary medicine in the U.S. Particularly, both amateur herbalists, professional healers, and physicians, have become aware of the use of herbs by Native American medicine. Many of the botanicals sold as dietary supplements today, have been used for centuries for the same purposes by Native American societies.

However, the commercialized supplements represent only a small fraction of the more the 2500 different plant species that have been discovered and used for their medicinal properties by Native Americans. We shall focus on the most common plants and their properties. This book is meant as an introduction to the native American herbal medicine and this chapter provides a brief explanation to the capital importance of the discoveries made by indigenous inhabitants of the North American continent for modern medicine.

It's an interesting perspective for an amateur or novice herbalist to know the history of the plants he/she wants to use both in traditional medical practices, as well as the current use in modern medicine and drugs.
However, if you want to jump right into the herbal dispensatory, you may skip this chapter and read on the basics of herbology in the next chapter and on the plants themselves in the second volume.

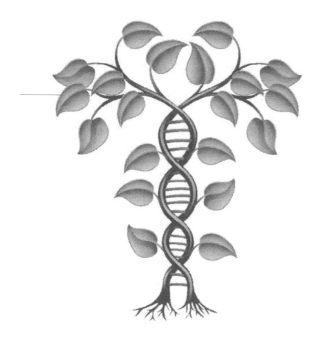

Brief introduction on Native American medicine

For centuries, Native Americans have harnessed the medicinal power of herbs. While written records of their herbal practices emerged only after the arrival of European explorers and their interactions with tribes like the Wampanoag, it is unfortunate that no pre-contact written accounts exist to precisely trace the origins of herbal healing among Native Americans.

As European colonists settled in the New World and pioneers traversed the plains, Native Americans generously imparted their knowledge of utilizing nature's medicines to promote well-being. This exchange of wisdom has bestowed upon us a rich legacy of healing. Remarkably, it is believed that at least two hundred of our present-day prescription drugs have their roots in Native American herbal remedies.

Presently, both synthetic reproductions of natural herbal compounds and the herbs themselves contribute to a plethora of over-the-counter medicines. As we delve into the subsequent subchapter, we will explore how Native American herbs have gained widespread commercialization as health supplements.

The indigenous peoples of America lived in symbiotic harmony with their surroundings, relying on the forests, plains, and coastal regions for sustenance. In various regions, they utilized wild plant species as sources of food. When weather and season permitted, a diverse array of game and fish served not only as sustenance but also as materials for clothing, tools, and adornments.

During springtime, people eagerly gathered various types of berries. Berries were highly valued for their medicinal properties and were used as a tonic or for specific treatments such as hemorrhage, high fever, and convalescence.
They were known to have a beneficial effect on blood health. In the autumn, cranberries were particularly popular and were considered tonics for the blood and liver. The roots of blackberries had astringent properties, while nuts provided essential nutrition and were used in nut breads or crushed for nut milks. Acorn and dandelion roots were roasted, pounded, and sprinkled over cooked roots to add flavor.

Pond lily roots were widely recognized as a food source across the continent, stretching from eastern Canada to the Pacific coast. Milkweed roots, collected with the morning dew still on the leaves, were used to prepare a unique root sugar that also held cultural significance. Some leaves and the white portions of hardwood ashes were used to produce salt. These natural alternatives added a diverse range of flavors and seasonings to their culinary practices.

In preparation for winter, apples, other fruits, and vegetables were stored in barrels or buried in pits. Some were sliced, strung together, and dried for future consumption.

Yucca leaves and Quillaja bark were used as natural alternatives for soap and shampoo. While the traditional indigenous way of life may have faded, it's important to acknowledge that many elements were adopted and assimilated by European colonizers. This included the cultivation of crops such as corn, squash, pumpkins, and tobacco, as well as the use of canoes and snowshoes. There also exists an idealized perception, only partially understood, of what represents the Native American way of life.

Our ancestors believed that the happiest state for a human is when their food is also their medicine. The Native American people were once in complete harmony with this belief, incorporating it into their daily lives in numerous ways.

Native American tribes acquired their knowledge of medicinal herbs through empirical means, often relying on trial and error. They would administer an herb to a patient, and if there was a noticeable improvement, that herb might be employed again. It is important to note that the application of herbs was not solely based on empirical evidence but also on the observation of a plant's color, shape, odor, and taste.

These characteristics played a significant role in determining the herb's intended use. For instance, red-colored plants were associated with promoting blood health, while yellow plants were employed in treating jaundice.

In cases where plants resembled the liver in appearance, they were believed to possess properties beneficial for addressing liver-related issues. This approach, known as the "doctrine of signatures," can be found in the traditional healing practices of various cultures. It revolves around the belief that a plant's physical attributes can offer clues about its therapeutic benefits.

An intriguing example illustrating the doctrine of signatures is ginseng (*Panax quinquefolium*). Due to its shape resembling male genitalia, it was traditionally used as an aphrodisiac and to enhance sexual potency. Native American tribes along the East Coast, including the Delaware, specifically utilized ginseng to promote male fertility.

It is also worth mentioning that visions and dreams played a significant role in guiding the use of herbs for specific conditions. Medicine men, in particular, might experiment with certain herbal medicines or combinations after receiving knowledge or guidance in a dream. Additionally, another frequently employed method for discovering herbs involved observing animals to discern which plants they consumed, as this provided valuable insights into potential medicinal properties.

Through these diverse approaches, Native American tribes accumulated a wealth of knowledge regarding the healing properties of herbs. Their understanding was rooted in careful observations of nature, and their deep connection to the natural world informed their practices and contributed to their profound expertise as healers.

From the earliest encounters, Europeans were deeply impressed by the remarkable vitality and stamina exhibited by Native Americans across different regions. Artists and photographers of that era consistently depicted them as alert, courageous, strong, and, in many ethnic groups, possessing a striking standard of beauty. Technical studies conducted later further confirmed their exceptional physical endurance. Archaeological evidence often fails to uncover bone deficiencies, cavities, arthritis, tuberculosis, and other ailments commonly found in modern times. Another perspective, gleaned from studies of early travelers and missionaries, reveals that Native Americans displayed robust health and relatively low disease prevalence.

Among the limited records available, only around eighty-seven different illnesses are mentioned. In their time, occurrences of cancer, tuberculosis, and heart conditions, which have become prevalent in our era, were infrequent. This figure of eighty-seven illnesses pales in comparison to our modern catalog of over 30,000 diseases, a number that continues to expand with each passing day.

Native American women often assumed the dual roles of mother and doctor during childbirth and resuming their daily activities within a few hours, following in the footsteps of their mothers before them.

In fact, the indigenous people of America were their own physicians in more ways than one. While civilization has led us to build empires around life insurance companies, medical research, welfare systems, and organizations for the elderly, Native Americans relied on nature for their protection and healing. They understood how to utilize the plant life around them to treat various ailments—it was medicine derived from the earth itself.

However, with the arrival of the white man, Native Americans were abruptly exposed to a new way of life that brought with it diseases against which they had not developed immunity. This led to the tragic loss of thousands of lives. Their self-sufficiency was shattered as they became dependent on the ways of civilization.

Despite these challenges, Native Americans never lost their profound knowledge of which plants were most beneficial and the optimal time for gathering them to achieve the most effective cures. They possessed exceptional skills in treating physical, surgical, and obstetric conditions, surpassing what modern medical teachings have come to offer. Their expertise in the healing arts was a testament to their deep connection with nature and the wisdom passed down through generations.

Vapor baths were widely employed by Native American healers to address a range of ailments. Patients would enter sweat lodges, where they would experience intense heat and moisture, promoting the elimination of toxins from their bodies. For treating fractured bones, splints made of several rods tied together at the ends were utilized. These splints were then covered with leaves and bound with deer skins. In cases of severe cuts and sprains, finely pounded herb roots were applied as poultices. Additionally, a wash made from an infusion of a specific root was used to treat sore eyes. Interestingly, substances derived from the coca plant, such as cocaine and Novocain, were employed by Native American healers to alleviate pain.

The Native American art of healing was deeply ceremonial in nature. Although their rituals may appear unfamiliar and lacking in meaning to us, they recognized that physical health often required spiritual support. Dancing, chanting, and other rituals were conducted in accordance with the condition or severity of the patient. In present times, our gestures of support, such as get-well cards, entertainment, flowers, and prayers, may be less physically oriented but are given with the same intention—to uplift the spirit. Their profound connection between health and spirituality was intertwined with their close relationship with the natural world, finding inspiration in the significance of nature, the Sun, Moon, Stars, Rain, Wind, and other elements that encouraged well-being.

Training as a Native American healer commenced at an early age, often through familial selection or signs of devotion, wisdom, and honesty. It was more than just a career; the healer was chosen based on their abilities. Trusted with the sacred secrets, rituals, traditions, and legends of their people, they attended ceremonial celebrations and critical meetings alongside the tribe's leader.

The trainee healer had to possess extensive knowledge of various herbal species, including their properties and uses. They understood their limitations and recognized that garden flowers did not hold the power to defy death. However, they knew which flowers had medicinal properties and could contribute to overall health and longevity. The healers utilized all the medicinal plants available in their region, adapting their practices to the unique flora and fauna of each locality. The principles of both modern medicine and natural healing still encompass elements such as strong steam therapy for inducing perspiration, isolation for contagious diseases, fasting for health, physiological adjustments, special diets, and, of course, the utilization of herbs.

As healers responsible for the well-being of all people, they transcended tribal restrictions and cared for the wounded and needy, embodying the principles of Hippocrates' art. Their expertise was rooted in a deep understanding of nature's offerings and their commitment to serving their communities.

The vast wealth of Native American herbal remedies is well-documented, with numerous resources attesting to their remarkable healing capabilities. Ethnobotanist Daniel A. Moerman, in his work "Native American Ethnobotany," documents an impressive 24,945 plants used therapeutically by Native Americans, highlighting their profound knowledge and utilization of the natural world.

In this book I have tried to include those herbs that have historically been used most frequently to treat the conditions listed in the third volume.

In discussing the healing herbs used by the Native Americans, the spiritual beliefs of Native American culture must first be emphasized. These beliefs are tightly, intricately, and unchangeably woven into the tapestry of a Native American's daily life.

For native people, medicine encompasses more than physical remedies like pills or surgeries. It's the combined healing of the spirit, heart, and mind. Medicine is not simply the physical cure, it's also a celebration of the greater power behind the cure.
It recognizes the interconnectedness of all aspects of a person's being and seeks to restore balance and harmony on multiple levels. Healing is a holistic journey that engages the individual's entire being and acknowledges the vital connection between humans and the natural and spiritual realms.

In addition to their medicinal and food uses, Native Americans have used the plants that grow wild in the fields and forests for weaving, dyeing, basket-making, and for making brushes, ropes, cords, pottery, and decorations. They have used herbs as hunting charms or basket charms and as flavorings and spices.

Herbs were also used in sacred ceremonies, to purify shamans, and to assist in visions and dreams. For example, the great Sioux medicine man and chief, Sitting Bull, had a vision three weeks before the Battle of Little Bighorn that all the white soldiers would fall in defeat and his people would triumph. This is, of course, exactly what happened when Custer and his men met Sitting Bull in battle.

Tobacco was one of the most important herbs for many tribes. It can have both positive and negative effects. According to the Traditional Native American Tobacco (TNAT) Seed Bank and Education Program, "When used improperly, such as when it is smoked in cigarettes, or otherwise ingested in a commercial form, tobacco is a deadly killer. When used properly, in very small amounts in traditional Native American ceremonies and prayer, tobacco (like sacramental wine in a Catholic mass) becomes a positive source of religious power." In addition to tobacco, herbs used in sacred ceremonies and pipe ceremonies include sage, lobelia, gentian, myrtle, magnolia, and slippery elm.

Herbs were of particular benefit in clearing the mind and soul and warding off evil spirits. When used in this way, herbs were often burned in smudges, bundles of herbs that are burned much like incense. Some of the most popular purifying herbs used to please the spirits and the human senses were aromatic, including cedar, juniper, mesquite, pinion, red willow, sage, and sweet grass.
Herbs were also smoked for pleasure, as well as for fighting respiratory disorders. A few herbs used for these purposes include angelica, bearberry, corn silk, coltsfoot, dogwood, deer's tongue, mullein, sumac, valerian, and yerba sante.

As mentioned earlier, herbs are used in sweat lodges to detoxify and cleanse the body. Native Americans have also used herbal mixtures in enemas to stimulate the removal of unwanted toxins through perspiration, bowel excretion, urination, or vomiting. In fact, Virgil Vogel, author of American Indian Medicine, notes that American Indians discovered the bulb syringe and the enema tube, using fish and animal bladders plus inserts constructed from reed and small hollow bones.

These Native American techniques were successfully used for centuries and are still in use today. Today, Navajo medicine leaders claim they can even cure people with cancer using routine colon cleansing and fasting, accompanied by sweating.

Enemas used by the Native Americans discarded undesirable toxins trapped in the intestines and worked metaphorically as a way to purify the body in a spiritual sense. Maintenance of a healthy colon is essential for optimal body balance.

The Native Americans have also used herbal laxatives to purge deadly toxins and as a preventive measure against illness. Enemas can be administered at home, or colonic therapy can be performed under the guidance of a trained chiropractor or naturopath.

Although there is a wealth of herbal knowledge present within the culture of American Indians, it is not always easy to encourage Native Americans to part with their herbal secrets. Many feel that Native Americans have been exploited enough through the centuries, and they do not want to perpetuate that exploitation. Others believe that the power of their healing systems might be weakened by sharing them with non-Indians, who might misrepresent the techniques. Many of the sacred songs and healing rituals were passed on during vision quests or initiations into secret societies; so naturally, Native Americans are not comfortable sharing this fragile, sacred information with those who might alter it or abuse it—especially when most who hold the knowledge had to undergo so much in order to attain it.

However, I strongly believe that sharing Native American healing secrets with non-Native Americans is the only way to keep them alive and protect them from extinction. This, then, is my goal: to celebrate the greatness of the Native American herbal healing traditions and to share this information with you so that you can take charge of your life for better health.

The healing properties of herbs

For centuries, Native Americans have used whole herbs for the treatment of disease; and while they knew that the herbs worked, it wasn't always known why. For example, teas of pine needles or rose hips were used to cure colds or flu. As we now know, it was the vitamin C and bioflavonoids in the pine needles and rose hips that possessed the healing action.
Today, science is identifying the healing properties contained in herbs, including vitamins, minerals, enzymes, and phytochemicals.

PHYTOCHEMICALS
Phytochemicals, the bioactive compounds found in plants, offer a plethora of positive effects on human health. These plant nutrients can be isolated and concentrated from herbs and other plants.
Flavonoids, for instance, have been linked to reduced risk of heart disease and certain types of cancers, while carotenoids, such as lycopene and beta-carotene, have been associated with promoting eye health and supporting a strong immune system. Phenolic acids, another group of phytochemicals, exhibit potent antioxidant properties that help combat cellular damage caused by free radicals, potentially lowering the risk of chronic diseases like diabetes and neurodegenerative disorders.
Following are some of the phytochemicals found in many of the herbs used by American Indians over the centuries.

Alkaloids

Alkaloids, remarkable compounds found in various Native American plants, including goldenseal and Oregon grape root, offer a wide range of positive effects on human health. These bioactive substances have been harnessed for centuries in traditional medicine due to their potent pharmacological properties. Alkaloids have shown promising results in providing pain relief, managing respiratory conditions, and even combating certain diseases by preventing yeast overgrowth, maintaining healthy bacteria in the gastrointestinal and urinary tracts, and supporting immune function. They serve as the foundation for numerous pharmaceutical drugs, highlighting their immense therapeutic potential. Ongoing research continues to unveil the incredible benefits that alkaloids can bring to human well-being, opening doors to new possibilities in natural medicine.

Anthocyanidins

Anthocyanidins, naturally occurring compounds found in bilberries, black currants, and raspberries, provide a wide range of health benefits. These plant-based compounds possess potent antioxidant properties, combating free radicals that contribute to degenerative diseases such as cardiovascular disease and cancer. Additionally, anthocyanidins support cardiovascular health by reducing plaque formation in blood vessels and promoting optimal blood flow. They also exhibit anti-inflammatory properties, aiding in the fight against inflammation and reducing the risk of edema. Furthermore, anthocyanidins have been associated with potential improvements in vision.

Chlorophyll

Chlorophyll, found in all green herbs, offers a range of health benefits. It exhibits antibacterial properties, aids in the healing of burns and wounds, and shows potential in fighting cancer. Additionally, chlorophyll serves as a good source of vitamin K. Its presence in green herbs highlights its potential contributions to overall health and well-being.

Diterpenes

Diterpenes, present in numerous herbs including rosemary, possess remarkable properties that contribute to health benefits. These compounds exhibit potent antioxidant effects, combat oxidative stress, and show potential as anticancer agents by inhibiting the growth and spread of cancer cells. Additionally, diterpenes are known for their anti-liver-toxin properties, supporting liver health.

Eleutherosides

Eleutherosides, a group of bioactive compounds found in Eleutherococcus senticosus, commonly known as Siberian ginseng or eleuthero, offer a wide array of positive effects on human health. These adaptogenic substances have been traditionally used in native herbal medicine for their potential to enhance physical and mental performance, boost energy levels, and support the body's ability to adapt to stress. Eleutherosides have also been associated with improved cognitive function, immune system modulation, and overall vitality. With their remarkable adaptogenic properties, eleutherosides hold promise as natural allies in promoting resilience, vitality, and well-being.

Essential Fatty Acids

Essential fatty acids, such as omega-3 and omega-6 fatty acids, are vital fats that are necessary for overall well-being, but cannot be produced by the body. They play a crucial role in maintaining the integrity of cell membranes and protecting the myelin sheaths that cover nerve fibers.

These fatty acids also promote the production of prostaglandins, which are hormone-like substances involved in various bodily functions such as metabolism, smooth-muscle activity, and nerve transmission. Additionally, they contribute to lowering blood cholesterol levels and enhancing the immune system. Many herbs, including saw palmetto, contain these essential fatty acids.

Flavonglycosides

Flavonglycosides possess potent antioxidant properties, effectively combating free radicals. These compounds also have the ability to dilate blood vessels, enhancing blood flow throughout the body. Additionally, flavonglycosides contribute to improved mental clarity, vision, and hearing. They have also shown potential in alleviating symptoms of depression. Ginkgo biloba is a rich source of these beneficial flavonglycosides.

Gingerols

Gingerols, the active constituents of ginger, possess antioxidant properties and contribute to the improved digestion of proteins and fats. These compounds also have soothing effects on the stomach, aiding in digestion and alleviating discomfort. Additionally, gingerols play a role in combating liver toxicity and reducing inflammation.

Ginkolic Acid

Ginkolic acid, present in Ginkgo biloba, is an additional antioxidant compound. It promotes improved circulation and mental clarity, aiding in cognitive function. This acid has also been utilized in the treatment of depression. Furthermore, ginkolic acid has been studied for its potential anti-cancer properties.

Glycyrrhizins

Glycyrrhizins, the protective phytochemicals found in licorice, offer various health benefits. These compounds possess antiviral and anti-inflammatory properties, contributing to the body's defense against viral infections and reducing inflammation. Additionally, glycyrrhizins have skin-protective properties. They are also known to inhibit tumor formation, making them potentially valuable in cancer prevention.

Hesperidin

Hesperidin, a flavonoid abundant in citrus fruits like oranges and lemons, has potent antioxidant properties, which help protect cells from oxidative damage and reduce inflammation in the body. Hesperidin has also shown potential in supporting cardiovascular health by promoting healthy blood flow and maintaining optimal cholesterol levels. Moreover, studies suggest that hesperidin may have anti-cancer properties and contribute to improved cognitive function.

Hypericin

Hypericin, a notable constituent found in St. John's Wort (Hypericum perforatum), is widely used for its antidepressant properties, with studies indicating its potential in alleviating symptoms of mild to moderate depression and anxiety. Hypericin also exhibits antiviral activity, making it valuable in combating certain viral infections. Additionally, this compound has shown promise in supporting wound healing and reducing inflammation.

Isothiocyanates

Isothiocyanates, bioactive compounds found in cruciferous vegetables such as broccoli, cauliflower, and kale, as well as in horseradish have been studied for their potent anticancer properties and have shown to inhibit the growth of cancer cells and promote their destruction. Isothiocyanates also demonstrate powerful antioxidant and anti-inflammatory activities, contributing to the prevention of chronic diseases such as heart disease and diabetes. Furthermore, they support detoxification processes in the body, aiding in the elimination of harmful substances.

Lactones

Lactones, present in kava kava root, offer protective effects against cancer by aiding in the elimination of carcinogens from the body.

Lipoic Acid

Lipoic acid, abundantly found in various edible plants, acts as a powerful antioxidant that helps eliminate heavy metals from the body. It offers protective effects against cancer and heart disease, contributes to normalizing blood sugar levels, and slows down the aging process. Additionally, lipoic acid plays a crucial role in energy production, making it a key factor in cellular metabolism.

Phenolic Acids

Phenolic acids, which can be found in berries, parsley, and all flowering plants, serve as antioxidants that effectively inhibit the formation of nitrosamines, which are known to be cancer-causing agents.

Phthalides

Phthalides, present in parsley, have the ability to detoxify carcinogens and stimulate the production of beneficial enzymes.

Polyacetylenes

Polyacetylenes, found in parsley, play a role in regulating the production of prostaglandins and offer protection against carcinogens.

Proanthocyanins

Proanthocyanidins, a class of flavonoid compounds abundant in elderberry and bilberry, as wellas various fruits, vegetables, and plants, have powerful antioxidant properties, protecting cells from oxidative damage and reducing the risk of chronic diseases such as heart disease and cancer. Proanthocyanidins also exhibit anti-inflammatory effects, and have been associated with supporting cardiovascular health, improving cognitive function, and promoting healthy aging.

Quercetin

Quercetin, a flavonoid widely present in the plant kingdom, exhibits various beneficial properties. As a naturally occurring antioxidant, it contributes to the body's defense against oxidative stress.

Quercetin possesses antihistamine and anti-inflammatory properties, making it valuable in managing allergic reactions and reducing inflammation. It also shows potential as an anticancer agent. Moreover, quercetin plays a role in stabilizing cell membranes and reducing capillary fragility.

Rosemarinic Acid

Rosemarinic acid, the active component of rosemary, offers several therapeutic benefits. It helps combat nausea, intestinal gas, and indigestion, providing relief for digestive discomfort. Additionally, rosemarinic acid has shown effectiveness in alleviating headaches.

Salin

Salin, also known as salicin, is a compound found in white willow bark. It possesses anti-inflammatory properties, making it effective in combating inflammation. Additionally, salin provides relief from pain and fever. Furthermore, it has shown efficacy in fighting the influenza virus.

Saponins

Saponins, a diverse group of naturally occurring compounds found in various plants, including ginseng root, licorice, black cohosh, yucca, and others, hold immune-modulating properties, helping to enhance immune function and defend against infections. Saponins also exhibit anti-inflammatory effects, which may contribute to reducing the risk of chronic diseases such as cardiovascular conditions and certain types of cancer. Additionally, these compounds have been linked to potential benefits for cholesterol management and digestive health.

Silymarin

Silymarin, a flavonoid complex derived from milk thistle (Silybum marianum), is well-known for its hepatoprotective properties, supporting liver health and aiding in the detoxification process. Silymarin has been studied for its potential in preventing and managing liver conditions such as liver cirrhosis and hepatitis. Additionally, it exhibits potent antioxidant and anti-inflammatory effects, contributing to overall cellular health and reducing the risk of chronic diseases. Furthermore, silymarin has shown promise in supporting skin health and promoting a healthy aging process.

Tannins

Tannins, which are widely distributed in plants, act as antioxidants and exhibit antiviral properties. These compounds also contribute to the strengthening of capillaries. Additionally, tannins offer protection against cancer, heart disease, and asthma.

Terpenes

Terpenes, commonly known as monoterpenes, are antioxidants present in several aromatic and medicinal plants.

Triterpenoids

Triterpenoids, found in licorice root and gotu kola, contribute to various health benefits. These compounds help prevent dental decay, combat ulcers, cancer, and liver toxicity.

ENZYMES

Enzymes, naturally occurring in herbs that have not undergone high-temperature exposure or alcohol processing, play a vital role in unlocking the potential of phytochemicals and other nutrients within these herbs. These enzymes are essential for activating and enhancing the absorption, effectiveness, and bioavailability of the beneficial compounds present in the herbs. In cases where the enzymes have been destroyed during the processing of herbal preparations, it becomes beneficial to supplement with enzymes alongside the herbs. Ideally, enzyme supplements should include a combination of proteases (which break down proteins), lipases (which break down fats), and amylases (which break down carbohydrates) to support optimal digestion and assimilation of herbal nutrients.

Native American herbal medicine and modern health supplements

Native American heritage brims with a profound legacy of utilizing herbal remedies, which has left an indelible mark on modern medicinal practices. Even today, numerous herbal supplements widely available owe their origins to the traditional wisdom of Native American healers. Among these revered botanical treasures are black cohosh (Cimicifuga racemosa), blue cohosh (Caulophyllum thalictroides), elderberry (Sambucus species), and juniper (Juniperus communis). What adds intrigue to this rich tapestry is the fact that Native Americans' exploration of medicinal plants has, at times, unveiled remarkable pharmaceutical discoveries. Remarkably, Taxol, derived from the Pacific yew tree (Taxus brevifolia), and etoposide phosphate, a derivative of podophyllotoxin found in May apple or American mandrake, now stand as vital treatments for various ailments.

Beyond their therapeutic significance, plants hold an integral role in Native American medicine. They are not only employed for diagnostic and curative purposes but also for physical and ritual purification, often preceding sacred ceremonies. In the realm of healing, plants stand as cherished allies. Within the vast tapestry of North American flora, encompassing over 17,000 plant species, Native American societies have derived medicinal value from more than 2,500 vascular taxa and over 2,800 taxa in total.

This knowledge has been a continuous pursuit for over a century, culminating in a comprehensive compendium published in 1986 and subsequently compiled into an esteemed online database (http://www.umd.umich.edu/cgi-bin/herb).

Yet, the quest to unlock the potential of medicinal plants remains alive and vibrant. Ethnobotanists persist in unearthing new discoveries and expanding upon the documented uses of these botanical treasures. Remarkably, specific applications of medicinal plants by Native Americans often exhibit remarkable consistency across diverse tribes and regions of North America. Their discerning selection of botanical remedies was driven by a profound understanding, with certain plant families commanding extensive usage while others were deliberately overlooked, reflecting a keen knowledge of nature's offerings.

Evidence suggests that Native Americans approached the use of botanicals as medicine in a manner akin to Western science. They employed different plant parts to treat specific ailments, combined various botanicals for targeted therapeutic purposes, and recognized certain toxic plants as both poisons and medicinal agents.

The historical records provide fascinating insights into how Native Americans approached the medicinal use of plants, showcasing a methodology akin to Western scientific principles. Their careful selection of plant parts for targeting specific ailments, blending different botanicals for personalized therapeutic purposes, and even recognizing the dual nature of certain toxic plants as both poisons and medicinal agents showcase their sophisticated understanding. Yet, it is important to acknowledge the spiritual aspect deeply intertwined with their healing practices.

Native Americans held a profound belief in the inherent power or "spirit" residing within plants, attributing their therapeutic effects to this spiritual essence. This spiritual connection added a dimension of reverence and respect to their utilization of botanicals for healing purposes. Consequently, adhering to specific rules during plant collection was considered vital in order to harness the plant's full potency.

Interestingly, while collection rituals may have carried religious significance rather than purely therapeutic intent, it is intriguing to observe similar instructions across geographically and culturally distinct tribes. For instance, both the Iroquois of the Northeast and the Salishan of the Northwest (Vancouver Island) emphasize gathering plants in the morning, collecting tree bark from the eastern side of the tree, offering tobacco, and reciting prayers. These shared practices hint at a cultural connection and a shared understanding of the importance of ceremonial collection. However, the precise details regarding collection procedures, specific plant parts used, and preparation methods may vary among tribes and are not consistently documented.

Despite the prevalence of medicinal botanicals in health food stores, supermarkets, and pharmacies, our understanding of their efficacy and safety is constrained by limited scientific research. The comprehensive investigation of these botanicals, especially those employed in Native American traditional medicine, remains a rarity.

Fortunately, several plant species used by Native Americans for medicinal purposes are not exclusive to North America but also thrive in other parts of the world. Consider species like Sambucus nigra, Sambucus racemosa, and Juniperus communis, which can be found in both North America and Europe.

Similarly, certain botanicals introduced to European settlers by indigenous North American populations, such as various Echinacea species and Lobelia inflata, have gained significant popularity in Europe. Conversely, settlers from different continents brought their native botanicals, which eventually found utility among Native Americans.

THE 7 TOP-SELLING HERBAL SUPPLEMENTS IN THE U.S., THEIR USES BY NATIVE AMERICANS, AND THEIR MODERN USES

Common name (Latin name)	Family	Native American tribes	Traditional Native American uses	Current uses
Ginseng (Panax quinquefolius)	Araliaceae	Cherokee, Creek, Delaware, Fox, Houma, Iroquois, Mohegan, Pawnee, Penobscot, Potawatomi	Tonic, expectorant; for fevers, tuberculosis, asthma, and rheumatism; as a strengthener	Immune function and stress
Garlic (Allium sativum)	Liliaceae	Cherokee	Stimulant, carminative, diuretic, expectorant, mild cathartic; for scurvy, asthma, and prevention of worms	Cardiovascular health and cholesterol lowering
Echinacea (Echinacea purpurea, Echinacea angustifolia, Echinacea pallida)	Asteraceae	Cheyenne, Choctaw, Dakota, Delaware, Fox Kiowa, Montana, Omaha Pawnee, Ponca, Sioux, Winnebago	Pain relief; for coughs and sore throats, fevers, smallpox, mumps, measles, rheumatism, and arthritis; antidote for poisons and venoms	Immune function
Goldenseal (Hydrastis canadensis)	Ranunculaceae	Cherokee, Iroquois, Micmac	Tonic; for fever, whooping cough, and pneumonia	Immune function
St John's wort (Hypericum perforatum)	Hyperiaceae	Cherokee, Iroquois, Montagnais	For fever, coughs, and bowel complaints	Antidepressant
Evening primrose (Oenothera biennis)	Onagraceae	Cherokee, Iroquois, Ojibwa, Potawatomi	For premenstrual and menstrual pain, obesity, and bowel pains	Antioxidant status: premenstrual and menstrual pain
Cranberry (Vaccinium macrocarpon)	Ericaceae	Montagnais	For pleurisy	Health of urinary tract

A prime example is Urtica dioica, commonly known as stinging nettle, originally from Europe and Asia, which quickly spread and became widely utilized by various Native American societies across North America. Native Americans employed different parts of the stinging nettle, both internally and externally, for purposes ranging from general tonics to the treatment of fevers and rheumatism.

Consequently, the current body of research on plant species utilized by Native American communities in North America often relies on studies conducted in other countries where the same species have been employed for similar medicinal purposes. These studies typically involve in vitro screenings of individual plants or their components, aiming to assess their potential antibacterial, antiviral, or anti-inflammatory properties. Exploring the traditional use of a botanical in treating wounds, fevers, infections, edema, or rheumatic diseases serves as a valuable foundation for investigating its potential anti-inflammatory effects. By building upon this traditional knowledge, researchers can uncover the therapeutic potential of these botanicals and contribute to our understanding of their medicinal properties.

Echinacea, a plant widely utilized by Native Americans for various purposes, has garnered more extensive research compared to many other medicinal botanicals. Over time, Echinacea purpurea has risen in popularity to become one of the most widely used medicinal botanicals in Europe and the United States, alongside its counterparts Echinacea angustifolia and Echinacea pallida, which are also commonly utilized.

Fascinatingly, different Echinacea species and the utilization of distinct plant parts give rise to significant variations in chemical compositions and biological activities. For instance, echinacoside, often utilized for standardizing Echinacea angustifolia and Echinacea pallida extracts, is absent in Echinacea purpurea. Furthermore, the extraction process, choice of solvents, and selection of plant parts impact the composition and potential effects of Echinacea preparations. Polysaccharides, known for their immune-stimulatory effects, are more likely to be found in aqueous extracts rather than alcoholic extracts.

In the United States and Europe, Echinacea is frequently combined with other medicinal botanicals, such as goldenseal. However, it is crucial to note that different Echinacea species and formulations may possess distinct properties and compositions, which should be clearly indicated on product labels. Unfortunately, the scientific literature often overlooks these differences, leading to potential confusion and misinterpretation of research findings.

While the consumption of botanical supplements continues to rise, our knowledge regarding the efficacy and safety of Native American medicinal botanicals remains limited due to the scarcity of scientific research. Most studies have focused on experimental animals, with a dearth of clinical trials involving human subjects. Nevertheless, the existing scientific data provide support for the potential of many of these plant species to address ailments traditionally treated by Native Americans, as they contain bioactive constituents known for their therapeutic properties.

Of particular significance is their potential in treating chronic inflammatory diseases, such as rheumatoid arthritis and systemic lupus erythematosus. Current therapies for these conditions often fall short in terms of efficacy and are accompanied by significant side effects. Exploring the therapeutic potential of Native American medicinal botanicals could offer promising alternatives in managing these challenging conditions.

It is essential to recognize that the effects of isolated chemical constituents derived from plant extracts may differ from those of the complex blend of bioactive molecules found in whole-plant extracts. Therefore, a shift in scientific approaches is necessary to comprehensively investigate botanical supplements. Rather than solely focusing on isolated compounds, we should embrace the holistic nature of these traditional remedies. New research methodologies that consider the historical use, anecdotal evidence, and potential therapeutic benefits of these botanicals are needed.

Further research is warranted to unlock the full potential of Native American medicinal botanicals. By adopting comprehensive and innovative research approaches, we can gain a deeper understanding of these botanicals and their applications in promoting health and well-being. This will enable us to harness their potential as valuable additions to our healthcare toolkit, aligning modern scientific principles with the ancient wisdom of Native American healing traditions.

Sourcing Herbs

Herbalism, contrary to popular belief, is not a mystical or otherworldly practice but rather rooted in scientific principles. Our ancestors possessed a profound understanding of health and the human body, far more extensive than commonly acknowledged in mainstream culture. The art of herbalism represents the accumulation of centuries' worth of wisdom derived from countless experiments and observations. Although certain aspects of herbalism still elude scientific explanation, it is essential to recognize that it is not reliant on "magic" or the supernatural.

Herbalists engage with plants because they harbor an array of vitamins, minerals, and organic compounds that serve to maintain their own well-being, and consequently, can contribute to the health of humans as well.

The efficacy of herbs as medicinal agents often hinges on the stage of growth and development at which they are harvested. The timing of their collection and extraction is critical, aligning with the plant's optimal susceptibility and known attributes. Whether it be the bounty of summer, the frigidity of winter, the blossoming of spring, or the fading hues of autumn, adhering to the plant's specific protocol becomes paramount.

Consider, for instance, Cascara, also known as Sacred Bark. Once carefully stripped from the tree during the appropriate season and transformed into a powder or tincture, its value and effectiveness increase with age. Conversely, Nettle proves to be an exceptional herb during its nascent growth, yet diminishes in potency as it matures. Another pivotal aspect when selecting a plant for its medicinal qualities lies in its natural habitat. If the herb is indigenous to the region or country where it is found, it is the appropriate choice.

Plants introduced from foreign lands may experience a diminishment or alteration of their inherent virtues unless they encounter in their new abode all the essential conditions they possessed in their native environment. It is evident that herbs are susceptible to the influences of soil, climate, and other factors, resulting in variations in their attributed medicinal properties. When administering a medicinal herb, it is imperative to possess knowledge regarding its precise curative effects on the human system.

It would be inaccurate to label herbs as "weak" or "gentle" drugs due to their complex nature. Instead, they hold a significant position within a comprehensive healthcare system that diverges from the mainstream Western model. The holistic herbal model focuses on proactive preventive care and, in the event of illness, prioritizes strengthening and fortifying the body's innate response mechanisms. Therefore, when engaging with herbalism, it is crucial to approach it with the utmost seriousness and to understand the optimal methods of sourcing and preparing these plants.

Whenever possible, it is advisable to eschew the notion of "using" herbs. The concept of "use" implies exploitation, which is an inadequate perspective. Instead, we should regard herbs as wise instructors, steadfast allies, and cherished companions, in harmony with the Native American tribes' perspective as illustrated by their ritualistic reverence for these botanical treasures. We do not "use" our human friends to merely assist us with physical tasks or event planning; rather, we collaborate with them. Similarly, we extend this sentiment to plants and strive to express it through our language and written discourse.

This represents just a small fragment of an ongoing endeavor to acknowledge and honor plants as autonomous living organisms, each with their own distinct needs and desires. While plants may not perceive or interact with the world in the same manner as we do, their undeniable life force enables them to respond to their surroundings. Books like "What a Plant Knows" by Daniel Chamovitz and "The Hidden Life of Trees" by Peter Wohlleben provide insightful explorations into the sensory perception and sensitivity of plants. As stewards and caretakers of the natural world, it is our responsibility to extract from plants only what is necessary, minimize waste, and actively work towards restoring plant habitats and populations.

By adopting such practices, we ensure the preservation of these sentient beings, allowing them to continue bestowing their invaluable gifts upon us for generations to come. In this spirit of dedication, we strive to emulate the Native American approach to wild foraging, drawing inspiration from their deep spiritual connection to nature.

Native American rituals for wild foraging

The act of gathering herbs and other plants is deeply intertwined with spiritual beliefs, which dictate the precise procedures and ceremonies to be followed. Phyllis Hogan, a renowned figure in the field of applied ethnobotany, has devoted nearly three decades to collaborating with sixteen Native American tribes, including the Navajo and Hopi, through her organization, the Arizona Ethnobotanical Research Association. Her extensive work involves documenting and comparing the various uses of plants among indigenous communities in Arizona.

In addition to her research endeavors, Phyllis also owns the Winter Sun Trading Company, a Flagstaff-based enterprise specializing in traditional herbs and American Indian art. As a practitioner associate in anthropology, an honorary position bestowed upon her by Northern Arizona University, she possesses exceptional expertise in the utilization of southwestern botanicals. Phyllis's insights into traditional gathering practices were shaped through her tutelage under the Navajo people.

According to Navajo teachings, it is customary to embark on herb gathering in the early hours of the morning. The process begins with the burning of juniper, with some of the resulting soot applied to one's skin, serving as a form of purification. A prayer is then offered to the sun deity, accompanied by the presentation of cornmeal as a symbolic offering to the plant. In this act, Phyllis introduces herself to the plant, expressing her intention to employ its healing properties. Subsequently, she seeks permission from the plant to collect its fellow plants and patiently awaits a sign or indication of consent.

Phyllis describes the granting of permission as a potential vibratory connection established between the gatherer and the plants. This connection may manifest through the rustling of the wind, intuitive sensations, or even melodic songs. Should the plant withhold permission, it is understood that the gathering should not take place on that particular day.

You don't pick the plant you are praying to, because it is your emissary to the plant world. You then give an offering to the earth, then the sky, then the four directions, starting with the east and going clockwise. And also honor the middle. We also put a little cornmeal on our heads. This is a connection to the spirit world and also a sign of purity."
She adds that some plants don't want to come, some pull easily and some won't. It is also important to never take more than you need and always leave at least one-fourth of what's there.
Rare and endangered plants should never be picked, and you should never pick in someone else's picking place. Some areas have been picked for thousands of years by the same clan members. Pickers show respect for the plant world, always wearing nice clothing and jewelry when gathering herbs. This is because they are meeting the deities and want to be recognized as someone of stature. Phyllis's favorite pastime is herb-gathering because she stops thinking of worldly problems during this time.

According to Phyllis, pickers only pick one type of plant per day. "This is because you must take responsibility for the plant and feed it with cornmeal or pollen again, then pray to welcome it." Once the plants are picked they are placed on clean sheets or other cloths and aligned with the herb, roots, leaves, and flowers pointing in the same direction as the other herbs, roots, leaves, and flowers. They are then fed cornmeal once again and welcomed, and told again why they are needed. They are then allowed to rest for a day; only one species of plant is picked a day. Before preparing the herbs, they are again prayed to and thanked for being here. Only then are they prepared into tinctures, extracts, or other forms.

Buying

Depending on where you live, you can find wonderful herbs in a variety of places! Check out your local health food store, nearby farms, or perhaps look in your neighbor's garden. You might be surprised to find that your regular grocery store carries high-quality herbs too, especially the ones commonly sold as produce. Don't forget to explore herb shops or reputable online retailers if physical access to herbs is limited.

Now, let's talk about prices. Remember, cheaper doesn't always mean better when it comes to herbs. Local small-scale producers often charge slightly higher prices, but their herbs are often of superior quality. It's worth starting with small batches and trying out different producers to find the ones that consistently offer the best quality. This way, you can decide if the investment is worth it for you.

When sourcing herbs, there are a few things to consider. Think about the quality of the soil where the herbs are grown, the farming practices used, and how the herbs are dried and processed. These factors can greatly influence the overall quality of the herbs you find.

So, keep an open mind and enjoy exploring different sources to discover the best herbs for your needs!
Soil quality plays a significant role as any contamination, such as heavy metals or pollutants, present in the soil can find its way into the plant matter. Knowing the origin of the herbs is crucial to assess whether the soil was clean. This concern applies to herbs grown in any location, but it is particularly relevant for those cultivated in regions with lax soil pollution regulations. Certain larger herb retailers, like Mountain Rose Herbs, conduct tests to ensure their products are free from soil-based contamination. Urban farms, although initially seeming less favorable, should not be dismissed outright. Engage in conversations with the producers, inquire about their soil quality, and most urban farms utilize clean soil and employ water filtration to ensure the safety of their produce.

Growing practices are equally important to consider. Questions regarding insect management, fertilizer usage, greenhouse or outdoor cultivation, and whether hydroponic or soil-based methods were employed are pertinent. While each approach has its pros and cons, the ultimate determinant of quality is the end result. Vibrant colors, robust aromas, and flavors indicate good quality.

The drying and processing phase can also impact the final product. Improper drying at excessively high temperatures or inadequate storage can compromise the quality of even the finest herbs. Significant browning in dried herbs is a clear indication of subpar drying techniques. This browning resembles the dried, browned leaf of a living plant and appears lifeless. For instance, consider St. John's wort as an example. When properly dried, it exhibits a deep-red mahogany brown, which is distinct from the undesirable brown-black color of basil leaves that have deteriorated in the refrigerator.

In conclusion, it is essential to familiarize yourself with the source of your herbs. Inquire about the growing practices, soil and water quality, and processing methods employed by the supplier. This not only enables you to make informed choices but also fosters a sense of community between herb growers (and food producers) and consumers. Understanding the origins of our herbs allows us to value them, appreciate the efforts of our farmers, and demonstrate care for our environment.

Wild Crafting

While the idea of venturing into the wilderness to harvest your own herbs may be enticing, it is often advised against. Overharvesting poses a serious threat to wild herbs, and in many cases, it is more sustainable and beneficial to opt for organically cultivated varieties instead of depleting wild populations.

It is of utmost importance to prioritize the preservation of certain herbs due to the imminent risk of extinction caused by overharvesting and habitat destruction. Specifically, woodland plants heavily rely on thriving forests for their growth and cannot be easily cultivated. Some examples of these vulnerable plants include goldenseal, osha, and black or blue cohosh, despite their endangered status, they unfortunately remain popular choices. However, there exists a plethora of alternative herbs that possess similar properties, rendering the purchase of these at-risk species unnecessary. For a comprehensive understanding of endangered herbs and those that should be avoided, I highly recommend visiting the website of United Plant Savers at unitedplantsavers.org. There, you will discover invaluable insights and information concerning this critical matter.

Furthermore, it is crucial to consider the social implications surrounding the production of herbs in addition to their ecological impact. Certain popular herbs should be approached with caution due to the potential exploitation of the communities from which they originate. Whenever a new "superfood" trend emerges from a distant location, it is essential to exercise prudence and reflect upon the broader context.

Let us consider the example of maca. Marketed as a plant that provides increased energy and possesses a delightful flavor, it has garnered considerable attention. However, it is essential to acknowledge that maca serves as a vital staple food for indigenous Peruvians residing in high-altitude regions. As demand from industrialized nations escalates, the price of maca rises, rendering it unaffordable for local communities. This situation sheds light on the intricate complexities entwined within the global herb trade.

In light of these challenges, it is imperative to emphasize the existence of our own local superfoods readily available to us. Plants such as cranberries, nettle, and dandelion leaves may not possess the same exotic allure, but they are equally nourishing and beneficial. By directing our focus towards these locally available options, we can actively support sustainable and ethically sourced herbs while simultaneously indulging in their remarkable health benefits. Let us celebrate the nurturing power of these local superfoods and make conscious choices that align with both our well-being and social responsibility.

Nevertheless, there is immense satisfaction in discovering and working with wild plants. To ensure safety for yourself, the plants, and the ecosystems they inhabit, here are some guidelines to follow when engaging with wild herbs.

WILDCRAFTING ETHICS AND GUIDELINES
Prepared by the Rocky Mountain Herbalists' Coalition

Wildcrafting
1. Never gather an endangered or threatened species. Check your local herbarium or botanical garden for a list of these plants. You may also contact the American Herbalist Guild for a national listing: AHG, Box 1683, Soquel, CA 95073.
2. I.D. positively before harvesting. Use identification keys and voucher specimens.
3. Ask permission and give thanks, acknowledge connection with all life, share your appreciation.
4. Leave mature and seed-producing plants—grandparent plants—within the stand and at the top of a hill to seed downslope. Work your way up.
5. If unsure, harvest no more than ten percent native whole plant and root, and thirty percent naturalized plant species or native leaves and flowers. Gather only from abundant stands. Harvest conservatively to insure maintenance and well-being of plant communities.

Site Selection
1. Obtaining permission: On BLM land, a free use permit may be obtained for a minimal charge if you are collecting small amounts. Both the U.S. Forest Service and BLM will tell you there is no picking (a) in or near campgrounds or picnic areas; (b) any closer than 200 feet from trails; and (c) on the roadsides.
2. Stay away from downwind pollution, roadsides (at least 50 feet), high-tension electric wires (may cause mutations), fertilizers in lawns and public parks, downstream from mining or agribusiness, around parking lots, and possible sprayed areas. Some BLM and Forest Service districts use routine spraying. This applies to private land as well, and you may need to ask about herbicides and pesticides.
3. Use discretion with fragile environments—one irresponsible wildcrafter can severely alter a rocky hillside or streamside ecosystem.

Gardening and Propagation Techniques

1. Using proper wildcrafting techniques will ensure minimal impact, increase harvest yields, and continue to provide plant food for wildlife. Do not harvest the same stand year after year, but tend the area as necessary. "Gardening" techniques that apply include thinning, root division, top pinching, and preserving a wide selection of grandparent plants to seed and guard young plants.

2. Be aware of erosion factors. If digging roots, replant or scatter seeds, and cover holes. Be mindful of hillside stands, replace foliage and dirt around harvested areas. Gathering foliage from nearby harvested plants and spreading it around may be necessary. Wearing hard-soled shoes may cause delicate hillside ecosystems irreparable damage.

3. If harvesting leaf, don't pull the roots. Flower pruning of certain plants will increase root yields as well as foliage.

4. Make seasonal observations on wildcrafted areas. Be mindful of your harvested stands and check different growth cycles. This will determine your real impact on the ecosystem. (One experienced wildcrafter in the northwest has observed that a healthy population will increase about 30% a year until it reaches stasis. Anything less than this could be considered degenerative.)

Suggested Gathering Times

- **Aerial or above ground parts:** When gathering the aerial or above ground parts of plants, it is best to do so in the mornings between 6 and 10 a.m., right before they start wilting in the sun. If you are harvesting leaves, they are often at their prime just before flowering. As for flowers, it is ideal to harvest them as they are beginning to bloom, allowing you to see the vibrant colors of the buds. In traditional practices, harvesting aerial parts aligns with the full moon phase or occurs near it.

- **Roots:** Harvest roots after the plant has completed its seeding phase. If possible, harvest in the early morning before the sun's rays reach them. For biennial plants, the ideal time to harvest the roots is either in the autumn of the first year or the spring of the second year, depending on the specific plant's life cycle. In traditional practices, the new moon phase is traditionally associated with root harvesting.

- **Bark:** When it comes to gathering barks from trees, it is best to do so during the spring or fall seasons. It is important not to strip the bark completely, as this can harm the overall health and survival of the tree. In cases where tree populations are dense, thinning the trees may be necessary. However, it is crucial to selectively remove trees, ensuring that the healthiest specimens are left behind. If you choose to harvest from smaller branches, be mindful of the potential risk of leaving the tree vulnerable to fungal rot. For many barks, the most active part is the inner bark, also known as cambium. It is advisable to focus on collecting the inner bark for its medicinal properties. To ensure sustainable harvesting practices, consider leaving short trunks for pollarding. This involves pruning the main stem of the tree to encourage new growth. Additionally, leaving low stumps for coppicing allows the tree to regenerate from the base, providing an ongoing source of harvestable material. The traditional time to harvest bark is during the three-quarter waning moon phase. This phase is believed to enhance the potency and effectiveness of the harvested barks.

- **Saps and Pitches:** Harvest saps and pitches in the late winter or the early spring.

- **Seed and Fruit:** Harvest when mature, with some exceptions such as citrus, unripe scarlet bean pods, etc.

Growing

Regardless of whether you live in an urban environment, cultivating your own herbs is an accessible option. Even without a yard, many herbs thrive in pots near sunny windows, making it possible to grow them indoors. If you're new to gardening or consider yourself inexperienced in plant care, there's no need to worry. Growing plants is like any other skill—it becomes easier with a little time and effort invested each day. Certain herbs are particularly beginner-friendly and can be readily found as seedlings or seeds at local garden centers. Mint, catnip, sage, and yarrow are excellent choices to start with. Mint and catnip, in particular, adapt well to indoor cultivation and can flourish in pots if outdoor space or safe soil is unavailable. If you want to ensure the safety and quality of your soil, you can have it tested through your local Extension Office.

They provide testing kits and offer valuable information about soil safety, including recommendations for the best fertilizer based on your soil type. Typically, this service is available for a nominal fee of around $10. Extension Offices also offer classes, gardening advice specific to your area, and a range of other services, often free of charge or at a low cost. You can find the Extension Office near you by searching for "county extension office."

While wild crafting herbs is ideal, it can be time-consuming. Growing your own herbs is a viable alternative, and most of the herbs you commonly use are worth cultivating. Here are 11 plants you might consider growing, as they are relatively easy to maintain, especially when starting with established plants instead of seeds or seedlings. These herbs are commonly found, inexpensive, and offer an enjoyable and rewarding gardening experience.

Certainly! Here are 11 herbs worth considering for your own cultivation. They offer various health benefits and are relatively easy to grow:

1. **Garlic**: Known for its infection-fighting properties and stimulating effects.
2. **Rosemary**: Rich in cancer-fighting antioxidants and serves as a stimulant.
3. **Basil**: Contains antioxidants and acts as an infection fighter.
4. **Mint**: A stimulating herb with digestive properties.
5. **Lemon balm**: Known for its relaxing qualities, often used as a tonic for mild depression, irritability, and anxiety.
6. **Fennel**: Possesses anti-inflammatory and analgesic properties, stimulates appetite, and aids in alleviating flatulence.
7. **Lovage**: Serves as a respiratory and digestive tonic, particularly beneficial for bronchitis.
8. **Oregano**: An antiseptic herb with anti-flatulent properties, stimulates bile and stomach acid, and aids in managing asthma symptoms.
9. **Cilantro** (Coriander): Effective in treating flatulence, bloating, and cramps, also acts as a breath freshener.
10. **Horseradish**: Exhibits perspirant properties and acts as a stimulant.
11. **Thyme**: Often used as a tea to prevent altitude sickness, possesses antiseptic qualities, serves as an inhalant for asthma management, and acts as a stimulant.

Cultivating these herbs will not only provide a convenient supply for culinary uses but also offer the opportunity to enjoy their medicinal benefits.

Embarking on the journey of growing herbs is as simple as taking that first step! To begin, you can purchase a seedling and place it in a pot filled with quality soil. Remember to provide it with a little water and make it a daily habit to check on your plant. Plants, like our beloved pets, are living beings, and with time, you'll develop a sense of understanding and connection with your herb. You'll learn to "hear" your plant's communication and respond to its needs, just like you do with your cat or dog. Embrace the joy of nurturing and learning from your herb as it thrives under your care.

Preparing Herbs

Herbal preparations

While modern technology has advanced the processes of distilling, extracting, purifying, and standardizing herbal extracts to a level beyond what is covered in this book, it is important to familiarize oneself with some basic herbal preparations to enhance the effectiveness of this guide. These simple techniques are particularly useful for beginners in the field of herbalism.

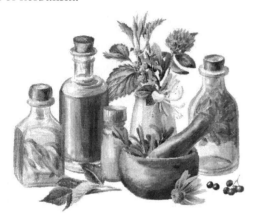

Tea: Select dried or fresh herbs useful to your particular condition (check out the second volume to discover them!). Common Native American herbs used in teas include sage, red clover, and yarrow.

For each cup of boiling water, use approximately one teaspoon of dried herb or two teaspoons of fresh herb. Place the herbs in a teapot or mug and pour the boiling water over them. Cover the vessel and let it steep for 5 to 10 minutes to allow the herbs to release their beneficial compounds.
Once the tea has steeped, strain it into a cup using a fine-mesh strainer or tea infuser. You can add natural sweeteners if desired.

Dosage: As a general guideline, use a ratio of one teaspoon of dried herb or two teaspoons of fresh herb per cup of boiling water. It's recommended to consume one to three cups of herbal tea daily.

Decoction: To prepare a herbal decoction, start by selecting dried roots, barks, or tougher plant parts known for their therapeutic benefits. Common Native American herbs used in decoctions include burdock root, black cohosh root, and willow bark.

Measure approximately one tablespoon of dried herb per cup of water. Place the herbs in a saucepan and add cold water in the ratio of 1:10 (1 part herb to 10 parts water).

Slowly bring the mixture to a boil over low heat. Once boiling, reduce the heat and let the decoction simmer for about 20 to 30 minutes. This longer cooking time helps to extract the medicinal compounds from the tougher plant material.

After simmering, remove the decoction from heat and allow it to cool for a few minutes. Strain the liquid using a fine-mesh strainer or cheesecloth, separating the liquid from the herb material.

Dosage: The recommended dosage for herbal decoctions can vary based on the specific herb and individual circumstances. As a general guideline, start with one cup of decoction per day.

Percolation: Percolation is a method that resembles making drip coffee. It involves a slow dripping of water or alcohol through a powdered herb mass. This process extracts the potent properties of the herb. An example of percolation is the act of slowly dripping hot water or alcohol through cayenne powder, resulting in a concentrated extract known for its strength. Even a single drop of this extract can have a powerful effect.

Dosage: For percolation, drip 100 milliliters of liquid through 10 grams of dried herb. This process can be repeated multiple times to further increase the concentration of the extract.

Tincture: To make a tincture, you'll need to chop the herbs and blend them with alcohol, although alternatives like apple cider vinegar or glycerin can also be used. The process starts with maceration, where the chopped herb is blended, often using a blender. For instance, diluting a volume of 190 proof alcohol, such as Everclear 95% alcohol, with an equal amount of water will result in approximately 50 percent alcohol content.

For dry herbs, the typical ratio is 1:5. This means blending 1 ounce of dried herb with 5 ounces of 50 percent (100 proof) alcohol. When using fresh herbs, a common ratio is 1:2, with 1 gram of fresh herb used for every cubic centimeter of 50 percent (100 proof) alcohol.

For example, you can take fresh-cut Echinacea flowers, chop them into small pieces, blend them, and cover them with 50 percent alcohol. After blending, allow the maceration to rest in the refrigerator for approximately four hours. Finally, strain the mixture and bottle it, creating a tincture ready for use.

Tinctures offer a concentrated form of herbal remedies and have a long shelf life. Keep in mind that specific herbs may require different ratios and maceration times. Check out the specific requirements for each herb in the second volume and specific recipes in the third volume

Double Extraction: To create a double extraction, follow these steps:

1. Fill a container, such as a 1-quart canning jar, with one cup of macerated plant material, such as Echinacea leaves and roots. Ensure that the maceration is completely covered with 8 ounces of 50 percent diluted Everclear. You can achieve a 50 percent alcohol concentration by adding an equal volume of water to an equal volume of Everclear. Seal the container.
2. Allow the blend to steep for several days to up to two weeks, preferably in a darkened cupboard or refrigerator. Remember to shake the container twice a day to facilitate the extraction process.
3. After the steeping period, strain the liquid using an effective strainer like a pair of pantyhose. For further clarification, pass the liquid through an unbleached coffee filter. Squeeze out any remaining liquid from the filter. This step yields the "single extraction."
4. Take the leftover herb material, known as the marc, and cover it with water. Simmer the mixture for thirty minutes, adding water as needed to prevent excessive evaporation. This step creates a decoction.
5. After simmering, strain the decoction and blend it with the tincture obtained in the previous step, resulting in a stronger "double extraction."

Note: To maintain an alcohol concentration of at least 25 percent (50 proof), avoid adding more water to the second extraction than the original amount of 50 percent alcohol used in the initial extraction. For instance, if you poured 10 ounces of 50 percent alcohol over the herb in the first step, do not exceed 10 ounces of water when preparing the second extraction.

Double extractions allow for a more comprehensive extraction of both water-soluble and alcohol-soluble compounds from the herbs, resulting in a potent herbal remedy.

Fomentation: Fomentations are a form of external herbal application, which involves creating a liquid infusion or decoction that is then applied externally to the affected area.

To prepare a herbal fomentation, you can start by selecting specific herbs based on their medicinal properties. Some Native American herbs commonly used in fomentations include:

1. Plantain (*Plantago spp.*): Known for its soothing and anti-inflammatory properties, plantain can be used in fomentations to support wound healing and relieve skin irritations.
2. Yarrow (*Achillea millefolium*): Yarrow, with its antimicrobial and anti-inflammatory properties, is often used in fomentations to aid in wound healing, reduce inflammation, and promote blood circulation.
3. Comfrey (*Symphytum spp.*): Comfrey is valued for its ability to promote tissue repair and alleviate inflammation. It can be used in fomentations to support the healing of bruises, sprains, and strains.

Here's a general process for making herbal fomentations:

1. Infusion or Decoction: Prepare a strong infusion or decoction of the chosen herb(s). For an infusion, steep 1 to 2 tablespoons of dried herb or 2 to 4 tablespoons of fresh herb in a cup of boiling water for 10 to 15 minutes. For a decoction, simmer the herb(s) in water for 15 to 20 minutes.
2. Straining: After the infusion or decoction is prepared, strain the liquid to remove any solid herb particles. You can use a fine-mesh strainer or cheesecloth for this purpose.
3. Temperature Adjustment: Allow the liquid to cool to a comfortable and safe temperature suitable for application to the skin. Make sure it is not too hot to avoid burns.
4. Application: Soak a clean cloth or towel in the herbal liquid, wring out the excess liquid, and apply it to the affected area. You can also use a compress by placing the soaked cloth on the area and securing it with a bandage or wrap.
5. Duration: Leave the fomentation on the affected area for 15 to 30 minutes, or as directed by a qualified healthcare practitioner. Repeat the application as needed throughout the day.

Poultice: Making Herbal Poultices

Poultices are a traditional method used in Native American herbalism to apply fresh herbs directly to the skin for localized healing effects. Here's a guide on how to make herbal poultices, including examples of Native American herbs commonly used.

To create a herbal poultice, follow these steps:

1. Select Fresh Herbs: Choose fresh herbs known for their medicinal properties. Some Native American herbs often used in poultices include:
   -Slippery Elm (*Ulmus rubra*): Slippery elm has mucilaginous properties, making it beneficial for soothing and healing skin conditions such as burns, rashes, and wounds.
   -Jewelweed (*Impatiens spp.*): Jewelweed is well-known for its ability to relieve skin irritations, including poison ivy rashes and insect bites. It has anti-inflammatory and antipruritic properties.
   -Sagebrush (*Artemisia tridentata*): Sagebrush is used by Native American tribes for its antimicrobial and anti-inflammatory properties. It is often applied as a poultice for treating skin infections, wounds, and bruises.
2. Pound and Macerate: Take the fresh herbs and pound them gently using a mortar and pestle or another suitable tool to release their juices. Alternatively, you can macerate the herbs by finely chopping or crushing them to create a moist herb mass.
3. Warm and Wet Application: Optionally, warm the herb mass slightly to enhance its soothing effect. Apply the warm, wet, and pounded or macerated herb mass directly to the targeted body part. Ensure that you prepare enough herb mass to cover the specific area requiring treatment.

4. Secure the Poultice: Use a clean cloth, gauze, or muslin to cover the herb mass and hold it in place. You can secure it with a bandage or wrap to keep the poultice in position.

5. Duration: Leave the poultice on the affected area for approximately 30 minutes to an hour. You can repeat the application several times a day as needed.

Poultices offer a direct and effective way to utilize the therapeutic properties of fresh herbs, promoting localized healing and soothing effects.

Powder: To create an herbal powder, simply grind the dried herbs into a fine powder using a mortar and pestle, grinder, or blender.

Once the herbs are ground into a powder, they can be used in various ways, including:

1. Topical Application: Apply the herbal powder directly to the affected area for localized healing effects. For example, powders made from herbs like calendula or chamomile can be used to soothe skin irritations and promote healing.

2. Oral Consumption: Herbal powders can also be consumed orally. They can be added to beverages, smoothies, or sprinkled over food.

3. Capsule Form: If preferred, the herbal powder can be encapsulated for easier consumption. Capsules provide a convenient way to take herbal remedies in a measured dose. The most common dosage is the 00 capsule which typically contain 500 to 1000 mg of the powdered herb

Remember to properly label and store your herbal powders in airtight containers away from moisture and sunlight to maintain their potency.

Oils and salves: To create herbal oils and salves, follow these steps:

1. Herb Infusion: Select either dried or fresh herbs for the preparation. In a heat-resistant container, immerse the herbs in a carrier oil, such as olive oil or lard. Simmer the mixture on low heat for a period of time to extract the active components of the herb into the oil. The specific duration can vary based on the herb and desired potency.

2. Straining: After simmering, strain the oil infusion using a fine-mesh strainer or cheesecloth to remove any solid herb particles, ensuring a smooth and clear oil.

3. Beeswax Addition: Return the infused oil to low heat and add warm beeswax. The beeswax helps solidify the oil into a salve consistency. The exact ratio of oil to beeswax can vary depending on the desired texture and consistency of the salve. Stir the mixture gently until the beeswax is fully melted and incorporated into the oil.

4. Cooling and Storage: Allow the blend to cool slightly before pouring it into clean, airtight containers or salve tins. Let it cool completely, which will cause it to solidify into a salve. Label the containers with the herb used and the date of preparation. Store the salve in a cool, dry place away from direct sunlight.

For example, to create a yarrow salve, immerse the aerial parts of the plant (flowers, leaves, and stems) in oil and simmer them. Blend the resulting infusion with warm beeswax and allow it to cool, resulting in a topical salve for wound treatment.

It's important to note that the quantity of herbs used in the preparation can vary. Lightly packing a pan with fresh leaves and flowers and covering them with olive oil or lard is a recommended method for yarrow salve, but other herbs might need more or less oil.

Essential tools

Creating high-quality herbal preparations does not require elaborate equipment or costly ingredients. In fact, you likely already have most of what you need in your kitchen.

Mason jars. The herbalist's best friends. Mason jars, made of heat-resistant glass, which makes them convenient even for brewing herbal infusions. They are also useful for creating tinctures, storing herbs, and serving various purposes in herbal practices.

Quart- and pint-size mason jars are particularly versatile and commonly used. However, if you require storage for larger quantities of dry herbs, you may opt for larger jars. It's worth noting that many store-bought foods are packaged in mason jars. These jars can be easily cleaned by handwashing or running them through the dishwasher, allowing for their reuse in herbal preparations.

Wire mesh strainers. Wire mesh strainers come in a variety of sizes, offering flexibility in herbal preparations. Fine mesh strainers are ideal for removing fine particles from liquid herbal extracts, while larger mesh sizes are suitable for straining herbs in poultices or decoctions, allowing for customization based on the specific herbal application. The range of sizes available in wire mesh strainers caters to the diverse needs of herbalists, ensuring effective filtration and optimal quality in herbal preparations.

Measuring cups and spoons. Having a set of measuring tools is highly beneficial for precise herbal preparations. Cup, tablespoon, and teaspoon measures are essential for accurately measuring ingredients. Additionally, graduated measuring cups with pour spouts are particularly useful, as they enable measurements as small as a quarter ounce.

Cheesecloth. Cheesecloth is a versatile material whose loose weave allows for excellent straining capabilities, making it ideal for filtering herbal infusions, decoctions, and tinctures to remove fine particulate matter. Cheesecloth is also commonly employed in the process of creating herbal sachets or bundles, where it securely holds herbs while allowing the aromatic properties to be released. Its lightweight and breathable nature make cheesecloth a valuable tool in herbal preparations, enabling the extraction of desired herbal qualities while maintaining clarity and purity. In a pinch, you can also use an old pantyhose for the same purpose.

Funnels. Small funnels are invaluable tools for transferring tinctures and other liquids into bottles with narrow openings. They facilitate the process by providing a controlled and precise way to pour the liquids without spills or wastage.

Bottles. Bottles play a crucial role in preserving the integrity and longevity of herbal preparations. When storing tinctures, it is advisable to opt for amber or cobalt blue glass bottles. These tinted bottles offer superior protection against light exposure, which can degrade the potency and efficacy of herbal remedies over time. The preferred choice is often the classic "Boston round" shape, but any amber or blue glass bottle can be utilized effectively. Building a collection of such bottles, including repurposing those from kombucha brands or other sources, helps create a sustainable and suitable storage solution for tinctures and other herbal creations. For convenient dosing, one- to two-fluid-ounce bottles are recommended, while larger sizes ranging from four to twelve fluid ounces are commonly employed for storage purposes. Sealing storage bottles with tight-fitting caps and employing dropper tops for dose bottles facilitate accurate dispensing of the tinctures, ensuring precise and controlled use.

Labels. It is important to label your herbal remedies promptly after making them. This ensures proper identification and prevents confusion. For labeling purposes, address labels can be sufficient for most needs. In a pinch, even a small piece of masking tape can serve as a makeshift label. The key is to have clear and easily readable labels that provide the necessary information about the remedy, such as the herb used, preparation date, and any specific instructions or dosage recommendations. Make sure to write clear instructions, that can be easily understood by everybody and not only you!

Blender. A standard kitchen blender is a versatile tool that can be utilized for various herbal preparations. It is suitable for a variety of purposes such mixing lotions and blending fresh leaves and soft plant matter. Make sure that the blender is thoroughly cleaned before and after each use to prevent cross-contamination and conform to hygienic standards.

Useful instruments

While the following tools are helpful in incorporating herbs into your daily routine, it's important to note that they are not essential for herbal practices. They can certainly facilitate the process, especially for those with busy schedules or limited time. However, if you don't have access to these tools, it should not discourage you from exploring and benefiting from herbal remedies. With a bit of creativity and resourcefulness, you can still engage in herbal preparations and incorporate herbs into your life using alternative methods and basic kitchen equipment. The most important aspect is your intention and willingness to learn and experiment with herbs.

French press. This is myfavourite tool for crafting herbal infusions. It enables the herbs to float freely in the water, allowing for optimal extraction of flavors and properties. It also provides a substantial surface area for the infusion process. With a simple press down, the filtered tea can be easily dispensed, ensuring a convenient and mess-free experience.

Thermos. When you're on the go or need to bring your herbal tea to work, having a reliable thermos is a very valuable asset. Opting for a thermos with a built-in filter in the lid can be particularly convenient. This design allows you to combine the herbs and water directly in the thermos right from the start, eliminating the need for a separate infuser or filter. It ensures that you can enjoy your herbal tea wherever you go, without the hassle of carrying additional equipment.

Press pot. While commonly used for coffee or strained tea, you can also use a press pot for infusing herbs directly. By placing the herbs directly into the pot, pouring in boiling water, and allowing them to infuse inside, you can create herbal beverages. The insulation of the pot helps maintain the desired temperature, keeping the infusion hot throughout the day. When ready to enjoy a cup of the infused herbal beverage, simply press the lever to dispense it. To prevent any herb particles from passing through the tube, it is advisable to hold a small mesh strainer under the spout to catch any residue.

Herb grinder. After so many years in the field I still use my trusted compact coffee grinder to grind herbs into powder for most of my daily preparations. However, for larger quantities of herb powders, you might want to invest in a larger and dedicated herb which can handle greater volumes and ensure consistent results.

Ingredients

For most of your preparations you will only need the selected herb and water, but for more complex preparations you'll do well to keep a few other ingredients on hand.
And speaking of water, not all water is made equal, so let's take a look at your options

Water. When it comes to herbal preparations, the water you choose can make a significant difference in the quality and effectiveness of your final product. Here are a few guidelines to help you select the most suitable water for your herbal concoctions:

1. Distilled Water: Distilled water is made by boiling water and then collecting the condensed vapor, leaving behind impurities and minerals. This clean and neutral water provides a blank canvas for your herbs to express their full potential.
2. Filtered Water: Using a high-quality water filtration system is another great option. These systems are designed to remove common contaminants like chlorine, heavy metals, and pesticides, while retaining essential minerals.
3. Spring Water: If you prefer a touch of natural goodness, spring water sourced from trusted springs can be an excellent choice. It contains minerals naturally present in the Earth, which can enhance the flavor and medicinal qualities of your herbal preparations. Ensure that the spring water you choose has been tested for purity to avoid any potential contamination.
4. Reverse Osmosis Water: Reverse osmosis is a water purification method that removes a wide range of impurities, including minerals. While this results in highly purified water, some herbalists prefer to have a minimal amount of minerals present in their preparations. If using reverse osmosis water, you may need to compensate for the lack of minerals by incorporating other mineral-rich ingredients into your recipes, especially if they are meant to be nutritive preparations.

Consider the specific characteristics and needs of the herbs you are working with when selecting the water. Additionally, ensure that the containers and utensils used in your herbal preparations are clean to prevent any contamination.

Alcohol. You are going to need alcohol for tinctures, some of the most effective and easiest herb preparations you will be able to make. Use 190 proof alcohol, such as Everclear 95% alcohol, if possible. In a pinch, you can also resort to vodka.

Apple cider vinegar. Always opt for apple cider vinegar (never white wine vinegar!). It is always your best choice for herb-infused vinegars, oxymels (which are a blend of vinegar and honey), and topical applications.

Honey. Opt for locally sourced honey whenever available, preferably in its unprocessed and unfiltered form. This not only supports the local economy but also ensures that the honey retains its natural enzymes, pollen, and other beneficial components due to minimal processing.
It is important to be mindful of the quality and authenticity of the honey you choose. Select honey from trusted and reputable producers to avoid potential contamination or adulteration.
It's worth noting that honey can vary in consistency, and different types of honey may be better suited for specific purposes. Liquid honey is generally easier to use in herbal honey infusions, while thicker honey may be more suitable for applications in first aid and wound care. Consider the desired consistency when selecting honey for different uses, keeping in mind its intended purpose.

Oils. Different oils can be used in herbal preparations depending on the specific purpose. Olive oil is a versatile option, while lighter oils like grapeseed or almond oil may be preferred for certain applications. Thicker oils such as shea butter or cocoa butter can be used for creating balms and ointments. Animal-derived oils like lard, tallow, or lanolin can also be utilized.

Beeswax. Salves often require the addition of wax to achieve a thicker consistency. Beeswax is commonly used and can be purchased in rounds or chunks, which can be cut down as needed. Alternatively, beeswax pellets are available, which may be easier to work with due to their smaller size.

Witch hazel extract. choose a variety made without alcohol. Alcohol-free witch hazel extract offers greater versatility, particularly for applications in first aid or wound care.

Rose water. Rose water has been traditionally used for skincare purposes and is also utilized as a food ingredient. Look for rose water in the food section of the grocery store. These rose waters are just as effective as the higher-priced alternatives typically found in the health and beauty aisle.
Even better, if you have the time and possibility, or if you grow enough roses, you can make your own rose water. There are few days in the year I enjoy more than when my kitchen is filled with the sweet intoxicating smell of roses.
The most common used rose varieties for rose water are aromatic rose varieties like Rosa damascena, Rosa centifolia, or Rosa gallica for their delightful scent and therapeutic properties.

However, I strongly recommend you use native varieties, here are just a few:
Native American wild roses encompass various species that are indigenous to North America. Some notable examples include:

1. *Rosa setigera* (Climbing Prairie Rose): Found in the central and eastern regions of North America, this climbing rose features pink flowers and thrives in open woodlands and prairies.
2. *Rosa woodsii* (Woods' Rose): Native to western North America, this shrub rose bears fragrant pink flowers and is often found in mountainous regions, meadows, and open forests.
3. *Rosa carolina* (Carolina Rose): Found in the eastern and central parts of North America, this wild rose species showcases fragrant pink flowers and is typically seen in wetland areas, swamps, and along stream banks.
4. *Rosa nutkana* (Nootka Rose): Native to the western regions of North America, this wild rose displays pink or white flowers and is commonly found in forests, meadows, and along coastal areas.
5. *Rosa arkansana* (Prairie Rose): Indigenous to the central and eastern parts of North America, this rose species features bright pink flowers and prefers open prairies and grasslands.

These are just a few examples of the many native wild roses found across different regions of North America. Each species exhibits its own unique characteristics, including flower color, fragrance, and preferred habitats. Exploring and appreciating these native wild roses can be a rewarding experience that connects you with the natural beauty of the continent.

Now, let's take a look at the process

Gather Petals: Pluck approximately two cups of fresh rose petals, gently removing them from the stems. This quantity will provide a concentrated infusion of the rose's aromatic compounds.

Simmer the Petals: Place the rose petals in a pot and cover them with distilled water. Bring the mixture to a gentle simmer over low heat. Allow the petals to simmer for about 30 minutes, allowing their essence to infuse into the water.

Cool and Strain: Once the simmering process is complete, remove the pot from the heat and let the mixture cool completely. Strain the liquid through a fine-mesh sieve or cheesecloth, separating the infused rose water from the spent petals. Discard the petals.

Storage: Transfer the strained rose water to a clean glass jar or bottle. Seal it tightly and store it in the refrigerator to maintain freshness.

Your homemade rose water is now ready not only to help in your herbalist preparation, but also enhance your culinary creations, skincare routines, or sensory experiences. From adding a delicate floral note to your dishes to soothing and refreshing your skin, the possibilities are endless. Enjoy the process of creating this fragrant elixir and savor the beauty and benefits of nature's botanical wonders in your own home.

Sea salt and Epsom salts. Adding a small amount of salt can enhance the effectiveness of herbal preparations used in baths, soaks, nasal sprays, and gargles. The addition of salt provides certain benefits, such as soothing irritated nasal passages, promoting sinus health, and assisting in the healing process of minor wounds or irritations. The salt acts as a natural saline solution, helping to cleanse and moisturize the affected areas. When preparing these remedies, incorporating a pinch of salt can contribute to their overall therapeutic properties.

Gelatin capsules. When it comes to making homemade herb capsules using herbal powders, the most commonly used size is "00" gelatin capsules. These capsules provide a convenient and efficient way to encapsulate herbal powders for personal use.

Safety Tips

Label everything. Label maker have a bad rep, but there is nothing more useful in keeping your natural medicine cabinet organized. Make sure to include the content, amount, recommended dosage, and most important of all, the date!

Start small. It is wise to start with small test batches and doses when experimenting with a new herbal remedy. By beginning with smaller quantities, you have the opportunity to assess how your body responds to the herb or preparation. Scaling up or adjusting the dosage can be done later if the remedy proves to be well-tolerated. This cautious approach allows you to identify any adverse reactions or sensitivities with minimal risk and waste.

Be cautious with pharmaceuticals. It is important to recognize that herbs and pharmaceutical drugs can interact with each other in various ways. These interactions can have both positive and negative effects. Positive herb-drug interactions may offer benefits such as reducing drug dosage or minimizing side effects. However, navigating herb-drug interactions requires careful consideration and attention. In the accompanying notes for each remedy, we highlight the major interactions to be mindful of. Nonetheless, it is highly recommended to consult with a knowledgeable herbalist or healthcare provider, particularly if you are taking multiple medications simultaneously. Their expertise can provide valuable insights into potential interactions and help ensure the safe and effective integration of herbs and pharmaceutical drugs in your healthcare regimen.

Use your senses. It is essential to carefully examine the herbs you are working with as well as the final product to ensure their quality and safety. Take the time to visually inspect the herbs for any signs of mold or contamination in your infused oil. When receiving dried herbs, carefully check for any bits of packaging material that may have found their way into the shipment.

Additionally, engaging your senses of smell and taste can provide valuable information about the potency of your herbs and remedies. These sensory cues can help you gauge the strength and effectiveness of the herbal preparations, allowing you to adjust the dosage accordingly.

By being attentive to the quality and characteristics of your herbs and remedies, you can ensure a higher level of safety and effectiveness in your herbal practice.

Make only what you need.
If you find a particular remedy that yields excellent results and you wish to have it readily available, that's wonderful—go ahead and make it a part of your routine. However, it is important to be mindful of the quantity you prepare. While having a gallon of nasal spray solution may initially seem convenient, it is unnecessary and may ultimately go to waste before you have the opportunity to utilize it all.

To avoid excessive amounts and maintain the freshness and effectiveness of your remedies, make only what you genuinely need. By preparing remedies in appropriate quantities, you can minimize wastage and ensure that each batch remains potent and useful. This approach promotes efficiency and allows you to maximize the benefits of your herbal preparations without unnecessary surplus.

Remember, the key is to strike a balance between having an ample supply and avoiding unnecessary excess, ensuring that your remedies remain fresh and effective for the desired period.

Begin with what's abundant. As you begin your herbal exploration, start with the herbs that are abundant in the wild or commonly grown. These readily available herbs are like the tried-and-true classics, and they will be your reliable allies on your herbal journey.

As you gain confidence and experience, consider exploring the local plants that thrive in your area. These plants have adapted to your specific environment and can offer unique benefits. By focusing on local herbs, you not only support the ecosystem but also establish a deeper connection with your surroundings.

Remember, you don't need to chase after rare and exotic herbs to find effective solutions. Nature has provided us with a wealth of powerful herbs that are readily accessible. Embrace the practicality and effectiveness of these herbs, and let them guide you on your path to wellness.

So, dive into the world of herbs and let the practicality of locally available plants be your guiding light. Enjoy the journey of discovering the herbal allies that nature has provided right at your doorstep.

Get the herb to the tissue. To harness the full potential of herbs, it's important to ensure that they reach the targeted area and come into direct contact with the affected tissue. Simply drinking herbal tea may not always yield optimal results. Instead, consider choosing a delivery method that facilitates the herb's action where it's needed most.

Let's explore a few examples to illustrate this concept. If you're dealing with a respiratory issue, a steam inhalation can effectively deliver the herb's properties directly to your airways. For skin-related concerns, applying a soak or poultice allows the herbs to directly interact with the skin, promoting healing and relief. In cases of intestinal troubles, consuming herbal powder in its intact form ensures that it reaches the lower intestine, where it can have the desired impact.

By selecting the appropriate delivery method, you maximize the effectiveness of the herbs and enhance their ability to address specific concerns. So, get creative and find the best way to let your herbs work their magic where they are needed most.

Four essential methods for the budding herbalist

Now that you have a grasp of the basic methods of preparing herbal remedies, let's delve into the four traditional methods employed by Native American tribes.

Native Americans typically used plants as medicines in four main ways, although this is not an exhaustive list: **infusions or decoctions** made by steeping the plants in water; **tinctures** created through extended immersion of the herbs in a combination of alcohol and water; **salves** made by transferring the medicinal properties of the herbs to an oil base; and **using the plants in their unaltered state**, such as chewing or consuming the root, or grinding the plant for direct use or encapsulation.

During the process of transforming the plant into a medicinal form, healers would offer prayers at each stage. They believed that by engaging in ceremony and prayer, they could invoke the spirit of the plant, infusing it with life force and transforming it into true medicine.

It is important to acknowledge and respect the spiritual connection between humans and nature. Even if you do not personally hold such beliefs, expressing gratitude to the Creator or Nature can help foster a deeper and more meaningful connection with the plants. This, in turn, can enhance the effectiveness of your treatments. When you approach your work with care, attention, and reverence, you are less likely to make mistakes and can utilize the gifts of the plants with greater focus and precision.

Remember, the art of herbal medicine is not solely about scientific explanations but also encompasses a profound appreciation for the interconnectedness of all beings. Embrace this holistic approach and allow it to guide your journey into the world of herbal healing.

Making Infusions and Decoctions

To create an infusion, simply submerge an herb in either cold or hot water (not boiling). It's important to use the purest water available, avoiding tap water. Opt for rainwater, water from healthy wells or springs, or distilled water for the best results.

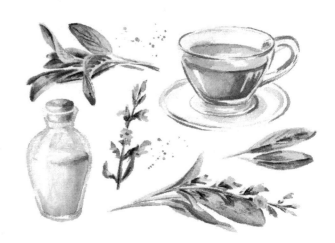

When selecting herbs for infusion, those with potent volatile oils, which have a strong fragrance akin to essential oils or perfumes, are ideally infused in cold water. On the other hand, other herbs thrive when infused in warm water.

By choosing the appropriate temperature and water quality, you can extract the beneficial properties of the herbs through infusion, allowing you to enjoy their healing effects in a gentle and natural way.

They should be left for a period of time, from fifteen minutes to overnight, depending on the herb, to allow the water to absorb the essential elements of the herb.
Glass or earthenware vessels are best for making infusions and decoctions.

Quart or pint canning jars are very good as they will not break from heat, and the screw cap keeps the nutrients from floating away in the steam.

Main'gans (Hot Infusion)
To prepare a nutritive infusion commonly used by women in menopause, follow these steps:

1. Combine equal parts (one pound each) of dried, cut, and sifted nettles, oat-straw, red clover, alfalfa, horsetail, and spearmint.
2. Take one cup of the herbal mixture and place it in a quart container. Fill the container with hot water and securely close the lid. Allow the mixture to steep overnight.
3. In the morning, strain the infusion to remove all the herbs, ensuring only the liquid remains. Drink the infused mixture throughout the following two days.
4. Remember not to keep the infusion for more than two days, as it may start to spoil.

As a general guideline, individuals weighing between 130 to 160 pounds are advised to consume 16 ounces (two cups) of the infusion per day.

This nutritive infusion harnesses the beneficial properties of various herbs to support overall well-being, particularly during the menopausal phase. Enjoy this nourishing blend and embrace the natural support it offers during this transitional period in life.

To achieve optimal infusion results, follow these general guidelines for different plant parts:

Leaves: Use one ounce of leaves per quart of water. Steep the leaves in hot water for approximately four hours, ensuring the container is tightly covered. If the leaves are tougher, they may require a longer steeping time.

Flowers: Use one ounce of flowers per quart of water. Steep the flowers in hot water for about two hours. Delicate or more fragile flowers may require a shorter steeping time.

Seeds: Use one ounce of seeds per pint of water. Steep the seeds in hot water for around thirty minutes. Highly fragrant seeds like fennel may need only fifteen minutes, while rose hips may require a longer steeping time of three to four hours.

Barks and roots: Use one ounce of barks or roots per pint of water. Allow the barks and roots to steep in hot water for approximately eight hours. However, certain barks such as slippery elm may require a shorter steeping time of one to two hours.

You will find specific instructions for the preparations of each plant in the second volume of these series, but in the meantime these few examples will illustrate the importance of choosing the right preparation for each plant and each part of the plant. Yarrow, for instance, can be quite bitter when prepared in hot water but is not bitter when prepared in cold water. The aromatic components of yarrow, and their corresponding antispasmodic properties, are soluble in cold water while the bitter components of the herb are not.
Cold infusions are prepared in the same manner as hot infusions but each herb will need to be immersed a period of time specific to itself. This can only be learned over time though many herbal books on the market can give guidance (see reference section for suggestions).

Decoctions, made by boiling herbs in water, can yield more potent results compared to infusions. The typical approach involves combining one ounce of herb with three cups of water, boiling steadily until the liquid is reduced by half.
When preparing decoctions, it is important to use a stainless steel or glass container, avoiding aluminum. The dosage can vary depending on the specific herb used, ranging from a tablespoon to a cup.
To maintain freshness and potency, decoctions should be refrigerated and consumed within a maximum of two days.

Tincturing Herbs
When preparing a tincture for internal use, you have the option to use either straight alcohol or a mixture of alcohol and water. Here's what you need to know:

- When using fresh plants for tincture-making, a general guideline is to combine one part plant with two parts 190-proof alcohol (95% alcohol). For example, if you have three ounces of fresh yarrow, you would combine it with six ounces of 190-proof alcohol in a jar, preferably a Mason jar.

- Allow the tincture to sit for a duration of two weeks, ensuring it is kept away from direct sunlight. After this period, decant the liquid by straining it and use a cloth to squeeze the herb to extract as much liquid as possible. The resulting tincture will be a combination of both water and alcohol, capturing the medicinal properties of the plant.

- When working with fresh plants, personal preferences may vary. Some herbalists prefer leaving the plants whole instead of cutting or chopping them into small pieces. While there is a belief among some herbalists that increasing the surface area of the plant exposed to alcohol results in a stronger tincture, it's important to experiment and find the method that works best for you and yields desired results.

- For dried plants, their moisture content decreases. You can find tables on the moisture content of various medicinal plants, which will help you determine the amount of water to add back when making a tincture. Generally, dried plants are tinctured at a five-to-one ratio of liquid to dried herb.
- Dried herbs should be finely powdered, often using a blender. It's recommended to store them whole until you need them. Let the tincture sit for two weeks, then decant it and extract the liquid from the herbal material.
- With fresh plants, you usually get as much liquid out as you put in. With dried material, especially roots, extract as much liquid as possible. Using amber jars for tincture storage helps protect the tincture from sunlight and preserve its integrity for many years.
- Herbal tinctures can be combined for dispensing, although some combinations may not work well. Many herbalists prefer tinctures due to their long shelf life and ease of use.

A Combination Tincture Formula for Upset Stomach
1. Ten milliliters each of yarrow, poleo mint (or peppermint), and betony.
2. Place in a one-ounce amber bottle with dropper.
3. Take 1/3 to 1/2 dropper as needed.

This mixture will usually quiet an upset stomach or nausea in seconds.

Making Oil Infusions for Salves
To create a soothing salve, you'll need to infuse the healing properties of the plant into an oil base and thicken it with beeswax. Follow these steps:

For dried herb infusion:
1. Grind the dried herbs into a fine powder.
2. Place the powdered herbs in a glass baking dish and cover them with your chosen oil, such as olive oil.
3. Stir the herbs well to ensure they are fully saturated, adding enough oil to cover them by about 1/2 to 1/4 inch.
4. Slowly cook the herb-infused oil in the oven on low heat for eight hours or overnight. Some herbalists prefer longer cooking times at lower temperatures.
5. Once the infusion is complete, strain the oil from the herbs by pressing them through a tightly woven cloth.

For fresh herb infusion:
1. Fill a mason jar with the fresh herbs and cover them completely with your preferred oil, ensuring they are fully submerged.
2. Allow the jar to sit in a sunny location for two weeks, letting the infusion process occur.
3. After the infusion period, press the herbs through a cloth to extract the infused oil.
4. Let the decanted oil sit for a day, allowing any water in the herbs to settle at the bottom.
5. Carefully pour off the oil, leaving behind any water or sediment.

Some herbalists may choose to begin the oil infusion by soaking the herb in a small amount of alcohol for 24 hours before adding the oil. After two weeks, when the oil is poured off, any water and alcohol will remain behind.

Once you have your infused oil, it's time to make the salve by adding beeswax. The ratio of oil to beeswax will depend on the desired consistency of the salve. Gently heat the infused oil and beeswax in a double boiler until the beeswax melts. Stir thoroughly to ensure a homogeneous mixture, then pour it into jars or tins to cool and solidify.

Remember to label your homemade salve with the ingredients used and the date of preparation. Enjoy the benefits of your nourishing herbal creation!
By following these steps, you can create an infused oil that forms the base for making salves.

Making Salves
To make a salve, combine the oil infusion with beeswax in a glass or stainless-steel cooking pan. Use about 2 ounces of beeswax per cup of oil. Heat the mixture gently on the stovetop until the beeswax melts. Test the consistency by placing a few drops on a small plate and letting it cool. Adjust the wax or oil amounts if needed. Pour the mixture into a jar and let it harden uncovered. Here's a formula for a wound salve:

1. Use a heavy pot made of glass or stainless steel.
2. Grind all herbs into a fine powder.
3. Add the powdered herbs to the oil in the pot.
4. Cook the mixture in the oven on a low setting (around 150 to 200 degrees Fahrenheit) overnight.
5. Allow the mixture to cool, then press the herbs in a cloth to extract all the oil.
6. Clean the pot and return the oil to it, reheating it slowly on the stovetop.
7. Measure about 4 ounces of beeswax (usually 2 ounces per pint of oil) and add it to the pot.
8. Stir in approximately 1/4 teaspoon of vitamin E.
9. Pour the salve into containers and label them.
10. Optional: Add essential oil for fragrance.

The combination of herbs used in the salve formula has specific healing properties. Comfrey root promotes rapid cellular healing and wound closure with reduced scarring. Echinacea, usnea, chaparral, and osha offer antibacterial, antifungal, and antiviral properties. Burdock is beneficial for the skin, while cranesbill helps to stop bleeding.

In some cases, when a wet dressing like a salve isn't suitable for a wound, you can directly apply the powdered herbs to the wound. The powdered herbs help to control bleeding, facilitate quick healing, and prevent infection. Once the wound starts to heal, using the wound salve continues to support the healing process.

Using Whole Herbs
Some herbs can be consumed directly when needed for their medicinal properties. Osha is a great example of this. It can be used to alleviate sore throats and upper respiratory infections caused by both viral and bacterial factors. Osha is quite potent, so it is typically consumed in small amounts when necessary. In certain cases, a combination of using the whole herb and taking tinctured herbs can be an effective approach.

Storing Herb

I f you don't dry and store your herbs properly, they will quickly use their effects.

Fresh herbs can lose intensity very quickly, so if you don't need to use them immediately, dry them immediately after you've sourced them.

To dry herbs, separate the leaves from the stems and spread them in free, single layers on a spotless, leveled surface. Bulkier plants might be dangled from a line in a dry zone, for example, a warm storm cellar or attic. Flies and different bugs might be attracted by your hanging herbs, so you might need to cover them with a cheesecloth. The time required for drying depends both on the herb and the earth in which it's being dried. Since herbs lose their strength so rapidly, the shorter the drying time frame the better. For most herbs, it takes about seven days. An herb is adequately dry when it despite everything has a smell yet is sufficiently dry to break. On the off chance that it disintegrates totally when you handle it, you dried it excessively long.

Roots, which ought to be completely washed before drying, take more time to dry than leaves and flowers— for the most part around three weeks. However picturesque is the image of a homestead kitchen with dried herbs handing from the rafters there are more efficient methods to preserve the freshness and potency of their herbal products. One such method is the use of mason jars, the go-to storage solution for a wide range of herbal preparations. Mason jars offer a multitude of advantages. They are available in various sizes, making them versatile for storing different quantities of herbs. The airtight seal provided by their tight-fitting lids helps to maintain the integrity of the herbs by preventing moisture and air from entering the container. Additionally, mason jars are affordable and easily accessible, making them a practical choice for herbal storage.

While dark-colored glass jars, such as amber or cobalt, are often recommended to shield the contents from light exposure, clear glass jars can be used as long as they are kept away from direct sunlight. Although light can potentially affect the quality of stored herbs, clear glass jars are still suitable for storage purposes. When it comes to the shelf life of herbal products, different types have varying longevity. Dried herbs, when properly stored in glass jars with tight lids, can retain their potency for anywhere between 1 to 5 years. Tinctures, which are concentrated herbal extracts made with alcohol, have a longer shelf life and may last up to 10 years if stored correctly.

However, it's important to note that oils and salves have a shorter lifespan compared to dried herbs and tinctures. Oils can turn rancid over time, which can affect their quality and effectiveness. As a result, oils and oil-based salves typically have a shelf life of around 6 months to 1 year. It is crucial to regularly check the aroma and appearance of oils to ensure they are still fresh. Lotions, on the other hand, have an even shorter shelf life due to their water content. The combination of oil and water creates an environment conducive to mold growth. As a result, lotions generally have a shelf life of 1 to 3 months. To extend the freshness of lotions, refrigeration is recommended.

To assess the viability of dried herbs or herbal products, trust your senses. A strong aroma, vibrant color, and potent flavor indicate that the herbs are still in good condition and suitable for use. By paying attention to these sensory cues and storing your herbal treasures in well-sealed mason jars, you can ensure that they maintain their quality and efficacy over time.

Drying

1. Dry most plants in shaded, well-ventilated areas, avoid wire screens and newspaper print. Research which plants dry better in the sun.
2. Don't wash leaf or flowers. Shake them to get bugs and dust off. If the quantities are manageable, tie bundles at the base of the stems in diameters of 1 1/2 inches or less. They may also be scattered loosely on screens to dry.
3. Barks: Scrape off the outer bark if appropriate. This is called Tossing.
4. Roots: Lay them out or string. Rinsing usually will not remove soil particles. A pressure hose is often required as well as hand brushing, especially with clay. Cut lengthwise for large heavy roots without aromatic properties.
5. All plant parts are dry when brittle. Pinch the lower part of hanging plants. Cut large sample root in half to see if center is dry.

Storage

1. Avoid light and excessive heat that could destroy aromatic properties and other valuable constituents. When totally dry, food grade plastic bags or fiber barrels or other containers that omit oxygen and moisture are desirable to preserve quality and potency as long as possible.
2. Label with dates and location.
3. Broken or crushed herbs lose their value more rapidly than whole, uncut herbs.

Sacred Medicine

I have left the most complicated matter for the last chapter of this first volume. Up until now I have spoken of Native American Medicine as matter-of-factly, scientifically-proven therapies and treatment. I talked about how herbal medicine was incorporated in pioneer and modern medicine and how we can utilize its wisdom to this day as herbalists and healers. This was by design, this book after all is meant for beginners and specialists alike, and spirituality cannot be forced upon anybody. One should come to it to his/her own accord. However, one should not forget that tribal medicine was not simply the decoction of herbs.

Although this book is about herbal healing, herbs are only one part of the overall Native American philosophy of health. At the heart of Native American healing is a trust and belief in a higher power—the Great Spirit, the Creator—and the role He plays in our everyday lives. Each tribe or nation has its own name for this Great Spirit. The Arapaho call It "Man Above," the Pawnees refer to It as "Ti-rá-wa," the Crows speak of It as "First Maker," and the Sioux call It "The Great Spirit" or "Mystery."

In our native tradition, we hold deep reverence for the gifts bestowed upon us by our Creator— the animals, plants, and water that form the fabric of nature. These sacred offerings provide us with sustenance, clothing, shelter, and the means to heal our bodies and spirits. It is our responsibility to care for and respect the natural world and to use these gifts only when necessary. We understand that as human beings, we are an integral part of the larger universe, lovingly crafted by the Creator. Every living creature, plant, rock, tree, mountain, and even water has a soul, and therefore, all of nature deserves our utmost respect and honor.

Our approach to medicine is rooted in spirituality, for we perceive the medicine man as a spiritual figure deeply connected to the community. Healing is not just a physical act but a ceremonial one as well. We recognize the importance of ceremonies in our healing practices, as they allow us to express our sacred feelings and reverence for the interconnectedness of all life.

In our modern times, it is crucial to periodically renew our connection to the sacred, as forgetting our place in the web of life can lead to disharmony and illness. We draw inspiration from the enduring practices of our ancestors, such as the Hopi people who still don ceremonial masks and engage in community rituals to restore their bond with the Earth. Through these ceremonies, we reaffirm our connection to the natural world and ensure its preservation for future generations.

Our ceremonies need not be elaborate; simplicity holds its own power. Each morning, we offer thanks to the Creator for the gift of life. We seek guidance and assistance from our plant relatives, and the act of smudging with sage purifies our spirits. These simple gestures of gratitude and respect contribute to our ongoing harmony with the web of life.

Throughout our diverse native cultures, we have developed various primary ceremonies and rituals that help us regain balance and harmony. The sweat lodge, sacred pipe ceremony, vision quest, and medicine wheel are some of the profound practices that guide us on our spiritual journey. In our sacred plant medicine practices, two ceremonies hold special significance and benefit— the sacred pipe ceremony and the medicine wheel.

The sacred pipe ceremony exemplifies the intricate beauty of our ceremonial practices. It is a profound act of uniting Heaven, Earth, and Man. This union holds profound teachings for our sacred plant medicine practices, revealing the interconnectedness of all beings and the wisdom inherent in the natural world.

Through our ancestral teachings and personal experiences, we recognize that our connection to the sacred must be continuously nurtured through ceremony. We acknowledge the ebb and flow of human nature, understanding that our connection to the sacred can fade if not actively maintained. Thus, we embrace the power of ceremony to renew our bond with the Earth and all its living beings.

As we walk this sacred path, we hold deep gratitude for the teachings passed down to us and for the opportunity to experience the profound unity between ourselves, the spirit world, and the elements of the Earth. It is through these ceremonies that we weave a vibrant, living fabric that celebrates the sacredness of all existence.

The medicine wheel incorporates an essential element of sacred plant medicine, the indigenous understanding that all of life is a circle, that each element of the life web sits together in a council of life, and that human beings travel around a great wheel as they progress through life.

Thus, the medicine wheel has particular relevance because it is a highly developed expression of the Earth-centered experience. It incorporates the belief that there are unique and specific stages of human development that transcend psychology and environment, and that plants have a specific place in helping at certain stages of travel around the wheel. Finally, herbs sometimes contain within themselves the power of a specific direction, and awareness of this power when working with plants can be of special benefit during healing ceremonies. Each of these ceremonies can utilize smudging: the sacred pipe always, the medicine wheel sometimes. So, before I go into detail on these two ceremonies, let's see what smudging is all about.

Smudging

Smudging is a sacred practice deeply ingrained in our traditions. It involves the burning of herbs to cleanse and purify ourselves, our surroundings, and ceremonial tools. The act of smudging marks a significant moment in time, signifying the transition into the sacred space of ceremony. Throughout history, our ancestors have used four main herbs for smudging: cedar, sweetgrass, sage, and wormwood.

To perform smudging, we take dried herbs and place them in a bowl or container. Igniting the herbs, we allow the flame to extinguish, creating a smoldering smoke. With great reverence, we use our hands or a feather to gently fan the smoke over our bodies, other participants, and the plants or tools present.

In our cultural beliefs, the herbs used for smudging possess profound qualities. They are believed to have the power to dispel negative energies and restore harmony and balance to our being. This sacred act of smudging creates a sacred space where we can connect with the spiritual realm and align ourselves with the natural flow of the universe.

By engaging in the ritual of smudging, we honor the ancient wisdom passed down through generations and invite the transformative energy of the herbs to envelop us. It is a practice of purification, cleansing, and renewal, allowing us to embark on our ceremonial journeys with a sense of clarity, reverence, and harmony.

The Sacred Pipe

The American Indian ceremonial pipe has been in use for centuries. The earliest pipes that have been found are simple tubes discovered in prehistoric mounds in Ohio. They are made of clay and alabaster. The earliest long stemmed pipes had bowls made in the shape of animal heads.
The use of ceremonial pipes spread along the Mississippi River and into the lakes and eastern plains around the 11th century. One of the first tribes observed by Europeans to use the pipe were the MicMac of Nova Scotia. The pipes have been used in holy ceremonies by Earth-peoples for at least a thousand years.
—JOHN FREESOUL

Most indigenous peoples of North America who use the pipe have legends of its creation or appearance in their culture. Some tribes received it as a gift from another tribe, others received it from holy people or supernatural beings who were sent by Creator to bring it to humans.
This gift of the pipe by the intervention of Creator through a sacred being or prophet is akin to the tablets given to Moses in Hebrew tradition, or the appearance of Christ in Christian tradition. In the ceremonial pipe, each component holds symbolic significance. The bowl represents the female, while the stem represents the male. The bowl is likened to flesh and blood, while the stem symbolizes bones. Metaphorically, the bowl represents the Earth mother, and the stem represents Father Sky. The channel that runs through the pipe stem and bowl represents the direct connection between all things and the spiritual realm. It represents the straight and narrow path that each individual walks to establish a relationship with the Spirit. Therefore, when the pipe is joined, all these elements come together as one. Duality fades away, and a sense of unity is embraced. The pipe ceremony serves as a symbolic reminder of the interconnectedness of all things and the profound relationship between humanity and the spiritual realm.

The tobacco that is smoked in the pipe is made from a variety of plants. There is often tobacco (Nicotiana), mullein (Verbascum), uva-ursi (Arctostaphylos), sage (Artemisia), raspberry (Rubus), red willow (Salix), and sometimes many other herbs. Whenever possible, the pipe carrier must pick the herbs. The plants should be picked in a specific sacred manner and prepared as smoke mixture by the pipe carrier. Prayers of thanks are offered to the plants who give themselves up to be smoked. When smoking the pipe, pinches of tobacco mixture are offered to the four directions, the plant kingdoms, the animal kingdoms, the elementals, Great Spirit, Creator, the Earth, the sky, humans, sun, moon, all those in Spirit, the rocks of the Earth, and sometimes many more. In this way, when the pipe is smoked, the whole universe participates.

With each puff of smoke a prayer is offered to be carried up to Creator, Great Spirit. The pipe is used in prayer for whatever is needed. There are some guidelines in addressing the integrity of these prayers—that the prayers honor all life, human and nonhuman, and the continuing existence of all relations, not just human. In this way the pipe is a major Earth-centered tool because it belongs to all life, not just humans. It represents and speaks with the life essence in all things. In this way, the pipe carrier is not the owner of the pipe but its keeper. The pipe carrier is a spokesperson for all life and the life force of creation. There are specific pipe ceremonies, depending on the lineage and culture of the pipe carrier, and the visions that have given rise to specific pipe ceremonies number in the hundreds or, perhaps, thousands. The pipe holds a versatile purpose in connecting with the spiritual realm and serving various needs. It can be used for communion with Spirit, providing a means to establish a profound connection with the divine. During challenging times, the pipe can offer solace, guidance, and strength. It becomes a source of support and wisdom to navigate through difficult circumstances. Additionally, the pipe can be utilized for healing purposes, offering a conduit for spiritual healing and restoration for those who are unwell.

The specific manner in which the pipe is used in these instances can vary greatly, as it is tailored to the specific needs and purposes of the moment. The rituals, prayers, and intentions associated with the pipe ceremony may differ depending on the circumstances and the individuals involved. The pipe ceremony is a deeply personal and sacred practice, shaped by the unique needs and intentions of the participants, allowing them to engage in a direct connection with Spirit, find solace, seek guidance, and experience healing.

Pipes are made from many materials besides the well-known pipestone; any soft stone will do. Alabaster and soapstone, for instance, are often used. The stems can be made of any wood that feels right. If one is called to the pipe, the correct form will soon present itself.

As the pipe carrier engages in the pipe ceremony over time, a deep relationship with the pipe is established. Eventually the pipe "awakens" and comes alive. An awakened pipe is a channel between the pipe carrier (the human community) and Spirit. Just as there is a spirit and soul in all things so, too, is there one in the pipe. The pipe carrier establishes relationship with the spirit of the pipe and through it acts as a sacred intermediary for the human community, the Earth, and for all life. Frances Densmore makes a reference to this event in her article "The Belief of the Indian in a Connection Between Song and the Supernatural." She notes:

On one occasion the writer was questioning Lone Man, a trusted Sioux informant and singer, concerning information received from a pipe. He was asked whether a spirit had entered into the pipe and gave the information. He replied that this was not the case, saying that under certain conditions a pipe might "become sacred" and speak to the Indian.

This living spirit of the pipe is and should be consciously evoked and related with by the pipe carrier when working with the pipe in ceremony. Almost all Earth-centered practitioners have some physical object of the Earth that is used for ceremonial purposes. These objects become a focus for communion with Spirit and an honoring of the soul and spirit essence in all creation. They often play a special part in Earth relationship and rites of passage for humans. It is a tool for balancing between the worlds and developing depth of Spirit for those on the Earth-centered path. Each part of the pipe ceremony represents communion with a sacred archetype of the universe. As years are spent in this communion one comes to understand these archetypes and to be in personal relationship with them. Through them one approaches closer to Creator and one's own true nature. The special power of the sacred, which comes from this process, can be evoked to help one's self, friends, family, and community during troubled times. When people work with sacred plant medicine they are consciously evoking the power of Heaven and Earth by calling on Creator in their prayers. Within the body of the practitioner of sacred plant medicine, the two are united in balance and sacred power is evoked when the plants are called on to become medicine. When one uses the pipe this process is enhanced.

The pipe is akin to many martial art forms that have their origins in Asia. These martial arts have at their center the act of joining Heaven and Earth in the body of the practitioner. This act is a unique one and central to any deep knowledge of sacred plant medicine. In the following detailed account of a generic pipe ceremony, the specific mindset necessary to each ceremonial stage is discussed. Each act deepens the joining of Heaven and Earth and then goes on from there to direct intention toward some expected outcome. This process is central to all forms of ceremony.

To truly understand ceremony and enter into that world, one should come to understand that certain states of mind, of power, exist for which there are few words in the English language. But indigenous tribes, closely connected to the sacred as a part of their cultural life, had well-developed terms for these things. This is especially true of the pipe.

Terminology of the Sacred

In all tribes, each had a specific term that was used to refer to the sacred. The term among the Sioux was *wakan*, among the Ojibwa, *manido*, among the Omaha, *wakanda*, among the Mandan, *ho'pinis*. These are similar to the Asian *tao*. The act of limiting those terms to mean "sacred" is somewhat incorrect, however. It means much more than that. The word refers to the sacred center of all things from which all things have come.

So, using Sioux terminology, and quoting Joseph Epes Brown, the degree of wakan a thing possesses *"is in proportion to the ability of the object or act to reflect most directly the principle or principles that are in Wakan-Tanka, the Great Spirit, who is One."*

The commonness of this concept among indigenous cultures in the Americas indicates a general sensitivity to perceiving manifestations of the sacred and a refined capacity to distinguish the degree of sacredness a thing possessed. As this characteristic was so fundamental to all things in indigenous life, understanding of the pipe or any other sacred object or ceremony would be impossible without it. Within each origin tale of the appearance of the pipe to native peoples, these particular terminologies are present, the meaning of which is culturally implied; thus, it is imperative to understand that which is not said as well as that which is said.

The Ceremony of the Sacred Pipe

The pipe as a sacred tool combines the most powerful elements of two processes. First it is equivalent to the Buddhist meditation process of working with a *koan*. *Koans* are statements designed to force one beyond the rational meaning of words into an awareness of a higher truth. The pipe, when worked with devoutly can, like a *koan*, stimulate one beyond this everyday normal reality into an awareness and understanding of deeper sacred truths. Second, the pipe is an act in which the inherent duality of the universe is made one. Each act in the pipe ceremony represents a specific sacred meaning. In other words, there is an underlying discrete and specific spiritual meaning that is evoked at that moment in the pipe ceremony. Though there are differing elements in pipe ceremonies, depending on the lineage and type of pipe being smoked, generally all pipe ceremonies are identical in essence.

Besides the pipe (bowl and stem) there are usually a number of other objects that go up to make a pipe bundle. There is the smoking mixture in its own container and a pipe tamper—usually a stick that is narrower at one end, used to pack the pipe before it is lit and during the smoking itself—and matches. There is also smudge, usually sage or wormwood; a container in which to carry it; a smudge bowl; and often a feather or bird wing to be used to waft the smoke onto the objects being smudged. There is usually an altar cloth or small rug on which everything is placed, and a container in which all these things may be kept. Then there are any other sacred objects that may be important to the pipe carrier and all of these, together, are carried within a ceremonial pipe bundle. When the pipe bundle is unpacked the altar cloth is laid down and the objects are laid out. Smudge is lit and everything is smudged, beginning with the people involved in the ceremony—the pipe carrier first. The pipe is usually smudged last—the stem first and then the bowl. When the stem and bowl are smudged many pipe carriers pass them across the smudge bowl north to south then west to east. The stem first and then the bowl are held, their opening to the lips, and smudge drawn through them so that they are purified inside and out. In this beginning element of the ceremony the mind has a chance to quiet itself, the participants to take on the proper attitudes and states of mind. This signals that what is to follow is a sacred thing, set off from what has gone before.

The next step is the joining of the stem and bowl. The bowl is held in the left hand, the stem in the right and both are held up to Creator and permission to smoke is requested. This is the first act that is koan-like in its nature. The pipe carrier acts as an intermediary for the manifestation of the sacred. It is through the carrier's training, directed intention, and sensitivity that the ceremony evokes all the power of the holy, that it is truly wakan. At this point one listens for permission to be granted; if it is, then, and only then, are the bowl and stem joined. At the moment of unity, the duality of the universe is made one. This act is central to the nature and purpose of the pipe. It is through this joining and the participatory smoking of the pipe that divisions, human and nonhuman, between people and cultures, between secular and sacred are transcended. All things become one.

The next step is the filling of the pipe. The bowl rests on the ground, the stem in the lap. Generally four pinches of tobacco are used to fill the bowl. With each pinch some portion of the web of life is invited to come into the circle and into the pipe. All life is brought into the process. A pinch of tobacco (smoking mixture) is taken between the thumb and first two fingers in the right hand, held up to Creator, and a prayer is said.

For example:
Creator, Grandmother Earth, all my relations
all the Spirits of this place
I ask that You come and join us now
There is a place for You in this pipe
A second pinch is taken and held up to Creator, the prayer continuing:
All the green relations
spirits of tree, and osha, and all the green growing things
I ask that You join us now
There is a place for You in this pipe
A third pinch is taken and held up to Creator, and again one prays:
All the animal relations
the two-leggeds, the four-leggeds, the wingeds, the swimmers and crawlers
I ask that You join us now
There is a place for You in this pipe
And finally, a fourth pinch is taken:
I call on the powers of the four directions, the stone people, fire, water, and air

All the star relations, all those who have walked this path before us
I ask that you join us now
There is a place for you in this pipe
As each pinch is taken and as each part of the life web is invited to come and join in the pipe ceremony, the pipe carrier is intently focused on the underlying meaning that is being evoked. The participation of these other members of our world is actual and literal. One must be able to feel them come and take a seat in the council circle of the pipe. Often many years of work are necessary to truly evoke these powers, to feel them actually come and take their place, to create dialogue and communication.

In the fourth step, prayers are placed in the pipe. If others are participating in the ceremony the pipe is passed to the left. The person takes the pipe and holds it, bowl in left hand, stem in right. Anything that person desires to pray for is voiced. For example: if one needs help with a certain thing, for others or oneself, to offer thanks for the help of Creator, to voice a pain that is carried, thanks for a joy felt, anything, it is offered at this time. The pipe is passed around the circle until it comes back to the carrier.

The fifth step is the lighting of the pipe. The pipe is lit, puffed vigorously until it is going well, then it is held up, stem first, for Creator to smoke. This is another portion of the ceremony that works with underlying meaning. The pipe carrier works with personal sensitivity, humility, and intention until the time when one can feel Creator actually come and smoke the pipe. After Creator smokes, the stem is lowered and offered to Grandmother Earth. When Grandmother Earth smokes the pipe it is offered to the Four Directions, one after another, until each one has smoked. Then, and only then, does a person smoke the pipe.

The sixth step is the smoking of the pipe. In this process, a person engages in a deeply interactive process with Creator. The smoke is drawn into the mouth, then into the lungs, and released into the air, whereupon it rises up. The prayers in the pipe take on a visible form. Further, they blend with the body; a portion of this sacred prayer remains in the body and a portion of the body intermingles with the prayer. As the prayer is spoken or offered, it transcends the physical realm and ascends to the Creator, merging with the essence of the entire universe. Through this process, the individual who utters the prayer becomes interconnected and united with all things.

The act of prayer serves as a reminder of our inherent unity and the power of our intentions to reach beyond ourselves and become an integral part of the greater whole. The process of smoking is continued until all the tobacco in the pipe is gone.
When the pipe is empty the carrier holds it up and thanks Creator and all things for the pipe:
Creator, I thank you for the gift of this pipe
and as I (we) go forward from one day to the next
from one pipe to the next
I (we) say "Yes, yes, yes, yes"
A-ho!

Then finally, the pipe is taken apart, cleaned, and put away.

The Medicine Wheel

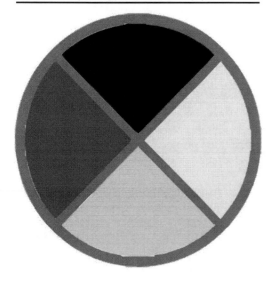

Is not the south the source of life, and does not the flowering stick truly come from there? And does not man advance from there toward the setting sun of his life? Then does he not approach the colder north where the white hairs are? And then does he not arrive, if he lives, at the source of light and understanding, which is the east? Then does he not return to where he began, to his second childhood, there to give back his life to all life, and his flesh to the earth whence it came? The more you think about this, the more meaning you will see in it.
—BLACK ELK

There are few permanent shrines in Earth-centered spiritual lineages. Two of these are the medicine wheel and the sweat lodge. Though the sacred circle is present in all cultures the medicine wheel, a specialized form of the sacred circle, is not. Some version of the sweat lodge is present on all continents and all cultures.

From William K. Powers' YUWIPI: Vision and Experience in Oglala Ritual, published in 1982 by the University of Nebraska Press.

Architecturally, the only permanent shrine in Oglala religion is the sweat lodge. It stands, sometimes wavering in the wind, in sharp contrast to the countless Christian churches that dot the reservation—little frame boxes with identical steeples and church bells that look as if they had all been constructed by a mission construction company. All are painted a sacramental white and have blue- or green-shingled roofs. It is as if they had come off an assembly line, just the way federally funded housing projects deliver prefabricated homes intact to the owner's land.
The sweat lodge is a perfect symbol for the Oglala religion; when not in use the structures look rather pitiful: a dome made of willow saplings stuck into the ground, bent over, and tied in place with cloth strips or rope. There is something exceedingly profane about them when not in use, in contrast to the white man's shrines and churches, which are perpetually sacred, set off from the rest of society in a feeble attempt to separate religion from the culture's social, political, and economic institutions. The sweat lodge reflects the Oglala principle of austerity and simplicity: the entire universe is a

cathedral: everything is permanently sacred unless desecrated by human foibles that cause disharmony between humans and the rest of nature. At this time a special ritual is required to reinstate a balance among all living things, and only then are special places like the sweat lodge temporally and spatially separated from the rest of the mundane world; it is only during the ritual itself that special rules of conduct are in force and require different behavior toward nature.

When not in use, the sweat lodge becomes a playground for children, who dodge in and out of the framework, stepping into the central hole where the heated stones are placed during the ritual. It is a stopping place for multitudes of dogs, who lift their legs and declare the sacred saplings, placed there in honor of the various aspects of Wakantanka, their special territory. It is a meeting place for ants, spiders, grasshoppers, and flies seeking refuge from predatory birds who alight on the willow frame during their morning feeding. The sweat lodge is often invaded by a recalcitrant cow or a frightened horse, and it tolerates all these intrusions, along with the constant battering of the wind against its desiccated skeleton. It is partly this tolerance that makes the sweat lodge potentially sacred: like humans, it is subject to the whims of nature and must abide by its relentless impositions.

Like the sweat lodge, the medicine wheel is usually an unimpressive structure. Most are simple circles of stones laid in a pattern on the ground. They are overgrown easily and, if left untended, cannot be found in a few years. But they have an ancient history, from Stonehenge to the 20,000 or so examples on this North American continent. They serve as a pattern for focusing awareness and as a way of relating to all living things. In the past, when people would encounter a place on the Earth where the sacred was manifesting itself, where hierophany was strong, they would often construct a circle of stones to mark it. In effect, the stone circle said, "This place is sacred. When you enter this place you enter a sacred space and time." In time, more stones would be added to the circle, rising as walls and more clearly defining sacred space. In some cultures, these would be roofed over and become churches. Sometimes, like the ancient shrine of The Mother of the Hunt in Bandolier National Monument in New Mexico, it would become a low wall. In other places there would be only a circle of stones. The medicine wheel is a powerful symbol that embodies the interconnectedness of all life. As we sit within the wheel and invoke the sacred, a profound council of life unfolds before us. In this sacred space, we can restore our connection with the diverse web of life that surrounds us. When we enter the medicine wheel, we open ourselves to the presence and wisdom of all living beings. The animals, plants, stones, and spirits all come together in this council, offering their guidance, teachings, and healing energies. We, as human beings, are just one thread in the intricate tapestry of life, and through the ceremony of the wheel, we have the opportunity to reestablish our bonds with all our relations.

In this council, the profound wisdom of the animal kingdom, the nurturing power of the plant realm, the stability of the stones, and the guidance of the spirit realm converge. It is a sacred space where all aspects of creation unite to guide us and restore harmony to the Earth. Through the medicine wheel ceremony, we reawaken our deep connections with the natural world and engage in the process of healing and restoration. We recognize that our well-being is intricately linked to the well-being of all beings, and by honoring this interdependence, we play an active role in healing the Earth and nurturing the sacred balance of life. As we embrace the teachings and energies of the medicine wheel, we embark on a profound journey of unity, understanding, and reverence. It is through this ancient ceremony that we reestablish our place in the circle of life, allowing the healing of the Earth to unfold once more, guided by the wisdom and interconnectedness that the medicine wheel represents.

The wheel of life, the medicine wheel, is a map for everything in the universe, a blueprint of the web of life. As Black Elk said, this wheel exists in all things. Within each of us, too, the medicine wheel exists as our inner council. A human cannot sit in relationship with all life if the life inside is in disarray and disharmony. It is important to understand how the medicine wheel exists inside you and to work to establish harmony in all its parts. From this starting place you can then move outward to larger and larger external circles, finally encompassing all of the universe.

The Medicine Wheel inside You

To embark on a journey within the sacred realm of the medicine wheel, find a quiet and comfortable place where you can sit without interruptions. Take a few deep breaths and allow yourself to relax. Close your eyes and visualize yourself walking along a serene path in a meadow. The gentle sounds of birds singing and grasses rustling in the wind surround you. As you continue walking, you come across a small hill that you ascend with ease. At the top, you notice a modest building with an open door. Curiosity guides you inside. Inside the building, you discover a spacious room adorned with an oval table and numerous chairs encircling it. Some of the chairs may be occupied by people, animals, or other beings, while others may be empty. Find a seat that calls to you, and as you sit down, observe the diverse members of your inner council gathering around the table. These are the various aspects of yourself that often go unnoticed in your daily life—the child, the wise parent, the one who challenges, the warrior, the sage, and many more. Engage in conversation and get to know each of them.

Over time, it is essential to cultivate a harmonious relationship with every member of your inner council, ensuring that no aspect of yourself is left outside the circle within you. This process may require patience and dedication, as some parts of you may initially harbor anger or resentment for being neglected. By working through these emotions and reaching a consensus with your inner council, you can make choices in your life that are embraced by all parts of yourself.

This integration leads to a profound sense of wholeness, a sacred completeness that permeates your being and influences your actions. Achieving this state of unity may take time, and it is recommended to engage with your inner council in daily dialogues for at least a year to establish a deep and genuine connection with them. This

practice of working with the inner council extends beyond the self and can be applied to external relationships as well. Just as members of your inner council take their places around the wheel, so too can community members, family, or the interconnected web of life find their positions within the wheel. By engaging with others in the same way, establishing relationships, balance, and harmony can be nurtured.

The importance of working with the inner council cannot be overstated when it comes to sacred plant medicine. When venturing into the sacred realms offered by these medicines, one delves into the very fabric of reality—the essence of who we believe ourselves to be, our perceptions of others and the world, and the profound truth that exists beyond our limited perspectives. This transformative process often entails years of introspection and restructuring of deep-rooted aspects of our personalities. It is necessary because our unconscious parts influence every facet of our lives. By unraveling and transcending fears, limitations, and obstacles within our psyche, we gain personal power and the ability to navigate life with greater clarity.

Working with plant medicines can initially blur the lines between projected emotions and genuine insights derived from the plants themselves. It takes considerable time and dedicated inner council work to distinguish between the two, a skill crucial in this field. Furthermore, sacred states induced by plant medicine can sometimes evoke fear or unsettlement. Therefore, maintaining balance and stability at all times is essential. Developing strong bonds with your inner council fosters this equilibrium and allows its members to act as allies during spiritually intense moments. Additionally, the members of your inner council have their unique ways of communicating with the plants, opening pathways to richer and more diverse wisdom when you have established a genuine friendship with yourself.

In the sacred practice of plant medicine, the profound journey within and the nurturing of relationships with the inner council are vital steps toward understanding oneself, transcending limitations, and deepening connections with the plant realm and the sacred forces of the universe.

Creating a Medicine Wheel

The ceremony of constructing a medicine wheel serves to restore the balance and harmony of all life. It is a sacred rite that transforms a simple circle of stones into a holy place, reminding us to live in harmonious relationship with the entire universe. As the wheel takes form, it becomes a vortex of energy, honoring the life forces and inviting all beings to join in the dance of life. By engaging in this ceremony, we acknowledge and return the gift of life bestowed upon us by the Creator and creation itself. The medicine wheel represents the unending spiral of interdependence, a mandala that encompasses the circle of existence.

Within the circle of stones, the medicine wheel not only demarcates sacred space but also represents the gathering of the Earth community in a unified council. Each of the four directions—north, south, east, and west—is symbolized by a gate, and at the center of the wheel, a larger stone signifies Spirit, the essence that resides at the core of all things. Each direction corresponds to a specific archetype, providing insights into how these archetypes manifest in human life.

The south represents the beginning of life, the season of spring when hope is born anew, and the vitality of life surges forth. It is a time of renewal, rebirth, and connection with nurturing caretakers. In the west, during adolescence, we grapple with our inner demons and embark on a journey of self-exploration. It is a transformative phase where we confront our shadows, seek our unique identities, and strive to find meaning and purpose. The west demands shedding that which no longer serves us, a process that can be painful yet essential for personal growth. Emerging from the west, we enter the north—the time of middle age—where we shoulder the responsibility of maintaining the status quo and nurturing the younger generations. It is a phase of caretaking and giving, embodying maturity and wisdom. Finally, the east signifies enlightenment and old age, a time of profound wisdom and the passing on of knowledge to the next generations. It is a period of deepening spiritual connection and preparation for the transition beyond this realm. These patterns of life repeat continuously, influencing our every action and experience.

To construct a medicine wheel, select a suitable location that resonates with you—a quiet corner of your yard or a serene space within your home. Offer prayers to the chosen place, perform a smudging ritual with sage to purify the energy, and declare your intention to create a wheel. The next step is to find stones in places that evoke a sense of well-being, preferably wild and natural areas. Pray for guidance and assistance as you search for stones—eight larger stones for the directional gates, a minimum of four stones between each gate, and a central stone representing the source of all things. Treat each stone with reverence, smudging and offering tobacco in exchange for taking it.

Once you have gathered all the stones, begin the ceremony with utmost reverence. Each stone has its own place within the wheel, so respectfully ask each stone where it wishes to be positioned and honor its choice. The wheel can evolve and grow over time, with the addition of more stones if desired.

Similar to the sacred pipe, each element of the medicine wheel carries specific meanings. It is important to engage in meditation and contemplation with each aspect of the wheel, deepening your understanding of their significance and establishing a profound relationship with them. This level of understanding allows the invocation of specific meanings and powers of the wheel for healing and desired outcomes.

In the realm of plant medicine, parallels can be drawn between certain plants and the sacred powers embodied in different aspects of the wheel. Some plants seem to encompass the power of the south or the north, while others embody the entirety of the medicine wheel. When working with these plants, their medicinal properties are invoked alongside the specific directional powers they

hold. This understanding can guide us when providing plant medicine to individuals.

For those who struggle to transition from the south to the west, resisting the development of their warrior spirit or confronting the darkness within, offering a plant associated with the west can aid their journey around the wheel in that direction. Similarly, individuals who have become overwhelmed by responsibilities and lost touch with their inner childlikeness may benefit from an herb representing the south, facilitating the restoration of balance.

As you deepen your connection with the essence of each direction, you will discern their presence within the plants you encounter and utilize for medicinal purposes. The medicine wheel and the plants intertwine, offering profound wisdom and healing to those who seek communion with the sacred forces of life.

Sweat Lodge Ceremony

For centuries, Native Americans have used sweat lodges and fasting as ways to benefit from the healing properties of detoxification. Of all the purification ceremonies in North America, the sweat lodge ceremony is the most widespread. The Lakota call the ceremony inikagapi, and the Chippewa called the sweat bath ritual a madodoson. The Apache called the sweat lodge itself taachi, while the Cheyenne called it vonhäom. Similar in action to a sauna, the sweat lodge's heat and moisture help detoxify the body—mentally, physically, and spiritually. The smoke in the lodge and the ceremonial rituals conducted there all contribute to the native healing process.

Sweat lodges have several health benefits:

- In the sweat lodge, healing can begin for many physical or emotional disorders. It is an opportunity to pray, speak, and ask for forgiveness from the Creator, as well as from other people who have been previously hurt.
- The cleansing heat increases body temperature, thereby increasing the body's enzymatic activity. This increased activity helps the body destroy viruses and bacteria and stimulates immune function. The famous Greek physician Hippocrates once said, "Give me a fever and I can cure any disease." Increased temperatures help the body to practically burn away bacterial and viral agents and illnesses.
- Physically, sweating helps detoxify the body by opening any clogged pores and allowing elimination of internal toxins, heavy metals, excessive urea, and metabolic by-products.
- As the body's temperature rises, endocrine glandular function is stimulated. This helps to cleanse the body and improve body function.
- The heat of the sweat lodge dilates the large blood vessels and capillaries which, in turn, stimulates increased blood flow to the skin and increases the rate at which the body's organs are flushed of toxins.

- The moist air of the sweat lodge improves lung function. Clogged respiratory passages are dilated, giving relief from minor respiratory problems and colds. Caution: Individuals with major respiratory problems and pneumonia should not use the sweat lodge.
- Hot water and steam created by pouring water over the rocks result in negative ion release. Positive ions are associated with tension and fatigue, as well as allergies, rheumatism, arthritis, insomnia, and asthma.
- Sweat lodges can improve metabolic function. By removing toxins and other waste products, as well as improving circulation, the digestion, absorption, and utilization of herbs and other nutrients can be improved.
- The sweat lodge can be a cleansing and regenerative experience, much like a rebirth. In his book Sweat, Mikkel Aaland observes, "The warm, dark, moist ambiance inside a sweat bath is easily likened to a womb, even the womb of Mother Earth, Herself."

Sweat lodges can be many different sizes and shapes and are constructed using materials found in the local environment. For example, tribes of the Southwest built circular subterranean sweat lodges in which individuals descended a ladder to the underground structure, which was encased in bedrock. Other tribes used mud, wood, or animal skins to build sweat lodges. Cedar planks were used in the far Northwest; buffalo skins covered the Plains Indians' sweat lodges, while skins or birch bark might cover frames made from willow poles in the Northeast. In the Southeast, sweat lodges might be dug into a hillside or built up into earth mounds. The polar Inuit Indians even used igloos as sweat lodges.

The sweat lodge typically holds ten to fifteen people comfortably and is light-tight to ensure that they are in total darkness. Usually, hot rocks are heated on a fire and then brought into the sweat lodge. The ceremony leader then pours water onto the rocks to produce steam to encourage sweating and cleansing and to stimulate spiritual healing. Prayers are then recited, songs are sung, and the spirits are called into the lodge in an effort to purify the participants. The door is rarely opened during a ceremony, because the heat and dark are important to help the participants focus on what they are doing.

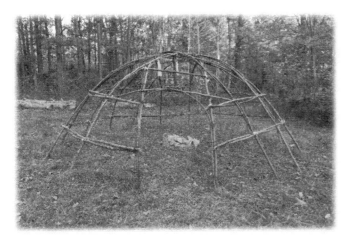

Do ~It ~Yourself Sweat Lodge

If a sweat lodge is not available, a sauna, such as those found at any health club, makes a good substitute. Or you can build your own sweat lodge. Follow the American Indian's example and use materials available in your own environment.

1. First find the proper location to build your sweat lodge. The sweat lodge should be located close to a cool clear stream, lake, or river, or the ocean, since there must be a location to cool the body after being in the sweat lodge or sauna. If this is not possible, you can use your shower or bath to cool down after the sweat lodge.
2. Dig the pit. The pit should be in the very center of the structure and should be about two feet deep and two to three feet wide. This hole is extremely symbolic and even holy. To the Plains Indians, it traditionally represents the center of the universe.
3. Gather poles to use for the framework. Willows and other saplings work well for this purpose. Although there is no set size for a sweat lodge, gather sufficient poles to construct a lodge two to four feet high in the center and about ten feet in diameter.
4. To make the framework, plant the ends of the poles into the ground, joining the ends in the center (much like a dome in appearance). Use leather string or rope to tie the ends together. Be sure to point the entrance of the lodge to the east toward Father Sun, who has tremendous power.
5. The next step is to cover the poles with material that will keep the heat in and the light out. Rather than the animal skins that used to be used to cover sweat lodges, you may need to use heavy duty canvas sheets.
6. To use the sweat lodge, you'll need to heat rocks. The best way to do this is in an outside pit. To the Creeks, the fire used to heat the rocks represents a portion of the sun and a symbol of the Creator. The stones used in the pit represent earth as both mother and grandmother and symbolize endurance, just as the earth endures.
7. Once the rocks have been brought into the sweat lodge and placed in the pit, water should be poured onto the rocks to produce steam. The water used in the sweat lodge represents the life-giving elements of air and water.
8. An offering should be made to the fire. Native Americans often used tobacco for this purpose.
9. Drinking herbal teas in the sweat lodge can help encourage healthy skin and sweating. Cayenne, elderberries, ginger, pepper, peppermint, sage, and wintergreen are the most commonly used options, since they are all warming herbs. Consume as much tea as you can while you sweat. This will also help replenish fluids the body loses during sweating.
10. Stay in the sweat lodge for about fifteen minutes.
11. After the sweat, wrap up in a blanket and cool in bed for thirty to sixty minutes. Then, plunge into a nearby stream, river, or other body of water. If this isn't possible, take a cold shower or bath instead.

For more information on the spiritual aspect of healing, see the following books:

- *American Indian Medicine* by Virgil J. Vogel (Norman: University of Oklahoma Press, 1970).
- *Earthway* by Mary Summer Rain (New York: Pocket Books, 1990).
- *The Medicine Men, Oglala Sioux Ceremony and Healing* by Thomas H. Lewis (Lincoln: University of Nebraska Press, 1990).
- *Secrets of the Sacred White Buffalo* by Gary Null (Paramus, NJ: Prentice Hall, 1998).
- *Shamanic Healing and Ritual Drama* by Åake Hultkrantz (New York: Crossroad, 1992).
- *Spirit Healing* by Mary Dean Atwood (New York: Sterling, 1991).

Conclusion

I hope you have enjoyed reading this book as much as I've enjoyed writing it, and I hope it will accompany you in your ongoing journey to the discovery of Native American herbs and their medicinal uses.

If you found this book useful and are feeling generous, please take the time to leave a short review on Amazon so that other may enjoy this guide as well.

I leave you with good wishes and hopefully a better knowledge of the plants around us and their amazing powers. This volume is part of a seven-books series on Native American Herbalism from foraging and gardening native plants to making herbal remedies for adults and children. Check out the other volumes to gain a deeper understanding of the amazing wisdom and knowledge of our forefathers and to improve not only your health, but the health of our land as well.

The Native American Herbalist's Bible 2

The Complete Field Book of the Wild Plants of North America

From Agave to Zizia. Find, Grow, and Discover the Traditional and Modern Uses of Forgotten Herbs

Linda Osceola Naranjo

Introduction

"All plants are our brothers and sisters. They talk to us and if we listen, we can hear them"
Arapaho prover

We live in a country where the cure for virtually any disease and ailment is within our grasp. In our forests, meadows, plains, and gardens grow small, seemingly insignificant flowers and herbs, plants that we don't look twice at, and trees of which we don't even bother to learn the name. Yet, they are the key to a better, healthier, and more sustainable way of life.

Our forefathers, more attuned with nature than we could ever imagine to be, understood that, and took carefully and sparingly the gifts that Nature offered to heal themselves and grow stronger.
We have lost that knowledge.
Only starting from the 1970s, a renewed interest in botanic medicine has uncovered the depth of the Native American knowledge of plants and their healing powers. The research has not only helped herbalists, but physicians and scientist as well that re-discovered substances that the Native Americans people knew about for hundreds of years.

This book is the extended edition of the best-selling *The Native American Herbalist's Bible: 3-in-1 Companion to Herbal* Medicine, offering four more volumes on gardening techniques, growing healing plants and wildflowers, and pediatric healthcare.
This is the unabridged companion to Native American herbs, their traditional and modern use, complete with appropriate doses and usage, gardening tips and techniques for both medicinal plants and wildflowers. The book is completed by a list of simple and effective recipes for the most common ailments for both adults and children.

You don't need to put at risk the delicate natural balance of your body and that of your loved ones by taking drugs and medications, if an easily available natural solution is just outside your door. Harvest carefully or grow your own herbs, learn to know your body and what works best for you, communicate with the nature surrounding you, and you will in a small way bring back a culture that for too long has been treated as inferior.

This book will teach how to find and treat the herbs the way the native American tribes did: from the forest to your herbalist table, but you will have to find your way to listen to your body and the plants around you.

To aid you in your holistic journey, we have decided to divide the book in seven handy volumes.

The first volume will give you a full theoretical approach to Native American medicine and the herbal medicines methods and preparations. I urge you to read it before tackling this field book, in order to understand fully the native way of thinking about nature and the world

This second volume is a complete encyclopedia of all the most relevant herbs used in traditional Native American medicine, complete with modern examples, doses, and where to find them, making it a very effective field guide.

The third volume is a "recipe book" of sorts: it offers easy herbal solutions to the most common diseases a budding naturopath can encounter. It is meant as a jumping point to find your own way to treat yourself and your fellow man and will come in handy even to the most experienced herbalist.

The fourth volume provides a complete theoretical and practical approach to Native American traditional planting techniques and how they can be implemented in modern gardens.

The fifth volume is the native gardener's almanac for medicinal herbs. Foraging is not always an option and a lot of herbs are handy to have in your garden: this volume will guide you through the herbs that you can and (should) have in your garden.

The sixth volume continues the guide to the plants you can plant in your gardens focusing on healing wildflowers, which are not only good for your health, but for the planet as well, and they are not bad on the eyes either!

The seventh volume focuses on native pediatric healthcare. Treating children is a very delicate undertaking, their physiology is more sensitive to external agents, especially drugs. Natural herbalist treatments are effective and gentle in treating common, less severe, pathologies and they won't needlessly weaken your child's immune system. The herbs listed in this last volume have been carefully researched to specifically treat children and their ailments, avoiding any allergic reaction and boosting their immune system.

Please keep in mind that, because herbs were the very first medicines, they can be very powerful. Do not gather herbs from the wild unless you know what you are doing. And please, grow your own herbs whenever possible; native herbs are becoming increasingly rare, and many are threatened with extinction. I have included only herbs which can be safely, legally, and ethically harvested. However, to ensure that their status remains so, please follow the guidelines for ethical harvesting discussed in the first book.
When you go out harvesting, observe the nature around you and beyond the guideline try to understand if what you are taking is freely given by nature, let your instincts and not only your rationality guide you.

May this knowledge bring you peace, wisdom, and health.

Definitions

For each plant in the following chapter, I will enumerate the effects, or rather the medical actions of herbs and herbal medicines. The definitions for these effects are listed alphabetically for a quick reference, should the reader need it.

Alterative: herbs that gradually restore the proper function of the body and increase health and vitality, without any immediate perception of this healthful alteration. Such as stinging nettle (*urtica diocia*), yellow dock (*rumex crispus*), dandelion (*taraxacum off. radix*).

Anodyne: pain-relieving. Such as *Valeriana off.* (Valerian) and *Atropa belladonna* (Deadly Nightshade)

Anthelmintic: antiparasitic herbs or preparations that expel parasitic destroy or expel worms from the digestive system. The term is synonymous with vermifuge and antiparasitic. Such as *Artemisia absinthium* (Wormwood).

Aperient: mild laxative. Such as *Juniperus communis* (Juniper).

Aromatic: a spicy stimulant with a strong and often pleasant odour. Such as *Pimpinella anisum* (Aniseed) and *Melissa officinalis* (Lemon Balm).

Astringent: causing the tightening of skin, mucosae, and other exposed body tissues. Such as *Rubus idaeus* (Red Raspberry) and *Quercus sp* (White/Red Oak).

Antibilious: preparations that counter disorders of the liver.

Antiemetic: to stop vomiting. Such as *Chionanthus virginicus* (Fringetree)

Antileptic: anticonvulsant, soothing.

Antiperiodic: preparations preventing the recurrence of certain symptoms.

Antirheumatic: herbs or preparations used in the treatment of inflammatory arthritis, rheumatoid arthritis, and others. Such as *Sambucus nigra/canadensis* (Black Elderberry) and dandelion (*taraxacum off. radix*).

Antiscorbutic: to cure or prevent scurvy.

Antiseptic: antimicrobial herbs or preparations to reduce the possibility of infection, sepsis, or putrefaction. Such as *Hamamelis virginiana* (Witch Hazel), *Capsella bursa-pastoris* (Shepherd's Purse), and *Quercus alba* (White Oak).

Antispasmodic: to prevent or soothe spasms or craps of the muscles. Such as *Viburnum prunifolium* (Black Haw) and *Passiflora incarnata* (Passionflower).

Carminative: herbs and preparations rich in volatile oils, that increase the peristalsis of the gastric and intestinal mucosae and relieve cramping by expelling gases. Such as *Pimpinella anisum* (Anise).

Cathartic: to accelerate defecation. Such as *Juglans nigra* (Black Walnut) and *Podophyllum peltatum* (May Apple).

Cephalic: related to the treatment of headaches.

Cholagogue: to stimulate the flow of bile from the liver. Such as *Hydrastis canadensis* (Goldenseal)

Condiment: to improve the flavour of foods.

Demulcent: herbs rich in mucilage that can soothe and protect irritated or inflamed internal tissue. Such as *Althea off.* (Marshmallow leaf or root) and *Glycyrrhiza glabra* (Licorice).

Deobstruent: to clear or open the natural ducts of the fluids and secretions of the body; see aperient.

Depurative: detoxifying; see alterative.

Detergent: cleansing herbs that contain saponins. Such as *Agave Americana* (Agave).

Diaphoretic: to stimulate perspiration and the production of sweat. Such as Eupatorium perfoliatum (Boneset) and *Sambucus niger* (Elderberry).

Diuretic: to increase the secretion and flow of urine. Stimulating diuretics such as *Arctostaphylos uva-ursi* (Bearberry) and *Juniperus communis* (Juniper) either irritate the kidneys or increase the flow of blood (caffeine) to the kidneys to increase the flow of urine. Osmotic diuretics such as *Agropyron repens* (Couch Grass) and *Althea officinalis* (Marshmallow) works as unmetabolized polysaccharides change the osmotic pull of the kidneys and increase the flow of water.

Emetic: herbs that induce vomiting; first aid treatment for poisoning. Such as Lobelia (*Lobelia inflata*) and Ipecac (*Cephaelis ipecacuahana*)

Emmenagogue: to stimulate and regulate menstrual flow and function. Such as Achillea millefolium (Yarrow), Actaea racemosa (Black Cohosh), and Caulophyllum thalictroides (Blue Cohosh).

Emollient: softens and soothes the skin. Such as *Plantago major/lanceolata* (Plantain) and *Aloe barbadensis* (Aloe).

Esculent: edible.

Expectorant: herbs that help the body to remove excess mucous from the lungs, or more generally a tonic for the respiratory system. Stimulating expectorants such as *Inula helenium* (Elecampane), *Glycyrrhiza glabra* (Licorice), and *Sanguinaria canadensis* (Bloodroot) work as chemical irritants to the mucosae of the bronchiole forcing the expulsion of the congested material.

Soothing or Relaxing expectorants such as *Tussilago farfara* (Coltsfoot) and *Verbascum thapsus* (Mullein) soothe bronchial spasms and loosen mucous secretion.

Febrifuge: Abates and reduces fevers. Such as *Sambucus nigra* (Elderberry) and *Filipendula ulmaria* (Meadowsweet).

Hepatic: herbs or preparations that aid the work of the liver. Such as *Taraxacum officinalis* (Dandelion root) and *Silybum marianum* (Milk thistle).

Laxative: to promote bowel movements. Stimulating laxatives such as *Cassia angustifolia* (Senna), *Rheum palmatum* (Turkey Rhubarb), and *Rhamnus purshiana* (Cascara) contain anthraquinones which stimulate the contractions of the muscle wall of the large intestine. Osmotic laxatives such as *Althea off.* (Marshmallow) bulk up the colon by drawing water and softening the stool.

Mucilaginous: soothe and protect irritated tissues in the body. Such as *Althea off.* (Marshmallow), *Plantago lanceolata* (plantain), and *Verbascum thapsus* (Mullein).

Nervine: a remedy that has a beneficial effect on the nervous system, either relaxant, stimulant, or tonic. Such as *Hypericum perforatum* (St. John's wort), *Humulus lupulus* (Hops), and *Lavendula off.* (Lavender).

Refrigerant: cooling. Such as *Borago off.* (Borage).

Rubifacient: to increase capillary circulation and produce redness of the skin. Such as *Bryonia alba/diocia* (White Bryony).

Sedative: to reduce stress and aid sleep. Such as *Gelsemium sempervirens* (Yellow Jasmine), *Piscidia erythrina* (Jamaican Dogwood) and *Eschscholzia california* (California Poppy).

Sialogogue: to increase the secretion of saliva. Such as *Rheum palmatum* (Turkey Rhubarb).

Styptic: an astringent applied externally. See Astringent.

Tonic: herbs and preparations that are generally invigorating and strengthening.

Vermifuge: See Anthelmintic.

Native American Herbs

Agave

Century plant *(Agave americana)*, blue agave *(A. tequilana)*, and others

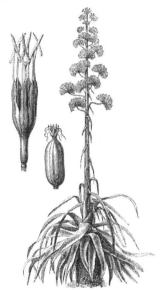

Habitat: Agave plants are native to arid and semi-arid regions, typically found in desert ecosystems with well-drained sandy or rocky soil. They are well-adapted to survive in dry and harsh conditions, often growing in areas with high sun exposure and limited rainfall. In the United States, agave plants can be found in states such as Arizona, California, New Mexico, Nevada, Texas, and parts of Utah, where the arid climates provide suitable habitats for their growth.

Identification: The grayish-green desert plant, reaching heights of up to 10 feet, showcases elongated, sword-shaped leaves that possess succulent characteristics. It exhibits flowers that emerge from a central fruiting spike. Often referred to as the American century plant, it acquired this name due to the misconception that the plant blooms solely once every 100 years. However, this belief is erroneous as the plant actually flowers at an advanced age, typically blooming once every 10 to 20 years. Following the emergence of its colossal flower spear, the mother plant eventually perishes. Actually, the term "American decade plant" might be more appropriate in describing this species.

Taste: sweet, comparable to honey.
Medicinal Parts: The leaf and the juice.

Solvent: Water, alcohol.

Effects: anti-inflammatory, diuretic.

Traditional uses: The Agave water, also known as juice or sap, is recognized for its anti-inflammatory properties and diuretic effects. Additionally, the consumption of fresh juice has been associated with an elevation in metabolism and an increase in perspiration.

Furthermore, the sap of the Agave plant holds medicinal value in the treatment and closure of wounds. A notable historical incident involves Cortez, who had accidentally embedded an axe halfway into his thigh. It is believed that he would have succumbed to the injury if not for the intervention of the Mesoamerican natives. They stemmed the bleeding and sealed the wound by applying a compress composed of adhesive agave leaf sap, honey, and charcoal. This compress was then secured with spiderwort stems.

Modern uses: The residual leaves of the Agave plant serve as a valuable resource for the production of steroid drugs, specifically hecogenin. One notable example is the drug Crinone, which is derived from Agave sisalana and prescribed as a hormone replacement therapy containing progesterone for specific pregnancy-related circumstances. Agave roots, on the other hand, contain saponins that possess foaming properties, making them suitable for the manufacturing of soap products. By grating and pressing agave roots, a foaming liquid soap can be obtained, which can be utilized for various cleaning purposes, including shampoo, dish soap, and laundry soap.

The sturdy fibers extracted from Agave leaves are widely used in rope and fiber production, particularly in the creation of sisal. Sisal is incredibly durable and finds application in elevator systems. The strong and coarse sisal cordage is woven, oiled, and wrapped around pulley systems within elevator shafts. As elevator cables pass through these pulleys, the lubrication provided by the oiled sisal fibers prevents friction buildup, enabling smooth vertical movement. Additionally, the sap of the Agave plant continues to be utilized for its demulcent and laxative properties.

Agave nectar, commercially processed from the plant, is marketed as a low glycemic index sugar or liquid sweetener. However, caution should be exercised when consuming agave sugar or nectar due to its high fructose content. High consumption of fructose can inhibit insulin release, promote fat formation and storage, and potentially contribute to insulin resistance and an increased risk of heart disease. It is important to be mindful of the potential health effects associated with agave sugar and nectar consumption.

Food: Agave plants, particularly Agave deserti found in the Sonoran Desert, have significant culinary uses. Indigenous communities like the Pima, Papago (Tohono O'odham), and Cahuilla tribes gather and dry the agave flowers, grinding them into flour for making tortillas. Each plant produces several pounds of flowers, providing a substantial food source. The Papago people also consume the flower stalks as a green vegetable, while various Native American groups bake or roast the roots and hearts of the agave to create traditional cakes and breads. The Navajo tribe utilizes baked and dried agave heads as a thickener for soups.

The heart of the agave plant, known as the "piña," can be roasted and eaten. Baking and mashing the piña is also the method used to extract its juices, which are then fermented and distilled into tequila.

In some bottles of tequila, you may find a small worm at the bottom, commonly known as the agave worm, maguey worm, or gusano. This worm serves as an indicator of the tequila's proof, added during the bottling process. If the alcohol content of the tequila is inadequate, the worm will deteriorate. However, if the worm remains intact and in good condition, it signifies that the tequila is of high quality.

Warning: The consumption of agave leaves can prove fatal for livestock, and they typically avoid consuming them unless faced with severe drought conditions or when no other forage is available.

Interestingly, humans have occasionally capitalized on the toxic nature of agave leaves in certain regions of Mexico. Indigenous communities devised a method to harvest fish by placing agave leaves, specifically from the A. lechuguilla species, in a stream. Fish swimming in the vicinity would inadvertently ingest the toxic water through their gills, resulting in paralysis and causing them to float to the water's surface. This enabled the collection of the immobilized fish. Importantly, the poison from the agave leaves did not render the fish unsafe for consumption, as the toxicity of the agave is not harmful to humans. If any uncollected fish drifted into clean water, they would eventually revive and swim away.

Alder

(Alnus rubra Bong.)

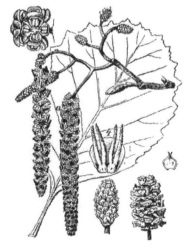

Habitat: Species ranges from California to Alaska east to Idaho. Moist areas. It forms thickets along waterways. In Colorado the primary species is Alnus tenuifolia and is common in the foothills to subalpine areas.

Identification: Alder trees are deciduous trees belonging to the genus Alnus. They are known for their distinctive features and valuable contributions to various ecosystems. Alder trees typically grow near water sources such as rivers, lakes, and wetlands, where they thrive in moist soil conditions. These trees possess a unique ability to enrich the soil through a process called nitrogen fixation, which involves capturing nitrogen from the air and converting it into a form that can be utilized by other plants.

Alder trees display a dense and bushy appearance with elongated leaves that are dark green in color. The leaves have serrated edges and a smooth, glossy texture, providing an attractive display during the growing season. The male and female flowers of the alder tree are separate but appear on the same tree. The male flowers are long, pendulous catkins that release pollen, while the female flowers are smaller and develop into cone-like structures.

Beyond their aesthetic qualities, alder trees play a crucial ecological role. Their ability to fix nitrogen enriches the soil and supports the growth of nearby vegetation. The dense foliage provides shade and shelter for various wildlife species, including birds, insects, and small mammals. They are also ideal habitats for bears. It is important to exercise caution when encountering such areas. Alder trees also contribute to stabilizing riverbanks and preventing erosion due to their extensive root systems.

Medicinal Part: The bark.

Solvent: Boiling water.

Effects: Tonic, Alterative, Astringent, Cathartic.

Traditional uses: Alder leaves were commonly used to cover the floors of sweat lodges, providing a natural surface. Additionally, switches made from alder branches were utilized to apply water onto the body and hot rocks during sweat lodge ceremonies. The ashes of alder were mixed with a chewing stick to form a paste, which was used as a teeth-cleaning agent.

Certain subspecies of alder, such as A. sinuata, had medicinal applications, including the use of their cones. The spring catkins of alder were crushed into a pulp and consumed as a cathartic to aid in bowel movement. The bark of alder was sometimes combined with other plants in decoctions, serving as a tonic. Decoctions made from the female catkins were employed in the treatment of gonorrhea. Poultices made from alder leaves were applied to skin wounds and infections.

In the Okanagan area of central Washington and British Columbia, the indigenous communities embraced the healing properties of alder through various preparations. To stimulate the appetite of children, an infusion of fresh alder shoots was employed. The infusion of alder leaves, brewed as a tea, was believed to alleviate itching and inflammation resulting from insect bites, stings, as well as exposure to poison ivy and poison oak. Informants from the Upper Tanana region shared that a decoction made from the inner bark of the alder tree was utilized to help reduce fever. Furthermore, an infusion created from the bark served as a cleansing agent for treating sores, cuts, and wounds.

Modern uses: Black alder (A. glutinosa), specifically, maintains its significance as a warrior plant in sweat lodge ceremonies, contributing to its continued reverence. This species, native to the Northern Hemisphere, holds cultural importance in Russia and eastern European countries, where it is utilized as a gargle to provide relief for sore throat and aid in reducing fever. Its traditional use in these regions showcases its enduring role in promoting wellness and supporting individuals in their healing journeys.

Furthermore, research indicates that certain compounds found in alder, such as betulin and lupeol, may possess inhibitory properties against tumor growth. These findings suggest potential therapeutic applications of alder in the field of oncology.

Dose and usage: Due to its high tannin content, alder can be utilized in various situations where tannin is effective. Internally, it can be used to address conditions such as diarrhea, gum inflammations, and sore throats. Externally, it can be employed as a wash for cuts, hives, poison ivy, swellings, and sprains. The infusion or tea made from the bark exhibits shrinking, clotting, and antiseptic properties, making it beneficial for wound care.

For optimal results, it is advisable to collect the bark during the spring or fall, although it can be used effectively at any time. Fresh or recently collected bark is preferred for use. When preparing for internal consumption, a strong decoction should be made, while a weaker one is suitable for external applications.

Food and other uses: The wood of alder trees is versatile and has been utilized for various purposes. It is known for its moderate strength, smooth texture, and attractive light brown color. Alder wood is commonly used in the production of furniture, cabinetry, and woodworking projects. Its durability and resistance to rot make it suitable for outdoor applications such as fencing, decking, and boat building

In the Northwest region, alder is considered a valuable resource for firewood, particularly for savory barbecue cooking. The bark and wood chips of alder are preferred over mesquite when it comes to smoking fish, especially salmon, imparting a distinctive flavor.

To smoke meat using alder, the wood chips should be soaked in water overnight to moisten them. Afterward, the moist chips can be placed on coals or charcoal to generate smoke for the meat. An observation from 1961 reveals that Native Americans in Alaska smoked fish, moose, and caribou along a 10-mile stretch of the Denali Highway for winter preservation. The hunting regulations at that time mandated that anyone shooting a caribou was required to provide a portion of the meat to the First People, who would then preserve it for winter consumption.

In the process of smoking fish, they would remove the skin, impale the fish on sticks, and suspend them above a smoldering alder fire until the fish became smoked and dry. Additionally, the ashes of alder were mixed with tobacco and smoked.

In regions with limited availability of hardwood, alder serves as a suitable fuel for home heating since it burns slower than pine. The bark of alder can be stripped and soaked in water to create an orange-to-rust dye.

During the early spring, the sweet inner bark of alder can be scraped and consumed fresh. It can be eaten raw or mixed with flour to create cakes, adding a unique taste to culinary preparations.

Aloe

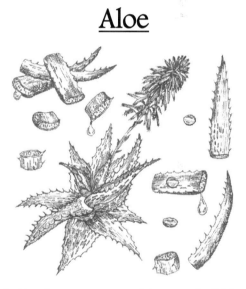

Habitat: Aloe is a genus comprising nearly 200 species, primarily native to South Africa. These plants are known for their succulent characteristics. The properties of Aloe have been recognized since ancient times by the Greeks, and it has been gathered on Socotra, an island in the Arabian Sea, for over 2,000 years. Aloe thrives in warm regions and can be found growing wild in places like Florida, USA. In terms of texture, Aloe is similar to succulent cacti.

Identification: Aloe plants typically exhibit elongated leaves that are deep brown or olive in color. The leaves often have pointed tips, but can also be blunt or have spine-like teeth. Some leaves may display blotches or mottled patterns. The stem of the plant is typically short, with a basal rosette arrangement of leaves at the base.

The flowers of Aloe are tubular in shape and can be red or yellow. They are borne on a stalk and are found in simple or branched clusters.

These characteristics may vary across different varieties of Aloe, with some species resembling trees and having forked branches. For instance, Aloe bainesii can reach heights of up to 65 feet and have a width of 5 feet at the base. Other species of Aloe are commonly cultivated in succulent gardens, including miniature varieties grown indoors. These plants require ample sunlight and careful watering.

It's worth noting that the term "American aloe" refers to Agave americana, which is not a species of Aloe.

Taste: peculiar and bitter.

Powder: bright yellow.

Medicinal Parts: The insipid juice of the leaves, which is a greenish translucent salve-like substance.

Solvent: Water.

Effects: Tonic, Purgative, emmenagogue, anthelmintic.

Medicinal uses: Aloes are highly effective for their cleansing properties for various organs and tissues such as the stomach, liver, spleen, kidneys, and bladder. They do not cause griping or discomfort and are known to be healing and soothing to all types of tissue, including blood and lymphatic fluids.

However, it is important to note that aloes should never be used during pregnancy or by individuals suffering from hemorrhoids, as it can cause irritation to the lower bowels. Aloes find application in cases of suppressed menstruation, dyspepsia (indigestion), skin lesions, liver ailments, headaches, and more.

It is always recommended to seek professional medical advice before using any herbal remedies, including aloes.

Dose and use: For constipation, aloes can be taken in powder form ranging from 0,5-2 grams, depending on age and specific conditions. To address obstructed or suppressed menstruation, a dosage of 5-10 grams twice daily is recommended. In the case of threadworms, aloes can be dissolved in warm water and used as an injection. The same mixture can also be taken orally for several days.

Externally, powdered aloes can be prepared into a strong decoction and applied to the nipples to aid in weaning a nursing child. The bitter taste of aloes creates an aversion that encourages the child to seek alternative sources of nourishment. Aloes also demonstrate cleansing properties when applied externally.

For wound care, a piece of white linen or cotton soaked in aloe water can be applied to fresh wounds or old wounds to promote rapid healing and closure. In cases where ulcers become more severe and produce discharge, a thick layer of aloe powder can be sprinkled over the open wound and secured with clean gauze. This should be repeated daily. The powder absorbs the unhealthy fluids while stimulating the growth of new, healthy tissues.

The fresh juice of aloes or a solution made from dried leaves is soothing for tender sunburns, insect bites, over-exposure to X-rays, and other emollient uses. It provides relief and comfort in such situations.

Warning: It is important to exercise caution and avoid giving aloes in cases of liver and gallbladder degeneration, as well as during menstruation, pregnancy, and hemorrhoids. While aloes are generally considered safe for use based on folk medicine practices, in complex or complicated cases, it is highly advisable to seek the advice of medical professionals or trained practitioners in the field. Their expertise can provide appropriate guidance and ensure the safe and effective use of aloes in specific situations.

Amaranth

Amaranthaceae: Redroot amaranth *(Amaranthus retroflexus)*, red amaranth *(A. cruentus)*, and others

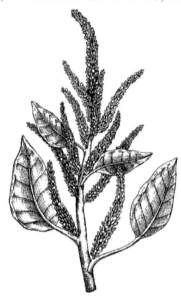

Identification: Tall, weed-like plant that typically reaches a height of 4 feet. It features grayish leaves that are arranged alternately along the stem. The flowers of amaranth are found within bristly and hairy bracts, located in the leaf axils of the upper part of the plant. As the stem ascends, the size of the leaves gradually diminishes, while the hairy flower bracts increase in size and density. The seeds are typically small, numerous, and black in color.

Amaranth possesses a taproot and a lower stem that exhibit a reddish hue, giving rise to its name. The leaves are ovate to rhomboid in shape and have a rough texture along the margins, which can be felt by touch. It flowers during the summer season and produces edible seeds in the fall.

Habitat: There are numerous species of amaranth that can be found growing on waste ground throughout the country, particularly along the edges of prairies and field margins. Additionally, they are extensively cultivated in Mexico and South America.

Medicinal Parts: Flowers and leaves. Edible seeds and shoots.

Solvent: Water.

Effects: Astringent.

Food: Native Americans have been eating amaranth seeds for thousands of years. The Apaches and Navajos used amaranth to make flour for bread, while the Aztecs and later the Tarahumara (Rarámuri) people of what is now Mexico would make pinole — toasted amaranth or cornmeal that is mixed with sugar, spices, and a bit of water and eaten as hot cereal or cooked into cakes. Amaranth flour, mixed with cornmeal, was made into dumplings, too, and the seeds were popped like popcorn.

In Mexico a traditional sweet treat called alegría (Spanish for "joy") — popped amaranth seeds mixed with honey and chocolate, sometimes with pumpkin or sunflower seeds added, too — is made in honor of the Day of the Dead and other celebrations. The recipe's origins go back as far as the Mayans and Aztecs. Amaranth has again become an important food for the descendants of those early Mayans, who grow the amaranth and make products from the seeds, including alegría, as a way to earn a livelihood and provide nutritious food for their families. Similar to its relative quinoa, amaranth is a highly nutritious grain that is abundant in protein and various other essential nutrients. It is also gluten-free, making it suitable for individuals with gluten sensitivities or celiac disease. A single cup of uncooked amaranth seeds provides approximately 26 grams of protein, 307 milligrams of calcium, 14.7 milligrams of iron, and 158 micrograms of folic acid. These nutritional benefits make amaranth particularly beneficial for children and pregnant women, who require adequate protein, folic acid, calcium, and other essential nutrients for healthy development. The value of amaranth has also been recognized by NASA, as they have recommended it as one of the most nutritious foods for consumption during space missions. Furthermore, various parts of the amaranth plant are edible. The young leaves, in particular, are a rich source of vitamin C and vitamin A. They can be enjoyed fresh in salads or steamed and served as a cooked vegetable. Additionally, even the roots of the amaranth plant can be cooked and used as an excellent addition to soups and casseroles, expanding the culinary possibilities and nutritional benefits of this versatile plant.

Amaranth could become an important food in a future affected by climate change. It's easy to grow in many climates (and with limited water), adapts well to different soils, and doesn't require much fertilizer (whereas other grain crops like corn generally need good soil, abundant water, and lots of fertilizer and pesticides). And because it's so packed with nutrients, it can help reduce the rates of malnutrition wherever it's grown.

Easy to grow and packed with nutrients, amaranth will likely be an important food in a future affected by climate change.

Traditional uses: Amaranth holds significant cultural and ritualistic value among Native Americans, who incorporate it into sacred ceremonies by mixing and consuming it alongside green corn. The astringent properties of the plant's leaves have been utilized in traditional medicine to address conditions such as profuse menstruation, while an infusion of the plant has been taken to alleviate hoarseness (Moerman, 1998).

During the pioneer era and in herbalist practices, amaranth was recognized for its astringent qualities and was often employed in the treatment of inflammations affecting the mouth and throat. Additionally, it was considered beneficial for managing conditions like diarrhea and ulcers.

These historical uses and observations of amaranth's therapeutic properties by Native Americans, pioneers, and herbalists shed light on its traditional medicinal applications for various ailments and further contribute to its significance in traditional healing practices.

Other uses: Excellent as a pink dye. Perfect for your bird feeder

Angelica
Apiaceae *(Angelica atropurpurea L.)*

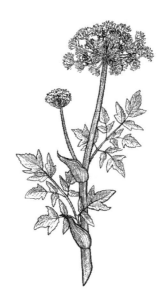

Identification: Angelica, a biennial plant known for its towering stature, can reach impressive heights of up to 9 feet. Its robust stem stands erect, displaying a vibrant purple hue. The plant's leaves are notable for their compound structure, consisting of three to five leaflets. Each leaflet possesses hollow petioles, while the emerging upper leaves are adorned with persistent sheaths that encircle the base of the petioles. Angelica flowers, forming in clusters reminiscent of umbrellas, exhibit a delicate greenish-white coloration.

One unmistakable characteristic of angelica lies in its captivating aroma. When the root is disturbed, its distinct fragrance, resembling a subtle blend of celery with its own unique angelica scent, permeates the air. The seeds and leaves also contribute to this aromatic symphony, albeit to a lesser extent. Notably, when the root is cut or handled, it imparts a smooth, slippery texture akin to that of a bar of soap.

The leaves of angelica are generously sized, featuring smaller leaflets nestled within their elongated ovals. Measuring approximately three to four inches in length, these leaves add to the plant's overall allure.
However, it is crucial to exercise caution during identification, as angelica bears a resemblance to the highly toxic water hemlock. Accurate recognition and differentiation are paramount before utilizing angelica for any purpose, ensuring the safe and beneficial use of this remarkable plant. Due to the resemblance between angelica and the highly poisonous water hemlock, it is crucial to ensure accurate identification before using angelica for any purpose.

Habitat: Northern tier of United States, typically east of the Mississippi River. Wet lowlands, along streams and rivers.

Medicinal Parts: Root, herb and seed.
Solvent: Boiling water.

Effects: Aromatic, Stimulant, Carminative, Diaphoretic, Expectorant, Diuretic, Emmenagogue.

Food: While there is limited literature on the edibility of A. atropurpurea, a similar Chinese herb called A. sinensis (dong quai) is consumed as root slices in stir-fries or soups. An interesting concoction known as a yin and yang cordial is made by combining 100 grams of A. sinensis root (typically available in Asian markets or drugstores), 100 grams of whole ginseng root and ½ liter of peppermint schnapps. The schnapps allows for the extraction of the saponins, including phytoestrogens, but mind that it will take least three weeks to make a medically viable tincture this way. This cordial is not only a very yummy cocktail, but it also regarded for its ability to balance yin and yang energies and boost overall energy levels.

In certain cultures, it is said that Laplanders consume cooked roots of A. atropurpurea. However, specific details or practices regarding its consumption are not widely documented.

Traditional uses: Angelica species have been widely utilized by over eighteen Native American tribes for their medicinal properties, incorporating them into their traditional healing practices. Decoctions of the A. atropurpurea root were employed to address various ailments, including rheumatism, fevers, chills, flatulence, and sore throats. Within sweat lodge ceremonies, angelica was administered to treat conditions such as arthritis, headaches, frostbite, and hypothermia. The crushed root was commonly applied externally as a poultice to alleviate pain, while the Creek Indians chewed, ingested, or smoked the root with tobacco to alleviate stomach disorders.

Among the Iroquois tribe, angelica infusions were utilized in steam baths to relieve headaches and frostbite. Poultices made from angelica root were applied to treat broken bones, and angelica tea served as a topical treatment for ulcers. Angelica also played a vital role as a purification herb, being added to sacred pipes and burned during healing ceremonies. It is important to distinguish that A. sinensis and A. atropurpurea are employed differently in Asian and Western traditions, and slight chemical variations exist between the plants. Unless otherwise specified, the following uses described primarily pertain to A. sinensis, which can be obtained as seeds or dried roots from various sources like herbs.com, health-food stores, and Asian markets.
In traditional Chinese herbal medicine, the root of A. sinensis is highly regarded as a warming tonic and a key female herb. It is employed to alleviate menstrual cramps and potentially enhance scanty menstrual flow. Furthermore, it is believed to possess antispasmodic properties and may help reduce angina symptoms. Similar to other members of the Apiaceae plant family, angelica contains calcium channel blockers, which are comparable to medications used in angina treatment. Chinese practitioners suggest that angelica improves peripheral circulation to the extremities of the body, promoting overall wellness and balance.

Modern uses: In German holistic medicine the 3 teaspoons of dried A. sinensis infused in water are often recommended to alleviate heartburn and indigestion. Similarly, A. sinensis is employed by European professionals to address colic.

In the United States, both A. sinensis and A. atropurpurea are utilized by naturopathic physicians. However, it is important to seek guidance from a holistic naturopathic practitioner for professional advice tailored to individual needs and conditions. Consulting with a qualified healthcare professional can ensure appropriate and safe usage of angelica species for therapeutic purposes.

Dose and usage: Angelica is highly valued by herbalists for its potential as a reproductive normalizer, as it is believed to help stimulate delayed menstruation and relieve cramps, both of a reproductive and intestinal nature. It is also known for its ability to normalize digestion, alleviate flatulence, and act as an expectorant during coughs and colds. Angelica is considered a diaphoretic and diuretic, making it useful in the treatment of urinary tract infections and as a urinary antiseptic. Additionally, it may offer some relief from joint inflammations.

The primary part of the plant used in herbal remedies is the root, although the seeds are also effective for addressing stomach nausea. In Europe, the stems and leaves of angelica are used candied as a dessert and are utilized to some extent in the liquor industry for flavoring purposes.

Angelica root offers versatile ways to enjoy its therapeutic benefits. For a convenient on-the-go option, simply carry a portion of the raw, whole root and nibble on it as desired. Alternatively, angelica can be used in tincture form, with a suggested dosage of thirty to sixty drops, up to four times a day. The seeds can also be tinctured (ten to thirty drops, up to four times a day), or chewed in their natural state.

To prepare a nourishing tea, steep two teaspoons of crushed angelica seeds in one cup of boiling water for thirty minutes. After straining, the infusion can be enjoyed in two tablespoons, up to four times daily. Alternatively, simmer two teaspoons of dried root in a pan with three cups of water until the liquid reduces to one and a half cups. Strain the liquid and take a quarter cup up to four times a day.

Notes: Angelica roots are used as a flavoring agent for vodka, gin, cooked fish, and various jams.

Veterinarian/Wildlife: The oil derived from the root of the angelica plant may attract fruit flies. Angelica itself is pollinated by a variety of insects, including bees, flies, and beetles. Additionally, the fruit of the angelica plant can be crushed and used as a decoction to create a wash that is believed to be effective in killing head lice.

Wild Anise
Apiaceae *(Myrrhis odorata L. Scop.)*

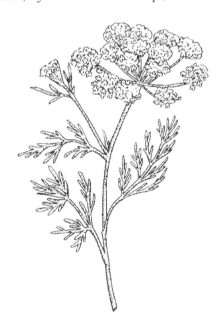

Identification: Caution should be exercised when dealing with wild anise, as it looks quite similar to hemlock, although it is much smaller even when fully grown, reaching a height of less than 3 feet. When the root of wild anise is broken, it emits a distinct anise seed smell. The plant has shiny, bright green leaves and produces small white flowers in umbels. Commonly known as sweet cicely, wild anise possesses a sweet aroma and flavor reminiscent of anise. The flowers typically appear in late spring to early summer. The fruit of the plant is pyramid-shaped, compressed at the sides, and can range in color from brown to glossy black, measuring approximately 1 inch in length. The leaves have a scent similar to lovage and taste like anise. They are short, feather- or fern-like, and are covered underneath with soft, hair-like bristles. The leaves have deep clefts, adding to their distinctive appearance.

Habitat: Wild anise is a forest dweller and can be found throughout the entire United States, excluding extreme desert and mountainous regions. It exhibits a preference for shaded environments.

Food: While the leaves and root of the plant are edible, it is important to exercise caution as it bears a resemblance to poison hemlock. It is crucial to accurately identify it before consuming it.

If wild anise is correctly identified, the root can be used as a spice to flavor cooked greens and baked goods, serving as a substitute for anise. The leaves can be added to salads to impart their unique flavor.

Additionally, the cooked root can be enjoyed cold or pickled, offering versatility in salads and soups. However, it is essential to ensure proper identification and proper preparation before incorporating it into any culinary preparations.

Traditional uses: Used as a blood purifier and expectorant for hundreds of years. Traditionally used to treat asthma and other breathing difficulties.

Modern uses: For centuries, wild anise has been employed as a blood purifier and expectorant in traditional herbal medicine. It has a long history of use in the treatment of asthma and other respiratory ailments, as it is believed to possess properties that support respiratory health and alleviate breathing difficulties.

Dose and usage: When harvesting wild anise, the leaves can be picked and incorporated into salads, adding their unique flavor to the dish. The root of wild anise is versatile and can be used for both culinary and medicinal purposes. It contains anethole, a volatile oil that imparts the characteristic anise-like flavor.

To prepare the root as a tea, it is recommended to macerate the root by soaking it in water, allowing the beneficial compounds to infuse. It is important to keep the pot or cup covered during preparation to prevent the loss of essential oils. For a potentially stronger infusion of aromatic and volatile oils, you can try keeping the macerated root in a stoppered bottle of water.

Balsam Fir

Pinaceae (*Abies balsamea* L. Mill)

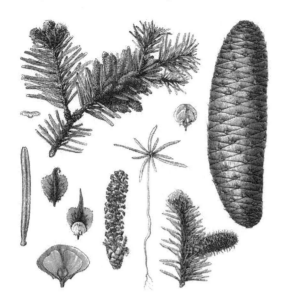

Identification: Evergreen tree that can grow up to 60 feet tall and has a spire-shaped growth habit. At higher altitudes, it may have a low, spreading, and mat-like form. The bark is smooth and contains resin pockets. Its flat needles are stalkless, reaching up to 1¼ inches in length, and have white stripes on the undersides. The needles are more rounded at the base. The cones are purplish to green, scaly, and about 4 inches long, being twice as long as they are broad.
Habitat: Canada south through the northern tier of the eastern United States. Moist woods and their fringes.

Medicinal parts: Resin, root, needles, and bark

Effects: Analgesic, antiseptic

Food: The needle infusion is a relaxing tea, traditionally considered a laxative.

Traditional uses: The resin of the balsam fir tree held significant importance for Native Americans, who utilized it for a wide range of medicinal purposes. The resin was applied topically to burns, wounds, sores, scrapes, insect bites, stings, and bruises, providing soothing relief and aiding in the healing process. Tea made from the balsam fir needles was a popular remedy for upper respiratory issues such as asthma, bronchitis, and colds. The leaves of the tree were stuffed into pillows, believed to possess general curative properties. Children would chew on the raw sap to alleviate symptoms of colds and sore throats. During sweat lodge ceremonies, balsam gum was applied to hot, wet stones, and the resulting smoke was inhaled to alleviate headaches. Steamed branches were utilized to address conditions such as arthritis (rheumatism). Additionally, a decoction of the balsam fir bark was used to induce sweating and aid in the treatment of acute infections.

Various Native American tribes, including the Algonquin, Woodlands Cree, Iroquois, Menominee, Micmac, Ojibwa, and Potawatomi, relied on tea made from the sap or bark of the balsam fir to alleviate symptoms of colds. The Ojibwa tribe also inhaled the smoke produced by the needle-like leaves as a remedy for colds.

The gum derived from the balsam fir tree proved effective in treating burns, wounds, and cuts by providing a protective coating. The Chippewa tribe found relief from headaches by inhaling the soothing steam generated by melting balsam gum. On the other hand, the Iroquois utilized the steam produced from a decoction of the balsam fir branches to alleviate symptoms of rheumatism and to aid in the process of childbirth.

Modern uses: The resin derived from bark blisters of the balsam fir is highly regarded for its antiseptic properties. It is commonly used as a key ingredient in various salves, lotions, ointments, and creams, including those specifically formulated to treat hemorrhoids. The resin is also incorporated into proprietary mixtures that are marketed for the treatment of diarrhea and coughs.

Dose and usage: To make a tea, cover one teaspoon of the bark with two cups of water in a pan and bring to a boil. Boil for thirty minutes and strain. Take a quarter cup a day.

Balsam Root

Asteraceae (*Balsamorhiza sagittata* [Pursh] Nutt.)

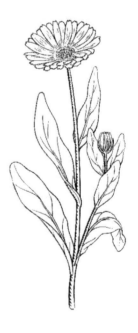

Identification: The balsam root (*Balsamorhiza*) encompasses several species, and one of them is Balsamorhiza sagittata. This particular species typically grows to a height of 1 to 2 feet and tends to form clumps. The plant features basal leaves with petioles (leaf stalks) and arrow-shaped leaf blades. The leaves have a hairy texture and feel rough to the touch, measuring between 8 to 12 inches in length. The flowers are yellow and have long stalks. They consist of up to twenty-two yellow ray florets that encircle the central yellow disc florets.

Habitat: Balsam root can be found in the foothills and higher elevations of the Rocky Mountains, ranging from Colorado northwards to Canada and westwards to British Columbia. It thrives in dry or well-drained areas, particularly on sunny slopes. This plant is abundant in various wilderness areas in Idaho, including the Bitterroots, as well as on the south-facing slopes of Rainbow Lake in the Absaroka/Beartooth Wilderness.

Medicinal parts: The whole plant.

Effects: Antiseptic, antibacterial

Food: The young leaves and shoots of balsam root are edible and can be consumed either raw or steamed. Similarly, the young flower stalks and stems can be eaten. The roots can also be peeled and eaten, but they have a bitter taste unless they are cooked slowly to break down the indigestible polysaccharide known as inulin. The roots can be cooked, dried, and later rehydrated in simmering water before eating. The seeds of balsam root can be eaten as a snack or pounded into a meal that can be used as flour. Roasted seeds can be ground into pinole, a type of traditional Native American flour. The Nez Perce tribe roasted and ground the seeds, forming them into small "energy balls" by adding grease.

Traditional uses: Balsam root (Balsamorhiza sagittata) holds significant cultural and medicinal importance among several Native American tribes. Various tribes, including the Nez Perce, Blackfoot, Cheyenne, and Shoshone, have utilized different parts of the plant for a range of traditional purposes. The Nez Perce tribe used balsam root extensively. They consumed the fresh roots, either raw or cooked, as a nutritious food source. The roots were also dried and ground into a powder, which could be stored and used as a flour substitute. Additionally, the Nez Perce tribe prepared a medicinal decoction from the roots to treat ailments such as coughs, colds, and gastrointestinal issues. The Blackfoot tribe employed balsam root for medicinal purposes as well. They brewed a tea from the plant's roots, which was believed to have diuretic and digestive properties. This tea was used to alleviate urinary tract problems, aid in digestion, and treat kidney disorders. Among the Cheyenne tribe, balsam root was utilized for its expectorant and cough-suppressant properties. A decoction made from the roots was consumed to relieve respiratory ailments, including coughs, congestion, and bronchitis.

The Shoshone tribe recognized the anti-inflammatory properties of balsam root. They would chew the plant's roots or prepare a poultice from them to reduce swelling, relieve pain, and treat skin irritations.
Additionally, several Native American tribes also made use of the sap or resin of the balsam root for various purposes. The sap was highly valued for its adhesive properties and was used as a natural glue or sealant by tribes such as the Nez Perce and Blackfoot. It was employed in the construction of tools, such as attaching arrowheads to arrows, and in repairing or waterproofing items like baskets and containers. The sticky sap was also used as a natural bandage to cover wounds and promote healing due to its antimicrobial properties.

Barberry
Berberidaceae (*Berberis canadensis* P. Mill.)

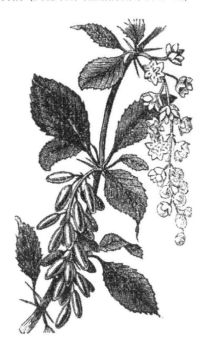

Identification: Thorny shrub, thorns to 1" in length. Grows to 7' tall, branches grooved, with tear drop–shaped, succulent leaves, alternate in whorled clusters; fruit round to ovate, scarlet color when ripe, tart tasting (sour). Flowers are yellow with six sepals hanging in clusters.

Habitat: Found in open woodland (dry) and edges of woods, northern tier of states from coast to coast; however, most prevalent east of the plains.

Medicinal parts: Berries, bark, and leaves
Solvents: Alcohol, water.

Effects: Tonic, purgative, antiseptic

Food: The berries of the barberry plant, can be cooked and juiced or dried and powdered to make mush. When the berries are ripe, they can be cooked to produce jelly. To extract the juice, the berries are cooked and then strained using a sieve, pantyhose, or cheesecloth. The resulting juice can be diluted and sweetened to taste. Additionally, the berries can be dried and pounded into a powder or paste, which can be cooked in a manner similar to hot cereal. These methods are just a few ideas to inspire you to incorporate barberries into health-conscious culinary creations.

Traditional uses: The barberry bush was highly valued by Native Americans, who made effective use of its various parts. The berries were consumed raw or transformed into jam, providing a source of nourishment and flavor. The root of the plant was utilized either raw or boiled as a seasoning and ingredient in stews. Additionally, the wood and bark of the barberry bush were employed to create a yellow dye.

Among the Cherokee tribe, a remedy for diarrhea involved scraping the outer bark of the plant, placing it in a gourd with water, and adding a hot stone to the mixture. The resulting tea was then consumed to alleviate the symptoms. Other tribes, such as the Micmac and Mohegan, used pounded bark on mouth sores, sore gums, and sore throats. The pounded roots, when placed in the mouth, induced salivation and were believed to promote healing. The Mohegan tribe utilized a decoction made from the berries to help reduce fevers. The Shinnecock tribe used decoctions of the bitter leaves as a liver tonic. These traditional uses demonstrate the wide range of applications for the barberry plant in Native American cultures.

Modern uses: Barberry contains an alkaloid called berberine, which has been found to possess potent antimicrobial properties. It has shown effectiveness against a wide range of microorganisms, including bacteria, fungi, protozoans, and viruses. The root of the barberry plant can be decocted to create a topical wash that is beneficial for treating cuts and bruises.

Furthermore, the root bark of barberry is a natural source of vitamin C. In traditional usage, the decoction of the root bark has been employed for alleviating mouth sores and sore throat, a practice observed in other species of the Berberis and Mahonia genera as well. Decoctions made from the leaves of barberry are utilized as a liver tonic, and it has been observed to increase bile flow in laboratory animals and stimulate peristalsis.

The plant has also been utilized in homeopathic and allopathic medicine to treat liver diseases. In addition to these uses, the root bark of barberry, when prepared as a decoction or infusion, can act as a diuretic, making it valuable in the treatment of urinary tract infections, gout, diarrhea, and arthritis.

Dose and use: To prepare tea from the berries, pour one cup of boiling water over one to two teaspoons of the ripe berries (either whole or crushed). Let steep for fifteen minutes and then strain. If using barberry roots, place half a teaspoon of the dried and powdered root bark in a pan with one cup of water. Bring to a boil and boil for twenty to thirty minutes. Remove from the heat, cool, and strain. You may want to sweeten with honey. Drink up to one cup per day of the tea, one tablespoon at a time.

The berries can also be used as an alcohol tincture to treat infections and colds.

Warning: It is important to note that excessive consumption or overdose of the root bark of barberry can lead to adverse effects. These may include diarrhea, kidney irritation, light stupor, nosebleeds, and vomiting.

Other uses: The berries of the barberry plant can be utilized to create a grayish-brown dye. This dye can be used to color various materials. Additionally, Native Americans found practical uses for the crushed berries as a means to waterproof their baskets. Applying crushed berries to the baskets helped to enhance their durability and resistance to moisture.

Bearberry

Ericaceae *(Arctostaphylos uva-ursi L. Spreng)*

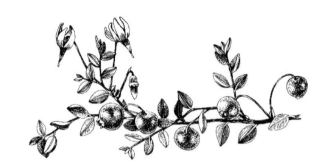

Identification: Bearberry, scientifically known as Arctostaphylos uva-ursi, is a trailing shrub that grows close to the ground, forming a low-lying and prostrate mat. The plant has dark, evergreen leaves that are leathery in texture and smooth-edged. The shape of the leaves is generally obovate or spatula-shaped, and they are less than ¾ inch wide. It is worth noting that the alpine variety of bearberry may have larger leaves compared to the typical variety. The fruit of bearberry is a dry red berry. In addition to its scientific name, bearberry is also commonly referred to as kinnikinnick or uva-ursi.

Habitat: Bearberrycan be found in the northern United States from the East to the West, as well as in various parts of Canada. It thrives in boggy and relatively dry areas, often growing at the base of pine trees, tamarack trees, and juniper shrubs.

Medicinal parts: The leaves.

Solvents: Alcohol, water.

Effects: Astringent, Diuretic, Tonic.

Food: The berries of bearberry, although dry, mealy, and lacking in flavor, have been traditionally used in various culinary preparations by Indigenous peoples. One common method is to cook the berries with animal fat or mix them with stronger-tasting foods such as fish eggs, particularly salmon eggs. The berries can also be dried and crushed into a flour-like meal. In the Northwest, Native American tribes used this meal as a spice to enhance the flavor of meat and organ meats.

Different tribes had their own ways of incorporating bearberry berries into their diets. For example, the Bella Coola Nation mixed the berries with fat and consumed them, while the Lower Chinook people dried the berries and combined them with fat for food. Many Native Americans boiled the berries along with roots and vegetables to create a nourishing soup. Another preparation method involves sautéing the berries in grease until crisp, then pounding them into a mash using a cheesecloth. This mash can be added to cooked fish eggs, mixed together, and sweetened according to taste. The aromatic and flavor-enhancing qualities of the berries make them a desirable addition to dishes featuring wild fowl and game.

Traditional uses: The traditional uses of bearberry encompass a wide range of applications by different cultures. The whole plant, including its aerial parts, was infused in water and mixed with grease obtained from animals such as geese, ducks, bears, or mountain goats. This mixture was then combined with glue made from the hooves of horses or deer. The resulting salve was used topically on sores, infants' scalps, and rashes. For oral health, an infusion of the aerial parts of the plant was used as a mouthwash to alleviate canker sores and soothe sore gums. Dried leaves and stems were ground into a powder and applied as a poultice to wounds. An infusion made from the leaves, berries, and stems served as a diuretic for cleansing the kidneys and relieving bladder complaints. Additionally, this beverage was believed to have analgesic properties, providing relief for back pain and sprains. The berries themselves were consumed or infused with the whole plant to address cold symptoms.

In certain cultures, such as the Kwakiutl peoples, the leaves of bearberry were smoked for their reported narcotic effects. Dried leaves were also crushed into a powder and applied to sores. Furthermore, a combination of bearberry leaves and tobacco was included in religious bundles for spiritual healing. Early pioneers utilized leaf infusions of bearberry as diuretics, astringents, and tonics.

Modern uses: Bearberry (Arctostaphylos uva-ursi) continues to find applications in modern times, building upon its traditional uses by Native American tribes. One prominent modern use of bearberry is in herbal medicine. It is commonly employed as a natural remedy for urinary tract infections (UTIs) due to its antibacterial properties. The leaves of bearberry contain compounds, such as arbutin, that have diuretic and antiseptic effects on the urinary system. Extracts or tinctures made from bearberry leaves are used to alleviate UTI symptoms and support urinary tract health. Bearberry is also utilized in the cosmetic industry. Its astringent properties make it a popular ingredient in skincare products, especially those targeting oily or acne-prone skin. Bearberry extract is known for its ability to help tighten pores, reduce excess oil, and promote a clearer complexion. It is often found in facial toners, serums, and creams.

Moreover, bearberry has been investigated for its potential antioxidant and anti-inflammatory properties. Research suggests that its bioactive compounds may have protective effects against oxidative stress and inflammation in the body.

Dose and use: The leaves of bearberry can be soaked in alcohol or brandy for one week or more. To prepare a tea, add 1 teaspoonful of the soaked leaves to 1 cup of boiling or cold water and drink 2-3 cups a day. The tincture of bearberry can also be taken, with 10-25 drops in water three or more times a day, depending on symptoms. The tea can be made without alcohol, similar to ordinary tea. Combining the tincture of bearberry with tincture of quaking aspen (Populus tremuloides) in specific amounts, such as 2-15 drops of quaking aspen and 10-20 drops of bearberry, has shown effectiveness as a diuretic and antibacterial, therefore I'd highly recommend it for urine tract infections.

Warning: Caution should be exercised when using bearberry (uva-ursi) during pregnancy or while nursing. Additionally, it is advised to avoid consuming acidic foods when using the tea to treat urogenital and biliary tract diseases. Prolonged use of uva-ursi may have negative effects on the liver and can cause inflammation and irritation in the bladder and kidneys. It is not recommended for use in children and individuals with high blood pressure.

Veterinarian/Wildlife: Bearberry is indeed used in some herbal formulas for horses. It is believed to have beneficial effects in certain areas, including joint health, fertility, and overall well-being. Uva-ursi is sometimes included in joint-rebuilding or joint-protecting supplements for horses, as it is thought to support joint function and reduce inflammation.

In addition, uva-ursi may be included in training mixes for horses to provide support for their overall health and performance during training sessions. It is believed to have potential benefits for endurance and stamina.

Furthermore, uva-ursi is sometimes incorporated into fertility boosters for horses. It is thought to support reproductive health and may be used to enhance fertility in breeding programs.

It is important to note that the use of herbal supplements and formulas for horses should be done under the guidance of a veterinarian or equine specialist who can provide appropriate advice and dosage recommendations based on the specific needs of the horse.

Black Cohosh
Ranuculaceae *(Actaea racemosa L. Nutt.)*

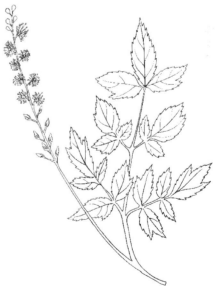

Identification: Black cohosh (Actaea racemosa), also known as black snakeroot, is a perennial herbaceous plant native to North America. It is easily recognizable by its tall, slender stalks and feathery compound leaves. The plant typically reaches a height of 3 to 8 feet (1 to 2.5 meters) and features deeply lobed, toothed leaflets that radiate from a central stem. The foliage has a dark green color and a glossy appearance.

In late spring to early summer, black cohosh produces long, slender flowering spikes that can reach up to 2 feet (60 centimeters) in length. The spikes are adorned with small, white or cream-colored flowers that are arranged in dense clusters. These flowers give off a faint, sweet fragrance and attract pollinators such as bees and butterflies.

After the flowers fade, black cohosh develops distinctive seed pods that contain small, shiny black seeds. The pods are elongated and cylindrical, giving them a resemblance to narrow cigars. When mature, the pods split open, releasing the seeds.

It is important to note that while black cohosh shares some similarities with other plants in the same family, such as blue cohosh (Caulophyllum thalictroides), it can be differentiated by its distinct leaves, flowers, and seed pods. Careful observation of these characteristics can help in accurately identifying black cohosh in the wild or in cultivation.

Habitat: Northern United States and southern Canada. Mostly found east of the plains in forests. Black cohosh prefers shady, woodland environments and can often be found growing in moist, rich soils. It is native to regions of eastern North America, including parts of the United States and Canada.

Medicinal Part: The root.

Solvent: Boiling water enhances the properties of the root but dissolves it only partially; alcohol dissolves it completely.

Effects: Alterative, Diuretic, Diaphoretic, Expectorant, Anti- spasmodic, Sedative (arterial and nervous), Cardiac stimulant (safer than Digitalis), Emmenagogue.

Traditional uses: Among the Cherokee, black cohosh was used to alleviate menstrual discomfort, regulate menstrual cycles, and address menopausal symptoms. It was believed to promote hormonal balance and provide relief from hot flashes, night sweats, and mood swings.
The Iroquois and Algonquin tribes utilized black cohosh for similar purposes. It was used by women to support reproductive health, ease menstrual cramps, and relieve the discomforts associated with PMS. During labor, black cohosh was employed to aid in childbirth by facilitating contractions.
The Ojibwe tribe also recognized the medicinal value of black cohosh. They used it as an analgesic and anti-inflammatory agent to alleviate muscle and joint pain, including conditions such as arthritis and rheumatism.

Modern uses: Commercial preparations containing black cohosh are commonly utilized for the treatment of premenstrual syndrome (PMS) and menopausal symptoms. It has shown effectiveness in alleviating uterine spasms, menstrual pain, hot flashes, mild depression, vaginal atrophy, and other menopausal discomforts.

Promising studies have supported the efficacy of black cohosh. For instance, a clinical trial conducted by Friede, Liske, et al. demonstrated that a proprietary black cohosh extract called Remifemin significantly reduced hot flashes and psychological disturbances in postmenopausal women. Another study by Jacobson found that a black cohosh preparation was effective in relieving symptoms such as hot flashes and sweating in breast cancer survivors undergoing premenopausal breast cancer treatment. Furthermore, research conducted by Wuttke et al. showed that black cohosh may contribute to increased bone formation in postmenopausal women.
Beyond its use in addressing female conditions, black cohosh continues to be employed by holistic health practitioners for the treatment of fever, arthritis, and insomnia.

Dose and use: To prepare a tincture of Black Cohosh, it is recommended to use fresh root or recently dried root. Mix 2 ounces of the root with 1 pint of 96 percent proof alcohol. Take 5-15 drops of the tincture four times a day. Alternatively, you can make a tea by adding 1 teaspoonful of the cut root to 1 cup of boiling water and drinking it three times a day. Another option is to add 15-30 drops of the tincture to 1 cup of water and sweeten it with honey. Externally, the bruised root was traditionally used by Native Americans as an antidote for snake bites. It was applied directly to the wound, and the juice was taken orally in very small amounts.

Warning: Caution should be exercised when using black cohosh for its medicinal benefits. It has been associated with potential risks, including rare cases of liver damage, allergic reactions, and interactions with certain medications. Pregnant and breastfeeding women should avoid its use. Mild side effects such as gastrointestinal discomfort and headaches have also been reported. It is advisable to consult with a healthcare professional before using black cohosh to ensure safe and appropriate usage.

Veterinarian uses: Black cohosh is used as an ingredient in some proprietary horse products, including those specifically formulated for fertility boosting. These products are designed to support reproductive health in horses and may contain a combination of herbs and other ingredients.

Black Haw

Viburnum prunifolium, (N.O.: Caprifoliaceae)

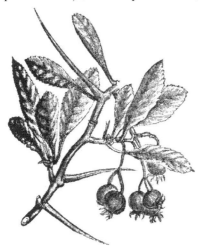

Habitat: Black haw is found in most of the North American states, more abundantly from New York to Florida.

Identification: Black haw is a shrub or tree that can reach heights of 10-25 feet, with a trunk diameter of about 10 inches. Its bark is irregular, transversely curved, and grayish-brown, sometimes turning brownish-red when the outer bark scales off. The inner surface of the bark is reddish-brown. The root bark has a cinnamon color and a bitter and astringent taste. The deep-green leaves are broadly elliptical or obovate, finely and sharply toothed, and smooth on the undersurface. They measure about 1-3 inches in length. The flowers appear in small white clusters from May to June, with each flower having 3-5 lobes. The fruit, known as Black haw, is edible but may be excessively sweet for some. The fruits are shiny black and grow on red stems.

Medicinal parts: Root bark (preferred), bark of stems and branches.

Solvents: Water, alcohol.

Effects: Diuretic, Tonic, Antispasmodic, Nervine, Astringent.

Uses: Black haw is considered a reliable remedy for expectant mothers at risk of abortion. It is recommended to start the preparation two or three weeks before the anticipated recurrence of the condition and continue it for about two weeks after any disturbance. If there are no further symptoms during the final weeks, it can be discontinued until after delivery.

In addition to its benefits for expectant mothers, a decoction of black haw is known to alleviate chills and fever. It is also effective in providing speedy relief from heart palpitations and is valuable in treating diarrhea and dysentery. It's worth noting that herbs with healing properties for the stomach and intestinal tract often prove effective for symptoms in the mouth and throat as well.

Dose: 1 oz. to 1 pint of boiling water, take one tablespoon three or four times a day; or 1 teaspoon of the tincture, three or four times a day. As a tea and decoction it is used for painful menstruation, excessive menstrual bleeding, cramps and hysteria. Sometimes associated with and used as a heart tonic, to improve blood circulation, kidney and bladder.

Bark decoction for cramps. Berries for ulcers. Leaves as tea and decoction.

Bloodroot

Papavaraceae *(Sanguinaria canadensis L.)*

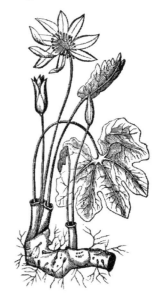

Habitat: Eastern forests south to Florida, west to Minnesota, and north to Manitoba. Damp, rich forests, along forest trails.

Identification: Bloodroot (*Sanguinaria canadensis*) grows to a height of 6 to 10 inches and features distinct lobed leaves that arise directly from the base of the plant. The leaves are rounded, palm-shaped, and have a bluish-green hue. Bloodroot produces solitary white flowers with eight to twelve petals, which appear in early spring. The flowers are ephemeral, lasting only for a short period before fading. The plant derives its name from the orange-red sap that exudes from its rhizome when cut or damaged, resembling the color of blood. The rhizome itself is thick, knotted, and covered in brownish scales. Overall, bloodroot is easily identifiable by its unique leaves, delicate white flowers, and the presence of the characteristic blood-red sap.

Medicinal parts: The root

Solvents: Water, alcohol.

Effects: Expectorant, antimicrobial, anesthetic

Traditional uses: Bloodroot has a rich history of traditional use among various Native American tribes. Indigenous communities recognized the medicinal properties of bloodroot and employed it for various purposes. The Cherokee used bloodroot as a topical application to treat skin conditions such as warts, tumors, and skin infections. They also used it as a wash for sore eyes. The Iroquois utilized bloodroot preparations as a remedy for rheumatism, respiratory ailments, and as an emetic to induce vomiting.

Modern uses: Today, bloodroot is primarily used in topical preparations and herbal remedies. Its active compounds, such as alkaloids and sanguinarine, have been studied for their potential health benefits. Bloodroot extract is commonly found in natural toothpaste and mouthwash products due to its antimicrobial properties, which help promote oral health and fight dental plaque. It is also used in certain topical salves and ointments for its potential antimicrobial and anti-inflammatory effects on the skin. However, it is important to note that bloodroot contains potent compounds and should be used with caution.

Warning: Bloodroot is a plant that holds potential dangers and should be approached with caution. While it has been used historically in certain traditional practices and herbal remedies, bloodroot contains toxic substances that can be harmful when ingested, applied topically, or used improperly. The plant's active compounds, such as alkaloids, can have adverse effects on the liver, heart, and nervous system. Moreover, bloodroot has been linked to skin irritation, burns, and even tissue damage if not used with extreme care. It is crucial to seek professional guidance and exercise great caution when dealing with bloodroot or any products derived from it to ensure personal safety and well-being.

Blueberry

Ericaceae *(Vaccinium spp.)*

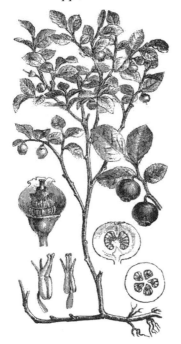

Habitat: Blueberries are native to North America and thrive in various habitats across the continent. They are commonly found growing in acidic soil in areas such as open woodlands, meadows, bogs, and mountainous regions. Blueberry plants prefer well-drained soil with high organic content and require a certain level of moisture to flourish. They often grow in clusters or colonies, forming dense thickets that provide shelter for wildlife. In the wild, blueberries can be found in regions ranging from low-lying coastal areas to higher elevations in mountainous regions. They are also cultivated in home gardens and commercial farms, with specific varieties adapted to different climate zones.

Identification: Blueberry plants (Vaccinium spp.) are small to medium-sized shrubs, typically reaching a height of 1 to 6 feet. They are characterized by their oval or elliptical-shaped leaves that are usually dark green and glossy, with serrated edges. The foliage turns vibrant shades of red and purple in the fall. Blueberry plants produce delicate, bell-shaped white or pink flowers in the spring, which give way to clusters of small, round berries. The berries start green and gradually ripen to shades of blue, purple, or black, depending on the variety.

Medicinal parts: Leaves and berries.

Solvents: alcohol and boiling water.
Effects: Diuretic, Refrigerant, Astringent.

Food: This highly nutritious fruit may be eaten fresh, dried, stewed, or as a jam or marmalade. Leaves can be made into tea.
We have energy bars; the Iroquois, and other Native American tribes, had pemmican. This high-energy food was a mixture of meat (often buffalo or fish), nuts and seeds, animal fat, and berries or other types of fruit.
They called these pemmican cakes, and they were a way to preserve food for winter and provide portable nutrition for hunting and other trips. Blueberries and other fruits were first dried like raisins, then added to the cakes. Our modern high-energy trail bars are really just a version of those early pemmican cakes — minus the meat and animal fat — usually with oats or other grains added.

Traditional uses: Blueberries have a long history of traditional use among Native American tribes for both culinary and medicinal purposes. For example, the Ojibwa tribe used blueberries as a food source, consuming them fresh or dried. The Chippewa tribe used the dried berries as an ingredient in pemmican, a traditional Native American food made from dried meat, fat, and berries.

In terms of medicinal uses, the Potawatomi tribe used blueberry tea to treat stomachaches, while the Chippewa used it to alleviate labor pains. The Iroquois and Mohegan tribes applied a poultice of mashed blueberries to treat burns and scalds. The Algonquin tribe utilized blueberry tea as a tonic to soothe the digestive system.

Michael J. Moerman, in his book "Native American Medicinal Plants: An Ethnobotanical Dictionary," also mentions the traditional uses of blueberries by different tribes. He notes that the Cherokee tribe used blueberry root tea to treat diarrhea, while the Iroquois and Ojibwa tribes used it to address dysentery and other gastrointestinal issues. Additionally, the Iroquois employed a decoction of blueberry roots as a blood purifier.

Modern uses: Blueberries have gained widespread recognition for their numerous health benefits, supported by both scientific research and the approval of Commission E. The use of fresh and dried blueberries, as well as dried leaves, is approved for treating various conditions such as diarrhea, inflammation of the pharynx, and mouth.

One of the key attributes of blueberries is their remarkable antioxidant properties. The high anthocyanin content in blueberries gives them their rich purple-blue color and serves as potent antioxidants, playing a crucial role in vascular health. These antioxidants help protect capillaries and promote better blood flow to vital areas of the body, including the brain, hands, feet, and eyes. Research suggests that blueberries have anti-atherosclerotic and antiplatelet aggregating effects, potentially contributing to cardiovascular health.

Blueberries have shown promise in benefiting specific conditions. They may provide support for individuals with glaucoma and night blindness due to their ability to enhance blood circulation and protect the delicate blood vessels in the eyes. Anthocyanins found in blueberries and bilberries, their European cousins, have demonstrated efficacy in the treatment of macular degeneration, a common age-related eye disease.

The impact of blueberries on vision has an interesting history. During World War II, bomber pilots consumed blueberries with the belief that they would improve their night vision. While some studies have confirmed benefits in reducing eyestrain and improving weak eyesight, the direct impact on night vision in healthy individuals is still under investigation.

In addition to their eye health benefits, blueberries have been found to induce the release of dopamine, a neurotransmitter associated with mood and cognitive function. This finding suggests that blueberries may provide adjunct nutritional support for conditions like Alzheimer's disease.

Dose and usage: Place two or three handfuls of Bilberry in a bottle and pour a good, real brandy over them. Secure with a good fitting cap or cork. The longer the tincture stays the more powerful a medicine will this berry spirit be. Violent, continuous diarrhea accompanied by pain, is stopped by taking 1 tablespoonful of Bilberry brandy in 1/4 pint of water; repeat every 8 or 10 hr. For diarrhoea, dysentery and similar complaints, a decoction of the leaves will bring relief.
Of the leaves, 1 teaspoonful to 1 cup of boiling water. In the Herbalist by J. E. Meyers: "A mixture of equal parts of Bilberry leaves, Thyme, and Strawberry leaves makes an excellent tea."

Consuming a daily portion of blueberries, approximately a fistful, can be beneficial during episodes of prolonged bowel discomfort, gas, or diarrhea. Additionally, drying the berries using a food dryer and storing them in the freezer can provide a remedy for winter stomach problems and serve as a general tonic for overall health.

Boneset
Asteraceae (*Eupatorium perfoliatum* L.)

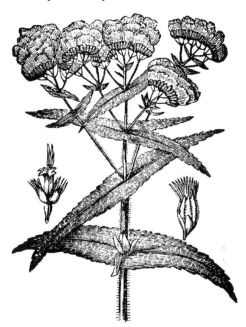

Identification: Perennial herbaceous plant that typically grows to a height of 2 to 4 feet. It features an erect, sturdy stem that is densely covered with coarse hairs. The leaves of boneset are opposite, meaning they grow in pairs along the stem, and they are characterized by their distinctive perfoliate arrangement. This means that the stem appears to pierce through the center of each leaf, giving the impression that the leaves are joined together around the stem.
The leaves of boneset are lanceolate in shape, with serrated edges and prominent veins. They have a rough texture and are a medium green color. The plant produces clusters of small, white flowers that bloom in late summer or early fall. The flowers are arranged in flat-topped clusters at the top of the stem, forming a rounded or slightly domed shape. The flowers are attractive to pollinators such as bees and butterflies.

Habitat: Boneset is commonly found in wetland areas, including marshes, swamps, and along the banks of streams or rivers. It thrives in moist, rich soil and can tolerate both full sun and partial shade. It is native to North America and can be found in various regions, including the eastern and central parts of the United States.

Medicinal parts: Leaves and whole aerial parts.

Solvents: alcohol and water.

Effects: Febrifuge, diaphoretic, tonic, laxative.

61

Traditional uses: Native American tribes such as the Cherokee, Iroquois, and Delaware utilized boneset for its medicinal properties. The plant was highly regarded for its ability to address a range of ailments.

One common traditional use of boneset was for treating fevers, particularly those associated with influenza and other viral infections. The plant was prepared as a tea or infusion, and it was believed to induce sweating and support the body's natural defense mechanisms. The Cherokee and Iroquois tribes used boneset tea to alleviate symptoms of colds, flu, and fevers, hence the plant's name.

Boneset was also valued for its potential to relieve digestive complaints. It was used to ease stomachaches, promote digestion, and alleviate constipation. Additionally, the plant was employed as a general tonic to strengthen the body and promote overall well-being. Traditional healers and herbalists in early American history also recognized boneset's potential as a mild pain reliever. It was used to alleviate headaches, body aches, and joint pain. Boneset was often prepared as a poultice or applied topically to soothe sprains, bruises, and minor injuries.

Modern uses: In modern times, boneset (Eupatorium perfoliatum) continues to be utilized for its potential health benefits. Scientific studies have explored its therapeutic properties, particularly in the context of immune support and the management of fever-related symptoms. Research published in the Journal of Ethnopharmacology (Volume 111, Issue 1, 2007) highlighted the immunomodulatory effects of boneset extract, indicating its potential in enhancing immune responses. Another study published in BMC Complementary and Alternative Medicine (Volume 14, Issue 1, 2014) evaluated the antiviral activity of boneset extract against influenza A virus, demonstrating its inhibitory effects on viral replication.

Additionally, boneset is occasionally used in homeopathic medicine, where it is believed to provide relief for fever and flu-like symptoms.

Dose and usage: Infusion: 1-2 tsp herb/cup water; to abate fever 1 cup every half hour as hot as possible.

Warning: Small doses of boneset can have laxative and diuretic effects, while larger doses may induce vomiting. However, it is important to note that boneset contains pyrrolizidine alkaloids, which can be potentially harmful to the liver. Therefore, never use boneset without consulting a licensed holistic health-care practitioner. They can provide guidance on the appropriate use and dosage of boneset, taking into account any potential risks and individual health considerations.

California Poppy
Papaveraceae *(Eschscholzia californica Cham.)*

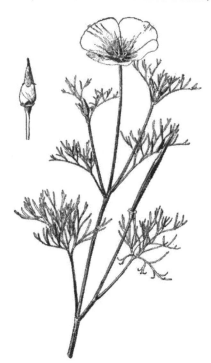

Identification: The California poppy is a flowering plant that can be annual or perennial, ranging in height from 15 to 40 inches. It has few bluish-green leaves that taper to a point and have a feathery or fernlike appearance. The plant produces brilliant yellow-orange solitary flowers that can reach up to 2 inches in width. The seed receptacle of the flower is cup- or bowl-shaped and contains several chambers filled with tiny seeds. There are hundreds of species of California poppy.

Habitat: The California poppy is native to regions stretching from California to British Columbia. It can be found in open areas, along roadsides, and in dry clearings. It is also commonly cultivated in gardens throughout the country, it's one of the easiest wildflower to grow (look it up in the sixth volume!)

Solvents: Boiling water.

Medicinal Part: Aerial parts, flowers, sap

Effects: Analgesic, anxiolytic, sedative

Traditional uses: The aerial parts of the California poppy are collected and dried for the purpose of creating a sedative infusion that promotes sleep. This herb has been historically utilized for its anxiolytic and antispasmodic properties, making it beneficial for addressing anxiety, nervousness, and muscle spasms. It is recognized for its warming and diuretic effects, and it also possesses analgesic properties. In traditional usage, it has been employed to alleviate nocturnal urination in children. Native Americans utilized the milky sap from the leaves as an analgesic to relieve toothaches, and placing the leaves under children at bedtime was believed to induce sleep. Additionally, the application of the white resin obtained from the seedpods was used to stimulate lactation in nursing mothers.

The Costanoan tribe applied the fresh plant as a poultice to treat headaches and applied the plant extract to relieve toothaches. They also used the dried plant in smoking mixtures to induce relaxation and sleep. The Ohlone tribe prepared a decoction of California poppy to alleviate pain, reduce anxiety, and induce sleep. They also used it as an eyewash to treat eye irritations and infections.

The Pomo tribe used the plant as a sedative and analgesic, employing it to relieve pain and promote relaxation. They also prepared infusions or decoctions of California poppy to address various ailments, including toothaches and colic in infants. The Shasta tribe incorporated the plant into their traditional medicine for the treatment of headaches, while the Maidu tribe used it to relieve general pain and discomfort.

In the Mendocino region, the roots of the plant were juiced and used to treat various ailments such as headaches, stomachaches, and toothaches. Nursing mothers in this area would wash their breasts with the juice of the roots to help reduce milk flow during the weaning process.

It is worth noting that some tribes regarded the California poppy as poisonous and refrained from its use. Among certain indigenous communities, such as the Yaqui, Gileño, and Pima tribes, the scattering of California poppy flowers, known as hoohi e's in the case of E. mexicana, took place ahead of processions during special ceremonial events. Similarly, women from the Cahuilla tribe adorned themselves with the pollen of the California poppy, applying it as eye shadow and body paint during significant occasions.

Modern uses: Indeed, Californidine, an alkaloid present in the California poppy plant, has been recognized for its potential as a sleep aid and sedative. However, it is important to note that the evidence supporting these effects is primarily based on animal studies, and further research is required to establish its efficacy in humans. Qualified holistic medicine practitioners may utilize Californidine as a component of sleep aid and sedative treatments, exercising caution and considering individual circumstances. In addition, homeopathic preparations incorporating California poppy may be employed under the supervision of trained professionals to address insomnia.

Warning: Don't use during pregnancy!

Gardening: The California poppy, renowned for its beauty, exhibits a robust growth habit with deep roots, making it an appealing addition to any garden. Notably, the plant produces edible seeds that can be incorporated into various baked goods, adding both flavor and visual appeal. It is important to note that in the state of California, picking this plant is strictly prohibited, as it holds the esteemed position of the state flower. Moreover, the California poppy plays a significant role in supporting wildlife, serving as a vital resource for various species. Due to its resilience and ability to thrive in diverse environments, it is frequently included in wildflower seed mixes utilized for ecological restoration projects and roadside plantings.

Cascara Sagrada (Buckthorn)

Rhamnaceae (*Rhamnus cathartica* L.; *R. purshiana* [DC.] Cooper)

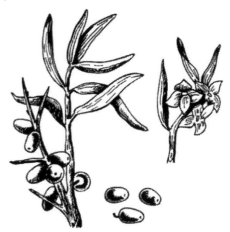

Identification: Cascara sagrada, scientifically known as Rhamnus purshiana, is a bush or small tree reaching heights of 4 to 20 feet.
It features a well-branched structure without thorns, and its foliage is densely packed. When mature, the bark takes on a gray-brown hue, adorned with gray-white lenticels. The leaves are thin, exhibiting hairiness along the ribs, and have a fully margined shape, ranging from elliptical to ovate, measuring approximately 2 inches in length. The plant produces numerous greenish-white flowers that form in axillary cymes. These flowers are small in size and consist of five petals. As the fruit ripens, it transitions to a red to black-purple color, enclosing two or three seeds. Another variation of cascara sagrada, known as Rhamnus purshiana (cascara buckthorn), grows taller, reaching up to 30 feet. Its leaves are characterized by twenty to twenty-four veins, and its white flowers cluster together.

Habitat: Cascara sagrada is native to the Pacific Northwest region of North America, including areas such as Oregon, Washington, and British Columbia. It thrives in moist, well-drained soils and is commonly found in forests, woodlands, and along streams. Cascara sagrada is a small to medium-sized deciduous tree that prefers shady habitats, often growing as part of the understory vegetation.

Solvents: Diluted alcohol, boiling water.

Medicinal Part: The bark and root.

Effects: Laxative

Traditional uses: The indigenous peoples, including the Coastal Salish, Nuu-chah-nulth, and Kwakwaka'wakw, utilized the bark of cascara sagrada for various medicinal purposes. The bark was commonly prepared as a tea or decoction and used as a natural laxative to relieve constipation and promote bowel movements. It was also employed to support digestive health, alleviate stomachaches, and cleanse the gastrointestinal system. The tribes valued cascara sagrada for its gentle yet effective properties in promoting regularity and overall well-being.

Modern uses: The bark extract of R. purshiana, known as cascara sagrada, possesses potent laxative properties. It has received approval from Commission E for the treatment of constipation. The laxative effects of cascara sagrada can persist for up to eight hours.

Warning: It is important to note that the use of cascara sagrada should never be employed to clear intestinal obstructions. While the bark infusion is regarded as a cleansing tonic, prolonged and excessive use of the herb may carry a potential risk of carcinogenicity. It is advised to use cascara sagrada under the guidance and supervision of a qualified healthcare professional, whether it be a physician or a holistic practitioner. Additionally, it should be noted that the berries of the plant are not suitable for consumption.

Dose and usage: Harvesting cascara sagrada involves carefully removing the outer bark from the trunk and branches of the tree, leaving the inner bark intact to allow the tree to continue growing. The best time for harvesting is typically in the spring or early summer when the sap is flowing. It is important to harvest from mature trees that are at least 10 years old to ensure sustainability and optimal potency.

After harvesting, the bark is typically dried and cured to enhance its medicinal properties. The curing process involves storing the bark in a cool, dry place for several months and up to three years to allow it to age and develop its characteristic laxative compounds and diminish its bitter components.

When using cascara sagrada, it is crucial to follow proper dosage and usage guidelines. It is recommended to start with a small dosage and gradually increase as needed. Generally, a typical dosage ranges from 1 to 2 grams of dried bark steeped in hot water to make a tea, taken once daily before bedtime. The tea should be steeped for about 10 to 15 minutes and strained before consumption. It is important to note that cascara sagrada should not be used continuously for more than one to two weeks without medical supervision.

Catnip
Lamiaceae *(Nepeta cataria L.)*

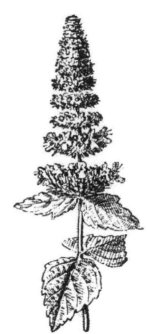

Identification: Catnip (Nepeta cataria) is a perennial herb belonging to the mint family. It typically grows to a height of 2 to 3 feet and has a square-shaped stem with opposite, heart-shaped leaves. The leaves are gray-green in color and have a soft, velvety texture. Catnip produces small, tubular, white or lavender flowers that bloom in clusters at the top of the stems. When crushed or bruised, the leaves and stems release a strong, aromatic scent that is attractive to cats.

Habitat: Catnip can be found throughout North America, spanning from border to border and coast to coast. It can be commonly seen in gardens, along roadsides, and in areas with disturbed or waste ground. Catnip is adaptable and can tolerate well-drained and dry conditions.

Solvents: Diluted alcohol, boiling water.

Medicinal Part: The Whole herb.

Effects: Carminative, Stimulant, Tonic, Diaphoretic, Emmenagogue, Antispasmodic

Traditional uses: The Mohegan and Iroquois tribes, utilized catnip for its medicinal properties. They brewed catnip tea to address various ailments, including colds, fevers, headaches, and stomach discomfort. Catnip was also employed as a natural remedy for insomnia, anxiety, and nervousness. Additionally, catnip leaves were often smoked or chewed for their calming and sedative effects. The herb was highly regarded for its ability to soothe digestive issues, relieve menstrual cramps, and promote relaxation.

Modern uses: Naturopaths have found catnip to be effective in treating colic and soothing upset stomach in children (Chevallier, 1996). It can be prepared as a tincture and used topically to alleviate rheumatic and arthritic joint discomfort. Catnip tea is known to stimulate the gallbladder and acts as a cleansing herb for the urinary system.

In combination with other herbs, catnip is often paired with elderflowers for the treatment of acute infections. Additionally, a combination of catnip, valerian root, and hops is commonly used as a sleep aid, as well as to reduce stress and promote relaxation.

Dose and use: Catnip Decoction: Infuse 1 to 2 teaspoons of dried catnip leaves in 1 cup of cold water for at least 45. Strain and drink up to 3 cups per day. Don't use warm water as its oil are volatile and reduced by heat. This preparation can help soothe digestive discomfort, relieve menstrual cramps, and promote relaxation.
Catnip Tincture: Take 1 to 2 teaspoons of catnip tincture, diluted in water or juice, up to three times per day. This form of catnip can help alleviate anxiety, nervousness, and promote restful sleep. Follow the instructions on the tincture bottle for specific dosage guidelines.
Catnip Essential Oil: Dilute 2 to 3 drops of catnip essential oil in a carrier oil, such as coconut oil, and apply it topically to the temples or pulse points for relaxation and headache relief. Always dilute essential oils before applying them to the skin.

Warning: Not to be used during pregnancy.

Veterinarian uses: Actinidine, an iridoid glycoside, is the cat-stimulating chemical of the plant.
Sprinkle dried catnip leaves on toys or scratching posts to entertain and stimulate cats. Monitor your cat's response to ensure they are not overly stimulated.

Cattail

Typhaceae *(Typha latifolia L.; T. angustifolia L.).*

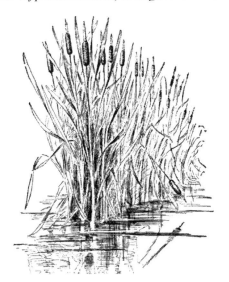

Identification: Cattail (Typha spp.) is a tall, perennial plant commonly found near wetlands, marshes, and the edges of bodies of water. It features long, erect stems that can reach up to 10 feet in height. The plant has long, lance-shaped leaves that grow in a vertical pattern, forming a distinctive tufted appearance. Cattails produce dense cylindrical flower spikes, known as catkins, which are composed of numerous small flowers. These catkins have a brownish color and can be seen protruding above the foliage during the flowering season.
Cattails are also characterized by their unique seed heads, which resemble a brown sausage-like structure. The plant's roots are thick and fleshy, often submerged in water or moist soil.

Habitat: It can be found throughout the United States, growing in various wet habitats such as the edges of lakes, slow-moving streams, marshes, shallow ponds, and any other areas with moist and nutrient-rich soil. They have a wide distribution and are adapted to thrive in diverse wetland environments across the country.

Dose and usage: Cattail roots are rich in polysaccharides, which can be extracted by beating the roots into water. The resulting starchy water can be used as a soothing wash for sunburned skin, providing relief and promoting healing. Additionally, the ashes of burned cattail leaves possess styptic and antimicrobial properties. They can be applied to wounds to help dress and seal them, assisting in the healing process and preventing infection. The use of cattail leaf ash can be beneficial in keeping wounds clean and promoting their proper closure.

Traditional uses: Indigenous North Americans have been weaving with cattail leaves for more than 12,000 years; the leaves thatched roofs and were woven into mats and baskets. Early settlers used cattail stems and leaves to weave rush seats for their chairs.
Cattails have also been a food plant since at least 800 CE; there are caves in Ohio where archaeologists found preserved evidence of cattails eaten in meals. The Blackfoot and the Northern Paiute tribes and early colonists roasted the seeds and dried the roots, then ground them into flour to make cakes, mush porridge, and bread. Other indigenous groups, like the Yuma, mixed the pollen with water and kneaded it into little cakes, which they baked. The juicy hearts of young spring shoots were eaten as a cooked vegetable, and immature green flower heads were boiled and eaten similarly to how we eat corn on the cob (it even tastes similar!)

Notes: Cattail pollen is very flammable and has a tendency to burst when ignited; in fact, it's been part of some formulas for making fireworks for at least 200 years. In the mid-1800s, miners and settlers found that they could wire the mature brown flower heads of cattail to sticks, dip them in oil or beeswax, and use them as slow-burning torches. This practice was later replaced with safer alternatives like miners' canvas caps that had a candle or lamp bracket, eliminating the need to use cattail torches. Today enthusiasts of primitive survival skills mix cattail fluff with oil or beeswax to shape a rustic, but useful, type of candle lighting.

Chamomile

Asteraceae *(Matricaria matricarioides; Chamomilla recutita L.; Chamaemelum nobile L.)*

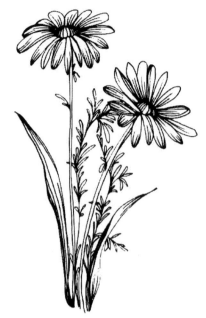

Identification: Wild chamomile, also known as pineapple weed, is a distinct variety of chamomile that differs from the cultivated herb chamomile. It is characterized by its small yellow flowers, measuring approximately ½" in width, which lack the white rays or petals found in chamomile. The plant has a prostrate and spreading growth habit, with many branches and deeply cut leaves. The rayless flowers of wild chamomile are highly noticeable and emit a pleasant scent reminiscent of pineapples, making them easily distinguishable from other chamomile species.

Habitat: It can be found in a wide range of habitats including roadsides, pathways, waste grounds, and both low-impact and high-impact soils. It is a common sight throughout the country, from east to west, with a particular prevalence along paths and roads in the Northwest and mountainous areas. The plant has adapted well to disturbed environments and can thrive in various conditions, making it a familiar presence in many regions.

Medicinal parts: Flowers and herb.

Solvents: Water, alcohol.

Effects: Stomachic, Antispasmodic, Tonic stimulant (volatile oil), Carminative, Diaphoretic, Nervine, Emmenagogue, Sedative.

Food: Tea made from fresh pineapple weed flowers is often preferred over dried flowers for its potent flavor and aroma. In comparison to chamomile, fresh pineapple weed is known to possess stronger characteristics. Although the leaves of pineapple weed are edible, they tend to have a bitter taste. Interestingly, Native Americans utilized dried pineapple weed by pulverizing it and combining it with meat and berries, employing its preservative properties.

Traditional uses: Wild chamomile, also known as pineapple weed (Matricaria discoidea), has a history of traditional uses by various indigenous cultures. For example, Native American tribes such as the Lakota, Blackfoot, and Ojibwe used the plant for its medicinal properties. The dried flowers and leaves were often brewed into a tea and used to alleviate digestive discomfort, including indigestion, gas, and stomachaches. The tea was also employed as a mild sedative to promote relaxation and reduce anxiety. Additionally, pineapple weed was applied topically as a poultice or wash to soothe skin irritations, rashes, and insect bites. Its pleasant aroma and calming effects made it a popular choice for promoting restful sleep. Pioneers found that consuming fresh flower tea of pineapple weed provided antispasmodic and carminative effects, aiding in digestion, preventing ulcers, and alleviating arthritis pain. It was believed to have a calming influence on the nerves. The warm tea was also used to alleviate toothache pain.

Modern uses: Research has shown that pineapple weed possesses anti-inflammatory and antioxidant properties, which may contribute to its effectiveness in treating various conditions. For instance, a study published in the Journal of Ethnopharmacology found that pineapple weed extract exhibited anti-inflammatory activity, suggesting its potential use in inflammatory disorders. Another study published in the journal Phytomedicine indicated that pineapple weed extract demonstrated significant antioxidant effects, supporting its role in protecting against oxidative stress.

In alternative medicine, pineapple weed is commonly used to alleviate digestive issues, such as bloating, cramps, and gastrointestinal discomfort. It is often brewed into a tea or taken in the form of herbal supplements. The herb's calming properties make it a popular choice for promoting relaxation, reducing anxiety, and improving sleep quality. Some practitioners also recommend using pineapple weed topically to soothe skin irritations, including rashes and insect bites.

Dose and use: Herbal Tea: Steep 1 to 2 teaspoons of dried pineapple weed flowers or leaves in 1 cup of hot water for 10 to 15 minutes. Consume up to 3 cups per day

Herbal Tincture: Follow the dosage instructions provided on the specific tincture product. Generally, tincture doses range from 2 to 4 milliliters (about 40 to 80 drops), taken up to 3 times per day. Dilute the tincture in water or juice before ingestion.

Topical Application: Create a strong infusion of pineapple weed by steeping the flowers or leaves in hot water. After cooling, apply the infusion topically to the skin using a clean cloth or cotton ball. This can be beneficial for soothing skin irritations and insect bites.

Bath: Infuse a handful of dried pineapple weed flowers or leaves in a muslin bag or directly in the bathwater. Allow the botanicals to steep for approximately 15 minutes before enjoying a relaxing bath. The aromatic qualities of pineapple weed can provide a calming and refreshing experience.

I use pineapple weed primarily for sinus congestion, here are a few helpful methods for it. Steam Inhalation: Add a handful of dried pineapple weed flowers or leaves to a bowl of hot water. Lean over the bowl, covering your head with a towel to create a tent, and inhale the steam deeply. The aromatic steam can help to relieve congestion and promote sinus drainage.

Herbal Compress: Prepare a strong infusion of pineapple weed by steeping the flowers or leaves in hot water. Soak a clean cloth in the infusion, wring out the excess liquid, and place it on your forehead or over your sinuses. Leave it on for several minutes to provide soothing relief and help alleviate sinus congestion.

Herbal Sinus Rinse: Prepare a saline solution using warm distilled water and a pinch of salt. Add a few drops of pineapple weed infusion to the saline solution and mix well. Use a neti pot or a bulb syringe to gently irrigate your sinuses with the solution. This can help flush out mucus and relieve sinus congestion.

Warning: It is important to note that while chamomile may have antiallergic properties for some individuals, it can also be allergenic to others, and in rare cases, it may even cause anaphylactic reactions. Individuals who are allergic to ragweed are advised to avoid using chamomile, both externally and internally. There have been reports of skin rashes and allergic stomachaches in some individuals after consuming or applying chamomile-containing products and cosmetics. If you have a known allergy to ragweed, it is possible to experience an allergic reaction from chamomile tea as well.

Corn
Stigmata maydis, L. (N.O.: Gramineae)

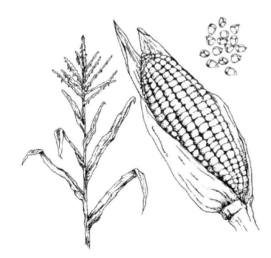

Identification: Corn, scientifically known as Zea mays, belongs to the grass family and is believed to have originated in the New World. It was cultivated in the Americas before Christopher Columbus's arrival. Columbus introduced corn to Spain, and initially, many people mistakenly believed it was brought from Asia. As a result, it was often referred to as Turkey corn or Turkey wheat. The silk of corn should be collected when the plant is about to release its pollen. Maizenic acid is considered the active principle of corn.

Solvents: Water, dilute alcohol.

Medicinal Part: The green pistils.

Effects: Diuretic, Demulcent, Alterative.

Uses: Corn silk, known as Stigmata maydis, is valued by herbalists and naturopaths for its medicinal properties. It is particularly used in cases where there are harmful deposits of brick dust in the urine and to address conditions related to cystic irritation caused by the accumulation of phosphatic and uric acid. Corn silk is believed to be beneficial for various inflammatory conditions of the urethra, bladder, and kidneys, which can lead to dysfunction and discomfort due to the retention of uric acid. Its use aims to promote proper urinary function and alleviate related symptoms.

Dose: A very effective herbal remedy for urinary complaints involves using a tincture of Corn silk (Stigmata maydis) in combination with Agrimony (Agrimonia eupatoria) tincture. It is recommended to take 15-30 drops of Corn silk tincture and 10-30 drops of Agrimony tincture in water between meals and at bedtime.

For more severe urinary issues, a stronger infusion can be prepared using 4 oz. of corn silk, 2 oz. of dandelion root (Leontodon taraxacum), and 1 oz. of golden seal (Hydrastis canadensis). To prepare the infusion, steep 1 teaspoonful of the herbal mixture in 1 cup of boiling water. This infusion can be consumed every three or four hours or as needed. Honey can be added for sweetness, according to personal preference.

If you want to learn more about corn and its paramount importance in Native American horticultural history, check out the 4th volume on traditional cultivation techniques.

Cranberry

Ericaceae *(Vaccinium oxycoccus L.)*

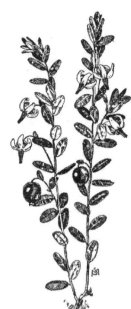

Identification: Cranberry plants are low-growing, evergreen shrubs that form dense mats or carpets. They have slender, creeping stems and small, elliptical to obovate leaves with a glossy dark green color and leathery texture. In late spring to early summer, they produce small, pinkish bell-shaped flowers on short, upright stalks. The flowers are followed by round berries that have a deep red color and a smooth, waxy skin when ripe.

Habitat: Cranberries can be found across the upper tier of states nationwide. They thrive in specific habitats such as the floors of sphagnum bogs, as well as in hummocks and wet alpine meadows. Cranberries can be found at elevations ranging from 6,000 to 7,000 feet, making them well-adapted to high-altitude environments.

Solvents: Water, dilute alcohol.

Medicinal Part: The bark.

Effects: Antispasmodic, Nervine, Tonic, Astringent, Diuretic.

Traditional uses: The berries and juice of cranberries have been traditionally used as a therapy for urinary tract infections due to their ability to acidify urine. They have also been attributed with the potential to help remove kidney stones and prevent the recurrence of urinary stones. Cranberries are a good source of vitamin C, which helps prevent scurvy.

Numerous Native American tribes, including the Mohawk and Inuit peoples, used cranberries both as a food source and as a medicinal plant. The fruit was used topically as a poultice to ease sore eyes, while the tea made from cranberries was employed to treat urinary tract infections. Cranberries' astringent properties were beneficial in reducing swelling and tightening and toning irritated mucosal tissue, both internally and externally, making it effective for various conditions such as infected wounds and ulcers. Additionally, tribal women used a tea made from the bark to alleviate discomfort during their menstrual cycles. Cranberry tea was also consumed by First Nation tribes to reduce swelling and discomfort in glands affected by mumps.

Modern uses: Research has shown that cranberries may be beneficial in the following areas:

Urinary Tract Infections (UTIs): Multiple studies have found that cranberry products can help prevent UTIs. A systematic review and meta-analysis published in the Journal of Urology analyzed various studies and concluded that cranberry products significantly reduce the risk of UTIs, particularly in women with recurrent UTIs (Jepson et al., 2017).

Cardiovascular Health: Studies suggest that cranberry consumption may have a positive impact on cardiovascular health. A study published in the American Journal of Clinical Nutrition found that cranberry supplementation improved blood pressure, lipid profiles, and markers of inflammation (Dohadwala et al., 2015).

Oral Health: Research has shown that cranberries may have benefits for oral health. A study published in the Journal of Periodontal Research found that cranberry juice reduced the growth of bacteria associated with gum disease (Nogueira et al., 2016).

Gastrointestinal Health: Cranberries have been studied for their potential effects on gastrointestinal conditions. A randomized controlled trial published in the World Journal of Gastroenterology demonstrated that cranberry extract improved symptoms and reduced disease activity in patients with ulcerative colitis (Vogt et al., 2014).

Dandelion

Asteraceae *(Taraxacum officinale G.H. Weber ex Wiggers)*

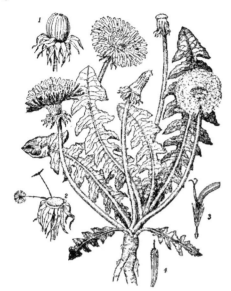

Identification: Dandelion (Taraxacum officinale) is a perennial herbaceous plant with a distinctive appearance. It typically grows to a height of about 6 to 24 inches (15 to 60 cm). The plant features a basal rosette of deeply toothed leaves that are generally hairless, with jagged edges that give them a unique shape resembling lion's teeth, hence the name "dandelion." The leaves grow directly from the base of the plant and can range in length from 2 to 10 inches (5 to 25 cm).

The dandelion produces bright yellow flowers that are composite in structure, consisting of numerous tiny florets clustered together. The flowerheads are borne on hollow stalks that rise above the basal leaves. Once the flowers have matured and been pollinated, they transform into globe-shaped seed heads known as "dandelion clocks" or "blowballs." Each seed head is composed of numerous white, fluffy parachute-like structures called pappus, which facilitate the wind dispersal of the dandelion's seeds.

The roots of the dandelion are long, thick, and taproot-like, extending deep into the ground. They are typically dark brown in color and contain a milky sap when broken.

Habitat: Common plant that can be found not only in yards but also in meadows, along trails, and in waste grounds. It is widely distributed in temperate regions around the world.

Food: The edible plant forager's best friend. Dandelion is a vitamin- and mineral-rich herb that can be enjoyed in various culinary preparations. The tender leaves can be torn into small pieces and mixed with other salad greens, along with herbs like thyme, fennel, and nasturtiums, to balance the bitterness.

The roots and leaves can be used to make a mineral-rich tea by gently simmering them. The fresh roots can also be chopped and simmered to create a stomach bitters. Early in the season, the fresh leaves can be cooked with olive oil, bacon, and lemon juice. As the season progresses, the leaves become more bitter, but pouring water on the plants before harvesting in late summer can help reduce the bitterness. Late-season bitter leaves can still be chopped and added to salads and flowers may be sprinkled over salads, rice dishes, vegetable dishes. Even if bitter, dandelion leaves can be an interesting (and healthy) addition to stir-fries, such as cooking them with tofu in oyster oil, cayenne, garlic, and beef strips.

Medicinal Part: The root.

Solvents: Boiling water, alcohol.

Effects: Diuretic, Tonic, Stomachic, Aperient, De-obstruent.

Traditional uses The Cherokee tribe used dandelion root infusions as a general tonic and digestive aid. They also applied poultices made from the leaves to soothe skin irritations and relieve joint pain. Additionally, the Cherokee and Iroquois tribes used dandelion root and leaf preparations to support healthy liver function and promote detoxification.

The Ojibwe tribe employed dandelion root infusions to treat digestive ailments, stimulate appetite, and alleviate stomach discomfort. The Mi'kmaq tribe used dandelion infusions to support urinary health and as a diuretic.

In addition to Native American tribes, dandelion has been used in traditional medicines in other parts of the world. In Traditional Chinese Medicine (TCM), dandelion is known as "Pu Gong Ying" and is used to support liver and gallbladder health, promote healthy digestion, and clear heat and toxins from the body.

In European traditional medicine, dandelion was valued as a diuretic, digestive aid, and blood cleanser. It was used to address conditions such as liver and gallbladder disorders, kidney stones, and skin problems.

Throughout history, dandelion has been regarded as a valuable herbal remedy for its potential diuretic, detoxifying, and digestive properties. It has been used to support liver health, aid digestion, promote urinary function, and address various ailments.

Modern uses: Studies have shown that dandelion extracts exhibit antioxidant properties, which can help protect against oxidative stress and reduce inflammation in the body. Some studies suggest that dandelion may have hepatoprotective effects, supporting liver health and promoting detoxification processes.

In alternative medicine, dandelion is often used as a diuretic to promote healthy kidney function and support urinary tract health. It is believed to help flush out toxins and excess fluids from the body. Some research has indicated that dandelion may have diuretic properties, although more studies are needed to confirm these effects.

Dandelion has also been investigated for its potential anti-inflammatory properties. Studies have shown that certain compounds in dandelion extracts may help reduce inflammation by inhibiting the activity of inflammatory markers in the body.

Moreover, dandelion has been traditionally used as a digestive aid and is believed to stimulate appetite, support healthy digestion, and relieve symptoms such as bloating and indigestion. Some studies have shown that dandelion may have a positive impact on digestive processes, including promoting the production of digestive enzymes and enhancing the movement of food through the digestive system.

Several studies have explored the potential cholesterol-lowering effects of dandelion. In a study published in the International Journal of Molecular Sciences, researchers found that dandelion root extract had the ability to reduce total cholesterol levels and improve lipid profiles in animals fed a high-cholesterol diet. Another study conducted on human subjects with high cholesterol levels demonstrated that dandelion leaf extract supplementation resulted in significant reductions in total cholesterol, LDL cholesterol, and triglyceride levels. Furthermore, dandelion has been studied for its potential anticancer properties. Research has shown that dandelion extracts may exhibit anti-proliferative and cytotoxic effects on various cancer cell lines, including breast, prostate, colon, and liver cancer cells. In a study published in Evidence-Based Complementary and Alternative Medicine, researchers found that dandelion root extract inhibited the growth of prostate cancer cells and induced apoptosis, a programmed cell death process.

Moreover, dandelion has shown promising results in preclinical studies regarding its potential anti-cancer effects. Researchers have observed that dandelion extracts can inhibit the growth and metastasis of cancer cells, as well as induce cell cycle arrest and apoptosis. However, further research is needed to better understand the mechanisms by which dandelion exerts its anticancer effects and to explore its potential clinical applications.

Dose: To utilize dandelion as a tincture, the recommended dosage ranges from 5 to 40 drops. For infusions, one can fill a cup with the green leaves, add boiling water, and allow it to steep for at least one hour, or even longer. The infusion should be consumed when it has cooled down, ideally three or four times a day. Another option is to add 1 teaspoon of the cut or powdered root to 1 cup of boiling water, steep it for an hour, and then drink it cold, three times a day.

Gardening tip: Having a selection of eight plants under lights or on a windowsill can indeed provide a sufficient supply of edible leaves for two people. Dandelion greens are a great addition to this selection, as they can be harvested and enjoyed year-round. By bringing the plants indoors during the winter, you can continue to have access to fresh dandelion greens even in colder climates. In southern latitudes where dandelions are available in yards throughout the year, the plant can be harvested directly from the yard for consumption. This allows for a consistent supply of dandelion greens regardless of the season.

Devil's club

Aralioideae (*Oplopanax horridus* Sm. Torr. & Gray ex Miq)

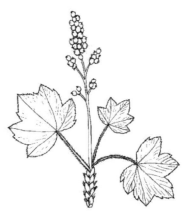

Identification: Devil's club, a member of the ginseng family, is characterized by its tall stems ranging from 6 inches to 12 feet in height, with a diameter of about an inch or less. The exterior of the stem is covered with numerous needle-sharp thorns, creating a striking and formidable appearance. One can envision it as a cane pole bristling with thousands of steel needles. As the plant grows, it maintains an upright posture until its height becomes too burdensome for the root system, causing it to bend and fall over. Along the length of the recumbent stem, new roots develop. Above the forest floor, the stem typically remains about five inches high. The wood of the plant emits a sweet aroma. The bright red berries of Devil's club are shiny and flattened in shape, adding a vibrant touch to its overall appearance.

Habitat: Primarily found in the northwest States, thriving in dark and moist old-growth forests. Due to its preferred habitat, it can be challenging to spot the plant as it blends in with the surroundings. Many people encounter devil's club for the first time while walking through such forests, unexpectedly stumbling over a recumbent stem and finding themselves immersed in a patch of the herb. This experience can be likened to falling into a scene reminiscent of a spooky movie, with its intense and eerie atmosphere resembling a thorny and foreboding blackberry patch.

Medicinal Part: The bark of the root, or even the whole stem.

Solvents: Boiling water, alcohol.

Effects: Hypoglycemic, Tonic, Hypertensive.

Traditional uses: Specific tribes known to have utilized devil's club include the Tlingit, Haida, Tsimshian, and other indigenous peoples of the Pacific Northwest. Among these tribes, devil's club was highly regarded for its medicinal properties. It was commonly used to treat a range of ailments, including arthritis, rheumatism, and other musculoskeletal conditions. The plant was often prepared as an infusion or decoction and used both internally and externally.

The Tlingit people, for example, would steep the bark and roots of devil's club to create a tea for relieving pain and inflammation associated with arthritis. Devil's club was also employed for its healing properties in treating respiratory conditions. The Tlingit and Haida tribes would make a decoction from the inner bark and roots of the plant and use it as a cough syrup or steam inhalation to alleviate symptoms of coughs, colds, and respiratory congestion.

Additionally, devil's club was revered for its spiritual significance and protective qualities. It was used in ceremonial practices, as well as for warding off negative energy and providing spiritual strength. The Tsimshian people considered devil's club to be a sacred plant and utilized it in rituals and ceremonies related to healing and protection. Moreover, the sharp thorns found on the stems and leaves of devil's club were utilized as effective hunting tools. The thorns were carefully harvested, sharpened, and attached to arrows or spears to increase their effectiveness in bringing down game. A decoction of the plat was also used as a wash to eliminate the human scent of the hunters and allow to get closer to the prey.

It is important to note that devil's club is a potent and potentially toxic plant, and its traditional uses were often carried out under the guidance and knowledge of experienced tribal healers.

Modern uses: Studies have indicated that devil's club contains various bioactive compounds with potential antimicrobial, anti-inflammatory, and antioxidant properties. For example, research has identified the presence of phenolic compounds, triterpenoids, and polysaccharides in devil's club, which are believed to contribute to its medicinal properties. In a study published in the Journal of Ethnopharmacology, devil's club extracts were found to exhibit antimicrobial activity against several strains of bacteria and fungi, including Staphylococcus aureus and Candida albicans. Another study published in the Journal of Natural Products demonstrated the anti-inflammatory effects of devil's club extracts, suggesting its potential use in inflammatory conditions.

Echinacea

Asteraceae (*Echinacea purpurea L.* Moench; *E. angustafolia* DC)

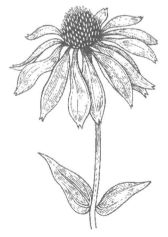

Identification: Echinacea, also known as purple coneflower, is a tall and erect perennial herb that reaches a height of approximately 3 feet. It is characterized by its large purple blossoms, which can measure up to 3 inches in diameter. The flowers are solitary and have rays that spread outwards, forming an umbrella-like or flat shape. The bracts surrounding the flowers are rigid and feature thorn-like tips. The leaves of echinacea are large and can be found in an opposite or alternate arrangement. They have smooth margins but a rough surface. When the rhizome (root) of echinacea is sliced, it reveals a yellowish center with black flecks and is covered by a thin bark-like skin.

Habitat: Echinacea can be found in various regions of the eastern and central United States, including meadows, prairies, and the fringes of fields and parks. It is also commonly cultivated in gardens across the country. In addition, echinacea is known to grow in specific states such as Arkansas, Texas, Montana, Wyoming, New Mexico, Kansas, Nebraska, and occasionally in Colorado. Its adaptability allows it to thrive in a range of environments within these regions.

Medicinal Parts: Dried rhizome, root, leaves, and flowers.

Solvent: Alcohol.

Effects: Diaphoretic, Sialagogue, Alterative.

Traditional uses: Echinacea, also known as purple coneflower, has a rich history of traditional use among Native American tribes across North America
The tribes of the Great Plains, including the Lakota, Dakota, and Pawnee, used echinacea for its immune-enhancing properties. Notably, echinacea was employed by a Lakota healer named Bear-with-White-Paw for conditions such as tonsillitis, abdominal pain, and toothaches.

It was also commonly used to treat infections, wounds, and snakebites. The Cheyenne tribe used echinacea root as a remedy for sore throat, toothaches, and coughs.

In the southern regions, the Choctaw and Creek tribes used echinacea for its antimicrobial properties. It was employed to address various infections, including those of the respiratory and urinary tracts. The Seminole tribe used echinacea as a blood purifier and for its potential to alleviate pain.

Among the Iroquois tribes, such as the Mohawk and Oneida, echinacea was used to support the immune system and treat colds, sore throats, and fevers. It was also utilized as a remedy for toothaches and mouth sores.

The Omaha, Ponca, and Osage tribes regarded echinacea as a sacred herb and used it in ceremonies to promote strength and healing. The Meskwaki and Menominee tribes used echinacea root as a treatment for rheumatism and as a general tonic.

Modern uses: In modern alternative medicine, echinacea has gained popularity for its potential health benefits. Several studies have explored its uses and efficacy. Research published in the Journal of Clinical Pharmacy and Therapeutics demonstrated the immune-stimulating effects of echinacea, supporting its traditional use as an immune system booster. Another study published in the Journal of Alternative and Complementary Medicine showed that echinacea extract reduced the severity and duration of common cold symptoms.

Echinacea has also been studied for its potential anti-inflammatory properties. A research article in the Journal of Ethnopharmacology demonstrated the inhibitory activity of echinacea against pro-inflammatory cytokines, suggesting its potential in managing inflammatory conditions.

Furthermore, research published in the Journal of Drugs in Dermatology explored echinacea's potential role in wound healing. The study found that echinacea extract promoted wound closure and increased collagen synthesis, indicating its potential use in promoting skin health.

Warning: Indeed, it is crucial to exercise caution and consult a healthcare professional before using Echinacea, especially during pregnancy. While a study involving 412 pregnant Canadian women indicated that the occurrence of malformations in babies was similar between the control group and the group that used Echinacea during pregnancy, it found that the Echinacea group had a higher incidence of spontaneous abortions. Specifically, the study reported 13 spontaneous abortions in the Echinacea group (Chow, Johns, and Mill, 2006).

Due to these findings, it is recommended that pregnant individuals consult with their physicians before using Echinacea or any other self-administered herbal therapy. It is important to note that individuals with allergies to the aster/daisy family or those with active autoimmune diseases should avoid Echinacea.

Dose and usage: I have personally used Echinacea tincture made from the flowers as a mouthwash to treat ulcers in my mouth and tongue. It has also been my go-to remedy for preventing colds and flu. Standardized commercial extracts are available in both solid and liquid forms with recommended dosages. Echinacea has shown remarkable benefits in speeding up tissue repair and healing, especially for torn ligaments and when included in healing salves.

Combining it with St. John's wort has been particularly effective in reducing scarring from surgeries and other wounds. In my experience, Echinacea tincture has been helpful in soothing and combating strep infections, specifically strep throat, by numbing the affected throat tissue and fighting the infection.

Veterinarian uses: Echinacea is utilized in pigeon racing formulas to promote health and cleanse the system after races. The vibrant flowers attract bees and butterflies, adding beauty to the surroundings. It is also incorporated in natural products designed to repair damaged nerves in horses. Herbalists often turn to Echinacea for treating acute infections in pets, recognizing its potential benefits for their well-being.

Elderberry

Caprifoliaceae *(Sambucus racemosa L.; S. cerulea Raf.; S. nigra L.; S. canadensis L.)*

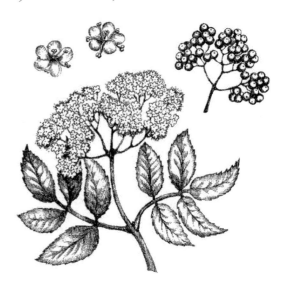

Identification: Elderberries are clump-forming shrubs with distinct characteristics. All four species have opposite pinnately compound leaves. Sambucus racemosa has five or seven leaflets per leaf, with smooth green surfaces and slightly hairy undersides. Sambucus cerulea leaves are shiny and may remain evergreen in certain regions. They are ovate or lance-shaped with pointed tips, sawtoothed edges, and a yellow-green color on top and hairy undersides. The fruits of S. racemosa are red and mature in summer, while S. cerulea bears blue fruits that also ripen in summer. Sambucus nigra, an introduced European variety, and Sambucus canadensis, the native eastern variety, are similar.

They can grow up to 25 feet in height and feature light brown to gray bark that is fissured and flaky. The branches are green with gray lenticels and can be easily broken. The compound leaves have oblong, ovate, serrated leaflets, with a matte green color on the upper surface and a light blue-green shade underneath. The white flowers form large rounded clusters, and the fruits are oval-shaped and range in color from black to deep violet.

Habitat: Elderberries are commonly found nationwide in various habitats, including woodlands, meadows, and along stream banks. They have a preference for moist, well-drained soil and can tolerate different soil types such as clay, loam, and sandy soil. Elderberry bushes thrive in regions with cool to moderate temperatures and are widespread in the eastern and central parts of the country. You can easily find it in nurseries and transplant it to your garden.

Medicinal Parts: The roots, inner bark, leaves, berries, and flowers.
Solvent: Water.

Effects: Emetic, Hydragogue, Cathartic, Diaphoretic, Diuretic, Alterative, Emollient, Discutient, Gentle Stimulant.

Food: Elderberries have a long history of culinary uses, with their deep purple-black berries being highly versatile in the kitchen. They are often used to make elderberry syrup, which can be enjoyed on its own or used as a topping for pancakes, waffles, or desserts. Elderberries can be cooked down into jams, jellies, and preserves, offering a rich and tangy flavor. They are also used to infuse beverages such as elderberry wine, cordials, and herbal teas. Elderberries can be incorporated into baked goods like pies, muffins, and cakes, providing a delightful burst of flavor. Additionally, elderflowers can be used to make elderflower cordials, syrups, and infusions, offering a delicate floral taste. I personally add it to maple syrup for a floral taste. I also make a great savory dip for wonton and other Asian culinary creations, mixing the juice with brown sugar, ginger, mustard, and soy.

Drying elderberries in a food dryer and subsequently freezing them is a great way to preserve them for culinary use during the colder months while also benefiting from their immune-boosting properties.

Traditional uses: The Cherokee tribe used elderberry as a remedy for ailments such as respiratory infections, fever, and rheumatism. They also believed that elderberry had protective properties against evil spirits. The Iroquois tribe utilized elderberry as a diuretic and a treatment for various conditions, including coughs, colds, and sore throats. They also used it as a topical treatment for wounds and inflammation. The Ojibwe tribe recognized elderberry as a powerful medicine for addressing fever, flu, and other respiratory illnesses. They also used it to alleviate pain and treat skin conditions. Additionally, many other tribes across North America incorporated elderberry into their traditional healing practices, recognizing its potential to boost the immune system and provide relief from various ailments.

Modern uses: Standardized extractions of elder flowers and berries are approved by the Commission E for treating cough, bronchitis, fevers, and colds. The recommended therapeutic dose for elder flower infusion is 1 to 3 teaspoons of dried flowers per cup of hot water. Over-the-counter elderberry extracts provide dosage instructions on the bottle. Both flower and berry extractions are commonly used to treat acute infections such as colds and flu.
Herbalist Michael Moore suggests that a tincture of elder flowers can have alterative and diaphoretic effects, stimulating the body's defense systems. Combining elderflower tinctures with mints may enhance their effectiveness and taste. Elderberries have mild laxative properties, but they also possess antidiarrheal and astringent properties. Research conducted by Erling Thom at the University of Oslo has shown that Sambucol, an over-the-counter elderberry preparation, can effectively treat and shorten flu symptoms when taken early during the episode. In Thom's study, 93 percent of the 60 patients responded positively to the treatment (Thom, E., 2002).

Dose and usage: The infusion of elder flowers is believed to have fever-reducing properties and can be used as a wash to soothe irritations. It is considered to have alterative, anti-inflammatory, and diuretic properties. The flowers and fruit of elderberry are commonly used to make tea for various purposes including treating influenza, colds, arthritis, asthma, bronchitis, improving heart function, reducing fevers, alleviating hay fever and allergies, and relieving sinusitis. The inner bark and leaves of elderberry, when taken as an expressed juice in doses of half to one fluid ounce, have reliable emetic effects. Lower doses can promote gastric secretions and fluid production. However, due to the potency of the bark, it is important to have proper knowledge and guidance before using it extensively. In general, herbal practice, the flowers and berries are more commonly used. Elderflower is particularly beneficial for upper respiratory inflammations such as colds, flu, and hay fever. Taking a tincture of elderflower (one dropperful, three times a day) can help alleviate mucous conditions in the upper respiratory tract, reduce inflammation, and promote healing. Steeping the flowers as a hot tea (using two teaspoons of fresh or dried flowers per cup of hot water) is considered a general stimulant for the body. When prepared in cold water with the same proportions, it is believed to have laxative and diuretic effects. The berries are also often used as a laxative by drinking a glass of diluted expressed juice with hot water twice a day. Elderflower and leaves are frequently used in salves to soften the skin and aid in general healing.

Warning: While elderberry is generally safe and well-tolerated by most individuals, it is important to exercise caution and be aware of potential risks. The leaves, stems, and unripe berries of the elderberry plant contain cyanogenic glycosides, which can be toxic if consumed in large quantities. Therefore, it is crucial to ensure that only ripe, cooked berries are used for consumption.
Additionally, individuals with underlying health conditions, such as autoimmune disorders or allergies, should consult with a healthcare professional before using elderberry supplements or products. It is also advisable to follow recommended dosages and guidelines provided by reputable sources, as excessive intake may lead to gastrointestinal distress or other adverse effects. Pregnant or breastfeeding women should seek medical advice before using elderberry. As with any herbal remedy, it is essential to use elderberry responsibly and consult a healthcare professional if there are any concerns or questions.

Wild Ginger

Aristolochiaceae *(Asarum canadense L.)*

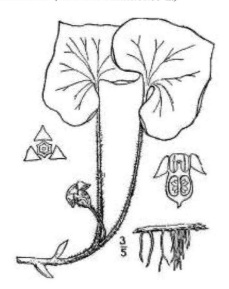

Identification: Wild ginger (*Asarum canadense*) is a low-lying colonial perennial herb with an aromatic root that emits a ginger-like scent. It features two dark-green, heart-shaped leaves, and both the stem and leaves are covered in fine hairs, giving them a hairy appearance. In May, a primitive red flower emerges beneath the leaves, typically found in Michigan. The plant grows from an adventitious rhizome and has a spreading growth habit.

Habitat: Wild ginger can be found across the entire United States, with the exception of extreme desert regions, southern California, and lower Florida. It thrives in rich soil and is commonly found in moist woods, where it serves as a ground cover in shady areas.

Food: For those adventurous in the culinary realm, an interesting experiment involves boiling the wild ginger root until tender and then simmering it in maple syrup, resulting in a unique and unconventional candy treat. The leaves of wild ginger can also be sampled for their distinct flavor. Additionally, crushed wild ginger root can be incorporated into salad dressings, adding a touch of its aromatic essence. When dried and grated, it can serve as a suitable substitute for Asian ginger in various dishes.

Medicinal Part: The root.

Solvent: Boiling water.

Effects: Stimulant, Carminative, Tonic, Diaphoretic, Diuretic.

Traditional uses: The root of wild ginger has a traditional use in treating colds and coughs, as it is believed to possess antiseptic and tonic properties. In traditional medicine, it has been included in various formulations to address conditions such as scarlet fever, nervousness, sore throat, vomiting, headaches, earaches, asthma, and convulsions. It is regarded as a versatile remedy with potential healing properties for a wide range of ailments.

Modern uses: The root of wild ginger is believed to have stimulating properties and is considered to be an appetite enhancer. Some herbalists utilize the root in tincture form, claiming that it can dilate peripheral blood vessels. However, it's important to note that the effectiveness of this use has not been substantiated by double-blind, placebo-controlled studies.

Ginseng

Araliaceae *(Panaxginseng C.A. Meyer; P. quinquefolius L.; Panax trifolius L.)*

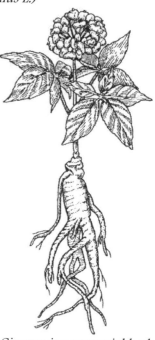

Identification: Ginseng is a perennial herb that grows up to 3 feet in height from a thick, fleshy root. It has a distinctive appearance with a short stem and a cluster of compound leaves at the top. The leaves are palmate, meaning they have multiple leaflets arranged like the fingers of a hand. The leaflets are oval or lance-shaped and have serrated edges. The stem of ginseng is smooth and typically reddish in color. In late spring or early summer, ginseng produces small clusters of greenish-white flowers. After flowering, it develops berries that turn bright red when ripe. The root of ginseng is the most prized part, often resembling the shape of a human body with branches resembling arms and legs. It has a gnarled and wrinkled appearance, with a yellowish-white color. The root has a distinct aroma and a slightly sweet, bitter taste. Ginseng is a slow-growing plant that prefers shady forest environments, typically found in cool temperate regions of Asia and North America.

Habitat: Ginseng is cultivated in various regions across the United States, from the East Coast to the West Coast. It can also be found growing wild in the Northwest and other forested areas in the eastern part of the country. However, it is considered rare in many of its former habitats. Ginseng thrives in shaded forests with a mature canopy and requires well-drained soil for optimal growth.

Medicinal Part: The dried root.

Solvent: Water.

Effects: Stimulant, Demulcent, Stomachic, Nervine, Aphrodisiac.

Traditional uses: Ginseng has a rich history of traditional uses among various indigenous cultures around the world, including the Native American tribes of the Iroquois Confederacy, Cherokee, and Ojibwe, as well as the Chinese, Korean, and Native Siberian peoples.

The Iroquois and Cherokee tribes considered ginseng to be a sacred plant with powerful healing properties. It was often used to treat ailments such as fatigue, weakness, digestive issues, and respiratory conditions. The Ojibwe tribe used ginseng as a general tonic to promote overall well-being and enhance vitality.

In traditional Chinese medicine, ginseng is considered one of the most important herbs. It is believed to strengthen the body, improve stamina, and boost the immune system. It has been used to support cognitive function, enhance physical endurance, and promote longevity. Ginseng is also known for its adaptogenic properties, helping the body adapt to stress and improve overall resilience.

In Korean traditional medicine, ginseng is used as a revitalizing herb to enhance energy, improve mental clarity, and promote overall vitality. It is often included in tonics and herbal formulations to address fatigue, boost immune function, and improve circulation.

Modern uses: Ginseng is often used by naturopaths as an adaptogen, a substance that helps the body adapt to stress and promote overall well-being. It is commonly used as an energy booster, cognitive enhancer, and immune system supporter. Several studies have demonstrated its potential in improving mental performance, reducing fatigue, and enhancing physical endurance.

One study published in the Journal of Psychopharmacology found that ginseng supplementation improved cognitive performance, particularly in tasks related to attention and working memory. Another study published in the International Journal of Sports Nutrition and Exercise Metabolism showed that ginseng supplementation enhanced exercise performance and reduced exercise-induced fatigue.

Ginseng has also been studied for its potential effects on various health conditions. Research suggests that ginseng may have a positive impact on blood sugar control, immune function, and cardiovascular health. For example, a study published in the British Journal of Clinical Pharmacology found that ginseng supplementation improved glycemic control in individuals with type 2 diabetes.

Some studies have investigated the potential anticancer properties of ginseng, with promising results. Research published in the journal Anticancer Research indicated that ginseng extracts demonstrated antitumor effects and inhibited cancer cell growth.

Dose and use: The typical recommended daily dose of ginseng root powder ranges from 1 to 2 grams. However, it is essential to refer to the specific product instructions or consult with a healthcare professional for the appropriate dosage. Ginseng can be consumed in various forms, including capsules, tablets, extracts, and teas, each with its recommended dosage. If using ginseng root in its raw form, it can be powdered for easier consumption. To powder the root, start with thoroughly dried ginseng root and break it into smaller pieces using a mortar and pestle or a sausage grinder, the root is too tough for a blender or a normal grinder. Store the powdered ginseng root in an airtight container

To prepare ginseng tea against nervous indigestion, combine 3 ounces of ginseng powder from 6-7-year-old roots with 1 ounce of honey and 60 drops of wintergreen. Blend the ingredients together. Use 1 teaspoon of the mixture for each cup of boiling water. Let it steep just below boiling point for approximately 10 minutes. Drink the tea while it is hot, preferably before each meal. Alternatively, you can steep dried ginseng leaves in hot water as you would with other types of tea.

Warning: Ginseng should not be used continuously for extended periods without breaks. Prolonged use or high doses of ginseng may lead to side effects such as headaches, insomnia, digestive disturbances, high blood pressure, and skin reactions. Ginseng may also interact with certain medications, including blood thinners, antidiabetic drugs, and immunosuppressants. Individuals with certain medical conditions, such as hormone-sensitive cancers, diabetes, cardiovascular disorders, and autoimmune diseases, should consult with a healthcare professional before using ginseng. Pregnant and breastfeeding women should also avoid ginseng due to its potential effects on hormone levels. It is advisable to seek guidance from a healthcare professional or licensed herbalist before initiating ginseng supplementation to ensure safe and appropriate use.

Gardening: Do not harvest ginseng, it's becoming all to rare in the wild. You can easily order ginseng roots online and plant them in your garden. Creating the ideal growing conditions is crucial for successfully cultivating ginseng in your garden. Ginseng thrives in shaded areas with rich, moist, and well-drained soil.
To mimic the natural environment of ginseng, consider planting it under the canopy of trees that provide shade. This not only protects the plants from direct sunlight, but also creates a favorable microclimate. Additionally, the trees contribute organic matter to the soil as their leaves fall, enriching it with nutrients.
Consistent moisture is essential for ginseng. Regular watering, particularly during dry periods, is necessary to maintain optimal soil moisture. However, it's important to avoid overwatering, as it can lead to root rot. Mulching around the ginseng plants helps retain moisture in the soil and suppresses weed growth.
Patience is key when growing ginseng. This herb is known for its slow growth, often taking several years to reach maturity.

Goldenrod

Asteraceae (Solidago canadensis L.; Solidago spp.)

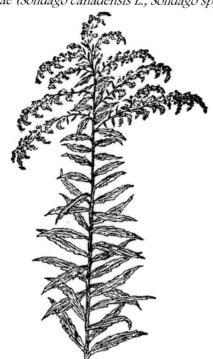

Identification: Goldenrod (Solidago spp.) is a perennial herbaceous plant belonging to the Asteraceae family. It can reach heights of up to three feet and displays clusters of bright yellow flowers with a sweet, slightly spicy fragrance. The lance-shaped leaves are serrated along the edges and may be smooth or slightly hairy. Goldenrod is widespread across North America and thrives in various habitats.

Habitat: Goldenrod is widespread across North America and thrives in various habitats, such as fields, meadows, roadsides, railroads, and vacant lots.

Medical Parts: The leaves and tops.

Solvent: Water.

Effects: Aromatic, Carminative, Stimulant, Astringent, Diaphoretic.

Food: I particularly enjoy using goldenrod blossoms in salads. The bright yellow flowers bring a subtly sweet and floral note to the dish, creating a visually appealing and flavorful ensemble.

Another practical way to incorporate goldenrod is by infusing it into beverages. You can add a few freshly plucked blossoms to a pitcher of iced tea or herbal infusions, imparting a delicate and refreshing essence to the drink.

Additionally, you can utilize goldenrod leaves as a seasoning or herbal ingredient. Finely chop the leaves and incorporate them into soups, stews, or sauces to infuse them with a distinctive herbal note and enhance the overall taste.

Traditional uses: Among the Cherokee tribe, goldenrod was highly valued for its diuretic properties, which aided in supporting kidney health and alleviating urinary tract discomfort. Infusions made from goldenrod leaves were used to address fever and respiratory ailments as well.

The Iroquois tribe recognized goldenrod as a useful remedy for digestive issues such as stomachaches and indigestion. They brewed goldenrod into teas, harnessing its soothing effects on the gastrointestinal system.

Within the Ojibwe tribe, goldenrod played a role in treating skin conditions. Poultices made from goldenrod leaves and flowers were applied topically to alleviate discomfort and promote the healing of rashes, sores, and burns.

The Navajo tribe found value in goldenrod's anti-inflammatory properties, specifically in the context of joint pain and swelling associated with arthritis. They incorporated goldenrod into salves and ointments for topical application.

Modern uses: Commission E recognized its diuretic properties, supporting kidney health and aiding in urinary tract discomfort

Beyond Commission E, modern research has further elucidated goldenrod's potential benefits. Studies have revealed its anti-inflammatory properties, suggesting its potential for managing inflammatory conditions. It has also shown antioxidant activity, which can help protect against oxidative stress and its associated health risks.

In terms of urinary health, goldenrod has been investigated for its diuretic effects and its potential in preventing urinary stone formation. These findings support its traditional use and provide a scientific basis for its modern applications.

Goldenrod has also shown promise as a natural antimicrobial agent. Research has demonstrated its inhibitory effects against various pathogenic bacteria, expanding its potential use in addressing microbial infections.

Dose and use: To prepare goldenrod tea, simply steep 1 teaspoon of goldenrod leaves in 1 cup of boiling water. This infusion can be consumed internally as a beverage.

Contrary to common belief, goldenrod is not the cause of autumn allergies; that distinction belongs to ragweed. In fact, goldenrod floral tea, made from fresh or dried flowers, is believed to have hypoallergenic properties and may help protect against allergens.

Additionally, dried goldenrod leaves and flowers can be used as a styptic to apply to wounds. This can help to stop bleeding and promote wound healing.

Other uses: A colorful garden addition (check out the 6th volume for more information). An infusion of the plant can be used as a yellow dye.

Goldenseal

Ranunculaceae (Hydrastis canadensis L.)

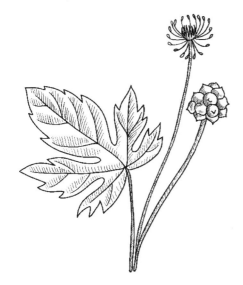

Identification: Goldenseal (Hydrastis canadensis) can be identified by its distinct characteristics. The plant features palmate, deeply lobed leaves that are glossy, dark green, and grow alternately along the stem. The stem is hairy and erect, typically reaching a height of 6-12 inches. In spring, a single white flower with three petals and numerous stamens emerges, eventually giving rise to small red fruits resembling raspberries.
The rhizome is thick, knotted, and displays a vibrant yellow-orange coloration.

Habitat: Goldenseal is native to the eastern United States and is commonly found in forested areas with wet and well-drained soil. It tends to grow in spreading colonies along banks in wooded areas. It is often found growing near ginseng plants. Goldenseal is also cultivated across the United States.

Traditional uses: Among the Cherokee tribe, goldenseal was traditionally used as a digestive aid. It was employed to support healthy digestion and address issues such as indigestion and stomachaches.

In the traditional practices of the Iroquois tribe, goldenseal was utilized for its antimicrobial properties. It was applied topically as a wash or poultice to cleanse wounds, soothe skin irritations, and promote healing.
Within the Appalachian traditions, goldenseal was considered a remedy for respiratory conditions. It was used to alleviate symptoms of respiratory infections, including sore throat and congestion.

Additionally, goldenseal has been valued by various Native American tribes for its immune-supportive properties. It was incorporated into herbal formulations to promote overall wellness and strengthen the body's natural defenses.

Chewing on dried goldenseal root was believed to be effective in treating whooping cough, and a decoction was used for relieving earaches. The root infusion, filtered through animal skin or cloth, was used as an eyewash. Additionally, goldenseal root steeped in whiskey was taken as a heart tonic. Traditional uses of goldenseal also include its application in cases of tuberculosis, scrofula, liver problems, and gall problems. Botanist Stephen Johnson has noted that the dried powdered rhizome of goldenseal acts as a hemostat and antimicrobial, promoting the formation of scabs over wounds and demonstrating beneficial effects.

Modern uses: A study published in the Journal of Ethnopharmacology in 2020 revealed the immunomodulatory effects of goldenseal extract, indicating its potential in enhancing immune function. Additionally, goldenseal's antimicrobial properties against harmful bacteria, including Helicobacter pylori, have been documented in a study published in the Journal of Medicinal Food in 2018. The herb's anti-inflammatory properties have also been investigated, with a study published in Planta Medica in 2017 highlighting its potential in managing chronic inflammation. Moreover, goldenseal has shown promise in supporting skin health, as demonstrated by research published in the journal Phytomedicine in 2016, which found its antimicrobial and wound-healing properties to be beneficial. Lastly, goldenseal extract has displayed significant inhibitory effects against respiratory pathogens, as indicated in a study published in MicrobiologyOpen in 2019, suggesting its potential in supporting respiratory wellness.

Warning: It is important to avoid taking goldenseal if you are pregnant or breastfeeding, as the plant alkaloids present in goldenseal may stimulate the uterus and there is limited data on the effects of these alkaloids on breast milk. Additionally, the extremely bitter taste of goldenseal may make it unpalatable for some individuals. At recommended dosages, goldenseal is considered non-toxic; however, consuming large doses of the active chemicals in goldenseal, such as berberine and hydrastine, can be potentially fatal. Excessive amounts of goldenseal may cause stomach discomfort, nervousness, depression, hypertension, reflex abnormalities, respiratory failure, seizures, paralysis, and even death. It is also worth noting that goldenseal may interfere with the activity of heparin, as observed with the isolated alkaloid berberine.

Dose and uses: Goldenseal indeed faces challenges in the wild due to overharvesting. It is cultivated in botanical gardens and widely grown in the United States and Canada to help protect the wild populations. While opinions on its usefulness may vary, there are other herbs that are considered safer, more effective, and more readily available for addressing similar health concerns. Some individuals prefer to rely on herbs like Echinacea, Siberian ginseng, and Astragalus for their health needs. In your personal experience, you have used a mixture of cinnamon, oregano, and goldenseal powder moistened with alcohol to treat athlete's foot by applying it to the affected areas. It's important for each person to explore and find the herbal remedies that work best for them.

Veterinarian uses: Goldenseal is included as one of the natural ingredients in Brain Cool, an herbal supplement for horses that is claimed to aid in nerve rebuilding. It is also used in various horse-related products such as training mixes, wound treatments, and fertility-enhancing formulas. These uses highlight the potential benefits and versatility of goldenseal in the context of horse health and well-being.

Gooseberry

Grossulariaceae *(Ribes cyosbati L.)*

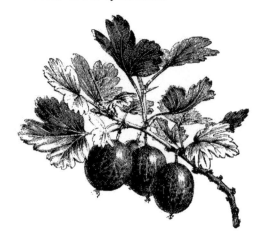

Identification: Gooseberry is a shrub that can either sprawl or grow erect, reaching a height of up to 5 feet. It has branches with spines and bears berries that can be either spiny or smooth-skinned. The leaves of the gooseberry plant are alternate, deeply cleft, and have a shape similar to that of a maple leaf. They have long hairy petioles and are divided into three to five lobes, measuring about 1 to 2.5 inches wide. The flowers of the gooseberry are pale greenish yellow or white, tubular in shape, and have a diameter of approximately 4 inches or slightly larger.

Habitat: Various species both east and west of the Mississippi River. They are typically found growing as undergrowth in forests, along forest edges, in bog fringes, and on mountain slopes. These plants have adapted to thrive in diverse habitats across their range.

Traditional uses: the Cherokee tribe of the southeastern United States valued gooseberries for their medicinal properties, utilizing them in decoctions to alleviate symptoms of diarrhea, dysentery, and sore throats. In the Great Lakes region, the Ojibwe people incorporated gooseberries into their diet and used the leaves for poultices to treat skin ailments. The Blackfoot tribe of the northern Plains region harvested the fruits and used the roots in a decoction for treating eye infections. The Navajo tribe prepared teas from gooseberry leaves and stems to address digestive issues. The Iroquois Confederacy of the northeastern United States and Canada incorporated gooseberries into their traditional dishes and applied gooseberry poultices for skin conditions.

The Kiowa Indians believed in the healing properties of gooseberries for snakebite, applying mashed berries as a poultice to draw out venom. In the Hidatsa tribe, young men used the juice of red or black currants mixed with clay as body paint for important tribal events, showcasing the cultural significance of these berries.

Modern uses: The root of currants and gooseberries has been traditionally used in decoctions or infusions for addressing uterine problems, specifically uterine prolapse. Some folk practitioners still continue to use it as an eyewash.

Gravel Root

Asteraceae *(Etrochium purpureum L. La Mont; E. maculatum L.)*

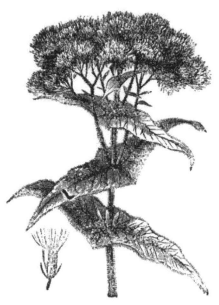

Identification: Gravel root is a perennial plant that can reach up to 5 feet in height in the northern range, and up to 10 feet in the southern states. It grows from a rhizome and has a stout stem with flower heads that form domed to flat tops. The flowers are pink to purple and have tubular-shaped disks. The leaves are lance-shaped and arranged in whorls, with up to seven leaves in each whorl. Each leaf is toothed, rough, and hairy to the touch. Another species closely related to gravel root is spotted Joe-Pye weed (*Eupatorium maculatum*). Joe Pye weed, also known as Eupatorium maculatum, is commonly found in southwest Michigan and holds historical significance in Native American healing practices. It was introduced to colonists by the Native American healer named Joe Pye, who utilized the plant to treat typhus fever caused by the Rickettsia bacteria. Interestingly, some tribes, including the Cherokees, used the hollow stems of E. maculatum as straws. This vibrant late-summer bloomer adds beauty to wildflower gardens and is a valuable addition to any natural landscape. Check it out in the sixth volume!

Habitat: Typically found in marshes, wetlands, the fringes of wetlands, seeps, and along lakesides in areas of damp ground. Its natural habitat is primarily in the eastern United States and eastern Canada. It thrives in moist environments and is well-suited to wetland areas.

Medicinal Part: The whole plant, especially the leaves.

Solvent: Boiling water.

Effects: Diuretic, Astringent.

Food: While gravel root is not edible, some American Indian tribes would use the ash of the root as a spice or a substitute for salt.

Traditional uses: Gravel root has a rich history of traditional use in various cultures. In colonial America, it was utilized to treat typhus, while Native Americans employed it as a revitalizing tonic, diuretic, and to relieve constipation. The aerial parts and roots were brewed into a medicinal tea to address infections, colds, and menstrual disorders. It was also used as a wash for infections and as a recovery tea for women after childbirth. Certain tribes, such as the Meskwakis and Cherokees, attributed additional properties to the root, considering it an aphrodisiac, a treatment for rheumatism and arthritis, and a diuretic. The root was even used as an antidote to poisoning by the Navajos. Gravel root holds a significant place in traditional medicine for its diverse range of applications.

Modern uses: Gravel root continues to be utilized by naturopaths for various therapeutic purposes. Hot infusions of the aerial parts are commonly employed to address conditions such as colds, fever, and arthritis. The plant is believed to possess antimicrobial properties and can help induce sweating, loosen phlegm, and promote coughing to facilitate the removal of mucus. Additionally, gravel root is used as a tonic to support overall well-being and as a laxative to assist in eliminating worms from the body. Its diverse range of applications highlights its potential as a natural remedy.

Warning: Not indicated for pregnant and lactating mothers

Hawthorn

Rosaceae *(Crataegus spp.: C. laevigata [Poiret] DC.; C. monogyna Jacquin Emend.; C. oxyacantha; C. douglasii Lindl; C. macrosperma Ashe)*

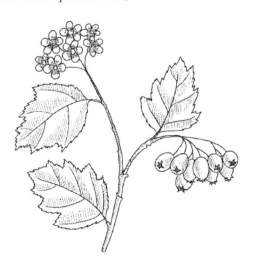

Identification: Hawthorn plants are characterized by their shrub to small tree form, reaching heights of 6 to 20 feet. They have multiple branches, often adorned with thorns. The leaves are yellow-green and glossy, typically three- to five-lobed, with lobes pointing forward and serrated edges. Hawthorn produces numerous white flowers that cluster at the ends of the branches. These flowers give way to small fruit with an apple-like appearance. The fruit can be ovoid or round, and it comes in red or black varieties, often having a mealy texture. Each fruit chamber contains a single seed.

Habitat: Hawthorn species can be found throughout the United States, spanning the country from east of the prairie. They typically thrive in damp woods and the fringes of forests. While they prefer some exposure to sunlight, they can adapt to varying light conditions.

Food: The fruit of hawthorn can be consumed by eating it directly, although it has a mealy texture and contains seeds. Despite this, its benefits for heart health make it worthwhile. The fruit can also be sliced, dried, and used to make a healthful drink by decocting or infusing it in water. It pairs well with green tea and can be gathered in August.

To prepare the berries, they are briefly immersed in boiling water, then cut in half, seeds removed, and dried using a food dryer. The dried berries can be added to hot cereals, used in tea, or incorporated into various recipes to add flavor and nutritional value.

Traditional uses: Hawthorn has been widely recognized for its therapeutic effects on heart conditions in both Europe and China. It contains bioflavonoids that improve blood circulation to the heart, brain, and extremities, as well as enhance coronary blood flow. It is also known to have hypotensive properties, helping to lower blood pressure. In Native American traditional medicine, hawthorn leaves were chewed and applied as a poultice to wounds and sores. The shoots were used to make an infusion for treating children's diarrhea, and the thorns were utilized as a counterirritant for arthritis. The Okanagan-Colville Nation even used the thorns in a unique practice similar to moxibustion in Chinese acupuncture, burning them close to the skin for heightened effects. Mouth sores were treated with a decoction of new shoots. These are just a few examples of the various uses of hawthorn in indigenous cultures, as documented in Moerman's Native American Ethnobotany.

Beyond its physical benefits, hawthorn has a rich history of being associated with emotional well-being. Celtic beliefs associated hawthorn with healing a broken heart, while ancient Greek wedding processions used hawthorn branches as symbols of hope. In the 1930s, Dr. Edward Bach developed flower essences, including hawthorn flower essence, to address emotional imbalances. Hawthorn flowers were specifically indicated for emotions related to the heart.

Modern uses: Hawthorn, particularly C. laevigata, has been extensively studied for its effects on cardiac and vascular function. It is believed to improve and protect the heart by dilating coronary blood vessels and promoting heart muscle regeneration.

The extract of hawthorn has shown potential antiangina effects and may benefit individuals with Buerger's disease, a condition characterized by arterial spasm. It is also used to treat tachycardia (rapid heartbeat) and is considered cholesterol-lowering and hypotensive.

The anthocyanidins and proanthocyanidin components of hawthorn are believed to work synergistically with vitamin C. European studies have shown that the standardized extract can improve exercise tolerance in patients with heart conditions. Other research suggests that the extract may alleviate leg pain caused by partially blocked coronary arteries.

In traditional Chinese medicine, dried hawthorn fruit is decocted and used to treat irritable bowel and gallbladder problems. The fruit is also considered antibacterial against certain strains of Shigella, a bacteria that causes dysentery. A decoction of dried fruit is used as an antidiarrheal and to help with dyspepsia.

A study conducted by Dr. Ann Walker at the University of Reading in the UK, published in the British Journal of General Practice, demonstrated that hawthorn extract can lower blood pressure in individuals with diabetes. The study found a significant reduction in diastolic blood pressure in patients taking hawthorn, with no observed interactions between the herb and other medications. Dr. Walker concluded that the blood pressure-lowering effect of hawthorn was real based on the study findings. It is important to note that hawthorn is not recommended during pregnancy and lactation. However, proanthocyanidins, a component of hawthorn, have been shown to be non-mutagenic in tests for carcinogenicity. Safety with berry extracts is well-established.

Dose and uses: In addition to hawthorn, garlic, ginger, ginkgo biloba extract, and cayenne are herbs known for their circulation-stimulating properties. Each of these herbs has unique bioactive compounds that contribute to their cardiovascular benefits. Garlic contains allicin, which promotes vasodilation and improves blood flow. Ginger has gingerol and other compounds that help relax blood vessels and reduce inflammation. Ginkgo biloba extract contains flavonoids and terpenoids that improve blood circulation and protect against oxidative damage. Cayenne contains capsaicin, which stimulates circulation and has a warming effect. Making a tea with the flower buds and new-growth leaves of these herbs in the spring can be a beneficial way to extract their active compounds. Hot water infusion can extract the bioflavonoids and other beneficial constituents that contribute to their hypotensive (blood pressure-lowering) and anti-angina effects.

Heal~all
Lamiaceae *(Prunella vulgaris L.)*

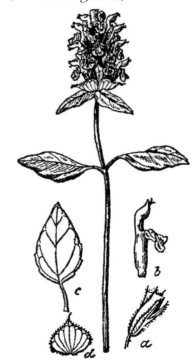

Identification: Heal all, also known as self-heal, is a perennial herb that usually reaches a height of 6 to 10 inches. It has a square stem that is erect when young but may later fall and creep along the ground. The leaves of heal all are ovate to lance-shaped, with toothed or sometimes entire margins, and they grow opposite each other on the stem. The flowers of heal all are clustered in a whorl at the end of the square stem and are typically blue to violet in color.

Habitat: Heal all can be found nationwide in various habitats such as waste grounds, lawns, edges of fields, margins of woods, and wetlands. It is a versatile plant that can thrive in diverse environments across the country.

Food Among the Cherokee tribe, heal-all was highly regarded for its culinary versatility. The leaves and flowers of heal-all were commonly used in salads and as a flavoring ingredient in soups and stews. The herb's mild, slightly minty flavor added a unique taste to dishes, enhancing their overall appeal.
Various First Nations across North America used the heal-all for a minty-tasting beverage that was quite com

The culinary uses of heal-all in Cherokee tradition and among the First Nations highlight the deep connection between food, culture, and well-being. The incorporation of this herb in traditional dishes not only added flavor and depth but also reflected a holistic approach to nourishment. Today, heal-all continues to be appreciated for its culinary value, both among Native American communities and in contemporary cuisine.

Please note that while heal-all has a long history of traditional use, it's essential to consult with a knowledgeable source or herbalist before incorporating it into your own culinary practices.

Traditional uses: Native American tribes, such as the Cherokee, utilized Heal-All as a tea infusion to treat fevers, sore throats, and mouth sores. They also applied it topically as a poultice for wounds and skin irritations. Among the Iroquois tribe, Heal-All was used in tea form to address digestive issues and respiratory conditions. The Chippewa tribe employed Heal-All as an infusion for headaches, fevers, and sore throats, while the Menominee tribe used it to alleviate stomachaches and promote overall healing. In Traditional Chinese Medicine (TCM), Heal-All, known as "Xia Ku Cao," is used to clear heat, cool the blood, and resolve toxicity, benefiting conditions such as sore throat, abscesses, and inflammation. European folk medicine also recognizes Heal-All for its use in respiratory ailments, digestive disorders, and skin irritations.

Modern uses: Research has shown that Heal-All possesses anti-inflammatory, antioxidant, antimicrobial, and antiviral properties. A study published in the Journal of Ethnopharmacology demonstrated that extracts of Heal-All exhibited strong antibacterial activity against various strains of bacteria, including those resistant to conventional antibiotics. Another study published in Phytomedicine found that Heal-All extracts showed antiviral activity against herpes simplex virus type 1 (HSV-1).

In alternative medicine, Heal-All is commonly used as a natural remedy for various conditions. It is believed to support the immune system, improve digestion, and promote overall wellness. Some practitioners utilize Heal-All as a topical treatment for skin conditions such as wounds, cuts, and eczema due to its potential wound healing and anti-inflammatory effects. It is also used as a herbal tea or tincture for respiratory ailments, sore throats, and digestive complaints.

Dose and uses: Just like the name says, it's a cure all!
To make a decoction, take 1 to 2 teaspoons of dried heal all herb and add it to 1 cup of water in a small saucepan. Boil, lower the heat and let it simmer for about 10-15 minutes. Strain the liquid and consume while warm. Take up to three times a day.
To make a heal all tincture, I recommend a 1:5 ratio of herbs to alcohol at 96%.
A heal all tincture may be used to support immune function. It can also be used topically on minor skin irritations, rashes, or insect bites to help reduce inflammation and promote healing. Some herbalists suggest that heal all tincture may aid in digestive issues such as indigestion, bloating, or stomach discomfort
Heal all decoction may be used as a mouth rinse or gargle to promote oral health. It is thought to have antimicrobial properties and can be used for minor mouth irritations or as a general mouthwash.
Furthermore, it may be used as a wash or compress for certain skin conditions, such as eczema, acne, or skin inflammation.

Honeysuckle
Caprifoliaceae *(Lonicera japonica Thunb)*

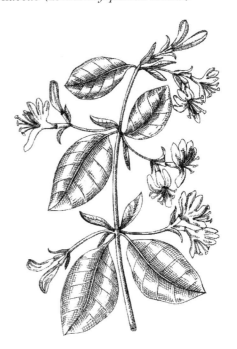

Identification: Honeysuckle encompasses numerous species of shrub-like or climbing vines. These plants bear elegant trumpet-like flowers in white or off-white, while certain species may have red flowers. The leaves are green and smooth, typically oblong and around 2 inches in length. The fruit of honeysuckle is a black spherical berry.

Habitat: Commonly found in the fringes of woods and have a tendency to be invasive along trails and edges of streams. They prefer to grow alongside woods rather than in open areas. In some cases, they can colonize and become dominant invasive species in areas of development or waste ground.

Traditional uses: Native Americans utilized various species of honeysuckle, including Lonicera dioica and Lonicera canadensis, for their medicinal properties. The floral tea derived from these species was used to treat conditions such as dysentery, acute infections like flu and colds, laryngitis, and enteritis. The tea was believed to have antimicrobial properties. Additionally, the tea was applied externally as a wash for edema, boils, scabies, and breast cancer. First Peoples also considered honeysuckle as a blood purifier. The traditional use of bark infusion suggests its potential in treating syphilis, gonorrhea, and urinary infections due to its antimicrobial properties.

Modern uses: Flower extracts of honeysuckle have been suggested to have potential cholesterol-lowering effects. Chemical extracts derived from the leaves have shown anti-platelet-aggregating properties, which could potentially help in preventing strokes, although further research is needed to establish conclusive evidence. Additionally, saponins found in the plant are known for their anti-inflammatory properties. However, it's important to note that more studies are required to fully understand and validate these potential health benefits of honeysuckle.

Hops
Cannabaceae *(Humulus lupulus L.)*

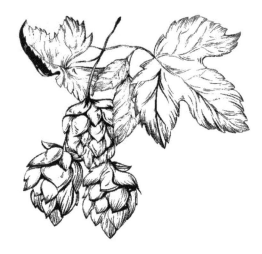

Identification: Hops are perennial climbing plants that belong to the Cannabaceae family. They have distinct features that aid in their identification. Hops typically have robust, twining stems that can reach impressive heights, often climbing up to 20 feet or more. The stems are covered in rough, textured bark and bear pairs of serrated leaves with three to five lobes. The leaves are deep green in color and have a rough texture.

The female flowers, known as cones or strobiles, which are the primary component used in brewing beer, are green and cone-shaped, consisting of papery bracts that enclose the small yellow lupulin glands responsible for the characteristic aroma and bitterness in beer. The cones emit a pleasant, distinct aroma when crushed.

Hops are dioecious plants, meaning they have separate male and female plants. The female plants produce the valuable cones used in brewing, while the male plants produce clusters of small, yellowish flowers. It is primarily the female plants that are cultivated for commercial use.

Habitat: Hops can be found in various habitats such as marshes, meadows, and edges of woods. While it is known to escape from cultivation, cultivated stands of hops are specifically found in northeastern Washington State, the Okanagan region of Washington and Canada, and northern Idaho.

Medicinal Parts: The strobiles or cones.

Solvents: Boiling water, dilute alcohol.

Effects: Tonic, Diuretic, Nervine, Anodyne, Hypnotic, Anthelmintic, Sedative, Febrifuge.

Traditional uses: Indeed, hops have been traditionally used for their calming and sedative properties. Pioneers would often place hops in pillows to promote better sleep and relaxation. Native Americans used it in a water extraction or infusion of hops has been used as a tea to help induce a sense of calm and relaxation. The aromatic compounds found in hops are believed to have mild sedative effects and can be beneficial for those seeking a natural sleep aid.

Modern uses: Hops have been approved by the German Commission E for treating nervousness and insomnia. Research has shown that the flavonoids found in hops exhibit antibacterial, antifungal, and antitumor properties. Hops are known to have diuretic effects and are commonly used in herbal teas to promote relaxation and induce sleep.
Studies have examined the use of hops in combination with other herbs like valerian, balm, and motherwort to improve sleep, particularly in individuals with alcohol-related sleep issues. Ongoing research, including studies conducted by the University of Chicago, is investigating the efficacy of hops as a sleep aid.
While early studies suggested a potential estrogenic effect of hop flower tea, subsequent research has yielded inconsistent results.

Warning: Contact with hops and its pollen has caused allergic reactions, in particular dermatitis upon contact.

Dose and uses: For a sleep aid, you can make a tea by adding about 1 teaspoon of dried hops flowers to a 6-ounce cup of hot water, allowing it to steep and cool before drinking.
To prepare a hot bath with hops, start by gathering a generous handful of dried hops flowers. Place the hops in a large muslin bag or a clean cloth and secure it tightly. Fill your bathtub with hot water and immerse the bag of hops in the bathwater. Allow the hops to steep in the water for at least 15 minutes, releasing their aromatic properties. You can also add a few drops of essential oils, such as lavender or chamomile, for a more relaxing experience. Soak in the bath for about 20-30 minutes, enjoying the soothing and calming effects of the hops-infused water. In a sweat lodge ceremony, hops can be used to create a fragrant steam. Start by heating up volcanic rocks in a fire outside the sweat lodge until they are red-hot. Carefully transfer the hot rocks into a pit or container inside the lodge. Sprinkle a handful of dried hops flowers onto the hot rocks. As the hops come into contact with the hot rocks, they will release their aromatic compounds, creating a pleasant and soothing scent. The steam generated from the hops-infused rocks will enhance the overall experience of the sweat lodge ceremony, promoting relaxation and a sense of well-being.

Additionally, hops can be used to enhance the flavor of cheap, watery beer. Simply add two hops into the open can or bottle and enjoy the improved taste.

Veterinarian warning: It is important to note that hops can be toxic to dogs, and ingestion of hops can be dangerous for them. Dogs have been known to experience serious health issues, including death, within a short period of time after consuming hops. Therefore, it is crucial to keep hops away from pets and to prevent them from accessing beer or any other products containing hops. If you suspect that your dog has ingested hops or is experiencing any symptoms of toxicity, it is recommended to seek immediate veterinary care.

Horsetail
Equisetaceae *(Equisetum hyemale L.; E. arvense L.)*

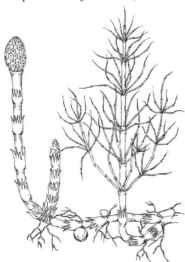

Identification: Horsetail (*Equisetum arvense*) is a perennial plant that can be easily identified by its unique appearance. It has hollow, jointed stems that resemble the tail of a horse, hence the name "horsetail." The stems are segmented and have a rough texture, resembling the texture of a pinecone or a bottle brush. The plant can grow up to 2 feet in height and has no true leaves. Instead, it produces thin, scale-like structures called "microphylls" that are fused together to form a sheath around the stem joints. At the tip of the stem, horsetail produces a cone-like structure that contains spores for reproduction.
The stems of horsetail are typically green and may have a slight brownish tint. They are erect and stand tall, with a distinctively vertical growth pattern. The plant spreads through an underground rhizome system, forming dense colonies in wet or marshy areas.
When touched, the stems of horsetail can feel rough and abrasive due to the presence of silica. This silica content gives horsetail a gritty texture, making it useful for polishing or scrubbing surfaces.

Habitat: Horsetail can be found nationwide in various habitats such as marshes, fens, bogs, streams, lakes, and rivers. It has a wide distribution across different regions in the United States.

Medicinal Parts: The leaves and root.

Solvent: Water.

Effects: Anodyne, demulcent, astringent.

Traditional uses: The Apache tribe used horsetail as a poultice to treat wounds, burns, and sores. The Chippewa tribe brewed horsetail tea to alleviate bladder and kidney ailments, as well as urinary tract infections. The Comanche tribe used horsetail to make an infusion for treating venereal diseases. The Creek tribe applied horsetail poultices to reduce swelling and inflammation. Among the Mexicans, traditional uses of horsetail include making infusions or decoctions for the treatment of kidney stones, urinary tract infections, and digestive issues. It has also been used externally as a wash for skin conditions and to promote wound healing.

Modern uses: Horsetail has been approved by Commission E for its external use in healing wounds and burns, as well as its internal use for treating urinary tract infections, kidney stones, and bladder stones. This regulatory approval acknowledges the effectiveness and safety of horsetail for these specific applications. Consequently, horsetail products can be found over the counter in various forms, including teas, capsules, and extracts.

Warning: Caution should be exercised when using horsetail, as an overdose of the herb may have toxic effects. It is important to use horsetail under the guidance and supervision of a knowledgeable holistic healthcare professional who can provide appropriate dosage instructions and monitor its usage.

Gardening: Horsetail is a fast-spreading plant that can thrive in various growing conditions, including both shade and sun. It can add an interesting touch to flower arrangements, although it tends to spread and wander through the garden.

Other uses: One unique use of horsetail stems is their high silica content, which makes them useful for cleaning pots and pans, particularly when camping. The abrasive quality of the stems can help remove stubborn residue from cookware.

Veterinarian uses and warnings: Horsetail ingestion by grazing animals has been associated with adverse effects such as weight loss, weakness, ataxia, and fever. However, the Meskwaki people reportedly fed horsetail to wild geese to make them gain weight within a few weeks.

Juniper

Cupressaceae *(Juniperus communis L.; Juniperus osteosperma [Torr.] Little)*

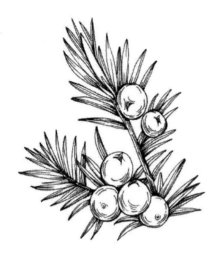

Identification: Juniper (*Juniperus spp.*) is a coniferous evergreen shrub or tree that belongs to the cypress family (*Cupressaceae*). It is characterized by its unique foliage, berry-like cones, and distinct aroma. Here is a description for identification:

Juniper typically grows as a dense, bushy shrub or a small to medium-sized tree, depending on the species. It has a conical or columnar shape with a straight trunk.

The leaves are needle-like, arranged in whorls of three, and have a sharp, pointed tip. They are usually dark green or bluish-green in color and may have a waxy coating, giving them a glossy appearance.

One of the most distinctive features of juniper is its cones, often referred to as "berries." These cones are actually modified scales that resemble small, fleshy berries. They start out as green and mature to a bluish-purple or black color. The cones are usually round or oval-shaped, and each contains one to three seeds.

In addition to its appearance, juniper is also known for its aromatic fragrance. When the foliage or cones are crushed, they release a strong, resinous scent that is often described as woody, spicy, or reminiscent of pine.

Habitat: Juniperus communis is found nationwide, spanning across various regions in the United States. Juniperus osteosperma, commonly known as Utah juniper, is primarily found in dry montane areas of the southwestern United States, including parts of Utah and Wyoming.

Medicinal Part: The ripe dry berries.

Solvents: Boiling water, alcohol.

Effects: Diuretic, Stimulant, Carminative.

Food: Juniper berries are commonly used in cooking to flavor a variety of dishes. They can be dried and cooked with game, fowl, lamb, goat, venison, duck, and turkey, adding a distinctive taste to the dishes. Juniper berries can also be ground using a pepper mill and used as a seasoning in bean soups, stews, and marinades. Additionally, they can be infused in hot water to make a tea. In the realm of beverages, juniper berries are often used to flavor gin, vodka, schnapps, and aquavit. It is important to use juniper berries in moderation, as consuming large amounts can be toxic, similar to excessive consumption of salt or pepper.

Traditional uses: The essential oil of juniper berries is sometimes diluted and applied topically to cleanse and purify the deeper layers of the skin. In traditional medicine, juniper berries have been used to stimulate menstruation and alleviate symptoms of premenstrual syndrome (PMS) and painful menstruation (dysmenorrhea). A traditional preparation involves boiling 1 teaspoon of berries in 1 cup of water for 3 minutes and allowing it to steep until cool. Some practitioners may also include juniper bark and needles in the tea. Juniper berries are believed to have antiseptic properties and can act as a diuretic, tonic, and digestive aid. They are particularly known for their strong antiseptic effects on urinary tract problems and gallbladder issues, although they should be avoided by individuals with kidney disease.

Modern uses: The essential oil of juniper berries has been recognized by Commission E for its use in treating dyspepsia (indigestion). A very small amount of the essential oil, one tenth of a milliliter, is typically used for this purpose. The diuretic properties of juniper berries extend to its extract, known as Odrinil, which also acts as a diuretic. Juniper berries have been suggested for the treatment of heart disease, high blood pressure, and edema (dropsy). In Europe, the berry extract is used to alleviate symptoms of arthritis and gout. Animal studies have shown that combinations of juniper berry extract with other substances have exhibited anti-inflammatory and anticancer activity, although these effects have not been proven in humans. Juniper berry extract has also been found to reduce blood sugar levels in diabetic rats. In a human trial, a combination of juniper oil and wintergreen oil (specifically Kneipp's Rheumabad) added to bath water was shown to reduce pain. Mice trials have suggested that the pharmaceutical dosage of juniper berry extract has anti-inflammatory properties. Juniper oil has been used as a diuretic and may have potential as an adjunct therapy for diabetes.

Dose: To prepare an infusion of juniper berries, typically several tablespoonfuls of the berries are softened by soaking (macerating) and then added to 1 pint of boiling water. The mixture is left to steep for 1 hour or more. Drink the infusion cold four times a day in the morning, noon, afternoon, and evening. The recommended dose of the tincture is 10-30 drops.

Warning: Juniper berries should be used with caution, as they may cause adverse reactions in some individuals. It is important to note that excessive consumption of juniper berries can lead to digestive upset, kidney irritation, and even kidney damage. Pregnant women and individuals with kidney or liver diseases should avoid the use of juniper berries altogether. If you experience any negative symptoms after using juniper berries, it is recommended to discontinue use and consult with a healthcare professional.

Gardening: Juniper can be easily transplanted to your garden, and the wild varieties, particularly the western ones, offer a bountiful supply of fruit. They can be a valuable addition to your garden and provide an abundance of berries for various uses.

Lady's Slipper

Cypripedioideae *(Cypripedium acaule Aiton)*

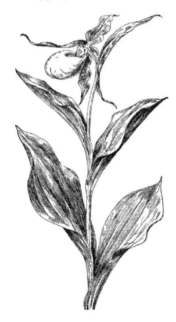

Identification: Lady's slipper is a perennial plant characterized by lily-like leaves that grow from a horizontal rhizome.
The leaves are stalkless, broad lance-shaped, and can reach up to 10 inches in length. They have a bright green color on the upper side and a pale shade underneath. The plant produces unique slipper-shaped flowers that resemble orchids. The flowers are typically pink, although white varieties are rare. Lady's slipper develops fruit capsules that turn brown as they mature.

Habitat: Northern United States and Canada. Upland pine forests, wet blackspruce sites. Occasionally open wetlands. More prolific in the northeastern states and southern Ontario. Grows along the north shore of Lake Superior. However, due to its habitat shrinking and over-harvesting is an endangered species and should not under any under circumstance be harvested in the wild.

Medicinal Part: The root.

Solvents: Boiling water, diluted alcohol.

Effects: Antiperiodic, Nervine, Tonic.

Traditional uses: Lady's slipper, specifically the horizontal rhizome, has been traditionally used for its medicinal properties. It is known for its styptic and astringent qualities. Native Americans regarded it as a versatile remedy for various ailments, including nervousness, colds, cramps, diabetes, flu, hysteria, menstrual problems, spasms, and inflammations. The rhizome was prepared as a decoction or tincture, and it was also used topically as a poultice. The harvest of the rhizome typically occurs in autumn, and it can be used either fresh or dried. In the past, the unique shape of the flower led to its association with aphrodisiac properties, following the belief of the Doctrine of Signatures. However, it's important to note that overharvesting of lady's slipper in the wild has led to its decline, and it is now protected in many areas.

Modern uses: Lady's slipper, due to its overharvesting and protected status, is no longer legally used. While its chemical constituents have not been extensively studied, it has been traditionally used to treat anxiety and insomnia. However, it's important to note that without proper scientific research and regulation, the safety and effectiveness of using lady's slipper for these purposes cannot be guaranteed.

Warning: Contact with pink lady's slipper may cause contact dermatitis.

Tips: Lake Superior Provincial Park is known for its beautiful display of pink lady's slippers during Memorial Day weekend. These stunning flowers adorn the park, creating a vibrant and captivating sight. It's a great opportunity to explore the park's natural beauty, and kayaking is a popular activity in the area.
However, it's important to note that lady's slipper species, including pink lady's slipper, are protected and should not be harvested illegally. It's best to appreciate these flowers in their natural habitat and refrain from picking or disturbing them.
Unfortunately, lady's slippers are difficult to relocate because of a complex symbiosis with soil fungi. Bees, moths, butterflies, gnats, and mosquitoes pollinate the orchids.

Lemon balm

Lamiaceae *(Melissa officinalis L.)*

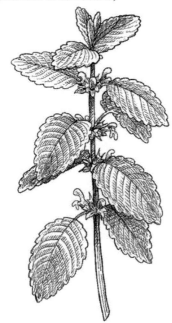

Identification: Lemon balm, also known as balm melissa, is a perennial herb with a pleasant lemon fragrance. It grows to a height of around 3 feet and produces small white flowers in clusters arranged in one-sided false whorls. The flowers have a tube-like corolla with two-lipped petals. The plant has square stems that can be hairy or hairless, and the leaves are oval to rhomboid-shaped, measuring about 3 inches in length. The leaves are abundant and emit a lemon scent when touched. Lemon balm blooms during the summer season, and its seeds are nut brown in color.

Habitat: Lemon balm is a popular garden plant that has a tendency to spread from garden to garden. It can escape cultivation and establish itself in roadsides and waste ground areas. It is widely available at garden stores and is considered a valuable addition to any herb garden. Its pleasant lemon fragrance and versatile uses make it worth growing and having in your garden.

Medicinal Part: The aerial parts.

Solvents: Boiling water, alcohol.

Effects: carminative, sedative, diaphoretic, febrifuge, antidepressant, mild analgesic, antispasmodic.

Food: Lemon balm is a versatile herb with various culinary uses. Its lemony and minty flavor profile adds a refreshing and citrusy twist to many dishes and beverages. Lemon balm leaves can be used fresh or dried, and they can be added to salads, soups, sauces, marinades, and desserts. They can also be steeped in hot water to make a soothing herbal tea. Lemon balm is often used as a flavoring agent in ice creams, sorbets, and herbal liqueurs. Its bright and aromatic qualities make it a popular choice for enhancing the flavor of fish, poultry, and vegetable dishes. Additionally, lemon balm leaves can be used to infuse oils, vinegars, and syrups, which can then be used in various culinary creations.

Traditional uses: Lemon balm has a rich history of traditional uses across various cultures. Native American tribes such as the Cherokee, Iroquois, and Mohegan utilized lemon balm for its medicinal properties. It was used to treat digestive issues, calm nerves, and promote relaxation. Lemon balm leaves were brewed into teas or made into poultices to alleviate discomfort from insect bites and skin irritations. In traditional European medicine, lemon balm was used for its calming and sedative effects, as well as to address digestive ailments. It was also employed as a topical remedy for cold sores and other viral skin infections. In Ayurvedic medicine, lemon balm was valued for its ability to balance the nervous system, improve cognitive function, and support overall well-being. Lemon balm continues to be cherished in herbal medicine traditions worldwide for its calming properties, digestive support, and as an ingredient in soothing teas and preparations for relaxation and sleep.

In Traditional Chinese Medicine (TCM), lemon balm, known as "Melissa" in Chinese, has been used for centuries. It is considered a cooling herb and is often used to address conditions related to excess heat and inflammation in the body. Lemon balm is believed to have a calming effect on the heart and spirit, making it useful for conditions such as restlessness, anxiety, and insomnia. In TCM, it is also used to soothe the digestive system, promote healthy liver function, and alleviate symptoms of indigestion and bloating. Lemon balm is often incorporated into herbal formulas and teas in TCM to balance and harmonize the body's energy. Its pleasant lemony aroma and taste make it a popular choice in both culinary and medicinal preparations in TCM.

Modern uses: A study published in the Journal of Psychopharmacology found that lemon balm extract significantly improved mood and cognitive performance in a group of healthy young adults. Another study published in the Journal of Ethnopharmacology demonstrated the anxiolytic and sedative effects of lemon balm, suggesting its potential as a natural remedy for anxiety and sleep disorders.

In addition, Commission E has approved the internal use of lemon balm leaves for nervous disorders, such as restlessness and sleep disturbances. Commission E also recognizes the topical use of lemon balm for cold sores (herpes labialis). Lemon balm is known to possess antiviral properties and may help in reducing the frequency and duration of cold sore outbreaks.

Furthermore, lemon balm has been studied for its potential role in supporting cognitive function. Research has shown that lemon balm may enhance cognitive performance, improve memory and attention, and have a positive impact on age-related cognitive decline.

Dose and uses: Make a cold infusion with lemon balm and other mints is particularly delightful. Simply fill a jar with various mint leaves and lemon balm leaves, add some thyme leaves and a couple of lemon slices, and refrigerate overnight. This infusion, especially with the addition of thyme leaves, is a great herbal remedy for mountain sickness.

Warning: While lemon balm is generally considered safe for most people when used appropriately, there are a few precautions to keep in mind.

Firstly, lemon balm may cause drowsiness or sedation, especially when used in higher doses or in combination with other medications or substances that have a similar effect. It's important to avoid activities that require alertness, such as driving or operating heavy machinery, if you experience excessive drowsiness after consuming lemon balm.

Secondly, individuals with thyroid conditions should use lemon balm with caution. Lemon balm has been found to have a mild effect on thyroid hormone levels, and it may interfere with thyroid medications or treatments. If you have a thyroid disorder, it's advisable to consult with your healthcare provider before using lemon balm.

Lastly, lemon balm may interact with certain medications, including sedatives, thyroid medications, and antiviral drugs. If you are taking any medications, it's important to speak with your healthcare provider to ensure there are no potential interactions.

Wild American Licorice

Fabaceae *(Glycyrrhiza lepidota [Nutt.] Pursh)*

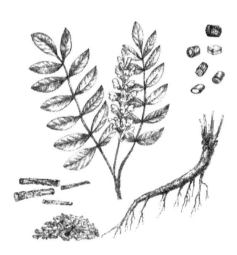

Identification: Member of the pea family with clusters of pealike flowers and compound pealike leaves. Grows in large colonies formed and connected by creeping rootstalks, which allows them to reach 5" in length. The leaves are made up of many smaller leaves along the leaf stalk (typical pea family) and are odd numbered, eleven to seventeen in number, with a single leaf at the tip. The plant stands one-and-a-half feet to three feet in height and has white to yellow-green, cloverlike blossoms. The seed pods of the plant are numerous and are a dark rusty brown and are burred, sticking easily to clothing. The burr-covered seed pods make this plant easily identifiable. The roots are the medicinal part of the plant and they are easy to harvest, growing fairly shallowly beneath the soil.

Habitat: Grows in moist, sandy soils along rivers and sunny stream banks. Ranges over the entire West and prairie states, with some extension into the East, but not Southeast. The plant likes to grow along irrigation ditches and slow-moving streams from 1,000 to 9,000 feet. It is often quite prolific when found, so harvesting an adequate supply of roots is not often a problem.

The tap roots as opposed to the runners are stronger and if you wish to spend time attacking the tough ground in which licorice grows, they may be the preferable harvest.

Taste: The American licorice is not sweet as is the European licorice. It tastes much more "pea-like." One of the benefits of the sweet variety of licorice is to make the rather strong taste of most herbal potions more palatable.

Medicinal Part: The dried root.

Solvent: Water, sparingly in alcohol.

Effects: Demulcent, Expectorant, Laxative, Pectoral.

Food: Warriors and hunters chewed the root as a sialagogue (produces saliva) to increase running endurance.

Traditional uses: The Cheyenne tribe used the dried, peeled roots of licorice to make a medicinal tea for the treatment of diarrhea and upset stomach. The Lakota tribe used the root as a medicine for flu, while the Dakota tribe made a topical medicine for earache by steeping licorice leaves in boiling water. The roots of the licorice plant were also chewed and held in the mouth to relieve toothache. The Blackfoot tribe prepared a tea from the roots to treat coughs, sore throat, and chest pain, and they also considered it to have antirheumatic properties and applied the foliage and wet, smashed roots to swollen joints. The Dakota tribe used an infusion of the leaves to treat earache.

Modern uses: Used as a flavoring agent and to sweeten tobacco. Holistic health practitioners use the herb in the same way as Asian licorice (Glycyrriza glabra) for ulcers, boosting the immune system, improving mental function, and stress reduction (no double-blind, placebo-controlled crossover studies have been done on wild licorice, G. lepidota, as of this writing).

Dose and usage: 1 lb. of Licorice root boiled in 3 pints of water, reduced by boiling to 1 quart, is an all-purpose decoction; a teaspoonful three times a day.

1 teaspoonful of the dried root to 1 cup of boiling water can be taken as an herbal tea, made fresh daily.

The root chewed raises the blood pressure in a matter of minutes.

Equal parts of tinctures of red root, echinacea, and licorice are used as an herbal flu shot of sorts. One dropperful of this mixture should be taken each hour at the onset of symptoms: it must be taken each hour to be effective.

Warning: Go gently, my friend. Glycyrrhizin in root raises blood pressure.

Lobelia

Campanulaceae *(Lobelia siphilitica L.; Lobelia cardinalis L.)*

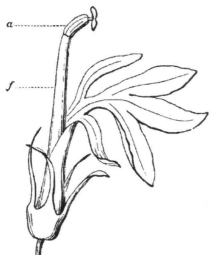

Identification: *L. siphilitica* is a perennial plant that grows to a height of 3 to 4 inches. It has oval-shaped leaves. The flowers are distinctive and birdlike, typically appearing in shades of blue to blue lavender, with a white-striped throat in the corolla. It should be noted that *L. cardinalis*, also known as cardinal flower, has similar birdlike features but is red in color and not as widely distributed as *L. siphilitica*.

Habitat: Lobelia plants thrive in moist to wet environments such as marshes, bogs, damp meadows, and along streams. They prefer partial shade or filtered sunlight and nutrient-rich, well-draining soil. Specific habitat requirements may vary between different lobelia species. Therefore, L. siphilitica can be transplanted to a moist, semishaded area in your garden. However, do not consume the plant, it's **highly toxic.**

Medicinal Part: Leaves and stems.

Solvent: Water.

Effects: Emetic, Stimulant, Antispasmodic, Expectorant, Diaphoretic, Relaxant, Nauseant, Sedative

Traditional uses: Lobelia has been used by various Native American tribes for its medicinal properties. For example, the Cherokee and Iroquois tribes utilized lobelia as a respiratory aid, using it to treat conditions such as asthma, bronchitis, and coughs. The Ojibwe tribe used lobelia as a purgative and to induce vomiting for various purposes. Additionally, the Penobscot tribe applied lobelia externally to alleviate toothaches and insect bites. Other tribes, including the Mohegan and Menominee, have also incorporated lobelia into their traditional healing practices for various ailments.

Modern uses: Lobelia has also gained attention as a potential aid in smoking cessation, although it should be noted that fatalities have been reported when used improperly. It has been recognized for its emetic, expectorant, and nervine properties. The root is believed to possess analgesic, anthelmintic, antispasmodic, and stomachic properties. A tea made from the roots has been used in the treatment of various conditions such as epilepsy, syphilis, typhoid, stomachaches, cramps, and worms. Additionally, a poultice of the roots has been applied to stubborn sores. The leaves of lobelia are considered analgesic and febrifuge. A tea made from the leaves has been used to address ailments such as croup, nosebleeds, colds, fevers, and headaches. Application of a poultice made from the leaves has been known to relieve the pain of headaches. Cardinal flower (L. cardinalis) shares similar traditional uses with L. siphilitica and L. inflata, although some sources suggest that it may have more modest biological activity.

In modern herbal medicine, lobelia is primarily used for its potential respiratory benefits. Research suggests that lobelia may have bronchodilatory effects, meaning it can help relax and open up the airways, making it beneficial for conditions such as asthma, bronchitis, and coughs. A study published in the "Journal of Ethnopharmacology" investigated the anti-inflammatory properties of lobeline, a key constituent of lobelia, and found that it exhibited potential anti-inflammatory effects.

Lobelia has also been explored for its potential analgesic properties. Some studies have indicated that lobelia extract may have mild analgesic effects, making it useful for managing minor pain and discomfort.

Warning: Lobelia is a **toxic** herb that should be approached with caution. Its active constituents can have strong effects on the body, and it is important to use it under the guidance of a qualified healthcare professional. Self-experimentation or misuse of lobelia can be risky and potentially harmful.

In homeopathy, very diluted and specially prepared microdoses of lobelia may be used, but even in this form, it is best to consult a trained homeopathic practitioner who can provide appropriate guidance and dosage recommendations.

Always prioritize your safety and consult a healthcare professional before considering the use of lobelia or any other potent herb or medication.

Mayapple
Berberidaceae (*Podophyllum peltatum* L.)

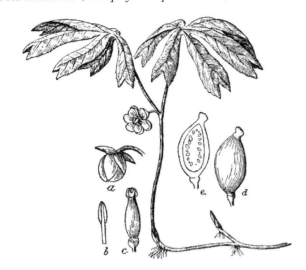

Identification: Mayapple, also known as American mandrake, is a perennial plant characterized by its distinctive umbrella-like appearance and cleft leaves. Each stalk of the plant bears two large leaves, each with five to seven lobes. A single white flower emerges from beneath the leaves, and the fruit of the plant ripens from mid- to late summer. It is important to note that the fruit is only edible when fully ripe.

Mayapple colonies can spread across the forest floor, creating a striking sight. The plant is valued for its unique appearance and can be found in various regions.

Habitat: Commonly found as an extensive ground cover in eastern forests and rich woods. Its ability to form dense colonies makes it a significant component of the understory vegetation in these habitats. The plant thrives in shaded areas with moist, well-drained soil, which is why it is often seen carpeting the forest floor in rich environments.

Medicinal Parts: Root and resin

Solvent: Boiling water and alcohol.

Effects: Cathartic, Purgative, Cholagogue, Alterative.

Food: Apologies for not adhering to the agreed-upon style. Here is a paraphrased version:
Ripe mayapple fruit is edible and can be enjoyed in various preparations such as marmalades, jellies, and beverages. However, it's important to note that **the rest of the plant and unripe fruit are poisonous** and should be avoided. Finding the ripe fruit can be challenging as not all plants produce abundant fruit, and there is often competition with wildlife for the available fruit. If one manages to obtain ripe mayapple fruit, it can be cooked and incorporated into recipes like pies, muffins, waffles, pancakes, or used to create jam or jelly. Native American tribes such as the Cherokee, Chippewa, Haudenosaunee, Menominee, and Meskwaki had their own traditional methods of utilizing the fruit, including drying and smashing it to create fruit cakes that could later be rehydrated with water and used as a sauce.

Traditional uses: Mayapple has a rich history of medicinal use among Native Americans, although it is important to exercise caution due to the plant's toxic nature. Native Americans utilized small doses of mayapple for various medicinal purposes. It was employed in the treatment of verrucae, which are warts caused by the papillomavirus. Additionally, mayapple was recognized for its emetic and purgative properties, serving as a potent laxative. The toxic root of the plant was used to eliminate intestinal worms, and the powdered root was applied externally to aid in the healing of slow-healing sores. It is worth mentioning that a small amount of fresh juice from the root was sometimes used to allegedly improve hearing, although this practice is not recommended. It is also noted that, regrettably, a potent extract from mayapple was historically used by certain Native Americans as a means of ending one's life. In more recent times, mayapple resin has been employed as a treatment for venereal warts, with injections administered for this purpose.

Modern uses: One notable research application of Mayapple is in cancer research, as mayapple contains compounds called podophyllotoxins, which have shown anticancer activity. Podophyllotoxin derivatives, such as etoposide and teniposide, derived from mayapple, have been used in chemotherapy to treat various types of cancer, including lung, testicular, and ovarian cancer.
Mayapple has also been explored for its potential antiviral properties. Studies have suggested that certain compounds in mayapple, such as podophyllotoxin, exhibit antiviral activity against viruses like herpes simplex virus (HSV) and human papillomavirus (HPV). However, further research is needed to fully understand the effectiveness and safety of using mayapple for viral infections. In traditional medicine practices, mayapple has been used as a purgative and for its potential effects on the liver. However, it's important to note that the use of mayapple in traditional medicine is generally not recommended due to its toxic properties and potential side effects.

Warning: Caution should be exercised when handling the plant, and it is advisable to seek medical supervision. The plant is highly toxic, and as such, it should not be used in herbal remedies. The toxic compounds present in the plant, including podophyllotoxin, can be absorbed through the skin, further highlighting the need for caution and medical guidance when dealing with this plant.

Gardening tip: The Menominees, Meskwaki, and Cherokee tribes used an infusion made from crushed mayapple plants to eliminate potato bugs and discourage crows from consuming newly planted corn seeds. Additionally, they soaked corn seeds and roots in a decoction of mayapple to protect them against fungal infections and pests. Some individuals today prepare a homemade insecticide for their gardens using mayapple roots. The process involves blending approximately 8 ounces of fresh root with 2 quarts of water, straining the mixture through cheesecloth or pantyhose, and using a garden sprayer to apply the resulting liquid. It is important to wear gloves when handling mayapple roots due to their toxic nature.

Maple

Aceraceae (*Acer spp.; A. saccharum; A. rubrum; A. macrophyllum; A. nigrum*)

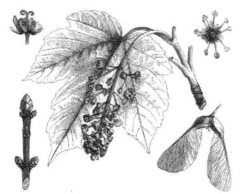

Identification: Maple trees have broad and rounded crowns. They vary in height, ranging from 30 feet to 150 feet, depending on the species. When young, the bark of maple trees is smooth, but it develops furrows as the tree ages. The leaves of most maple species are typically three-lobed, with red maple leaves having distinct red petioles. Maple seeds are notable for their helicopter-blade appearance, allowing them to be carried by the wind. The sugar maple leaf is recognized for its resemblance to the leaf depicted on the Canadian flag. Some common maple species include sugar maple (Acer saccharum), red maple (Acer rubrum), bigleaf or Oregon maple (Acer macrophyllum), and black maple (Acer nigrum).

Habitat: Maple trees, including species such as sugar maple, red maple, bigleaf maple, and black maple, are widely distributed throughout the United States and southern Canada. They can be found in a variety of habitats, including wet woods and dry woods. Sugar and red maples are typically more prevalent in the eastern region of the United States, particularly east of the Mississippi River. Bigleaf maple, on the other hand, is native to the Northwest region. Black maple shares a range with sugar maple in the eastern United States but is more restricted to the upper Midwest.

Medicinal Parts: The inner bark and leaves.

Solvent: Boiling water.

Effects: Astringent, Deobstruent, Tonic.

Food: Maple syrup is perhaps the most well-known culinary use of maple. It is derived from the sap of maple trees and is used as a natural sweetener in a variety of dishes and beverages. Maple syrup is often drizzled over pancakes, waffles, and French toast, but it can also be used as a topping for ice cream, yogurt, or oatmeal. It can be incorporated into glazes for meats, added to baked goods for flavor, or used as a substitute for sugar in recipes.

To tap a maple tree and collect its sap for maple syrup production, here is a general process:
1. Identify a mature maple tree, preferably a sugar maple or black maple.
2. Choose a suitable tapping location on the tree, usually about 2-3 feet above the ground.
3. Drill a small hole into the tree trunk, at a slight upward angle, using a specialized tapping tool or drill bit.
4. Insert a spout or spile into the hole, ensuring a tight fit.
5. Place a collection container, such as a bucket or plastic tubing, beneath the spout to catch the dripping sap.
6. Monitor the sap collection regularly, as the flow varies depending on weather conditions.
7. Once you have collected a sufficient amount of sap, it can be processed into maple syrup through boiling and filtering.

Traditional uses: Maple syrup is not only a delicious sweetener but also a rich source of glucose and various minerals, making it a more nutritious alternative to refined white sugar. The fresh sap of maple trees, before it is processed into syrup, is considered a tonic that is rich in minerals. Native Americans, such as the Iroquois, used different parts of the maple tree for medicinal purposes. They would prepare a compound by steeping the leaves in water, which was consumed as a blood purifier. Infusions of the bark were used as an antiseptic eyewash, and decoctions of the inner bark were made as cough remedies and expectorants. These traditional uses highlight the medicinal properties associated with different parts of the maple tree.

Modern uses: Maple syrup not only serves as a flavorful and natural sweetener but has also been utilized in cough syrups for its taste and sweetness. Interestingly, maple syrup contains a lower sugar content compared to honey. Additionally, maple sap contains polyphenols, which are beneficial plant compounds, as well as abscisic acid, a phytohormone that may assist the pancreas in insulin production. However, further research is needed to establish the potential antidiabetic properties of these components found in maple syrup. A study conducted at the University of Rhode Island in 2010 suggests the need for additional investigations in this area.

Milkweed

Asclepiadaceae (*Asclepias speciosa*)

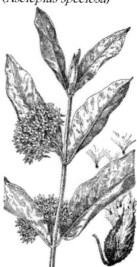

Identification: Milkweed is a perennial herbaceous plant that can reach a height of 2 to 6 feet (0.6 to 1.8 meters). It features tall, upright stems with opposite leaves that are broad and ovate in shape. The leaves are thick and have a slightly fuzzy texture.

Milkweed produces clusters of showy flowers that are usually pink, purple, or white, and they attract pollinators like bees and butterflies. The flowers develop into elongated seed pods that contain numerous small seeds, each attached to a silky parachute-like structure called a "coma." This allows the seeds to be dispersed by the wind. The plant also contains a milky sap that is toxic and can cause skin irritation, so caution should be exercised when handling milkweed. In herbal medicine, three main species of milkweed are commonly used: common milkweed (Asclepias speciosa), inmortal (Asclepias asperula), and pleurisy root (Asclepias tuberosa). While each species has its own specific uses, they also share certain similarities in their effects on the body.

Habitat: Milkweed species can be found in a wide range of habitats across the United States. They are commonly found along the edges of cornfields, waste grounds, roadsides, railroad, meadows, dunes, deserts, and gardens. Various species of milkweed are distributed nationwide.

The common milkweed (Asclepias speciosa) is prevalent in the western regions of the country. While its distribution may be scattered and inconsistent, it often forms large colonies when found.

The inmortal milkweed (Asclepias asperula) primarily grows in the desert southwest, extending into western Nebraska and Arkansas. It is well adapted to the arid conditions of these regions.

Food: Native Americans had various culinary uses for Asclepias syriaca, also known as common milkweed. The shoots of the plant were prepared in a similar manner to asparagus. They were harvested before the milky sap appeared, simmered in two changes of water (this softens the bitterness of the shoots), and then sautéed in oil. The flower buds, when harvested before they open, were cooked similar to broccoli. I'd recommend to put them shortly in boiling water like with the shoots.

The flower buds and seedpods of common milkweed were prepared by boiling water and pouring it over the pods. After steeping for five minutes, the water was poured off. This process was repeated with a second boil of water. The once-steeped pods were then stir-fried in olive oil or butter. The flowers could also be dried and stored for later use in soups and stews. They were sometimes diced, sweetened, and made into marmalade.

It's important to note that these culinary uses specifically refer to *Asclepias syriaca*. Make sure to identify it correctly before consuming. Other milkweed species may be toxic, and it is not recommended to experiment with them unless guided by an expert.

Traditional uses: The Cherokee people utilized milkweed in several ways. They would use the roots as a diuretic by boiling them and consuming the liquid to increase urine flow. The stems of milkweed were made into cordage and used for weaving baskets, nets, and ropes.

The Iroquois tribe used the fibers from the milkweed stems to create fine, strong threads for sewing and making fishing nets. They also extracted the milky sap from the plant and applied it topically to treat warts and corns.

The Ojibwa tribe employed milkweed in the preparation of a poultice by crushing the leaves and applying them to burns, sores, and wounds to promote healing. They also used the plant as a medicinal herb to treat respiratory ailments and as a laxative.

The Menominee tribe utilized milkweed as a source of food. They would harvest the young shoots and cook them as a vegetable, incorporating them into various dishes. The shoots were also preserved for later use by drying and pounding them into a powder.

Modern uses: Research suggests that milkweed extracts may possess anti-inflammatory and antioxidant properties, making them potentially beneficial for conditions such as arthritis and oxidative stress-related diseases. However, further studies are needed to fully understand the extent of its therapeutic effects.

In homeopathic medicine, milkweed has been used to address a range of conditions, including digestive disorders, respiratory ailments, and skin conditions. Homeopathic practitioners believe that milkweed can stimulate the body's self-healing mechanisms and restore balance.

Herbalist Michael Moore, known for his extensive knowledge of medicinal plants, viewed milkweed as an underutilized plant with potential therapeutic value. He highlighted its historical uses for respiratory ailments, including asthma, bronchitis, and coughs. Moore recommended milkweed as a valuable expectorant and bronchial relaxant.

Dose and usage: Milkweed is a versatile and beneficial plant with various uses. The young shoots, resembling asparagus, can be harvested and prepared for consumption. However, it's important to be cautious of the bitter milky sap, which contains cardiac glycosides.

The root of milkweed is primarily employed as an herbal remedy for respiratory ailments. It helps to alleviate bronchial congestion, promote expectoration, and expand the bronchial passages. This makes it valuable for conditions such as asthma, bronchitis, pleurisy, and chronic respiratory problems like emphysema and cystic fibrosis.

Milkweed also possesses diuretic properties and can induce sweating. It's crucial to avoid excessive consumption, as it may lead to nausea and vomiting. To determine the appropriate dosage, it's recommended to start with a low amount, such as 15 drops of milkweed tincture, taken three to four times a day. Gradually increase the dosage until a slight sense of nausea is felt, and then slightly reduce it to find the suitable level for individual tolerance.

The resin of milkweed can be collected from the leaves and stems. By cutting and collecting from the top of the plant and progressively working down, the white resin can be scraped. Allow the wound to dry and form a protective layer before collecting more resin lower down. Collected resin can then be oxidized and dried in a glass or stainless-steel dish, occasionally stirring or turning it for thorough drying. It's important to note that this process does not harm the plant as long as sufficient growth is left for its survival. The resin can be topically applied to remove warts.

Warning: Milkweed contains toxic compounds and should not be used without proper knowledge and precautions. The plant's sap, leaves, and other parts may cause adverse effects if ingested or come into contact with the skin. It is important to correctly identify milkweed species and exercise caution when handling or consuming any part of the plant. Milkweed toxins can cause gastrointestinal distress, nausea, vomiting, and allergic reactions in some individuals. The severity of these effects may vary depending on the individual's sensitivity and the amount consumed or exposed to. Ingesting large quantities of milkweed can be potentially harmful and may require immediate medical attention.

Other uses: The fiber from milkweed seeds and the fine hairs surrounding the seeds were utilized as batting for life jackets. The flowers of milkweed have a pleasant fragrance and could potentially be a source of sugar. The strong and fibrous stems of the plant can be processed to make cordage, while the pulp of the plant can be chopped, shredded, boiled, and used to create paper. These various uses demonstrate the versatile nature of milkweed and the resourcefulness of those who utilized it.

Gardening tip: Furthermore, milkweed is a vital plant for the survival of monarch butterflies and other pollinators. Harvesting milkweed from natural habitats can disrupt their populations and ecological balance. If you are considering using milkweed for any purpose, it is recommended to cultivate it responsibly in a controlled environment or seek sustainably sourced alternatives Milkweed plants are not only valuable for their uses and medicinal properties but also serve as beautiful additions to gardens. They have an exotic appearance and are known to attract various pollinators such as bees, butterflies (including monarchs and fritillaries), and hummingbirds. If you're fortunate, you may even spot monarch caterpillars crawling over the milkweed leaves, as they rely on milkweed as their primary food source. However, it's important to be aware of milkweed bugs (*Oncopeltus fasciatus*), black and yellow sucking insects that can be found on the underside of the leaves. To know more check out the sixth volume of the series!

Mullein
Scrophulariaceae (*Verbascum thapsus L.*)

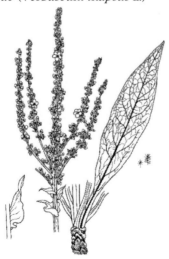

Identification: Mullein plants have a distinctive appearance characterized by a tall and stout stem that emerges from a cluster of large, woolly leaves at the base. As the stem grows, smaller leaves continue to appear along its length. The flowers of mullein are yellow in color and densely packed on a spike located at the top of the stem. The leaves of mullein are ovate and can grow up to 15 inches in length. They are covered with gray hair, giving them a fuzzy texture. The basal leaves are larger and clasp the stem, while the upper leaves are smaller and less dense.

Habitat: Found growing in various locations across the country, including waste grounds, along roadsides, fields, railroad rights-of-way, and montane areas. It has a wide distribution and is capable of thriving in diverse habitats.

Medicinal Parts: The leaves and flower, Culpeper also used the root also.

Solvent: Boiling water.

Effects: Demulcent, Diuretic, Anodyne, Antispasmodic, Astringent, Pectoral.

Traditional uses: The Cherokee tribe traditionally used mullein leaves to make a soothing tea for respiratory ailments, coughs, and congestion. They also used the leaves as a poultice or smoked them to alleviate joint pain and inflammation. The Iroquois tribe employed mullein leaves as a poultice for treating bruises, wounds, and inflammation. They also brewed a tea from the leaves to address respiratory conditions such as coughs, asthma, and bronchitis. The Mohegan tribe utilized mullein as a traditional remedy for earaches. They would infuse the flowers in oil and use the oil as ear drops to alleviate pain and discomfort.
The Meskwaki tribe used mullein roots as a diuretic to promote urination and address kidney and bladder-related issues. They also used the leaves as a poultice for wounds, boils, and skin infections.
The Navajo tribe used mullein leaves to make a tea that was consumed to soothe chest congestion, coughs, and sore throats.
Additionally, the Blackfoot tribe used mullein root tea for intestinal issues.

Modern uses: In modern herbal medicine, mullein has gained recognition for its potential benefits. Scientific studies have explored its respiratory-supporting properties, demonstrating its ability to reduce cough severity and frequency. Mullein extracts have also shown anti-inflammatory and analgesic effects, making it valuable for addressing conditions such as arthritis and joint pain. Furthermore, mullein has been used topically to promote wound healing and address skin infections.
Commission E has approved the internal use of mullein flowers for respiratory conditions like bronchitis and dry cough. Additionally, it recognizes the external use of mullein flowers for skin inflammation.

Dose and uses: For respiratory support, an infusion can be made by steeping 1-2 teaspoons of dried mullein leaves or flowers in 1 cup of hot water for 10-15 minutes. This infusion can be consumed up to three times a day.

For topical application, fresh mullein leaves or flowers can be crushed and applied directly to insect and spider bites. Leave the poultice on the affected area for about 15-20 minutes, then rinse with cool water.

For earaches or swimmer's ear, a homemade ear oil can be prepared by infusing fresh mullein flowers and garlic cloves in olive oil over low heat for several hours. Once cooled, a few drops of the oil can be placed in the affected ear.

Gardening tips: To add mullein to your yard, you can easily transplant a first-year growth that consists of a basal rosette of fuzzy leaves. Dig out the plant carefully, ensuring that you preserve the root system, and transplant it to your desired location. In the following year, the biennial mullein plant will bloom, adding its distinctive and attractive flowers to your yard.

Nettle

Urticaceae *(Urtica dioica L.)*

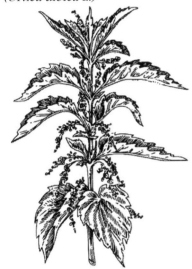

Identification: Nettle is a perennial plant that can grow up to 5 feet tall. It has an erect growth habit with a square, grooved stem that is covered in stinging hairs. The leaves of nettle are dark green, rough, and hairy, and they are typically heart- to oval-shaped with toothed edges.

The plant produces numerous green flowers, which are borne in the leaf axils and eventually develop into green seeds. Nettle plants can have both male and female flowers on the same plant, or they may have separate male and female plants.

Habitat: Nettle can be found in a wide range of habitats across the United States. It is commonly found along the edges of fields, stream sides, wetlands, marshy areas, fringe areas, wastelands, and roadsides.

Medicinal Parts: The roots and leaves.

Solvent: Boiling water.

Effects: Diuretic, Astringent, Tonic, Pectoral.

Food: Nettle shoots, especially the young ones in the fall and spring, are commonly harvested and prepared by steaming, sautéing, or stir-frying. They can be a delightful addition to various dishes. One popular recipe involves creaming nettle into soup, which provides a rich and flavorful result.

In addition to using the young shoots, older nettles that have hardened during the summer can also be utilized. The hardened shoots can be boiled with other herbs like rosemary, celery, thyme, onions, leeks, and lovage to make a savory broth. After simmering for around twenty-five minutes, the plant materials can be discarded, and the resulting broth can be used in various cooking preparations, providing a savory and aromatic flavor.

Traditional uses: Native American tribes utilized nettle for its medicinal properties. For instance, the Cherokee used nettle as a diuretic and to support healthy kidney function. They also used nettle as a remedy for allergies, arthritis, and skin conditions. The Iroquois used nettle to treat diarrhea, coughs, and colds, as well as to stimulate hair growth. The Navajo used nettle as a traditional food source and believed it had purifying and revitalizing effects on the body.

In traditional Russian medicine, nettle was widely used for its medicinal properties. It was commonly used as a blood purifier and to support overall health. Nettle tea was consumed to alleviate symptoms of hay fever, allergies, and urinary tract infections. It was also used topically to soothe skin irritations and promote hair growth.

In other medical traditions, nettle has been used for various purposes. In Ayurveda, nettle is believed to have a cooling and detoxifying effect on the body. It is used to support healthy digestion, promote joint health, and balance the doshas. In traditional European herbal medicine, nettle has been used for its diuretic properties, to support joint health, and as a general tonic for overall wellness.

Modern uses: Commission E has approved the use of nettle root for supportive therapy in lower urinary tract complaints, such as benign prostatic hyperplasia (BPH). Studies have shown that nettle root extract may help improve symptoms associated with BPH, including urinary frequency, nocturia, and urine flow rate.

Nettle leaf has been traditionally used for its potential anti-inflammatory and antiallergic effects. Studies suggest that nettle leaf may help reduce allergic symptoms, such as hay fever, by inhibiting the release of histamine and other pro-inflammatory compounds. It may also have a positive impact on allergic rhinitis symptoms, such as nasal congestion and itching.

Furthermore, nettle leaf has been investigated for its potential benefits in managing osteoarthritis. Studies have shown that nettle leaf extract may help reduce pain and improve joint function in individuals with osteoarthritis.

In addition to these uses, nettle has been studied for its potential antioxidant, antimicrobial, and anti-inflammatory properties. It has also been explored for its effects on blood sugar regulation, wound healing, and skin health.

Furthermore, sodium formate, an analog of formic acid found in stinging nettle and ants, has been found to significantly increase the effectiveness of a metal-based cancer treatment called JS07. In fact, the combination of sodium formate and JS07 was found to be fifty times more effective than using JS07 alone, as demonstrated by research conducted at the University of Warwick.

Dose and usage: According to the book "Identifying and Harvesting Edible and Medicinal Plants" by Brill and Dean, consuming nettle tea and nettles as food may promote clearer and healthier skin, potentially providing therapeutic benefits for conditions such as eczema. Consumption of nettles is also believed to improve the color, texture, gloss, and overall health of hair. The aerial parts of the plant can be infused as a tea and used for urinary tract infections, kidney and bladder stones, and rheumatism. Nettle root tincture is employed for irritable bladder and prostate complaints.

Nettle tonic is known for its strong yet gentle action on the body. Herbalists consider it a whole-body tonic as it supports the functions and overall health of various body systems. It has been used for a wide range of purposes, including promoting good digestion, providing relief from allergies due to its antihistamine properties, and addressing respiratory and skin conditions. Nettle tonic is also believed to nourish the blood. While the aerial parts of the plant are commonly used, a tea or tincture made from the roots can be taken internally to specifically support men's prostate health.

Notes: If fresh nettle is not available, freeze-dried nettle can be a suitable alternative. Nettle is an easily cultivated plant that can be grown in a garden, providing edible leaves for up to nine months. When harvesting, focus on the new-growth leaves at the top of the plant. Interestingly, when you pick the stem, it often bifurcates and produces two new growth sprouts, effectively increasing your crop. If you encounter the stinging sensation from nettle, you can try rubbing mullein leaves or the juice of spotted touch-me-not (jewelweed, Impatiens capensis) on the affected area to alleviate the discomfort.

Veterinarian uses: Nettle juice combined with nettle seeds can be used as a beneficial hair tonic for domestic animals.

Oak
Fagaceae *(Quercus spp.)*

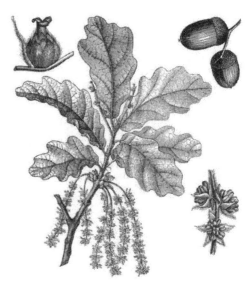

Identification: A visit to an arboretum is an excellent way to learn how to identify different oak species. The arboretum provides labeled trees that make it easier to visually recognize and differentiate between various oak species.

This knowledge will be valuable when foraging for nuts during the winter. Acorns come in different sizes and have varying tastes. Oak leaves also exhibit variations in their shape, with lobed, cut, pointed, or rounded characteristics that differ across species.

Habitat: Oaks can be found in a wide range of habitats across the country. They can be seen in yards, wood lots, forested areas, and even along roadsides. The adaptability of oaks allows them to thrive in diverse environments, making them a common sight in many different landscapes.

Effects: astringent

Medicinal part: Bark and oak galls, which contain the most tannins.

Food: The diverse species of oak trees produce acorns with varying degrees of bitterness. Oaks with rounded leaf lobes, such as white oak (Q. alba), bur oak (Q. macrocarpa), swamp chestnut oak (Q. michauxii), chestnut oak (Q. prinus), and chinquapin oak (Q. muehlenbergii), tend to have sweeter acorns in the eastern United States. In the western United States, Gambel's oak (Q. gambelii), blue oak (Q. douglasii), and Oregon white oak (Q. garryana) are known for their bittersweet acorns.

To reduce the bitterness of acorn meat, it is essential to leach out the tannins, which contribute to the bitter taste. One method involves blending the acorn meat with water (using 2 cups of water for every cup of nut meat) and then straining and pressing the water out of the nut meat using cheesecloth, pantyhose, or a clean cloth. This process helps remove the bitter compounds and makes the acorn meat more palatable.

In traditional Native American methods, acorns were prepared by shelling, cracking, or smashing them and then soaking them in a skin bag placed in a stream for a day or two. This soaking process helped remove the bitter tannins present in the acorns. Thinly chopping the acorn meats and drying them was another technique used to attenuate the bitter taste, making them more suitable for consumption.

The prepared acorn mash can be incorporated into various culinary applications, such as topping baked potatoes, mixing into tomato sauces, or incorporating into baking recipes. Additionally, acorns can be enjoyed as a snack on their own. The traditional methods of processing acorns have been used for generations to unlock their nutritional value and turn them into delicious and versatile ingredients.

Traditional uses: Oak trees have been highly valued by various indigenous tribes for their versatile uses. Different oak species hold specific significance and uses among different tribes. For example, the white oak (Quercus alba) has been traditionally used by several Native American tribes for its medicinal properties. The Cherokee used the bark and inner wood of white oak to make a decoction for treating diarrhea, sore throats, and fevers. The Mohegan tribe utilized the inner bark as a remedy for lung ailments.
Similarly, the acorns from oak trees were a vital food source for many tribes. Native Americans developed methods to process and prepare acorns to remove the bitter tannins and make them edible. The Miwok tribe in California gathered acorns from black oak (Quercus kelloggii) and blue oak (Quercus douglasii) trees. They would grind the acorns into a fine meal and leach out the tannins by rinsing the meal with water. This process created a nutritious and staple food source that could be used in various recipes.

Oak bark and leaves were often employed in traditional medicine for their astringent, anti-inflammatory, and antiseptic qualities.

The Cherokee tribe used the bark of the white oak (Quercus alba) as a poultice to treat skin inflammations, wounds, and sores. The inner bark of the black oak (Quercus velutina) was utilized by the Delaware tribe to create an infusion for managing diarrhea and dysentery. The Pomo tribe used a decoction of the bark and leaves from blue oak (Quercus douglasii) as a remedy for sore throats, colds, and coughs.

Some tribes also utilized oak bark infusions as a wash or gargle for various ailments. The Iroquois tribe made a decoction of oak bark (Quercus spp.) to relieve sore gums and mouth inflammations. The Navajo tribe prepared an infusion of oak bark to treat internal hemorrhages. Other oak species held cultural significance and ceremonial uses among different tribes. The Hopi tribe considered the Gambel's oak (Quercus gambelii) as a sacred tree associated with spiritual rituals and healing practices. The Apache tribe utilized the leaves and bark of Emory oak (Quercus emoryi) as part of religious ceremonies. Additionally, different tribes had specific uses for oak wood in crafting tools, furniture, and ceremonial objects. The Iroquois used oak wood for creating intricate masks, while the Tlingit tribe in Alaska crafted bentwood boxes from red oak (Quercus rubra) for storing food and other belongings.

Modern uses: Oak bark extract, derived from species such as Q. robur or Q. petraea, has been recognized by Commission E for its medicinal properties. It is approved for the treatment of various conditions including bronchitis, cough, diarrhea, mouth and throat sores, and inflammations of the skin.
Moreover, ongoing research is exploring the potential use of certain chemicals found in oak bark as a cancer therapy. These studies aim to investigate the anti-cancer properties and potential benefits of these compounds.

Dose and uses: A decoction can be prepared using 1 ounce of oak bark in 1 quart of water, boiled down to 1 pint. This decoction can be taken in wineglass doses and used as a gargle for sore throat. Oak is commonly used as a strong infusion or tea for various conditions such as gum inflammations, skin abrasions, sunburn, bleeding wounds, diarrhea, dysentery, and hemorrhoids. To prepare an infusion, one teaspoon of oak bark powder can be boiled gently in a cup of water for fifteen minutes and applied topically to the affected area. For bleeding wounds, the powdered herb (leaves, twigs, bark, or galls) can be directly applied to the affected area, sometimes in combination with powdered antibiotic herbs like usnea or echinacea.
Gum inflammations can be treated effectively with a tincture of oak bark, while other complaints can be addressed with a strong infusion or tea. In cases of diarrhea or dysentery, drinking the tea (prepared as described above) three to six cups a day can be beneficial. Additionally, using the tea as an enema has shown positive results for these conditions. In the past, oak enemas were commonly used for the treatment of severe dysentery.
It is worth noting that some Indigenous tribes have used moldy acorn meal scraped off and applied to boils, sores, and other inflammations as a traditional remedy.

Oregon Grape

Berberidaceae *(Mahonia aquifolium [Pursh] Nutt.; M. nervosa [Pursh] Nutt.)*

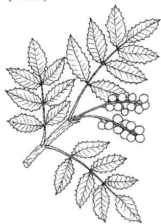

Identification: Oregon grape (*Mahonia aquifolium*) is a perennial shrub native to western North America. It is characterized by its dense clusters of small yellow flowers and its dark blue-purple berries. The plant typically grows to a height of 2 to 6 feet (0.6 to 1.8 meters) and features holly-like leaves with spiky edges. The leaves are pinnately compound, meaning they are divided into multiple leaflets. The plant also produces small, grape-like clusters of berries that turn dark blue-purple when ripe.

Habitat: Oregon grape is native to western North America and can be found in various habitats across the region. It is commonly found in forests, woodlands, and mountainous areas, particularly in the Pacific Northwest. Oregon grape thrives in well-drained soils and is often found growing in shady or partially shaded areas. It is adaptable to different soil types, including loamy, sandy, and clay soils. This plant is well-suited to the moist, cool climate of the region and can be found at various elevations, ranging from sea level up to mountainous slopes.

Food: Oregon grape (Mahonia aquifolium) has a long history of culinary uses among Native American tribes in the Pacific Northwest. The berries of the plant were traditionally used as a food source in the late summer by tribes such as the Nez Perce, Coeur d'Alene, and Salish. The berries have a tart and slightly bitter flavor, similar to cranberries, and were commonly used to make jams, jellies, and sauces. They were also mixed with other fruits to enhance their flavor. The berries were harvested when ripe and used fresh or dried for later use. In addition to the berries, the young shoots and leaves of the Oregon grape plant were sometimes used as a salad green or cooked as a vegetable. However, it's important to note that while the berries and shoots have culinary uses, other parts of the Oregon grape plant, such as the roots and bark, are generally not consumed due to their strong bitter taste.

Traditional uses: The Nez Perce tribe used the root bark of Oregon grape as a poultice to soothe skin inflammations, such as rashes, eczema, and psoriasis. It was also applied topically to treat cuts, wounds, and skin infections. The root was considered effective in promoting wound healing and reducing inflammation.

The Salish tribe utilized the root bark as a remedy for digestive issues. They prepared a decoction from the root, which was consumed to ease stomach problems, improve digestion, and alleviate indigestion.

Among the Coeur d'Alene tribe, Oregon grape was used to address a variety of health conditions. The root bark was brewed into a tea or decoction and consumed to treat fever, liver ailments, and gastrointestinal discomfort.

In addition to these specific uses, Oregon grape was also recognized for its potential antimicrobial and anti-inflammatory properties. The plant contains an alkaloid compound called berberine, which has shown antimicrobial activity against certain bacteria, fungi, and protozoa. This compound is believed to contribute to the plant's traditional use in addressing infections.

Modern uses: Mahonia aquifolium extractions are commercially available in the form of ointments to treat dry skin, unspecified rashes, and psoriasis. These ointments utilize the properties of Mahonia aquifolium to alleviate symptoms associated with these skin conditions. There is limited research on the potential appetite-stimulating effects of Mahonia aquifolium, and further investigation is needed in this regard. In homeopathic doses, Mahonia aquifolium has been used for liver and gallbladder problems, although the effectiveness of these uses is not well-established.

Regarding the treatment of psoriasis, three human studies have shown that the application of Mahonia aquifolium extract (in the form of a 10 percent cream or ointment derived from the leaves and root) is effective. Participants in these studies reported positive results, with the Mahonia aquifolium extract being rated as comparable to or better than the standard prescription alternative, Dovonex cream.

Warning: Caution should be exercised when using Oregon grape (Mahonia aquifolium) as a medicinal herb. It contains alkaloids that may interact with certain medications and can cause digestive upset or skin reactions. Consult a healthcare professional before use, especially if taking medications or during pregnancy and breastfeeding. Use responsibly and discontinue use if any adverse reactions occur.

Other uses: A decoction of the root and bark makes a bright yellow dye.

Pasque Flower

Ranunculaceae (*Pulsitilla spp.*)

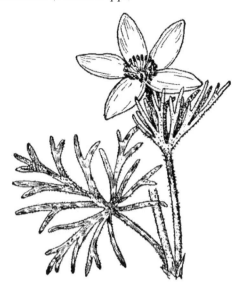

Identification: Across all thirty-three species the plant characteristics are similar: finely dissected leaves, hairy stems, and bell-shaped flowers. The biggest variable is height; species range from 3" to 9". Showy parts of the flower are the sepals. The lilac-colored pasque flower (Pulsitilla patens) is characterized by its soft, hairy down covering and typically produces only one or two flowers from its small root. Seed heads are plumed.

Medicinal Parts: Plant and flower.

Effects: Tonic, Sedative, Nervine

Habitat: Found in the prairie and mountain meadows. Pictured specimen from the Cloud Peak Wilderness, Bighorn Mountains, Wyoming.
Food: Not edible, highly toxic. May slow heart and cause cardiac arrest.

Traditional uses: Used historically by the Blackfoot nation to induce uterine contractions leading to abortion. Also believed to speed difficult childbirth. The Dakotas call it hokshi-chekpa wahcha (twin flower). The Lakotas call it hoksi' cekpa (child's navel). Blackfeet call it napi (old man). Omaha and Ponca call it te-zhinga-makan (little buffalo medicine). It was one of the sacred power medicines of the Omahas and Poncas and esteemed very highly. Among the latter two tribes, the right to use the pasque flower was limited to the medicine men of the Te-sinde gens.

Modern uses: Used as a homeopathic preparation or in combination homeopathically for a variety of ailments to include colds, coughs, and digestive problems. The olfactory essence of the flower is used in aromatherapy and reported to relieve shyness.

Warning: May slow heart and cause cardiac arrest.

Passionflower

Passifloraceae (*Passiflora incarnata L.*)

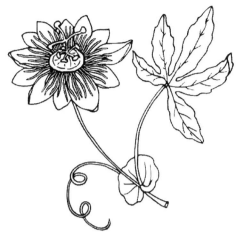

Identification: Perennial vine with a woody stem that can climb to heights of 35 feet or more. The mature bark of the vine is longitudinal and striated. The leaves are alternate, with petioles, and have serrated edges with fine hair on both the top and bottom surfaces, although the underside of the leaf is typically hairier. The leaf blades may have floral nectaries, which are small bumps on the surface. The flowers of the Passionflower are single and wheel-shaped, with petals resembling spokes, and they can be quite striking, reaching widths of up to 5 inches.

Habitat: Passionflower (Passiflora) vines grow in various habitats, including open areas and forest edges. While many species are native to tropical or subtropical regions, some can also be cultivated in temperate gardens. Passionflower has a wide distribution worldwide, with numerous species found across seven climatic zones. It is often introduced and can be found growing wild in the southeastern United States.

Medicinal Parts: Plant and flower.

Solvent: Diluted alcohol.

Effects: Anodyne, Nerve sedative, Diuretic, Antispasmodic.

Food: The leaf and flower tea of the plant exhibits mild sedative properties. The fresh fruit can be consumed raw, juiced, or used to make a beverage. In Mexican cuisine, it is mixed with cornmeal or flour to create a gruel-like dish. Native Americans have a tradition of eating the leaves. To prepare the leaves, they are usually parboiled and then pan-fried in vegetable oil or animal fat.

Traditional uses: Among the Cherokee, the leaves, stems, and flowers of passionflower were used to make a tea that was believed to alleviate anxiety, induce sleep, and calm the mind. The Choctaw used the leaves and roots of the plant as a sedative to treat nervousness and insomnia. They also employed the roots to relieve headaches and the flowers to soothe skin irritations. The Creek tribe used passionflower as a general analgesic, applying poultices made from the leaves and roots to reduce pain and inflammation.

In traditional Mexican medicine, passionflower, known as "flor de la pasión," was highly regarded for its calming and sedative effects. The aerial parts of the plant, including the leaves, stems, and flowers, were commonly used to make infusions or tinctures. It was employed to treat various nervous disorders, including anxiety, insomnia, and epilepsy. Passionflower was also utilized as a traditional remedy for menstrual pain and to promote healthy digestion. The leaves and stems were often used for their calming and sedating properties, while the flowers were valued for their soothing effects on the nervous system and skin. The roots were considered particularly useful for relieving pain and headaches.

Modern uses: Commision E recognized its calming and relaxing properties, making it useful for reducing symptoms of anxiety and stress. Passionflower is also used as a sleep aid, promoting restful sleep and helping with insomnia. Additionally, it is sometimes used as a complementary treatment for conditions such as depression, anxiety disorders, and ADHD. Passionflower has been reported to alleviate symptoms of premenstrual syndrome (PMS) and provide support during substance withdrawal. It may also help with digestive issues such as indigestion, stomach cramps, and irritable bowel syndrome (IBS).

Notes: According to the Doctrine of Signatures, passionflower's appearance is associated with its potential aphrodisiac properties. Passionflower does contain betacarboline harmala alkaloids, which are monoamine oxidase inhibitors (MAOIs) and have been found to possess antidepressant properties. While the flowers generally contain only small amounts of these chemicals, the leaves and roots of certain species have been historically used to enhance the effects of psychoactive substances.

Veterinarian uses: Mild sedative for cats and horses

Peppermint
Lamiaceae *(Mentha spp.: M. piperita L.)*

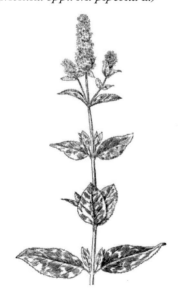

Identification: There are numerous American plants belonging to the mint family, sharing common characteristics such as a square and erect stem. When the leaves of these plants are crushed, they often emit a pleasant aroma. They tend to have an aggressive and spreading growth habit.
The height of these plants can range from 8 inches to 30 inches. They have a spreading rhizome as their root structure. The leaves are typically lance-shaped, although they can also be ovate or roundish, and they usually have serrated edges. The flowers are densely arranged in whorls, forming either a terminal spike or clusters in the leaf axils. The flower colors vary among species, with shades of white, violet, and blue being common. Peppermint (Mentha piperita) is the most well-known species within this family.

Habitat: Peppermint (Mentha piperita) can be found nationwide in various habitats. It is commonly found around water bodies, such as shorelines, stream banks, and the dunes of the Great Lakes. It can also be found in or around mountain passes, areas affected by blowdowns, avalanche slides, and wet meadows. Peppermint has adapted to thrive in diverse environments across the United States.
Medicinal Parts: Leaves and stems.

Solvent: Water.

Effects: Aromatic, Stimulant, Stomachic, Carminative.

Food: Peppermint is a versatile herb that is used in various culinary preparations. It can be used to make refreshing teas, added to salads and cold drinks, and used as a flavoring agent in sautéed vegetables. In the culinary traditions of the subcontinent and the Middle East, peppermint is an essential ingredient, adding its unique flavor to many dishes. Historical references, such as those from the Romans, indicate the use of mint, including peppermint, to flavor wines and sauces. Mint, including peppermint, can enhance the flavors of Mexican bean soups and chilled soups, offering a delightful taste experience in a range of culinary creations.
A warning for gardeners: Grow mints in a buried steel container to prevent their unabated spread.

Traditional uses: Peppermint (Mentha × piperita) has a diverse range of traditional uses across cultures worldwide. In Native American traditions, various tribes such as the Cheyenne, Chippewa, and Navajo utilized peppermint for its medicinal properties. It was often employed to ease digestive discomfort, alleviate headaches and migraines, and serve as a general remedy for various ailments.
In Traditional Chinese Medicine (TCM), peppermint, known as Bo He, is valued for its ability to clear heat, expel wind, and soothe the liver. It has been incorporated into formulas to address symptoms like headaches, fever, sore throat, and coughs.
Throughout Europe, peppermint has a rich history in folk medicine. It was relied upon to relieve digestive issues such as bloating, indigestion, and flatulence. Peppermint tea was commonly used to alleviate menstrual pain and promote relaxation.

In Middle Eastern and Mediterranean cultures, peppermint tea is a popular beverage valued for its refreshing and digestive properties. It is often consumed after meals to soothe stomach discomfort and aid digestion.

In Ayurvedic medicine, peppermint is considered a cooling herb that helps balance the Pitta dosha. It is utilized to relieve digestive problems, support respiratory health, and promote mental clarity.

Modern uses: Peppermint (Mentha piperita) has been widely studied for its modern uses and therapeutic properties. Numerous studies have demonstrated its effectiveness in various applications. For instance, a study published in the Journal of Gastroenterology found that peppermint oil capsules can effectively reduce symptoms of irritable bowel syndrome (IBS), such as abdominal pain, bloating, and gas. Another study published in Phytotherapy Research showed that peppermint oil may help relieve tension headaches when applied topically.

Peppermint oil has also shown potential antimicrobial properties. A study published in Food Chemistry demonstrated its effectiveness against various pathogens, including bacteria, fungi, and viruses. Additionally, peppermint oil has been studied for its potential anti-inflammatory effects. A review published in the Journal of Molecular Sciences highlighted the anti-inflammatory properties of peppermint oil, suggesting its potential use in managing inflammatory conditions.

In alternative medicine, peppermint is commonly used as a natural remedy for various ailments. It is often used to alleviate digestive issues, such as indigestion, nausea, and stomach cramps. Peppermint tea or oil is also used for its calming and soothing effects, promoting relaxation and relieving stress. Furthermore, peppermint oil is frequently utilized in aromatherapy for its invigorating scent and potential benefits in improving focus and mental clarity.

Warning: It's important to exercise caution when using mint oils in high concentrations, as they can potentially cause skin irritation and burns. Care should be taken to use them appropriately and follow recommended dilution guidelines.

Peppermint is contraindicated for individuals with ulcers, gastritis, and acid reflux due to its ability to relax the esophageal sphincter. This relaxation can allow stomach acid to flow back into the esophagus, exacerbating symptoms of acid reflux.

Notes: Mints such as peppermint, spearmint, and mountain mint offer not only their aromatic leaves but also their edible flowers, which can enhance the flavors of salads and desserts. For a delightful combination, try garnishing sliced pears with mint blossoms. Beyond their culinary uses, mints have long been valued as carminative herbs, known for their ability to relieve gas and digestive discomfort.

If you experience gallbladder pain or suffer from a spastic colon, you may find relief in mint lozenges, such as Altoids, which are readily available at an affordable price. These lozenges, infused with mint extracts, can help alleviate the discomfort associated with these conditions. Furthermore, individuals dealing with irritable bowel syndrome (IBS) may also find some relief by using mint lozenges, as they can help soothe the symptoms of this condition.

Pine

Pinaceae *(Pinus spp.: P. strobus L.; P. edulis L.)*

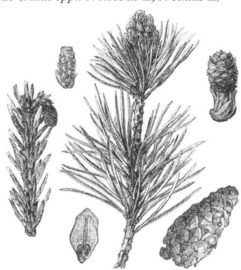

Identification: White pine (Pinus strobus) is an evergreen tree characterized by its medium to long needles, which grow in clusters of five. These needles have a light green color and are marked by a single white stripe. On the other hand, pinyon pine (Pinus edulis) is a shorter and more compact plant that thrives in dry alpine regions of the four-corner region, extending north to Canada. It is particularly abundant on the eastern side of Flaming Gorge, found in both Wyoming and Utah. The cones contain the delicious pine nuts often used in the preparation of pesto and other culinary dishes.

Habitat: White pine (Pinus strobus) is primarily found in the eastern United States. Pinyon pine (Pinus edulis) can be found in dry plateaus stretching from Mexico all the way up to Canada. Scotch pine (Pinus sylvestris), on the other hand, is often planted as an ornamental tree in yards, fencerows, and fallow fields.

Medical Parts: Inner bark or sprigs.

Solvent: Boiling water.

Effects: Expectorant.

Food: Seeds from pinecones may be eaten. Pinyon pine provides the most notable seeds used in pesto.

Traditional uses: The sap of pine trees has styptic properties and can effectively seal wounds, which made it a valuable treatment for gunshot wounds, cuts, scrapes, and lacerations among pioneers and First People. Additionally, pine needles were known to contain antiscorbutic properties, which helped prevent scurvy. This historical knowledge led to the tradition of brewing pine needle tea as a remedy.

Modern uses: The oil extracted from the needles of Scotch pine shoots has been approved by Commission E for its various medicinal uses. It is known to help prevent infections and is used in the treatment of blood pressure problems, colds, coughs, bronchitis, fevers, oral and pharyngeal inflammations, and neuralgias. Many species of pines and firs, including Scotch pine, contain vitamin C in their needles, particularly the end needles. This natural source of vitamin C provides the antiscorbutic effect traditionally associated with these trees in the wilderness.

Dose and uses: Pine needles are a valuable source of vitamin C and simple carbohydrates, providing quick energy when made into a sun tea. This makes it an excellent choice for backpackers in the wilderness, as pine trees are abundant in North America. In fact, pine needles contain five times more vitamin C than lemons do when compared by weight. For a refreshing tea, white pine needles can be crushed and added to a gallon jar of water along with mountain mint, lemon thyme, lemon balm, and the juice of half a lemon. Allow the mixture to infuse in the refrigerator for six hours, creating an uplifting beverage. Another invigorating and anti-infective tea can be brewed using various pine needles, along with lemon balm, mint, fennel, and lime juice. This cold infusion is made overnight by stuffing the leaves into a gallon jar, filling it with pure water, and refrigerating for twelve hours before enjoying. For a delightful treat, try making pinyon pine nut ice cream. Chop pine nuts and mix them into vanilla ice cream, allowing the flavors to infuse overnight. This delicious dessert is a favorite in Guanajuato and Dolores Hidalgo, Mexico.

Plantain

Plantaginaceae *(Plantago lanceolata L.; P. major L.; P. maritima L.)*

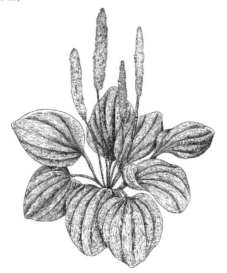

Identification: Plantain, also known as Plantago, is a perennial herbaceous plant characterized by its low-growing rosette of broad, oval-shaped leaves that arise from a central base. The leaves have prominent parallel veins and can vary in size, ranging from a few centimeters to several inches in length. The plant produces tall, slender spikes that bear small, inconspicuous flowers with greenish or brownish hues. As the flowers mature, they develop into small capsules containing numerous tiny seeds.

Plantain leaves have a distinct ribbed texture and are often slightly hairy. They grow in a basal rosette pattern, meaning they radiate from a central point at ground level. The leaves may have smooth or slightly toothed edges, depending on the species. Some varieties of plantain, such as broadleaf plantain (Plantago major), feature broader leaves, while others, like ribwort plantain (Plantago lanceolata), have narrower and more elongated leaves.

Habitat: Plantain is typically found in open fields, lawns, meadows, and disturbed areas. It is adaptable to various soil types and can tolerate both dry and moist conditions. This hardy plant can be found in different regions around the world, including North America, Europe, Asia, and Australia.

Medicinal Part: The whole plant.

Solvent: Water.

Effects: Alterative, Astringent, Diuretic, Antiseptic.

Food: The leaves of plantain are often used in cooking and are consumed in various cultures around the world. In Caribbean and African cuisine, plantain leaves are used as natural wrappers for cooking and steaming various dishes. The leaves provide a unique flavor and impart a subtle herbal essence to the food.

In some traditional recipes, plantain leaves are used to wrap foods such as tamales, sticky rice, or fish, adding a distinct earthy flavor and aroma. The leaves can also be used to make tea by steeping them in hot water, creating an herbal infusion with a mild, pleasant taste.

Plantain leaves are sometimes used as a natural ingredient in salads, particularly in Southeast Asian cuisines. The young and tender leaves can be harvested and added fresh to salads, bringing a slightly bitter and herbaceous flavor to the dish.

Additionally, plantain leaves are sometimes used as a natural food preservative due to their antimicrobial properties. They can be used to wrap and store certain foods, helping to extend their shelf life.

Traditional uses: Among Native American tribes, the Iroquois used the root of plantain to make a decoction for treating urinary conditions, while the Cherokee used it as a diuretic and to alleviate stomachaches. The Ojibwa tribe utilized the leaves as a poultice for insect bites and wounds, as well as a remedy for skin conditions. The Navajo used plantain as a wash for treating poison ivy and as a topical application for cuts and sores.

In European folk medicine, the leaves of plantain were used for their healing properties. The Anglo-Saxons believed that plantain had magical powers to protect against evil spirits and venomous creatures. The leaves were often chewed and applied as a poultice to soothe insect bites, stings, and skin irritations.

In traditional Chinese medicine, plantain seeds were used to clear heat and toxins from the body, and the leaves were brewed into a tea for its detoxifying and cooling effects.

The versatility of plantain extends beyond its medicinal uses. In some cultures, plantain leaves were woven into mats, baskets, and clothing. The young shoots and flowers were also consumed as a vegetable in culinary preparations.

Modern uses: Studies have indicated that plantain possesses antimicrobial and anti-inflammatory properties. Research published in the Journal of Ethnopharmacology showed that plantain leaf extract exhibited antibacterial activity against various strains of bacteria, including those resistant to conventional antibiotics. Another study in the Journal of Medicinal Food found that plantain leaf extract demonstrated anti-inflammatory effects, inhibiting the release of pro-inflammatory compounds.

Plantain has also shown promise in supporting wound healing. A study published in the Journal of Wound Care investigated the efficacy of a plantain-based ointment in healing venous leg ulcers. The results indicated significant improvements in wound closure and reduction in ulcer size among the study participants.

Furthermore, plantain has been studied for its potential antioxidant and antidiabetic properties. Research published in Food Chemistry demonstrated the antioxidant activity of plantain leaves, which may help protect against oxidative stress and cellular damage. In a study published in the Journal of Ethnopharmacology, plantain extract exhibited antidiabetic effects by lowering blood glucose levels and improving insulin sensitivity in animal models.

Prickly Pear

Cactaceae *(Opuntia spp.)*

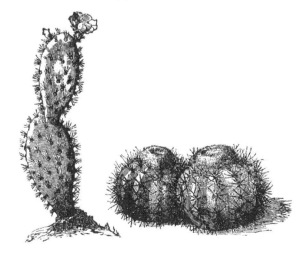

Identification: This cactus is a desert and arid land species that spreads and grows with large oval pads ranging from 4 to 10 inches in size. The pads are covered in thorny leaves of various sizes. The flowers of this cactus are yellowish in color. The fruits it produces vary in color, typically ranging from white to red to purple. They are approximately 2 inches in length and 3 to 4 inches wide.

Habitat: Various species of prickly pear cactus can be found across the United States, from coast to coast. They typically thrive in dry and sometimes sandy areas, as well as limestone hills and badlands. Along roadsides, you can spot them in eastern Colorado, much of Wyoming, Utah, and other arid regions of the western states.

Food: In Mexican cuisine, the green pads of the nopal cactus (Opuntia ficus-indica) are commonly used. They are harvested, cleaned, and prepared by removing the spines and outer skin. Nopales are then diced or sliced and added to dishes such as tacos, salads, soups, and stews. They provide a tangy, slightly acidic taste and a crisp texture.

The fruit of the prickly pear cactus, also known as tunas, is a popular ingredient in both Mexican and Native American cuisines. The red or purple fruits of the Opuntia genus are harvested when ripe and can be enjoyed fresh or used in various preparations. Native American tribes, such as the Hopi and Navajo, have incorporated prickly pear fruit into traditional dishes. They are used to make jams, jellies, and syrups, providing a vibrant and sweet flavor profile. Prickly pear fruit is also juiced and used as a base for beverages, including refreshing drinks and cocktails.

Among Native American tribes, different species of prickly pear hold cultural and culinary significance. For example, the Apache tribe traditionally used the fruit of Opuntia phaeacantha in their diet, consuming it fresh or dried for later use. The Comanche tribe used the pads of Opuntia engelmannii as a food source, cooking them and incorporating them into various dishes.

Traditional uses: Among Native American tribes, such as the Apache and Navajo, the prickly pear cactus was highly regarded for its medicinal properties. The Apache tribe used the prickly pear pads to address digestive issues like indigestion, stomachaches, and diarrhea. They would cook the pads and consume them as a remedy for these ailments.

The Navajo tribe utilized the mucilaginous gel extracted from the prickly pear pads topically to promote wound healing. The gel was applied directly to wounds and burns to soothe and protect the affected area, as it was believed to possess healing and antimicrobial properties.

Some tribes, including the Zuni and Hopi, recognized the prickly pear fruits as beneficial for blood sugar regulation. They consumed the fruits in their raw form or processed them into juices or teas to support healthy blood sugar levels.

In Mexican traditional medicine, the prickly pear cactus was used as a diuretic to promote kidney health. The fruits and pads were consumed to support proper kidney function and alleviate urinary tract issues.

Prickly pear is also known for its anti-inflammatory and antioxidant properties, which have been recognized by various traditional medicinal systems. These properties were believed to help reduce inflammation, alleviate pain, and support overall health.

Modern uses: Studies have shown that prickly pear has potential health benefits due to its rich nutrient profile and bioactive compounds. The fruit of prickly pear is a good source of vitamins, minerals, and antioxidants, which can support overall health and well-being. It has been studied for its potential effects on blood sugar control, lipid metabolism, and antioxidant activity.

Research has also suggested that prickly pear may have anti-inflammatory and anti-ulcer properties, which can help alleviate digestive disorders and promote gastrointestinal health. Additionally, prickly pear extract has been investigated for its potential hepatoprotective effects, meaning it may help protect the liver from damage and support liver health.

Furthermore, prickly pear has been traditionally used for its diuretic properties, helping to increase urine production and promote kidney health. It has also been studied for its potential anti-cancer properties, particularly in relation to its antioxidant and anti-inflammatory effects.

In Andrew Chevallier's Encyclopedia of Medicinal Plants, prickly pear is mentioned for its use in traditional medicine. It has been used to treat various ailments such as diabetes, high cholesterol, inflammation, and digestive disorders. It is often consumed in the form of fruit juice, extracts, or supplements.

Dose and uses: The flowers of prickly pear cactus have astringent properties and can be applied as a poultice over wounds. When prepared as a tea, the flowers are taken for stomach complaints, including diarrhea and irritable bowel syndrome. The ash from the stems can be applied to burns and cuts for its healing properties.

Southwestern holistic practitioners have reported success in using sliced Opuntia pads, with the moist side down, to apply over wounds, bites, stings, and envenomations. This traditional practice is believed to be effective in treating scorpion and recluse spider bites, providing relief and promoting healing.

Gardening tip: The prickly pear cactus can be successfully grown in gardens and is a hardy plant that provides a summer supply of edible flower petals. Having this plant readily available is beneficial due to its antiseptic and sealing properties, which can be useful for various purposes.

Evening Primrose

Onagraceae *(Oenothera biennis L.)*

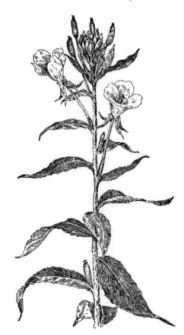

Identification: Evening primrose, scientifically known as *Oenothera biennis*, is a biennial plant that exhibits distinctive features. In the first year, it forms a low-growing rosette of lance-shaped leaves near the ground. In the second year, tall, erect stems emerge, reaching heights of up to six feet or more. These stems often display a reddish tint and are covered in fine hairs.

The leaves are alternate, growing singly along the stem. They are lance-shaped, narrowing to a pointed tip, and measure between two to six inches in length. The edges of the leaves are smooth, and they are typically covered with delicate hairs.

The flowers bloom in the evening, they emit a sweet fragrance to attract moths and other pollinators. The flowers have four petals arranged in a cross-like shape, resembling a miniature hibiscus flower. Usually pale yellow but occasionally white, each flower has a prominent tubular structure at the center that holds the reproductive organs.

Evening primrose follows a biennial life cycle. It germinates from seeds in the first year, forming a rosette of leaves close to the ground. In the second year, tall stems develop, bearing the distinct flowers. After flowering, the plant produces seed capsules that contain numerous tiny seeds. These capsules eventually mature and burst open, dispersing the seeds for future growth.

Habitat: Native to North America, evening primrose thrives in various habitats, including open fields, meadows, prairies, and disturbed areas. It prefers well-drained soil and is commonly found in areas with full or partial sun exposure.

Food: The root of the evening primrose, particularly from the first-year plant, is edible. The new leaves of both the first and second-year plant can be consumed in salads or stir-fries. However, it's important to note that the leaves are tough and require cooking to make them more palatable. The seeds can be extracted from the seed capsule, which resembles a small dried okra pod. The immature seed capsule can be cooked and eaten.

Traditional uses: Among the Ojibwe tribe, evening primrose was valued for its medicinal and nutritional properties. They used the roots to create poultices for wounds and incorporated the seeds and leaves into soups and teas. The Cherokee tribe recognized evening primrose seeds as a valuable food source and used them as a thickening agent in soups and stews. They also employed evening primrose preparations for soothing gastrointestinal discomfort. The Iroquois Confederacy brewed evening primrose roots into a tea to address digestive issues, coughs, and fevers. They also used it as a poultice for skin conditions. Similarly, the Blackfoot tribe utilized evening primrose for medicinal purposes, preparing decoctions for various ailments.

Modern uses: Evening primrose oil, derived from the plant's seeds and rich in gamma-linolenic acid (GLA), holds promise for various health conditions. In pharmacology, studies have explored its effectiveness in managing inflammatory skin conditions such as atopic dermatitis and eczema. Research published in the International Journal of Molecular Sciences in 2019 indicated the potential of evening primrose oil in improving symptoms and reducing inflammation in these conditions. Additionally, evening primrose oil has been studied for its potential benefits in menstrual and hormonal health.

A randomized controlled trial published in the British Journal of Obstetrics and Gynaecology in 2010 demonstrated that evening primrose oil supplementation reduced breast pain and tenderness in women with cyclic mastalgia. In alternative medicine, evening primrose is often used as an herbal remedy for a range of conditions, including hormonal imbalances, arthritis, and diabetic neuropathy. While further research is needed to fully understand its mechanisms and optimal usage guidelines, evening primrose remains a subject of interest for both conventional and alternative medicine practitioners.

Warning:
Before incorporating evening primrose or evening primrose oil into your healthcare routine, it's advisable to consult with a qualified healthcare professional.

While evening primrose is generally considered safe for most individuals, it may interact with certain medications, particularly anticoagulants or blood thinners, and increase the risk of bleeding. Individuals with epilepsy or seizure disorders should use evening primrose with caution, as there have been isolated reports suggesting it may potentially trigger seizures. Additionally, allergic reactions to evening primrose have been reported, although they are relatively rare. If you experience any adverse reactions or symptoms after consuming or using evening primrose, such as skin irritation or gastrointestinal discomfort, discontinue use and seek medical attention.

Veterinarian uses: Seeds of evening primrose can be a great addition to bird feeders, attracting various birds such as finches and sparrows. The seed-laden capsules of the plant provide a nutritious food source for these birds. Evening primrose oil, which contains omega-6 essential fatty acids, is utilized as a component in certain pet supplements, including Healthy Coat Skin & Coat Tabs from Doctors Foster and Smith. These supplements are formulated to support the health and condition of the skin and coat of pets.

Purslane
Portulacaceae *(Portulaca oleracea L.)*

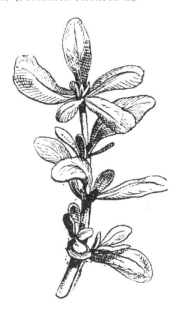

Identification: This low-growing plant is a spreading, fleshy annual with many branched reddish stems. Its leaves are approximately 1" long, thick, fleshy, smooth, and shiny, with an ovate or teardrop shape (resembling a spatula). The flowers are small and inconspicuous, with a yellowish color, and they appear within the leaf rosettes. Purslane blooms from June through November.

Habitat: Found nationwide, both in gardens and waste ground.

Food: Purslane, a common garden plant, is a versatile and nutritious plant that often grows as a volunteer creeper. It can be consumed directly from the ground, added to salads, or chopped and used in soups. One of the notable benefits of purslane is its high content of omega-3 essential fatty acids. Native Americans traditionally incorporated purslane leaves into their diet, both raw and cooked. They would boil it in soups and alongside meats. Today, it can be enjoyed by chopping it into salads, adding it to salad dressings, or even using it as an ingredient in turkey stuffing. In Mexican cuisine, purslane is often eaten raw with meat and green chiles, or cooked with onions, carrots, beans, and chiles. Additionally, purslane can be dried and reconstituted as a food source during the winter months.

Traditional uses: Purslane has been traditionally used as a poultice and skin lotion due to its soothing properties. The decoction of the whole plant was employed as a treatment for worms, while the juice was considered a tonic and used for relieving earaches. Purslane was also believed to possess antidotal properties against certain herbal toxins. Infusions made from the leaf stems were used to alleviate diarrhea, and mashed purslane plant was applied as a poultice to soothe burns and bruises. Additionally, a decoction of the entire plant was used as an antiseptic wash. In terms of internal use, purslane was consumed to alleviate stomachaches.

Modern uses: Purslane is valued for its culinary uses, with its leaves and stems adding a refreshing, tangy flavor to dishes like salads, stir-fries, soups, and sandwiches. Purslane's antioxidant and anti-inflammatory properties have been studied, showing potential benefits in reducing oxidative stress and inflammation in the body. Additionally, it has been explored for its potential positive effects on cardiovascular health, wound healing properties, and gastrointestinal health.

Gardening tips: Purslane can often be found in commercial bags of garden manure, and it can be beneficial to spread it in your garden. By midsummer, you will likely see purslane thriving. Personally, I enjoy adding the succulent leaves to my salads and actively encourage the growth of this plant in my garden. It not only provides a natural and tasty addition to my meals but also serves as a great source of omega-3 fatty acids. If you are not inclined to eat purslane, another option is to add it to your mulch pile. The worms in your compost will certainly appreciate it!

Veterinarian uses: In Mexico purslane is used as an important addition to the feed for wildlife and domestic animals, especially free-range chickens, since it provides essential fatty acids.

Red Clover

Fabaceae *(Trifolium pratense L.)*

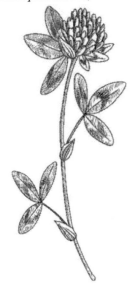

Identification: Red clover, a perennial plant, displays a tri-foliate arrangement with V-shaped markings on its leaflets. The leaflets themselves are ovate in shape and have finely serrated edges. The vibrant flowers of red clover range from pink to red and form dense terminal clusters in a dome-shaped or rounded configuration. This plant typically reaches a height of 12 to 18 inches as it grows.

Habitat: Commonly found in meadows, pastures, and open fields, red clover prefers well-drained soil with moderate moisture levels. It is often seen growing in full or partial sunlight, displaying its iconic pink to purple flower heads atop its slender stems.
This adaptable plant has become naturalized in many regions and is known for its ability to fix nitrogen in the soil, benefiting both itself and surrounding plant species.
Medicinal part: flower and leaves.

Solvent: Boiling water.

Effects: Alterative, antispasmodic, expectorant

Traditional uses: Among the Cherokee tribe, red clover was traditionally used as a remedy for respiratory ailments. It was employed to alleviate coughs, colds, and bronchial congestion, often prepared as an herbal infusion.

The Iroquois tribe valued red clover for its potential to promote women's health. The plant was used to address menstrual irregularities and symptoms associated with menopause. It was often consumed as a tea or incorporated into herbal preparations.
In the traditional practices of the Ojibwe tribe, red clover was employed as a blood purifier. It was believed to cleanse and strengthen the blood, promoting overall wellness. The plant was used in various forms, including teas, poultices, or salves.
Additionally, the Navajo tribe recognized the potential dermatological benefits of red clover. It was used topically to soothe skin irritations, such as rashes, burns, and insect bites. The plant was often prepared as a poultice or added to bathwater.

Modern uses: One notable area of study is red clover's potential to alleviate menopausal symptoms. Research suggests that its isoflavones, such as genistein and daidzein, may have estrogen-like effects, which could help regulate hormonal imbalances. Clinical trials have shown promising results in reducing the frequency and severity of menopausal symptoms.
Red clover has also been investigated for its potential impact on bone health, particularly in postmenopausal women who are at a higher risk of osteoporosis. Some studies suggest that red clover's isoflavones may contribute to improved bone mineral density and a reduced risk of bone loss. However, further research is needed to establish its efficacy in this regard.
In terms of cardiovascular health, researchers have examined red clover's potential benefits. Studies indicate that its isoflavones may have a positive impact on cholesterol levels by helping to regulate lipid profiles. This may contribute to a reduced risk of cardiovascular diseases. However, more research is required to determine the precise mechanisms and long-term effects.

Red Root

Ceanothus spp.

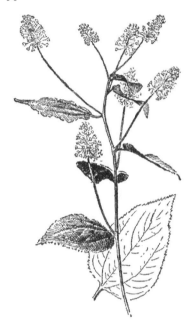

Identification: Red root is a genus of shrubs and small trees belonging to the Rhamnaceae family, with approximately thirty-five native species in North America. In California, red root often grows as small trees, while in Colorado, the common species is Ceanothus fendleri. This particular type of red root is commonly found as a scruffy ground cover with semithorny characteristics, spreading across sizable areas. The seed pods exhibit a vibrant dark reddish color, similar to the hue of the tincture derived from the roots. These triangular pods are relatively small, about half the size of a pea.

Prior to pod formation, the branches produce small clusters of fragrant white flowers, although California varieties may display lilac, pink, or purple flowers. Harvesting the plant can be painful due to the numerous sharp thorny projections on the stems. The outer bark of the root is dark to black in color, and when scraped with a fingernail, it reveals a bright reddish inner bark. The potency of the herb is often indicated by the intensity of this inner bark's red color. The root is best harvested in the spring or fall when the reddish color is most pronounced. When at its most potent, the core of the root may have a slight pinkish tinge, which can be observed throughout the entire root.

The root is characterized by its woody nature and is best cut into two-inch pieces when fresh. Once completely dried, the root becomes extremely hard, making it challenging to cut into smaller pieces.

Habitat: Members of the red root genus can be found thriving on dry and sunny hillsides, spanning from coastal scrub lands to open forest clearings. They have a wide distribution range, ranging from near sea level to elevations of up to 9,000 feet (2,700 m). These plants are abundantly distributed throughout the Rocky Mountains, extending from British Columbia in the north to Colorado in the south. They can also be found in the Cascades of Oregon and California, as well as the Coastal Ranges of California. In the case of Ceanothus fendleri, it is commonly found in pine forests within the altitude range of 4,900 to 9,800 feet. These forests provide a typical habitat for this particular species of red root.

Medicinal part: the root.

Solvent: Boiling water.

Effects: Astringent, Expectorant, Sedative, Antispasmodic.

Traditional uses: According to a translation of the Catawba uses of red root: *"Red root is good indeed. It is a good medicine root for the mouth of a child. When the little one's mouth is sore, wash with it. The roots of red root will prove good when nipples become sore. Using the red root make it up into medicine. You will be better and the little child will be better."*

Modern uses: Red root, with its high content of prussic acid, known as "Ceanothine," is recognized for its remarkable properties, particularly in relation to the lymph system. It plays a significant role in aiding the lymph system's efficient processing of waste cells, leading to a reduction in the duration of colds and flu. Herbalists have noted that red root may contribute to an increase in T-cell count, making it a valuable addition to the treatment of immune system disorders, including AIDS. Its unique properties make red root a beneficial herb for supporting immune health.

Dose and usage: Red root has been found to be beneficial in the treatment of inflamed tonsils, sore throat, and enlarged lymph nodes in various parts of the body. For inflamed tonsils or a sore throat, it is recommended to take the herbal tincture orally, allowing it to mix with saliva and trickle directly down the throat onto the affected areas.

The recommended dosage is 30 drops of the tincture per 150 pounds of body weight, taken three times a day for chronic conditions, and up to six times a day during acute episodes. This dosage regimen can help alleviate symptoms and promote healing.

Wildlife: Red root is a favorite food among deer, particularly the Arizonan mule deer. During the summer, it can make up to 10% of their forage.

Sagebrush

Asteraceae *(Artemisia tridentata Nutt.)*

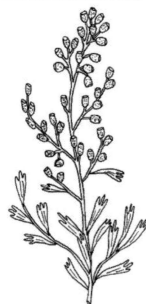

Identification: Sagebrush is a gray and fragrant shrub that can grow up to 7 feet in height. It has distinctive wedge-shaped leaves that are lobed with three teeth and broad at the tip, tapering towards the base. The flowers of sagebrush are yellow and brownish, arranged in spreading, long, narrow clusters. They typically bloom from July to October. The plant produces hairy achenes as seeds. Sagebrush is often recognized for its aromatic scent.

Habitat: Commonly found in dry areas of various states in the western United States, including Wyoming, Washington, Montana, Texas, New Mexico, California, Idaho, Oregon, Colorado, and other locations. It thrives in these arid regions and is well adapted to the dry and rugged landscapes of the West.

Food: The seeds of sagebrush can be consumed in different forms for various purposes. They can be ground into flour and used as a source of sustenance in survival situations. Additionally, the seeds have been utilized to add fragrance and flavor to liqueurs.

Traditional uses: Sagebrush was used for smudging and sweeping to cleanse and purify individuals from negative energies and evil spirits. The leaves of sagebrush were brewed into a tea to address infections, provide relief during childbirth, and as a soothing wash for sore eyes. When soaked in water, the leaves were applied as a poultice to promote healing of wounds.
The tea made from sagebrush leaves was also employed to alleviate stomachaches. In sweat baths, the branches of sagebrush were used as switches. The infusion of sagebrush was employed to treat ailments such as sore throats, coughs, colds, bronchitis, and headaches. It was also used as a wash for sores, cuts, and pimples. Internally, the decoction of sagebrush was believed to have anti-diarrheal properties and was consumed to relieve constipation. Native Americans also rubbed the herb over their bodies to hide the human scent when hunting.

Modern uses: It still has a role of paramount importance in Native American religious rituals, including smudging, sweeping, sweat lodge, and generally as a disinfectant. Studies have shown that Gram-positive bacteria are sensitive to the oil of A. tridentata.

Other uses: Sagebrush can be a valuable addition to a hot bath, hot tub, or sweat lodge. Adding this herb to your bathing experience can provide a fragrant and disinfecting cleanse, as well as promote relaxation. In desert regions, sagebrush is often the primary source of firewood.

Veterinarian uses: Sagebrush is known for its repellent properties against moths and fleas. In traditional usage, a decoction of the herb was applied to the wounds of domestic animals to help keep pests away.

Sassafras

Lauraceae *(Sassafras albidum [Nutt.] Nees)*

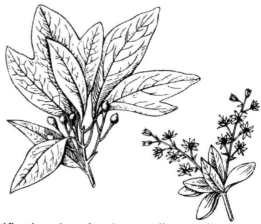

Identification: Sassafras is a small to medium-sized tree that can reach a height of 50 feet. The distinctive leaves of sassafras are mitten-shaped and irregular in appearance. The twigs and roots of the tree emit a pleasant and aromatic scent reminiscent of root beer. The flowers of sassafras are yellow-green in color. It is worth noting that the branches and twigs of the tree are fragile and can break easily.

Habitat: Located along edges of woods, in dry, well-drained areas along oak and hickory in Eastern forests and Midwestern and prairie states.

Food: Dried spring leaves of sassafras are commonly used as a spice called filé in Cajun cuisine, particularly in dishes like gumbo. To use the dried leaves, simply crush them into a powder and sprinkle it as a seasoning. The leaf powder can also be spread on various savory dishes such as pasta, soup, and cheese.
Additionally, the roots of sassafras can be used to prepare a tea by peeling the root, discarding the peel, and boiling the pith.

Traditional uses: Extracts from the sassafras plant were commonly used to produce perfume and root beer. The oil derived from the roots was once utilized as an antiseptic, although its use was discontinued in 1960 when the USDA deemed it unsafe due to its safrole content, which is considered a carcinogen. In traditional healing practices, a decoction made from the roots was consumed as a tonic and blood purifier to alleviate various conditions such as acne, syphilis, gonorrhea, arthritis, colic, menstrual pain, and upset stomach. Additionally, a tea made from the bark was used to induce sweating.

Modern uses: Sassafras is not scientifically proven to have medicinal effects, and it is important to exercise caution when consuming sassafras products due to the toxic effects of safrole. The dried leaves of the plant are used in small amounts as a spice, and chewing on a twig can provide a refreshing taste, but it is not recommended to use it excessively. Recent evidence has shown that safrole, a component found in sassafras oil, is being added as an adulterant to the drug Ecstasy in Cambodia.

Warning: Sassafras oils, due to its active component safrole, may be carcinogenic.

Other uses: When camping, you can utilize sassafras twigs as a makeshift toothbrush, commonly known as a chew stick. By chewing on the end of the twig until it becomes bristly, you can then use the bristles to clean your teeth and gums. Slippery elm twigs, which are abundant in antioxidants, can also serve as excellent chewing sticks. The flavor of these twigs is refreshing, and their sap acts as a mild sialagogue, stimulating the production of saliva.

Saint John's Wort

Hyperacaceae *(Hypericum perforatum L.)*

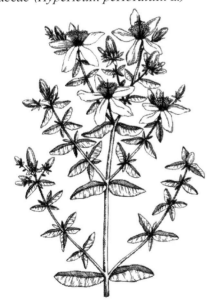

Identification: St. John's Wort typically grows as a perennial plant, reaching an average height of 1 to 3 feet (30 to 90 centimeters). The plant has numerous erect stems covered in small, oblong-shaped leaves that grow in pairs along the stems. The leaves are dotted with translucent glands, which give them a perforated appearance when held up to the light.

During the summer months, St. John's Wort blooms with bright yellow flowers. Each flower consists of five petals with numerous stamens, giving it a vibrant and eye-catching appearance. The flowers often have tiny black or dark red dots along the edges of the petals.

When observing the plant closely, you may notice that the stems exude a reddish sap when broken or bruised. This characteristic is more apparent in the flowering tops and leaves of the plant.

Habitat: St. John's Wort can be found across the country on roadsides, waste grounds, fields, prairies, and along stream banks and riverbanks. It is a versatile plant that is also cultivated in gardens, resulting in numerous garden varieties of St. John's Wort.

Traditional uses: One notable area of study is St. John's Wort's potential as an antidepressant. Numerous clinical trials have explored its effectiveness in reducing symptoms of mild to moderate depression. The herb's active constituents, including hypericin and hyperforin, are believed to play a role in modulating neurotransmitters in the brain, such as serotonin, dopamine, and norepinephrine.

In addition to its antidepressant properties, St. John's Wort has been investigated for its potential anxiolytic effects. Studies suggest it may have a role in reducing symptoms of generalized anxiety disorder and stress-related conditions. However, further research is needed to establish its efficacy and safety in these areas.

Topically, St. John's Wort has shown potential in aiding the treatment of certain skin conditions, such as mild burns, wounds, and inflammation. Research has indicated its potential for wound healing and anti-inflammatory effects when applied as an ointment or infused oil.

Furthermore, St. John's Wort has been studied for its potential in managing neuropathic pain, which is characterized by nerve damage. Preliminary research suggests that its active components may possess analgesic properties, potentially providing relief from conditions such as diabetic neuropathy and sciatica. However, more studies are required to establish its effectiveness and optimal dosing.

It is important to note that St. John's Wort may interact with certain medications, including antidepressants, birth control pills, and anticoagulants. Therefore, it is crucial to consult with a healthcare professional before incorporating St. John's Wort into your regimen, especially if you have underlying medical conditions or are taking medications.

Warning: While Saint John's Wort (Hypericum perforatum) may have potential therapeutic benefits, it is important to be cautious and aware of its risks. This herb can interact with certain medications, potentially reducing their effectiveness. It may also increase photosensitivity, making your skin more susceptible to sunburns. It's important to consult with a healthcare professional before using Saint John's Wort, especially if you are taking medications or have a history of photosensitivity. Start with a low dosage, monitor your body's response, and discontinue use if needed. Remember, herbal remedies are not a substitute for professional medical advice.

Seneca Snakeroot
Polygalaceae *(Polygala senega)*

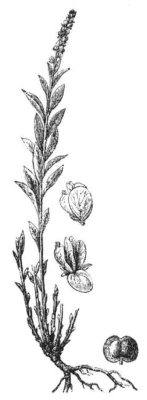

Identification: Seneca snakeroot, also known as Milkwort, is a perennial plant characterized by its firm, hairy, branching root with a thick bark. It produces several annual stems that are erect and smooth, typically reaching a height of 8-14 inches. The leaves are alternate, lanceolate in shape with a sharpish point, and smooth in texture. The plant bears small white flowers with five sepals and three petals. The capsules of the flowers are small, two-celled, and two-valved. Seneca snakeroot is commonly found in rocky woods and on hillsides, and it typically blooms in July.

Habitat: Seneca Snakeroot (Polygala senega) is a perennial herbaceous plant that thrives in open woodlands, forest edges, and prairies across eastern and central North America. It can be found in regions spanning from the eastern United States, including states such as Virginia, West Virginia, Pennsylvania, and New York, extending northward into parts of Canada.

Within the Polygala genus, Seneca Snakeroot is one of the most well-known species. It boasts a distinctive appearance, featuring tall stalks topped with clusters of small, white flowers and a basal rosette of lance-shaped leaves. Its ability to adapt to various habitats and climates allows it to flourish in a range of ecosystems throughout its distribution.

Effects: expectorant and antispasmodic

Medicinal Part: The root.

Solvents: Water, dilute alcohol.

Traditional uses: In the early eighteenth century, the Scottish physician Tennant learned about the use of Seneca snakeroot from the Senega Indians for treating snake bites. Intrigued by its potential, Tennant investigated the herb and discovered that an infusion of the dried roots could effectively stimulate salivation.

Among the Ojibwa people, Seneca snakeroot is known as bi'jikiwuk', which translates to "buffalo medicine". When used medicinally by the Ojibwa, it is often combined with one to seven other herbs, resulting in a combination also referred to as bi'jikiwuk. Seneca snakeroot is considered the key herb in this preparation, as it is believed to be essential for its efficacy. Bi'jikiwuk' was highly regarded as a war medicine among the Ojibwa, believed to enhance strength and possess potent healing properties. It was customary for Ojibwa warriors to chew the herb and spray it on their bodies and equipment.

Seneca snakeroot was also believed to have the power to counteract negative influences directed towards an individual. It was taken four times a day throughout one's life and was thought to enhance vitality and personal power.

Dose and usage: Use it for colds and flu, for croup, pleurisy, chronic catarrh, asthma, and coughs. The poultice can be used as an anti-inflammatory for rheumatism and swellings. The root tea also induces sweating and is a moderately good diuretic.

Slippery Elm
Ulmaceae (*Ulmus rubra* Muhl.)

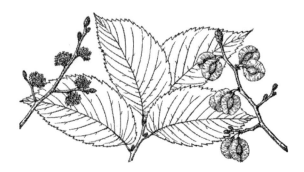

Identification: Slippery Elm (Ulmus rubra), a notable tree species, exhibits distinctive botanical characteristics that aid in its accurate identification. This medium to large-sized deciduous tree is indigenous to eastern North America and commonly thrives in environments such as moist forests, stream banks, and bottomlands.

The bark of Slippery Elm serves as a key identifying feature. It showcases a reddish-brown to grayish-brown hue and possesses deep furrows, contributing to its rugged appearance. Notably, the inner bark of Slippery Elm exhibits a mucilaginous quality, rendering it slippery and gel-like when moistened. This unique attribute has earned the species its common name and also makes it a valuable resource in traditional herbal medicine practices.

The leaves of Slippery Elm are alternate, simple, and ovate in shape, with serrated edges. Their upper surface displays a dark green coloration, while the underside appears paler. During the autumn season, these leaves undergo a remarkable transformation, turning into vibrant shades of yellow, thereby augmenting the visual splendor of the landscape.
Mature Slippery Elm trees produce inconspicuous flowers arranged in clusters. These flowers eventually develop into small, flat, winged seeds that facilitate dispersal via wind.

Habitat: North America, predominantly east of the Missouri River in forests and fields.

Effects: Demulcent, emollient, expectorant, diuretic, astringent

Medicinal Part: The inner and outer bark

Solvents: Water, dilute alcohol.

Traditional uses: The inner bark of slippery elm has been traditionally used to prepare infusions for treating gastritis and ulcers. The bark extract is known for its antioxidant properties and its ability to provide a mucilaginous and demulcent effect, making it useful as an emollient. Externally, the extract is often applied as a wound dressing, particularly for burns, and it has also been used to alleviate symptoms of gout, rheumatism, and arthritis. Internally, it has been employed for treating gastritis and ulcers in the stomach and duodenum. However, it's important to note that the outer bark of slippery elm was historically used for inducing abortions, which is not recommended or supported by modern medical practices.

Modern uses: Slippery Elm (Ulmus rubra) has been the subject of scientific research and trials, revealing potential modern uses in various areas. The mucilaginous inner bark of Slippery Elm has garnered attention for its potential benefits in several applications.
One area of research focuses on Slippery Elm's potential to soothe digestive discomfort. Studies suggest that the mucilage in its bark may help protect the stomach lining and provide relief for conditions such as gastritis, gastric ulcers, and irritable bowel syndrome (IBS). Although further research is needed, preliminary findings indicate Slippery Elm's potential in supporting gastrointestinal health. Slippery Elm has also been studied for its potential as a natural demulcent and expectorant for respiratory ailments. Research suggests that it may alleviate coughs, sore throats, and respiratory irritation.

The soothing properties of Slippery Elm could help reduce throat inflammation and temporarily alleviate coughing. Additionally, its mucilage content may assist in reducing mucus production, aiding in clearer airways. Furthermore, Slippery Elm has been explored as a topical remedy for skin conditions. Its mucilaginous properties have shown potential in providing relief for skin irritations, burns, and minor wounds when formulated into creams or ointments. However, further research is required to confirm its efficacy and potential side effects.

Dose and usage: Slippery Elm is commonly available in various forms, including powder, capsules, lozenges, and teas.
For gastrointestinal support, Slippery Elm powder is often mixed with water to create a soothing gel-like consistency. A typical dosage ranges from 1 to 2 teaspoons of powdered bark mixed with an appropriate amount of water, consumed two to three times per day. It is important to drink plenty of water after ingestion to ensure proper hydration.

When using Slippery Elm for respiratory concerns, lozenges or teas are commonly utilized. Lozenges should be dissolved slowly in the mouth as needed to relieve sore throat or cough symptoms. Teas can be prepared by steeping 1 to 2 teaspoons of Slippery Elm bark in hot water for 10 to 15 minutes before straining and consuming.

Usnea
Parmeliaceae (*Usnea spp.*)

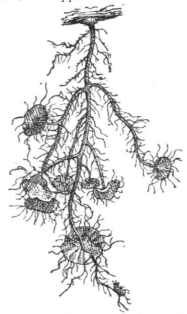

Identification: Usnea is a type of parasitic epiphyte known as a tree lichen. It is a symbiotic organism composed of both a fungus and an algae. It can be found hanging from conifers in the form of numerous hairlike structures. Usnea lichens have a light gray-green color and can be identified by carefully separating the outer mycelia sheath to reveal a tough, white central core or cord. This central core is unique to Usnea and distinguishes it from other clinging lichens. Usnea is sometimes referred to as "old man's beard" due to its appearance.

Habitat: Forests of the Pacific Northwest and in the broader north temperate climate zone of the West; worldwide in moist and damp habitats.

Medicinal Part: The whole plant.

Solvent: Water.

Effects: Carminative, Mucilaginous, Demulcent, Antiseptic.

Traditional uses: Among the Navajo tribe, Usnea has been traditionally used for its antimicrobial properties. The lichen was often collected and prepared as a tea or decoction, which was then applied topically to treat wounds, cuts, and skin infections. The Navajo people recognized Usnea's ability to support healing and prevent infection, incorporating it into their traditional medicine practices. The Ojibwa tribe also recognized the therapeutic potential of Usnea.

They utilized the lichen as a natural remedy for respiratory ailments such as bronchitis and sore throats. Usnea was prepared as a decoction or infusion, and the resulting liquid was consumed orally to alleviate coughs and soothe irritated airways. Its mucilaginous properties were thought to provide a soothing effect on the respiratory system. Similarly, the Salish tribe employed Usnea for its antimicrobial and wound-healing properties. They would gather the lichen and create poultices or salves, which were applied externally to wounds, burns, and skin infections. The Salish people valued Usnea as a natural remedy to promote healing and prevent bacterial growth in skin-related ailments.

Modern uses: Research on Usnea has revealed its antimicrobial properties, particularly against a variety of bacteria and fungi. Several studies have demonstrated its effectiveness against common pathogens, including Staphylococcus aureus and Candida species. These findings suggest that Usnea may have applications in the treatment of infections, both topically and internally. Moreover, Usnea has shown promise as an immune-modulating agent. Some studies have indicated its potential in stimulating immune system activity and enhancing the body's defense mechanisms.

This immunomodulatory effect may contribute to its traditional uses for respiratory conditions and support overall immune health. In pharmacological research, Usnea has been explored for its potential antioxidant and anti-inflammatory properties. Studies have suggested that Usnea extracts possess significant antioxidant activity, which can help combat oxidative stress and protect cells from damage. Additionally, its anti-inflammatory properties may have implications for managing inflammatory conditions and supporting overall well-being. In recognition of its therapeutic potential, Usnea has received approval from Commission E for its traditional uses in supporting respiratory health, promoting wound healing, and as an antimicrobial agent.

Dose and usage: Usnea can be utilized in various forms for different applications. When powdered or used in its whole form, it can be applied topically to skin infections with favorable outcomes. It can also be tinctured in alcohol, consumed whole, or infused as a tea for internal issues ranging from tuberculosis to acute bacterial infections. As a douche, it has been employed to treat trichomonas and yeast infections.

Herbalists commonly rely on usnea for the management of fungal infections, acute bacterial infections, lupus, trichomonas, mastitis, varicose and tropic ulcers, second- and third-degree burns, plastic surgery, athlete's foot, ringworm, urinary tract infections, colds, flu, bronchitis, pleurisy, pneumonia, tuberculosis, sinus infections, staphylococcus, dysentery, and streptococcus.

Other uses: Usnea lichen has been utilized by campers as a stuffing material for mattresses and pillows, providing a soft bedding layer under sleeping bags. In addition, historical accounts mention that Nitinaht women used usnea as sanitary napkins and as diaper material for babies. These uses demonstrate the versatility and resourcefulness of usnea in various practical applications.

Valerian

Valerianaceae *(Valeriana sitchensis Bong.; V. officinalis L.)*

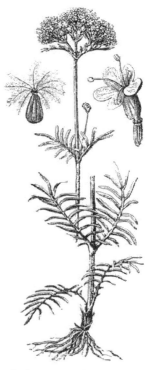

Identification: Valerian typically grows to a height of 3 to 5 feet (0.9 to 1.5 meters) and features a cluster of small, fragrant flowers at the top of sturdy stems. The flowers can range in color from white to pink, creating a visually appealing display. The plant's leaves are feather-like, with pairs of lance-shaped leaflets that grow in an opposite arrangement along the stem. The most distinctive feature of Valerian is its strong, pungent odor.

The roots of the Valerian plant emit an earthy scent that is often described as musky or reminiscent of dirty socks. This unique aroma, which is particularly noticeable when the roots are harvested or disturbed, sets Valerian apart from other plants.

If cultivating Valerian in a garden, it is recommended to provide well-drained soil and ample sunlight. The plant can be propagated through seeds or root divisions, and it may take up to two years for the roots to reach their full potency.

Habitat: Valerian (Valeriana officinalis) thrives in moist and fertile habitats such as damp meadows, marshes, and riverbanks. It prefers partial shade but can tolerate full sun in cooler climates. Valerian's habitat requirements include well-drained soil, access to water sources, and relatively low competition from other plants. This herbaceous perennial is naturally found in temperate regions of Europe, Asia, and North America.

Medicinal Part: The root.

Solvent: Water.

Effects: Antispasmodic, Calmative, Stimulating Tonic, Nervine.

Traditional uses: The roots of Valeriana sitchensis, a specific species of valerian, were traditionally used by decocting them in water to create a remedy for pain, colds, and diarrhea. Additionally, a poultice made from the root was applied topically to treat cuts, wounds, bruises, and inflammation, providing soothing relief.

Modern uses: Only few people still use Valeriana sitchensis in traditional ways, while Valeriana officinalis is commonly used by herbalists today. In a double-blind study, an aqueous extract of Valeriana officinalis root showed significant relaxing effects on individuals with poor or irregular sleep patterns and smokers. It is often combined with other herbs such as hops (Humulus lupulus) and skullcap (Scutellaria lateriflora) for enhanced benefits. Valerian is considered a nerve tonic by herbalists and is often used in combination with other herbs such as skullcap, blue vervain (Verbena hastata), mistletoe (Viscum album), gentian (Gentiana lutea), and peppermint (Mentha piperita) to increase its effectiveness. Valerian's effect on gamma amino butyric acid (GABA) may help reduce blood pressure and alleviate mild depression. This chemical is also found in evening primrose seeds and various tomato varieties.

Dose and uses: Valerian is well-known for its stress-reducing and tension-relieving properties, making it a popular choice for individuals dealing with insomnia.

Watercress

Brassicaceae *(Nasturtium officinale L.)*

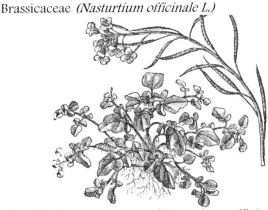

Identification: Watercress (Nasturtium officinale) is a perennial aquatic herb displays small, rounded leaves with slight lobes along slender stems, a characteristic that aids in its identification. The leaves showcase a vibrant green hue and possess a distinct peppery flavor, owing to the presence of compounds like glucosinolates.

During its flowering period, watercress produces delicate white flowers that are arranged in loose clusters at the stem ends.

Habitat: Watercress is typically found in aquatic habitats, such as streams and ponds, where it thrives in shallow water or moist soil. Its trailing or floating stems and emergent leaves contribute to its adaptive nature.

Medicinal Parts: Leaves, root.

Solvent: Water.

Effects: Tonic, Stimulant, Blood purifying.

Food: One of the simplest and most satisfying ways to enjoy watercress is in a fresh salad. Its vibrant green leaves add a refreshing element, while its peppery bite provides a delightful contrast to milder ingredients. One of my easy go-to salads includes crispy watercress leaves, juicy tomatoes, creamy avocado slices, and a tangy vinaigrette, creating a burst of flavors and textures that dance on the palate.

Watercress also lends itself beautifully to soups and stir-fries. Adding a handful of watercress to a pot of vegetable or chicken soup infuses it with a unique peppery essence, elevating the overall taste and transforming a humble dish into a culinary delight. In stir-fries, watercress adds a vibrant pop of color and a delightful peppery kick, perfectly complementing other ingredients such as mushrooms, garlic, and ginger.

You can also make a homemade watercress pesto. Blending together fresh watercress, toasted pine nuts, garlic, Parmesan cheese, and a drizzle of olive oil created a vibrant and flavorful sauce. This vibrant green pesto is a delightful companion to pasta dishes, spreading its herbaceous and peppery goodness with each bite.

Traditional uses: Watercress has a long history in the pharmaceutical record, with references dating back to Hippocrates. It has been described as a heart tonic, stimulating expectorant, and digestive aid. Watercress is known for its beneficial effects on respiratory health and is often used to alleviate symptoms of coughs, colds, and bronchitis. It is also recognized for its ability to relieve gas and promote healthy digestion. As a diuretic, watercress helps release fluid retention and supports kidney and bladder health. In Mexican tradition, watercress is revered as a spring tonic and is often dampened and grilled over charcoal for consumption.

Modern uses: Watercress is indeed a nutrient-rich plant, packed with vitamins, minerals, and beneficial compounds like isothiocyanates. Including watercress in your diet, such as in 8 ounces of V8 cocktail juice, can contribute to your daily vegetable intake and provide essential nutrients. The isothiocyanates found in watercress have been associated with potential cancer-protective effects. Additionally, watercress has been approved by Commission E for its traditional use in treating coughs and bronchitis.

Gardening notes: It is true that watercress growing in the wild can be exposed to potentially contaminated water sources. Therefore, if you plan to consume watercress, it is recommended to grow it in your own garden or obtain it from a trusted and reliable source. If you relocate it to your garden, it will purify itself in a few weeks.

Wildlife: Watercress mats can indeed provide habitats for various aquatic organisms, including snails, insect larvae, and frogs. The presence of these creatures can attract fish, making watercress mats an interesting spot for anglers, especially in a trout stream.

White Poplar

Salicaceae *(Populus spp.: P. balsamifera L.; P. tremuloides Michx.; P. deltoides Bartr. ex Marsh)*

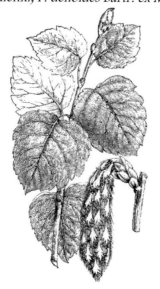

Identification: White Poplar (Populus alba) is a deciduous tree with distinctive features for identification. It can grow tall, reaching heights of 50 to 80 feet (15 to 24 meters). The leaves are broadly triangular, deeply lobed, and have a silvery-white underside. The bark is smooth and starts off grayish-green, aging to gray or white with shallow furrows. In spring, small inconspicuous flowers form in long catkins. White Poplar prefers well-drained soils and is commonly found in open fields, meadows, and along riverbanks.

Habitat: Poplar species, including Eastern Cottonwood (Populus deltoides), Black Poplar (Populus nigra), White Poplar (Populus alba), Quaking Aspen (Populus tremuloides), and Bigtooth Aspen (Populus grandidentata), have diverse habitats and distributions across the United States. Eastern Cottonwood is found in the eastern and central states, while Black Poplar occurs in localized regions. White Poplar has naturalized in various states.
Quaking Aspen has a wide distribution from Alaska to Mexico, and Bigtooth Aspen is native to the eastern U.S. Poplars adapt to different environments, including bottomlands, floodplains, open fields, and riparian areas.

Medicinal Parts: Leaves, bark, buds.
Solvent: Boiling water (soak buds in alcohol, then boiling water will expel their properties).
Effects: Tonic, Diuretic, Stimulant, Febrifuge.

Food: Balsam poplar cambium, also known as the inner bark, can be consumed raw and is known to be edible. In certain traditional practices, the cambium was boiled, dried, and pounded into a flour-like consistency. This flour was then mixed with corn flour (masa) and/or wheat flour to make bread. Shoots, leaf buds, and catkins of the balsam poplar tree are also edible and are often simmered in water to enhance their flavor, the are also an excellent source of vitamin C.

Traditional uses: Balsam poplar was highly valued by Native Americans, who regarded it as a panacea or cure-all plant. The decoction of the inner bark was used as a tonic to invigorate the body and as a remedy for colds. It was also believed to help cleanse the system after acute infections. The maceration and decoction of the bark were applied as a wash to treat rheumatism. Pioneers, on the other hand, collected the reddish resin that covered the new-growth leaf buds. They dissolved and thinned this resin using an alcohol solvent to create a salve. This salve was then applied to wounds to promote healing and relieve inflammation.

Modern uses: The bark of White Poplar contains various compounds, including salicin, which is a precursor to aspirin. It has been historically used for its analgesic and anti-inflammatory properties. White Poplar preparations, such as infusions or tinctures, have been employed to alleviate mild pain, reduce inflammation, and support general well-being.
In addition, White Poplar has received recognition from the Commission E for relieving mild joint pain and supporting the body's natural inflammatory response.

Although scientific research on White Poplar is limited, preliminary studies have shown promising results. Some studies have indicated the potential anti-inflammatory and antioxidant properties of White Poplar extracts, which may contribute to its traditional uses for pain relief and supporting overall health.

Warning: Do not use poplar if you are allergic to aspirin or other salicylates.

Other uses: Poplar is generally not considered a preferred choice for firewood due to its lower energy content and tendency to produce more smoke and sparks compared to other hardwoods. While poplar tree sap can be tapped, it contains relatively low sugar content, requiring more boiling to produce a sweet syrup compared to other tree species.
Dead and dying poplars are a favorite place to find oyster mushrooms.

Willow
Salicaceae *(Salix spp.: S. alba L.; S. nigra Marsh)*

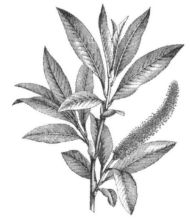

Identification: Willow trees or shrubs can vary in size, ranging from 10 feet to over 100 feet tall. They have lanceolate leaves with fine teeth along the edges. The male flowers are yellow, while the female flowers are green and densely clustered in catkins. The white willow (S. alba), also known as weeping willow, has branches that droop, while the black willow (S. nigra) is erect and large with branches that shed. Both species thrive in moist soil conditions and are often associated with wetlands.

Habitat: Willows can be found across the United States, extending north to the Arctic region. They are commonly found in various habitats such as marshy areas, mountain streams, thickets, lakeshores, and along streams and rivers.

Medicinal Part: The bark.

Solvent: Boiling water.

Effects: Aphrodisiac, Tonic, Astringent, Detergent.

Traditional uses: The use of willow bark as a natural remedy can be traced back to Native American tribes such as the Cherokee, Iroquois, and Mohegan. These tribes traditionally employed willow bark for its analgesic (pain-relieving) and antipyretic (fever-reducing) properties.
The Cherokee tribe, for instance, recognized the value of willow bark as a pain reliever. They would brew a decoction of willow bark and use it to alleviate headaches, muscle pain, and joint discomfort. The infusion was also consumed to reduce fevers and ease general discomfort associated with illnesses.

Similarly, the Iroquois tribe utilized willow bark to address various ailments. They would prepare a tea from the inner bark and use it to relieve headache pain and alleviate fever symptoms. The Iroquois also employed willow bark topically, applying it as a poultice or wash to soothe skin irritations, rashes, and burns.
Among the Mohegan tribe, willow bark was valued for its medicinal properties. It was commonly used as a natural pain reliever for headaches, toothaches, and general body aches. The Mohegan people would chew on the bark or create infusions for internal or external applications.

Modern uses: The extraction of willow bark, which contains salicin, has been approved by Commission E for the treatment of pain and rheumatism. However, it should not be used by individuals who are allergic to salicylates, as it may cause an allergic reaction.

Warning: Numerous scientific studies have examined the effects of aspirin in double-blind, placebo-controlled, and double-crossover trials, providing substantial evidence for its therapeutic benefits. In contrast, the specific effects of salicin from willow extraction have not been extensively studied using the same rigorous research methods. It is important to note that the infusion or decoction of willow contains a variety of compounds in addition to salicin. Recent research indicates that willow has the ability to accumulate cadmium, a toxic metal, in its tissues when present in the soil. This is a characteristic observed in all species of willow. Considering these factors, I would opt for a simple aspirin.

Gardening tip: Take caution when gardening near or under a willow tree, as its shallow and extensive root system can compete with nearby plants for water and nutrients. This may result in the distress of neighboring garden plants. Additionally, when a willow tree dies, it's important to note that its widespread root system will have depleted the soil of nutrients. Before replanting the area, it is advisable to replenish and improve the soil to ensure optimal conditions for new plant growth.

Witch Hazel

Hamamelidaceae *(Hamamelis virginiana L.)*

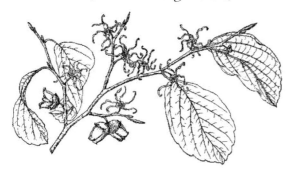

Identification: The leaves of witch hazel are alternate, simple, and broadly ovate with wavy or toothed edges. They typically measure 3 to 6 inches (7.6 to 15.2 centimeters) in length and turn vibrant shades of yellow, orange, or red during the autumn season. The leaves provide an attractive visual display throughout the year. The flowers bloom during late fall or winter, usually from October to December, when other plants are dormant. They have four narrow, ribbon-like petals with a distinctive crimped appearance. Their color varies from pale yellow to bright orange, creating a striking contrast against the backdrop of the dormant winter landscape. The bark is smooth, grayish-brown, and marked with shallow furrows, providing an interesting texture to the shrub's overall appearance.

Habitat: Witch hazel shrubs are typically found in woodland areas, forests, and along the edges of streams or wetlands, primarily east of the Mississippi River in coastal forests. They prefer moist, well-drained soils and can tolerate both partial shade and full sun..

Medicinal Part: The bark and concrete juice.

Solvent: Boiling water and alcohol.

Effects: Stimulant, Expectorant, Diuretic, Antiseptic, Disinfectant.

Traditional uses: The Potawatomi tribe recognized the medicinal properties of witch hazel and utilized it in their traditional healing practices. They made poultices from the bark and leaves of witch hazel, applying them externally to alleviate skin irritations, inflammation, and minor wounds. The Potawatomi also used witch hazel decoctions as a natural remedy for sore throats and respiratory ailments.

The Mohegan tribe valued witch hazel for its astringent properties. They extracted the tannins from the bark and used them as a wash or compress for skin conditions such as rashes, bruises, and insect bites. The Mohegan people also employed witch hazel as an eyewash to relieve eye discomfort and inflammation.

Among the Iroquois tribe, witch hazel was considered a sacred plant with multifaceted uses. They utilized various parts of the plant for medicinal purposes. The bark was brewed into a tea that was consumed to alleviate stomachaches, cold symptoms, and fevers. Witch hazel leaves were used in poultices and compresses to relieve pain, reduce swelling, and soothe skin irritations. Additionally, the Iroquois burned the twigs of witch hazel during spiritual ceremonies and purification rituals.

The Cherokee tribe valued witch hazel for its astringent and anti-inflammatory properties. They incorporated it into their traditional medicine to treat skin conditions, minor wounds, and hemorrhoids. Witch hazel extracts were also used as a mouthwash for oral hygiene and to alleviate toothaches.

Modern uses: Witch hazel water, derived from the leaves and bark of the plant, is known for its astringent properties. It is used as a natural toner to cleanse and tighten the skin, helping to reduce the appearance of pores and control excess oil. Witch hazel water is also valued for its soothing effect on skin irritations, such as minor cuts, burns, and insect bites.

Several studies have explored the potential benefits of witch hazel in dermatological applications. Research has indicated that witch hazel extracts possess anti-inflammatory, antioxidant, and antimicrobial properties, which may contribute to its effectiveness in promoting skin health and combating certain skin conditions.

Additionally, witch hazel has been investigated for its potential use in oral health. Studies have shown that witch hazel extracts may help reduce oral bacteria, gingivitis, and periodontal inflammation. These findings suggest that witch hazel could have a role in maintaining oral hygiene and supporting gum health.

Furthermore, witch hazel has been studied for its potential use in the management of certain digestive issues. Research has suggested that witch hazel extracts may possess anti-inflammatory and antispasmodic properties, which could help alleviate symptoms associated with gastrointestinal disorders such as diarrhea and irritable bowel syndrome (IBS). However, more research is needed to fully understand its effectiveness and optimal dosage in this regard.

Other uses: Traditionally, the twigs of witch hazel have been used to create divining rods for the practice of dowsing, also known as "water witching." This technique involves seeking out locations with underground water sources before digging or drilling water wells. Witch hazel branches, along with willow and peach tree branches, were commonly used for this purpose by early Americans.

The process involved holding a flexible Y- or L-shaped twig in front of a person as they slowly moved across the area where groundwater was being sought. If the twig inclined downward or exhibited any twitching movements, it was believed to indicate the presence of water beneath the surface.

Wormwood

Asteraceae *(Artemisia campestris L. subsp. caudata [Michx.] H.M. Hall & Clem.)*

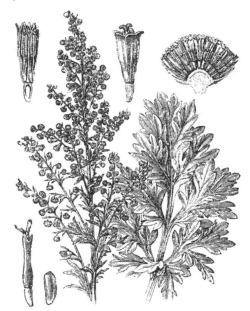

Identification: Artemisia species comprise numerous plants found worldwide. A. campestris is not aromatic, unlike many other artemisias. It is a biennial, a second-year flowering plant or a shortlived perennial. First-year leaves are a basal rosette, each leaf up to 4" long and 3" wide. Leaves are deeply divided with narrow, linear lobes; color is grayish blue. Upper mature (second-year) leaves have a green undersurface and whitish-green top. On the mature plant, leaves get smaller and more deeply cut or linear toward the top of the plant. Leaves are hairy at first and become smooth as they mature. Stems are branched, light green to red in color. Young stem ends are matte with fine hairs.

The cobweblike hairs disappear as the stem grows. Also known as dune wormwood or field sagewort. Many species of wormwood, also known as mugwort, are called "sage." This is a misnomer as they are not related to the sage family and cannot be used interchangeably.

Habitat: In Michigan, frequently found in Great Lakes dunes area. Widely dispersed, however, from coast to coast and south to Texas and north into Canada. Away from dunes, search on dry roadsides, sides of hills, and other dry, sandy areas.

Medicinal Parts: The tops and leaves.

Solvents: Diluted alcohol, water (partially).

Effects: Tonic, Stomachic, Stimulant, Febrifuge, Anthelmintic, Narcotic.

Food: Not edible. The leaves of Artemisia species are often made into bitter teas to treat indigestion. Absinthe from other Artemisia species is used to flavor vermouth and other spirits, to include the cordial absinthe.

Traditional uses: Tewa nation people chewed and swallowed juice to relieve gas and upset stomach. Leaf infusion also used to treat fever and chills (see Moerman, p. 93).

The herb has traditionally been used as a smudging agent. The green plant is cut and gathered together in a bundle and wrapped with small string and allowed to dry. The end is lit and used as a "smudge wand" in ceremonial smudging. The plant is also used, dry or moistened, in the sweat lodge. The plant is placed on the hot stones in the center of the lodge and the resulting vapor inhaled.

Numerous people and holistic practitioners have used the plant as medicine for thousands of years, particularly popular in Europe and China.

Modern uses: Thujone and artemisinin are anthelmintic, that is, they kill intestinal worms (including the malaria falciparum) and other parasites. In Europe wormwood (Artemisia) is used as a stomach bitter and digestive (an after-dinner drink, such as vermouth or absinthe, relieves indigestion). Artimisinin, a synthetic derivative from sweet wormwood (Artemisia annua) is used to control malaria and other parasites. Tu Youyou, who discovered this use, was awarded the Nobel Prize in 2015. A recent clinical trial showed artimisin 97 percent effective against noncomplicated cases of malaria (see ncbi.nlm.nih.gov/pmc/articles/PMC1887535).

Dose and usage: A rounded teaspoon of the dried plant in a cup of hot water, allowed to steep for fifteen minutes, is useful to promote sweating in feverish states or to increase scanty menstruation.

Wormwood tea, though bitter, is a good remedy for stomach indigestion. It has also been traditionally used, as its name suggests, in cases of intestinal worms. Michael Moore suggests two cups a day for at least two weeks, making sure its use is constant.

Warning: Thujone is a GABA antagonist—in large amounts it blocks gamma amino butyric acid, which can lead to seizures and even death. Artemisia chemistry is toxic in large enough dose, and the amount of Artemisia extract used in alcoholic drinks is government controlled.

Veterinarian/Wildlife: Wormwood extracts are used to treat worm infestations in domestic animals. There may be benefits for using Artemisia as a companion plant among vegetable and flowers. It is an attractive and unusual houseplant and garden plant.

Yarrow

Asteraceae *(Achillea millefolium L.)*

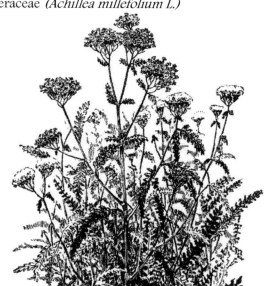

Identification: Yarrow typically grows to a height of 1 to 3 feet (30 to 90 centimeters) and features finely divided, fern-like leaves. The leaves are alternately arranged along the stem and have a feathery appearance, with numerous small leaflets densely packed together. The leaflets are narrow, elongated, and often have serrated edges, giving them a lacy and intricate look.

When in bloom, yarrow produces clusters of small flowers at the top of the stems. The flowers have a flat-topped or rounded shape and come in a variety of colors, including white, yellow, pink, or shades of purple. They are composed of numerous tiny individual florets that create a visually appealing display.

Yarrow has a characteristic aroma, often described as a pleasant and aromatic scent reminiscent of chamomile or a mix of flowers and herbs.

Habitat: Yarrow is a hardy plant that thrives in a range of environments. It can be found in meadows, open fields, along roadsides, and in other sunny locations with well-drained soil. Yarrow has the ability to adapt to different soil types, including sandy or clay soils.

Medicinal Part: The herb. Though some people prepare only the flowers as medicine, I commonly use the whole plant but leave the root. The root may be used with effectiveness but I prefer to leave it so that it can continue to produce new plants each year.

Solvents: Water, alcohol.
Effects: Astringent, Alterative, Diuretic, Tonic.

Traditional uses: The Cherokee tribe recognized the medicinal properties of yarrow and utilized it for various purposes. They would brew a tea from the leaves and flowers of yarrow and use it to treat fevers, relieve respiratory congestion, and alleviate stomach discomfort. Yarrow was also employed topically as a poultice or wash for wounds, cuts, and skin irritations.

The Iroquois tribe valued yarrow for its medicinal qualities as well. They prepared infusions from the leaves and flowers of yarrow and used it to address digestive issues, including stomachaches and indigestion. Yarrow was also used as a diaphoretic to induce sweating during fevers and to promote general detoxification. Among the Ojibwe tribe, yarrow was valued as a ceremonial herb. It was believed to possess spiritual properties and was used in smudging ceremonies to purify and cleanse spaces. The Ojibwe people also used yarrow medicinally as a tea for various conditions, including respiratory ailments and digestive discomfort.

Modern uses: Research has shown that yarrow possesses antimicrobial, anti-inflammatory, and wound-healing properties. Studies have demonstrated its effectiveness in promoting the closure of wounds and reducing inflammation. Yarrow extracts have been explored for their potential in treating various skin conditions, including dermatitis, eczema, and acne. Yarrow has also been studied for its potential in managing digestive disorders. Research suggests that yarrow may possess antispasmodic and anti-inflammatory effects on the gastrointestinal system. Studies have indicated its potential use in alleviating symptoms associated with conditions such as irritable bowel syndrome (IBS), gastritis, and indigestion. In addition, yarrow has shown promise as an analgesic and anti-inflammatory agent. Studies have revealed its potential in reducing pain and inflammation, which may be attributed to the presence of bioactive compounds such as flavonoids and sesquiterpene lactones. Furthermore, yarrow has been investigated for its antimicrobial properties, including activity against various bacteria and fungi. Research has highlighted its potential as a natural alternative to conventional antimicrobial agents.

Dose and usage: Yarrow, when prepared as a hot tea, can work wonders in stimulating perspiration. Personally, I've found the tincture to be quite effective in settling the stomach, especially when paired with other herbaceous companions like betony and poleo mint. This remarkable herb has a rich history of aiding the body during fevers, making it a valuable ally. Its bitter tea also aids digestion and possesses anti-inflammatory properties, which may help protect against infections. When you find yourself exposed to infective organisms or infected individuals, incorporating yarrow into your routine could be beneficial.

While yarrow's blood pressure-lowering effects are modest, I've discovered that combining it with passion flower can enhance its impact. Not only does it help promote digestion, but it also tones the stomach. This can be particularly beneficial for individuals experiencing conditions such as hiatal hernia, where the stomach loses its natural tone and protrudes through the esophagus or develops a tear in the muscle wall.

Fresh yarrow leaves are truly remarkable when it comes to curbing bleeding. Simply placing them on small to medium-sized cuts can facilitate clotting and promote healing. When it comes to managing heavy menstrual flow, a soothing cup of yarrow tea or a dropperful of the tincture taken every three hours can work wonders in reducing the intensity. Leaves and stems can also be smudged all over the body in warm summer evenings as a mosquito repellent. I prefer using lard for oil extractions from yarrow due to its deep-penetrating properties, although other plant-based oils like olive oil can also be used.

Warning: It's important to note that consuming yarrow tea or applying the herb topically may cause photosensitivity, making your skin more sensitive to light. Additionally, the tea may contain a small amount of thujone, which is a compound known to be a carcinogen and liver toxin. As with any herbal remedy, there is a potential for allergic reactions, so it's important to be aware of any adverse effects and discontinue use if necessary.

Other uses: Yarrow's distinctive flavor is highly valued in the realm of mixology, where it is often employed to elevate the taste of gin and other spirits, making it a sought-after ingredient among enthusiasts. This versatile herb is also an excellent addition to any garden, with its beautiful foliage and delicate flowers. Interestingly, yarrow has even found its way into the world of brewing, where it is sometimes regarded as a "secret" ingredient that adds a touch of complexity to fine beers. The whole aerial parts of the plant can also be utilized to preserve fish by stuffing them into the cleaned body cavity.

Yellow Dock

Rumex crispus

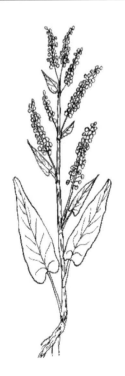

Identification: Yellow dock is characterized by its curly-edged leaves, which can reach a length of one foot, and they grow alternately along the stem. The plant exhibits a captivating transformation in the fall, as its foliage turns a striking rust-red color.

During the winter months, the dead stalks remain intact, along with the heavy seed panicles located at the top of the stem, making it easily identifiable. The root of the yellow dock resembles a carrot in shape and has a reddish-brown outer appearance, while the inner part ranges from yellowish to orange. The intensity of the root's yellow color corresponds to the potency of the plant's medicinal properties.

The yellow compounds found in the root are the primary medicinal substances, and their concentration increases as the root becomes more yellow. It is important to note that yellow dock plants growing in water are not suitable for medicinal purposes, so it is best to gather them from drier embankments and open meadows.

Habitat: Nationwide, along yards, streamsides, vacant lots, and roadsides.

Taste: The yellowish spindle-shaped root has scarcely any odour, but has an astringent, bitter taste.

Medicinal Part: The root.

Solvents: Water, alcohol.

Effects: Alterative, Astringent, Laxative, Antiscorbutic, Tonic.

Traditional uses: Yellow dock root has been valued by Native American tribes for its medicinal properties. One notable use was the application of mashed root to the skin as a treatment for arthritis. The Cherokee tribe specifically utilized the juice of the root to address issues of diarrhea. Additionally, an interesting remedy involved rubbing the throat with a crushed leaf to alleviate sore throat discomfort. In cases of diarrhea, the cooked seeds were consumed to help control the condition. The dried and powdered root was recognized for its styptic properties, making it effective in stopping bleeding. Early pioneers regarded yellow dock as an excellent blood purifier and a rejuvenating tonic, often turning to it as a remedy for various ailments during the spring season.

Modern uses Research suggests that yellow dock may possess laxative and mild diuretic properties, which can aid in promoting regular bowel movements and relieving constipation. Some studies have indicated that yellow dock extracts may enhance digestive function by stimulating bile flow and promoting liver health.

Yellow dock has also been studied for its potential antioxidant and anti-inflammatory effects. Research has shown that certain compounds found in yellow dock, such as anthraquinones and phenolic compounds, exhibit antioxidant activity and may help reduce oxidative stress in the body. Additionally, yellow dock has been investigated for its anti-inflammatory properties, which may have implications for managing inflammatory conditions.

Furthermore, yellow dock has been explored for its potential antimicrobial and antiviral activities. Studies have highlighted its inhibitory effects against various bacteria and viruses, suggesting potential use in combating certain microbial infections.

Warning: It is important to exercise caution when consuming yellow dock leaves due to their high tannin and oxalic acid content. These chemicals, when consumed in excess, may have potential negative effects on the kidneys and can impact bone density. Therefore, it is advisable to limit the consumption of yellow dock leaves to avoid any potential health risks.

Food: Young leaves of yellow dock can be prepared by steaming, sautéing, or stir-frying. However, it is important to note that the leaves can be bitter, so it is recommended to exercise moderation in their consumption. One method to reduce bitterness is to steam the leaves first and then sauté them in olive oil. The inner pulp of the flowering stem can also be consumed after cooking, and to minimize bitterness, the pulp can be squeezed out from the skin. Additionally, the seeds of yellow dock can be gathered and eaten.

Yew
Rhamnaceae *(Taxus brevifolia)*

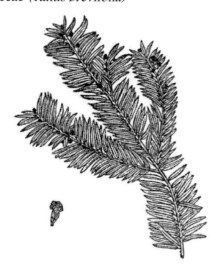

Identification: Yew is an evergreen shrub that can grow up to a small tree reaching a height of 50 feet. It has papery bark that is reddish-purple to red brown in color. The branches of yew hang down in a drooping fashion. The leaves, which are in the form of flat needles, are arranged in opposite rows along the branches. The flowers of the yew are small cones, and the fruit is a scarlet, berry-like structure with a fleshy cup surrounding a single seed.

Habitat: Yew trees (Taxus spp.) are primarily found in the Pacific Northwest region of the United States, including states like Washington, Oregon, and northern California. They thrive in diverse habitats such as forests, woodlands, and mountains. Yews prefer well-drained soils and can tolerate shade.

Food: According to Moerman's research on Native American ethnobotany, Karok and Mendocino tribes consumed the ripe fruit of the yew plant. However, it is important to emphasize that all other parts of the plant, including the seed, are toxic. Therefore, it is advised to **avoid eating any parts of the yew plant due to its toxicity.**

Traditional uses: Native Americans indeed had various traditional uses for the American yew (T. brevifolia). The wet needles of the plant were used as a poultice to apply over wounds, believed to have healing properties and alleviate pain. The needles were considered a potent tonic and were boiled for use in treating injuries. Additionally, bark decoctions were utilized by Native Americans to address stomachaches. In certain tribes like the Okanagan and other northwestern coastal tribes, yew berries were consumed by women as a form of contraception. The Quinault people prepared a decoction from the bark and consumed it in small doses to relieve conditions such as arthritis, tuberculosis, and kidney disease. The Cowlitz Indians utilized poultices made from the yew needles to apply externally on wounds. It is important to note that the leaves of the yew plant are toxic and should not be ingested internally.

Modern uses: Taxine, a toxic compound derived from the American yew (T. brevifolia), has found utility in the field of cancer treatment. The drug paclitaxel, derived from taxine, has shown promising anti-cancer properties. By impeding cell proliferation, it holds potential as a therapy for leukemia, cervical cancer, ovarian cancer, and breast cancer. Ongoing clinical trials are underway to further investigate the efficacy of this drug in combating cancer.

Warning: Both species can induce abortion. **All parts of the plant are toxic.** Unless guided by an expert, avoid eating any part of this plant.

Notes: The yew tree held significant cultural and spiritual importance for many Native American tribes in North America, symbolizing protection, strength, and masculinity. Its wood was highly revered and used in the creation of sacred items such as spirit poles, shaman's rattles, and drum frames. Similarly, in Europe, the yew tree has been regarded as sacred for centuries. The European species of yew, T. baccata, was among the nine sacred woods used by the Celts, who would burn it in ceremonial fires as part of their rituals.

Yucca

Agavaceae (*Yucca* spp.: *Y. filamentosa* L.; *Y. glauca* Nutt.; *Y. baccata* Torr.)

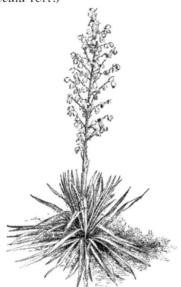

Identification: Yucca plants are medium to large perennials, ranging from 2 to 20 feet in height. They have strong, expansive rootstocks and tend to grow in clumps or colonies. The leaves of yucca plants are swordlike in shape and radiate out from basal rosettes. They have a waxy or shiny green appearance and are long, tough, and fibrous. The flowers of yucca plants are white or cream colored, and they can be cup, bell, or bowl shaped. These flowers are borne on tall woody spikes that extend well above the leaves. Yucca plants typically bloom from May through July. They are also known by various other names such as Adam's needle, Spanish bayonet, or Joshua tree.

Habitat: Found in in prairies, high plains, sandy blowouts, California coastal hillsides, and deserts.

Food: The white flowers of yucca plants are not only beautiful but also edible. They can be used in various culinary preparations, such as folding them fresh into frittatas or omelets, garnishing plates with them, or shredding them onto salads. Additionally, some species of yucca produce edible fruits, with Y. baccata being notable for its large and succulent fruits. While the taste of these fruits may be relatively bland, they are rich in health-protecting flavonoids.

Traditional uses: According to folklore, yucca root decoction is believed to have the ability to restore hair when applied topically.
Among the Navajo (Diné) tribe, yucca fibers hold immense importance. They skillfully extract the strong and durable fibers from the leaves of the yucca plant, utilizing them in the creation of intricate baskets, mats, sandals, and other woven goods. The art of yucca fiber weaving is passed down through generations, representing both practical and artistic expressions of Navajo craftsmanship.

For the Hopi tribe, yucca roots have long been valued for their medicinal properties. The Hopi people traditionally grind yucca roots into a paste and apply it as a poultice to treat a range of skin ailments, including skin irritations, cuts, and wounds. Yucca is recognized for its potential antimicrobial and anti-inflammatory effects, contributing to its use in promoting healing and soothing various skin conditions.

The Apache tribe has a rich history of utilizing different parts of the yucca plant for sustenance. Edible yucca flowers, fruits, and seeds are gathered and consumed as a source of nutrition. Apache people consume the flowers and fruits either raw or cooked, appreciating their distinct flavors. The seeds are often ground into a meal and incorporated into traditional culinary preparations, adding texture and taste to various dishes.

Modern uses: In Europe, dried and ground yucca leaves, as well as extracts from the plant, are available for medicinal purposes. The root and leaf extracts of Yucca filamentosa, which contain steroid saponins, are still used for liver and gallbladder issues. It is important to note that excessive intake of steroid saponins may lead to stomach upset and nausea, although the scientific evidence supporting these uses is limited. The saponins in the plant have the ability to lyse bacteria and produce suds, making it a traditional shampoo still used by Native Americans.

Zizia Aurea

Zizia Aurea (Apiaceae)

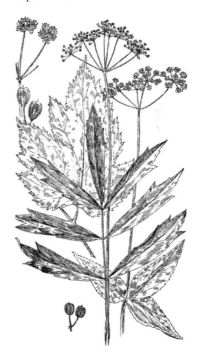

Identification: Golden Alexanders typically grows to a height of 1 to 3 feet (30 to 90 centimeters) and forms clumps of erect stems. The stems are smooth, sturdy, and often have a reddish tinge. The plant produces compound leaves that are pinnately divided into multiple leaflets. The leaflets are lanceolate to ovate in shape and have toothed edges.

When in bloom, Golden Alexanders produces vibrant and showy golden-yellow flower clusters known as umbels. These umbels are composed of numerous small flowers with five petals each. The flowers attract pollinators such as bees and butterflies, enhancing the plant's aesthetic appeal and ecological significance. Flowers give way to 3 – 4 millimeter long, oblong, green fruit capsules. The leaves as well as the fruit slowly turn light purple in the autumn.

Habitat: Golden Alexanders prefers moist to mesic habitats and can be found in various environments, including wet meadows, prairies, open woodlands, and along stream banks. It has a wide distribution across North America, spanning from the eastern United States to parts of Canada

Food: The flowers can be used in salads, and the green stems can be cooked like broccoli.

Medicinal parts: Flowers, leaves, and root.

Solvents: water

Effects: febrifuge, anesthetic

Traditional uses: Native Americans have a long history of utilizing Golden Alexander for its medicinal properties. The pulverized root of the plant was employed to alleviate sharp pains, while a tea made from the leaves and flowers was specifically used to address "female disorders." Additionally, poultices made from the root were applied to reduce inflammation and treat various types of sores.

Dose and usage: A decoction of the root, steeped for at least 15 minutes in simmering water should be taken warm at least four times a day to act as a febrifuge.

Conclusion

I hope you have enjoyed reading this book as much as I've enjoyed writing it, and I hope it will accompany you in your ongoing journey to the discovery of Native American herbs and their medicinal uses.

If you found this book useful and are feeling generous, please take the time to leave a short review on Amazon so that other may enjoy this guide as well.

I leave you with good wishes and hopefully a better knowledge of the plants around us and their amazing powers. This volume is part of a seven-books series on Native American Herbalism from foraging and gardening native plants to making herbal remedies for adults and children. Check out the other volumes to gain a deeper understanding of the amazing wisdom and knowledge of our forefathers and to improve not only your health, but the health of our land as well.

The Native American Herbalist's Bible 3

The Lost Book of Herbal Remedies

The Ultimate Herbal Dispensatory to Discover the Secrets and Forgotten Practices of Native American Herbal Medicine

Linda Osceola Naranjo

Introduction

The wilderness, the dew drops, the pollen...
I become a part of it.
Navajo Chant

We live in a country where the cure for virtually any disease and ailment is within our grasp. In our forests, meadows, plains, and gardens grow small, seemingly insignificant flowers and herbs, plants that we don't look twice at, and trees of which we don't even bother to learn the name. Yet, they are the key to a better, healthier, and more sustainable way of life.

Our forefathers, more attuned with nature than we could ever imagine to be, understood that and took carefully and sparingly the gifts that Nature offered to heal themselves and grow stronger. We have lost that knowledge. Only starting from the 1970s, a renewed interest in botanic medicine has uncovered the depth of the Native American knowledge of plants and their healing powers. The research has not only helped herbalists, but physicians and scientist as well that rediscovered substances that the Native Americans people knew about for hundreds of years.

The mountains, I become a part of it...
The herbs, the fir tree, I become a part of it.
The morning mists, the clouds, the gathering waters,
I become a part of it.

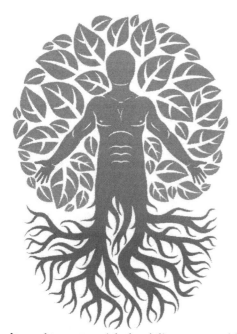

You don't need to put at risk the delicate natural balance of your body by taking drugs and medications, if an easily available natural solution is just outside your door. Harvest carefully or grow your own herbs, learn to know your body and what works best for you, communicate with the nature surrounding you, and you will in a small way bring back a culture that for too long as been treated as inferior.

This book will teach how to find and treat the herbs the way the native American tribes did: from the forest to your herbalist table, but you will have to find your way to listen to your body and the plants around you.

This book is the extended edition of the best-selling *The Native American Herbalist's Bible: 3-in-1 Companion to Herbal* Medicine, offering four more volumes on gardening techniques, growing healing plants and wildflowers, and pediatric healthcare.

This is the unabridged companion to Native American herbs, their traditional and modern use, complete with appropriate doses and usage, gardening tips and techniques for both medicinal plants and wildflowers. The book is completed by a list of simple and effective recipes for the most common ailments for both adults and children. You don't need to put at risk the delicate natural balance of your body and that of your loved ones by taking drugs and medications, if an easily available natural solution is just outside your door. Harvest carefully or grow your own herbs, learn to know your body and what works best for you, communicate with the nature surrounding you, and you will in a small way bring back a culture that for too long has been treated as inferior.

This book will teach how to find and treat the herbs the way the native American tribes did: from the forest to your herbalist table, but you will have to find your way to listen to your body and the plants around you.

To aid you in your holistic journey, we have decided to divide the book in seven handy volumes.

The first volume will give you a full theoretical approach to Native American medicine and the herbal medicines methods and preparations.

The second volume is a complete encyclopedia of all the most relevant herbs used in traditional Native American medicine, complete with modern examples, doses, and where to find them, making it a very effective field guide.

This third volume is a "recipe book" of sorts: it offers easy herbal solutions to the most common diseases a budding naturopath can encounter. It is meant as a jumping point to find your own way to treat yourself and your fellow man and will come in handy even to the most experienced herbalist. You can use it on its own for a quick solution to a pressing ailment, but if you have the time and interest, it is recommended that you read the two previous books to gather more precise information on the herbs and the native ways of healing, communing with nature, and understanding your body. This extended edition also offers a seventh volume on pediatric healthcare, please refer to it if you are crafting herbal remedies for children.

The fourth volume provides a complete theoretical and practical approach to Native American traditional planting techniques and how they can be implemented in modern gardens.

The fifth volume is the native gardener's almanac for medicinal herbs. Foraging is not always an option and a lot of herbs are handy to have in your garden: this volume will guide you through the herbs that you can and (should) have in your garden.

The sixth volume continues the guide to the plants you can plant in your gardens focusing on healing wildflowers, which are not only good for your health, but for the planet as well, and they are not bad on the eyes either!

The seventh volume focuses on native pediatric healthcare. Treating children is a very delicate undertaking, their physiology is more sensitive to external agents, especially drugs. Natural herbalist treatments are effective and gentle in treating common, less severe, pathologies and they won't needlessly weaken your child's immune system. The herbs listed in this last volume have been carefully researched to specifically treat children and their ailments, avoiding any allergic reaction and boosting their immune system.

I am happy to guide through a life-changing journey in search of lost knowledge, amazing healing plants, and carefully crafted herbal remedies and I hope it will help you nurture a stronger relationship with the nature surrounding us and the many gifts it bestows upon us.

Please keep in mind that, because herbs were the very first medicines, they can be very powerful. Do not gather herbs from the wild unless you know what you are doing. And please, grow your own herbs whenever possible; native herbs are becoming increasingly rare, and many are threatened with extinction.

Choosing the right herbs and herbal combinations for your health needs is most important for you. Follow three easy steps to identify and satisfy your herbal and nutritional needs:
1. Identify the injury or disorder that is affecting you.
2. Identify the areas of your health status and specific needs that require additional support.
3. Choose the most appropriate treatment program from this book that fits your needs. This should include herbs, enzymes, vitamins, minerals, and phytochemicals.

As always, if you are pregnant or nursing, if you suffer from a chronic condition such as heart disease or diabetes, or if you are currently taking medications of any kind, please consult with your physician or a well-trained herbal specialist before self-treating. Herbs and other supplements can alter the way your body utilizes other medicines. They can sometimes improve the efficacy of medicines and, at other times, interfere with the absorption or action of a particular drug.

If you have any questions about the appropriateness of any treatment, seek the services of a well-trained health-care professional. This book and the formulas contained herein are not intended to replace the services of a well-trained health-care professional.

Abscess and Gingivitis

An abscess represents a localized accumulation of purulent matter, commonly known as pus. While its occurrence is not limited to specific anatomical sites, the skin and oral gums serve as frequent host locations. The characteristic features of an abscess include tenderness, pain, inflammation, swelling, erythema, and occasionally, an associated pyretic response. These abscesses cmcrgc as a result of microbial infection, necessitating the typical course of treatment involving antibiotics. Nonetheless, the herbal realm provides a compelling and safe alternative, devoid of the potential adverse effects associated with antibiotic usage.

Relevant tissue states: heat (inflammation), dampness, laxity
Relevant herbal actions: anti-inflammatory, antimicrobial, astringent, vulnerary

Supportive Herbs

- Barberries
- Calendula flower
- Chamomile flower
- Echinacea
- Goldenrod leaf and flower
- Licorice root
- Meadowsweet flower
- Oregon grape root
- Plantain leaf
- Rose
- Sage leaf
- Self-heal leaf and flower
- Thyme leaf
- Uva-ursi leaf
- White Oak
- Yarrow leaf and flower
- Yerba Mansa

It can be very painful to have an abscess—a fluid-filled blister or infection—in the mouth. Gingivitis is an inflammation of the gums that can lead to loose teeth. Resist the urge to poke and prod at the gums too much—if you make them bleed, bacteria can move deeper. Treat your gums gently! Antimicrobial, astringent, anti-inflammatory, and wound-healing herbs fight infection and restore healthy tissue.

Herbal mouthwash

Makes 8 fluid ounces (16 to 20 swishes)

While saltwater works well on its own, adding herbs makes it much more effective. Adjust the amounts of each herb according to taste.
Swish with ¼ to ½ fluid ounce of mouthwash after brushing, and swish well, getting between the teeth and throughout the mouth, for 2 to 5 minutes.

- 4 fluid ounces water
- 1 teaspoon sea salt
- 1 fluid ounce tincture of uva-ursi
- 1 fluid ounce tincture of yarrow
- ½ fluid ounce tincture of calendula
- ½ fluid ounce tincture of plantain
- ½ fluid ounce tincture of self-heal
- ¼ fluid ounce tincture of licorice
- ¼ fluid ounce tincture of meadowsweet

1.In a jar with a lid, combine all the ingredients. Cover the jar, label it, and shake well. This is shelf stable.
2.Use this mouthwash every time you brush—twice a day is best.

Skin~abscess~fighting tea

30 drops echinacea tincture (See Part One for directions for tinctures.)
60 drops yerba mansa tincture
1 cup warm water

1. Combine all the ingredients.
2. Take up to five times per day to stimulate the immune system and help eliminate the infection.

Topical wash for abscesses and gingivitis

To create a potent herbal infusion to address a gum abscess, you will need the following ingredients:
- 1 to 2 teaspoons of barberries
- 1 tablespoon of white oak bark
- 1 teaspoon of echinacea root
- 1 teaspoon of granulated Oregon grape root
- 2 cups of boiling water

Follow these steps to prepare the infusion:
1. Combine the barberries, white oak bark, echinacea root, and granulated Oregon grape root in a glass container.
2. Pour the boiling water over the herbs, ensuring they are fully submerged.
3. Allow the herbs to soak in the boiling water for 3 to 4 hours.
4. After the infusion period, strain the liquid to remove the herbal residue.

To utilize the infusion:
1. Use the herbal infusion as a wash.
2. Repeat this process three times a day.
3. If specifically targeting a gum abscess, swish the liquid around in your mouth for several minutes before spitting it out.
By following these steps, you can harness the therapeutic potential of this herbal infusion, as it aids you on your journey towards alleviating the discomfort of a gum abscess.

Acne

Acne is an inflammatory skin condition that commonly affects adolescents (because of increased glandular activity during the teen years). Acne occurs when the sebaceous glands, which are located just beneath the skin, become inflamed. These glands secrete an oil called sebum, which acts to lubricate the skin. Acne results when the pores of the skin become clogged by the sebum. Acne can occur any time in life and may be due to allergies, high-sugar or high-fat diets, heredity, the use of oral contraceptives and other drugs (such as cortisone), hormone changes, and stress.

Relevant tissue states: heat (inflammation), dampness (oily)
Relevant herbal actions: anti-inflammatory, antimicrobial, astringent, circulatory stimulant, liver stimulant, lymphatic

Supportive Herbs

- Burdock
- Calendula flower
- Chamomile flower
- Dandelion root
- Echinacea
- Elder
- Ginger root
- *Gingko Biloba*
- Ginseng
- Licorice
- Milk thistle seed
- Rose
- Sage leaf
- Self-heal leaf and flower
- St. John's wort leaf and flower
- Thyme leaf
- Yarrow leaf and flower
- White Willow Bark

To cope with chronic skin problems, it's important to treat the issue from both the inside and the outside. Topical applications (compresses, poultices, and steams) of astringent, anti-inflammatory, and antimicrobial herbs will clear and tone the skin directly. Internal preparations (tea, tincture, capsules) of liver-stimulating, circulatory-stimulant, and lymphatic herbs support the health and nourishment of skin tissue from beneath.

Skin toner

Makes 12 fluid ounces (90+ applications)

The acidity and probiotics from the vinegar combine with the astringency of the witch hazel and rose to gently but effectively tonify the skin, reducing blemishes and protecting against breakouts. Be consistent; results will begin to show after a few days to a week of use. This simple skin toner is a key part of Katja's vibrant skin protocol.

(Though she's 44 years old, everyone thinks she's a decade younger.) If your skin is sensitive, reduce the amount of apple cider vinegar.

4 fluid ounces apple cider vinegar (preferably raw, unfiltered)
4 fluid ounces nonalcoholic witch hazel extract
4 fluid ounces rose water, or strong, well-strained rose petal infusion

1.In a small nonreactive bowl, stir together the vinegar, witch hazel, and rose water. This mixture is shelf stable. Store in an airtight container.
2.Apply this toner once a day after washing your face. If your skin tends toward dryness, rub a few drops of oil (rosehip or olive) into the skin afterward.
3.Apply this toner a second or third time during the day if your acne is persistent, but don't scrub too hard or use harsh soaps—just rinse gently with water first.

Acne-fighting tea

1 cup Oregon grape root tea
50 drops yellow dock tincture

Combine the ingredients. Take up to one-third of the mixture three times daily.

Acne wash

1 cup horsetail tea
30 drops gotu kola tincture

Combine ingredients in a glass container with a lid. Use as much as needed to wash the skin, three times daily.

Facial steam

Makes 2 cups dried herb mix (4 to 8 steams)

For an active breakout, especially one that is oily, a steam is a great way to effectively deliver circulation-enhancing, inflammation-reducing, and bacteria-eliminating herbal action right into the pores.

½ cup dried chamomile flower
½ cup dried sage leaf
½ cup dried thyme leaf
½ cup dried yarrow leaf and flower
½ gallon water

1.In a small bowl, stir together the chamomile, sage, thyme, and yarrow. Store in an airtight container.

2.Clean your face with gentle soap and water.

3.Make and execute an herbal steam: In a medium pot over high heat, boil the water. Place the pot on a heat-proof surface, someplace where you can sit near it, and make a tent with a blanket or towel. Add ¼ to ½ cup of the herb mixture to the water. Position your face over the steam and remain there for 5 to 20 minutes. (Bring a tissue; the steam also clears your sinuses!)

4.Follow with spot applications of raw or herb-infused honey.

Aging

We all yearn to lead a long and vibrant life, where the passage of time leaves us looking forever young. However, aging is an undeniable part of our journey, as our body's functions gradually decline. This natural process is characterized by wrinkles, joint discomfort, fatigue, and changes in hair color or loss. Certain lifestyle factors, such as an unhealthy diet, lack of exercise, excessive sun exposure, smoking, and drug use, can accelerate this aging process. These factors contribute to increased activity of free radicals, unstable molecules that cause damage to our cells' DNA and disrupt their normal functioning.

Thankfully, nature provides us with a range of herbs that act as antioxidants, effectively combating the presence of free radicals. Antioxidants have the remarkable ability to neutralize these unstable molecules, safeguarding our cells from their harmful effects. By incorporating these antioxidant-rich herbs into our lives, we can enhance our body's defense mechanisms and strive to maintain a balanced state, promoting the well-being of our cells as we navigate the natural process of aging.

Supportive Herbs:
- Ginkgo biloba
- Ginger
- Parsley
- Milk thistle
- Black currants
- Elderberries
- Horsetail

Anti-aging tea 1

Ingredients:
- ½ cup Ginkgo biloba tea
- ½ cup ginseng tea

1. Combine the Ginkgo biloba tea and ginseng tea.
2. Take one-third of a cup of this blended tea three times daily.

Ginkgo biloba tea is renowned for its memory-enhancing properties, while ginseng tea provides a notable boost in energy levels. By blending these two herbal teas, you can confidently enjoy their unique benefits, supporting your overall well-being.

Anti-aging tea 2

Ingredients:
- 5 drops of cayenne tincture
- 30 drops of burdock tincture
- 15 drops of goldenseal tincture
- 10 drops of ginger root tincture
- ½ cup of slippery elm tea (refer to page 72)
- 1 cup of warm water

Recipe:
1. Combine all the ingredients.
2. Take 2 to 3 tablespoons of this mixture three times per day to improve circulation and tighten your skin.

This potent blend of cayenne, burdock, goldenseal, and ginger root tinctures, combined with the soothing effects of slippery elm tea, provides a powerful solution. Incorporating this mixture into your daily routine will effectively improve circulation and tighten your skin.

Allergies

Allergies are a common immune system response to substances that are typically harmless to most individuals. When a person with allergies comes into contact with an allergen, their immune system identifies it as a potential threat and initiates a defensive reaction. This reaction leads to the release of chemicals, such as histamine, which trigger various allergy symptoms.

Allergies can manifest in different ways, affecting different parts of the body. Respiratory allergies, such as hay fever or allergic rhinitis, primarily affect the nose, sinuses, and lungs, leading to symptoms like sneezing, nasal congestion, itching, and coughing. Skin allergies, such as contact dermatitis or hives, can cause itching, redness, swelling, and rashes on the skin. Food allergies may result in digestive symptoms, such as nausea, abdominal pain, diarrhea, or more severe reactions like anaphylaxis. Allergies can also affect the eyes, causing redness, itching, and watery eyes.

Common allergens include pollen, dust mites, pet dander, mold spores, certain foods, insect stings, and various medications. Each individual may have different sensitivities to specific allergens, and the severity of allergic reactions can vary from mild discomfort to life-threatening situations.

Allergies can have a significant impact on daily life, affecting sleep, productivity, and overall well-being. They can be managed through various approaches, including avoidance of allergens, medications to relieve symptoms, and immunotherapy to desensitize the immune system.

It is important for individuals with allergies to identify their specific triggers and work with healthcare professionals to develop a personalized management plan. Allergies can be disruptive, but with proper understanding, prevention, and treatment, individuals can effectively minimize their impact and lead a more comfortable and symptom-free life. By turning to herbal remedies, individuals grappling with allergies can find support and comfort in managing allergic reactions.

Relevant tissue states: heat (inflammation), laxity (of the mucous membranes)
Relevant herbal actions: antihistaminic, anti-inflammatory, kidney supportive, liver stimulant

Supportive Herbs
- Agrimony
- All-heal leaf and flower
- Barberry Root
- Calendula flower
- Goldenrod leaf and flower
- Goldenseal
- Ground Ivy
- Marigold
- Milk thistle seed
- Mullein leaf
- Nettle leaf
- Oregon grape root
- Oxeye daisy
- Pearly everlasting flowers
- Plantain leaf
- Yerba sante

Allergic reactions to pollen, dust, or pets are primarily due to excessive histamine production, which ignites the inflammation underlying the runny nose, itchy eyes, and excessive phlegm. Histamine isn't all bad, though; it's a necessary part of sleep regulation, brain function, and even sexual response! Antihistaminic herbs are ideal because, while they help relieve allergy symptoms, they won't overshoot the mark and suppress histamine so much they cause adverse effects.

When trying to resolve allergies, we also must support the liver and kidneys. Among other things, the liver produces histaminase—an enzyme that breaks down histamine. So, when it's sluggish or overworked, histamine builds up and the inflammatory response worsens. The kidneys also help clear inflammatory instigators from the system, so giving them extra support helps reduce allergic symptoms.

Allergy relief tea

Makes about 3 to 4 cups dried herb mix (enough for 18 to 22 quarts of tea)

Nettle and goldenrod contain the antioxidant quercetin, which, according to a 2006 study by Shaik et al., stabilizes mast cells and prevents the release of histamine. Meanwhile, mullein supports the mucous membranes in the lungs and sinuses, reducing phlegm and mucus and quelling cough. Calendula and licorice improve liver function. Feel free to add some honey to your tea—especially if it's raw, local honey! Unfiltered honey helps reduce allergic response because it contains some pollen grains. Introducing these to the body through the oral route helps it become less reactive to them when you inhale pollen in the springtime.

1 cup dried nettle leaf (see Tips)
1 cup dried goldenrod leaf and flower
½ cup dried mullein leaf
½ cup dried calendula flower
½ to 1 cup marshmallow leaf (optional)
2 to 4 tablespoons dried licorice root

1.In a medium bowl, mix together all the herbs, including the marshmallow (if using, for a dry constitution). Store in an airtight container.
2.Make a long infusion: Prepare a kettle of boiling water. Measure 2 to 3 tablespoons of herbs per quart of water and place in a mason jar or French press. Pour in the boiling water, cover, and steep for 8 hours, or overnight.

3.Drink a quart or more every day, especially in the month before and during your personal peak allergy season. The earlier you start, the less you'll suffer.

TIP: Omit the nettle leaf and increase the goldenrod if you take blood-thinning pharmaceuticals.
TIP: Want a quick fix? No time for tea? The simple combination of freeze-dried nettle leaf capsules and milk thistle seed capsules offers quick relief from allergy. Choose a high-quality brand, and take 2 of each (with plenty of water) every 4 hours.

Quick allergy tea

1 teaspoon barberry root
1 teaspoon Oregon grape root
1 cup water

1. Combine the herbs in a pan and cover with the water.
2. Bring to a boil. Reduce heat and simmer for 30 minutes. Strain.
3. Take one-third cup three times daily.

Flower decoction

1 teaspoon oxeye daisy leaves
1 teaspoon pearly everlasting flowers
1 teaspoon yerba sante leaves
3 cups boiling water

1. Combine the herbs in a glass container and cover with the water; steep for 30 minutes; strain.
2. To use, take one-half to one cup every six hours.

Nettle tea

2 tablespoons nettle leaves
1 teaspoon Oregon grape root
2 cups boiling water
1. Combine all the herbs in a glass container and cover with the water; steep for 30 minutes; strain.
2. Take one-quarter cup three times a day.

Anemia

Anemia, a common condition, can disrupt the vitality of your body. It occurs when there is a decrease in healthy red blood cells or a decrease in hemoglobin, which is responsible for carrying oxygen. There are different types of anemia, including iron-deficiency anemia, vitamin deficiency anemias, and anemia of chronic disease.

The symptoms of anemia can have a significant impact on your daily life. Fatigue, weakness, and feeling out of breath with minimal exertion are common experiences. You may notice pale skin, dizziness, headaches, and an irregular or rapid heartbeat. These symptoms can affect your overall well-being and make it challenging to perform regular activities.

Diagnosing anemia involves a blood test to measure the levels of red blood cells, hemoglobin, and other related factors. Treatment options depend on the underlying cause. For iron-deficiency anemia, dietary changes to include iron-rich foods or iron supplementation may be recommended. Vitamin deficiency anemias may require specific vitamin supplementation or dietary adjustments. Anemia of chronic disease often involves addressing the underlying condition and managing its effects on red blood cell production.

Supportive Herbs
- Barberry
- Oregon Grape Root
- Nettle

Anemia tea

2 teaspoons barberry root
2 teaspoons Oregon grape root
4 tablespoons nettle leaves
2 cups cold water

1. Combine the herbs in a glass container.
2. Cover with the water.
3. Soak overnight.
4. Strain.
5. Take up to one-half cup three times daily.

Arthritis

Arthritis, a condition that brings inflammation and stiffness to the joints, affects people of various ages, with older individuals being more susceptible. The two primary types of arthritis are osteoarthritis and rheumatoid arthritis.

Osteoarthritis, often associated with the wearing down of joint cartilage over time, causes pain, stiffness, and limited joint mobility. It's like a gradual erosion that takes its toll on the body. On the other hand, rheumatoid arthritis is an autoimmune disease where the body's immune system mistakenly attacks joint linings, resulting in inflammation, pain, swelling, and potential joint deformity. It's like an internal battle gone awry.

Living with arthritis means encountering a range of symptoms that can vary depending on the type and severity of the condition. Joint pain, stiffness, swelling, redness, and limited range of motion become constant companions. These symptoms can have a significant impact on daily life, making even simple tasks and physical activities challenging to carry out.

Timely diagnosis and appropriate management are vital for effectively dealing with arthritis. Collaboration with healthcare professionals is crucial in developing a personalized treatment plan that caters to individual needs and aspirations. Regular monitoring and adjustments to the treatment approach may be necessary to effectively manage arthritis symptoms and maintain overall joint health.

Apart from the following herbs, there are other beneficial herbs for arthritis, including bilberry, black currant, nettle, and vervain. These herbs offer potential benefits in managing arthritis symptoms, adding to the arsenal of natural approaches available to those

Supportive Herbs
- Balsam Bilberry
- Black Cohosh
- Black Currant
- Blue Vervain
- Cascara Sagrada
- Cayenne
- Chamomile
- Devil's Claw
- Feverfew
- Mullein
- Nettle
- Sarsaparilla
- White willow bark
- Wild Cherry
- Yucca

Arthritis milding tea

2 teaspoons of devil's claw tuber
3 teaspoons of white willow bark
1 teaspoon of feverfew herb
2 teaspoons of yucca root
2 teaspoons of sarsaparilla root
3 cups of cold water

Combine the specified herbs in a glass container and cover them with cold water. Let the mixture soak overnight. Drain the liquid the next day and consume one-half cup of the infused liquid three times daily.

Quick analgesic arthritis tea

25 drops black cohosh tincture
90 drops wild cherry bark tincture
90 drops mullein tincture
1 cup warm water

1. Combine the above herbs in a glass container and cover with the water.
2. Take one-third of the mixture three times daily.

Nightly arthritis tea

1 teaspoon of black cohosh root
1 teaspoon of chamomile flowers
1 teaspoon of cascara sagrada bark
2 cups of water

Combine the above-mentioned herbs in a glass container. Cover them with water and stir well to ensure thorough mixing. Take 1½ teaspoons of the herb mixture and steep it in 1 cup of boiling water for 10 minutes. Strain the liquid. Consume one cup of this herbal infusion in the evening, just before going to bed.

Arthritis ointment

1 pound of petroleum jelly
1 tablespoon of Canada balsam
2 tablespoons of cayenne
2 tablespoons of chamomile

1. Melt the one-pound quantity of petroleum jelly in a double boiler.
2. Add the herbs to the melted petroleum jelly and stir. Heat the mixture for 2 hours.
3. Remove the mixture from the heat and strain it by pouring it through a cheesecloth, ensuring all the liquid is released by gently squeezing the cloth.
4. While still warm, pour the ointment into glass containers and allow it to cool.
5. Apply the ointment topically, massaging it into the affected area until fully absorbed, as needed for arthritis pain relief.

Asthma

Asthma, a distressing lung disease, leaves an unforgettable impression when you witness a child struggling to breathe. The wheezing sound and the ensuing panic as oxygen deprivation turns the skin blue are harrowing experiences. But, this common condition can affect individuals of all ages, characterized by inflammation of the trachea and bronchial tubes. The resulting narrowing of airways hampers the airflow, leading to shortness of breath, difficulty breathing, coughing, wheezing, and a sensation of tightness in the chest. Asthma attacks can vary in duration from a few minutes to several days, and in severe cases, they can pose a life-threatening risk.

While the exact cause of asthma remains elusive for many, some individuals experience asthma attacks triggered by allergies to molds, pollen, and other allergens. Certain foods and drugs can also induce asthma symptoms. Cold and damp weather, exposure to dust, smoke, or other irritants, and even infections can act as asthma triggers. Regrettably, asthma rates are on the rise in our country, potentially influenced by the presence of irritants in our polluted air.

Herbal allies
- Blue Vervain
- coltsfoot
- Echinacea
- Elecampane
- Ginseng
- Goldenseal
- Horehound
- Indian Root
- Passionflower
- Pleurisy root
- Wintergreen
- Yerba sante

Quick-acting asthma tea

1 teaspoon elecampane root
2 teaspoons horehound herb
1 teaspoon blue vervain leaves
2 cups water

1. Combine the herbs in a pan and cover with water.
2. Bring to a boil; reduce heat and simmer for about 20 minutes; strain and cool.
3. Drink up to two cups a day, a mouthful at a time.

Soothing tea

2 teaspoons powdered Indian root
2 teaspoons granulated echinacea root
2 teaspoons elecampane root
2 cups water

1. Combine the herbs in a pan and cover with the water.
2. Soak for several hours; strain.
3. Take one-half cup two times daily.

Back Pain

Back pain affects most of us at some time in our lives. It can be a dull ache or a sharp burning and stabbing. Sometimes back pain is accompanied by pain that radiates down your leg. This is called sciatica and is a sign that pressure is being placed on the nerves of the spinal cord. Sometimes back pain can be so severe that it limits your activities and renders you bedridden. Often, relaxing the muscles of the back can relieve back pain.
Back pain can have many causes—injury, spasms, sciatica (nerve pain), disc problems, and so on. Long-term resolution requires figuring out what exactly is the root of the problem, but in the meantime these herbs and formulas will relieve pain and release tension, allowing you to move more freely.

Relevant tissue states: tension (spasms), heat (inflammation)
Relevant herbal actions: analgesic, anti-inflammatory, antispasmodic, relaxant

Supportive Herbs
- Barberry
- Black Cohosh
- Black Currant
- Black Haw
- Blue Cohosh
- Blue Vervain
- Devil's claw
- Echinacea
- Feverfew
- Ginger
- Goldenrod leaf and flower
- Meadowsweet flower
- Mullein root
- Solomon's seal root
- Wild lettuce

Spine's fine tincture

Makes 4 fluid ounces (40 to 120 doses)

These warming, relaxant, analgesic herbs quell the spasms responsible for most back pain, regardless of whether the pain is acute or chronic, muscular or connective, etc. If you have infused oil made from fresh goldenrod or ginger, use it as a massage oil after you apply this formula topically. For help sleeping, take 1 to 4 drops of tincture of wild lettuce by mouth—this will also contribute more pain-relieving action.

1 fluid ounce tincture of Solomon's seal
1 fluid ounce tincture of ginger
½ fluid ounce tincture of goldenrod
½ fluid ounce tincture of meadowsweet
½ fluid ounce tincture of mullein root (see Tip)
½ fluid ounce tincture of St. John's wort (optional; see Tip)

1.In a small bottle, combine the tinctures. Cap the bottle and label it.
2.Take 1 to 4 drops by mouth 3 to 5 times per day.
3.Additionally, squirt 1 to 4 drops into your palm and rub it into the back muscles.

TIP: If the vertebral discs are impinged or worn away, increase the mullein root to 1 fluid ounce. It specifically supports these tissues. If sciatica or other radiating nerve pain is present, include the tincture of St. John's wort (unless you are taking pharmaceuticals). It regenerates damaged nerve tissue.

Warming compress

Makes 1 compress
This simple application provides immediate relief.

16 fluid ounces water
½ cup dried ginger (see Tip)
¼ cup Epsom salts

1.In a small pot with a tight-fitting lid over high heat, combine all the ingredients. Cover and bring to a boil. Reduce the heat and simmer for 5 minutes. Meanwhile, fill a hot water bottle.

2.Soak a cloth in the hot tea, holding it by a dry spot and letting it cool in the air until hot but comfortable to the touch.
3.Lie down and place the wet cloth over your back. Cover with a dry cloth and lay the hot water bottle on top. Get comfortable and let it soak in for 10 to 20 minutes. You should feel warmth, relaxation, and relief from pain.
4.Repeat as often as desired.

TIP: Have pain, but no dried ginger? If all you have on hand is fresh ginger from the grocery store, you can use that, too—sliced, chopped, or grated.

Sciatic pain tea

2 teaspoons crampbark
2 teaspoons kava kava root
2 cups water

1. Combine the herbs in a pan and cover with water.
2. Bring to a boil; reduce heat; simmer for 30 minutes.
3. Cool and strain.
4. Take up to one cup per day. This tea can help relieve sciatic pain.

Analgesic daily tea for back pain

1 teaspoon coltsfoot leaves
2 teaspoons St. John's wort leaves
2 cups boiling water

1. Combine the herbs in a glass container and cover with boiling water; steep for 15 to 30 minutes; strain.
2. Take one-half cup in the morning and one-half cup at night.

Soothing back pain tea

1 teaspoon chopped valerian root
2 teaspoons white willow bark
2 cups cold water

1. Combine the herbs in a pan and cover with the water.
2. Soak overnight; strain.
3. Take up to one cup a day, a tablespoon at a time.
This tea can help relieve pain caused by nerve irritation.

Bedsores

A bedsore, also called a decubitus ulcer, is an area of damage to the skin that can occur when pressure is applied to an area of the body for a prolonged period of time. The pressure restricts blood flow to the area and also causes irritation, leading to sores.

Skin ulcers are raw, open sores that occur when the top layer of skin cracks and peels away. They are marked by swelling, redness, pain, heat, and inflammation. They may also be infected and full of pus. Bedsores are very common in individuals in casts, as well as those confined to wheelchairs or to bed. In fact, the most common sites for bedsores are the lower back, the buttocks, and the heels. Some authorities estimate that treating bedsores and other decubitus ulcers costs the nation over $1 billion every year.

Herbal remedies
- Burdock
- Echinacea
- Evening primrose
- Marigold
- Nettle
- White Oak

Bedsore topical wash

2 teaspoons marigold flowers
1 teaspoon granulated echinacea root
1 tablespoon white oak bark
2 cups water

1. Combine the herbs in a glass container and cover with the water; soak overnight; strain.
2. Use as a wash periodically throughout the day.

Bites and Stings

Most of us have been bitten or stung by mosquitos, bees, wasps, ants, spiders, ticks, or even more exotic creatures, such as snakes or jellyfishes. We call it a "bite," but most insects and other creatures puncture the skin rather than actually take a bite. It is the substance the animal leaves in the wound and not the wound itself that usually does the damage.

Bites and stings frequently cause localized itching, pain, swelling, and redness. If untreated, any bite or sting can fester and become infected. Even though itching may be severe, resist the urge to scratch, as a secondary infection could result.

Native Americans have had thousands of years to practice using herbs on snakebites. Some of the most helpful herbs for this condition include echinacea and Seneca snakeroot. Whether it's mosquitoes, black flies, or fire ants, most bug bites are fairly simple: We just need to reduce the inflammation. Bee and wasp stings are a bit more intense: Here, our goals include drawing out the venom, if possible, reducing inflammation, and helping the immune system cope with the venom that has entered the body. Watch for anaphylaxis! If someone stung or bitten is having difficulty breathing, seek help immediately.

Note: If you are stung by a bee or other pest and begin to feel weak, or if you notice any swelling anywhere on the body, call a physician immediately. You may be allergic to the sting and need emergency medical attention. Needless to say, if you are stung by a rattlesnake or other venomous snake, get immediate medical care.

Relevant tissue states: heat (inflammation)
Relevant herbal actions: anti-inflammatory, astringent, lymphatic, immune stimulant

Supportive Herbs

- Echinacea
- Seneca snakeroot.
- Black currant
- Ginger
- Ginkgo biloba
- Licorice
- White willow
- Peppermint leaf
- Plantain leaf
- Rose
- Self-heal leaf and flower
- Yarrow leaf and flower

Cooling compress

Makes 1 compress

Peppermint's menthol provides a cooling sensation to the skin, while at the same time increasing blood circulation and dispersing the irritants from the bite or sting site.

16 fluid ounces water
½ cup dried peppermint leaf
¼ cup Epsom salts

1.In a small pot with a tight-fitting lid over high heat, combine all the ingredients. Cover and bring to a boil. Remove from the heat.
2.Soak a cloth in the hot tea, holding it by a dry spot and letting it cool in the air until hot but comfortable to the touch.
3.Apply the cloth to the bite or sting.

Bug bite relief spray

Makes 8 fluid ounces (number of applications varies by use)

If you regularly walk through clouds of mosquitoes or black flies or live in an area infested with chiggers, you'll want this cooling, itch-relieving spray stocked for when you come inside.

4 fluid ounces nonalcoholic witch hazel extract or apple cider vinegar
2 fluid ounces tincture of rose
1 fluid ounce tincture of self-heal
1 fluid ounce tincture of yarrow

1.In a bottle with a fine-mist sprayer top, combine all the ingredients. Cap the bottle and label it.
2.Liberally spray wherever you've been bitten.

Topical wash for bites and stings

2 teaspoons comfrey leaves
2 tablespoons marshmallow leaves
1 tablespoon dried yarrow
1 cup boiling water

1. Combine the herbs in a nonmetallic container and cover with boiling water.
2. Steep for 15 to 30 minutes; strain.
3. Use as a topical wash.

Skin soothing ointment

1 pound petroleum jelly
4 teaspoons dried agrimony leaves
4 teaspoons dried marigold flowers

1. Melt petroleum jelly in a double boiler.
2. Stir in the herbs and heat for 2 hours until the herbs begin to get crispy.
3. Strain by pouring through cheesecloth.
4. Squeeze the cloth to release all the liquid.
5. While warm, pour the ointment into clean glass containers. Use as needed.

Bronchitis

Bronchitis is an inflammation of the bronchial tubes that can range from a mild case (much like a bad cold) to a severe case, leading to pneumonia. Bronchitis may be accompanied by a fever, severe coughing, thick sputum, difficulty breathing, chills, and a sore throat. Bronchitis usually is caused by an infection but can also occur after inhaling dust, smoke, or other irritants. Repeated bouts of bronchitis can lead to chronic bronchitis, in which the bronchial tubes may become permanently damaged.

When you have a lung infection, don't suppress the cough—it's a vital response! Our goal is to cough when it's productive, so all the irritating or infectious material is expelled as you cough up phlegm, and to reduce the amount of unproductive coughing. If you can't bring up the phlegm, you may find a simple cough developing into pneumonia because of the mucus buildup.
(True pneumonia is a serious condition—seek higher care. Meanwhile, take elecampane and garlic—they're your strongest allies for this problem.)

Infection-instigated coughs are usually wet, and the herbs we discuss here assume that's the case. The goal is to get it just a little on the moist side—nice and productive—so you can expel that phlegm.
As with any respiratory condition, an herbal steam is a great remedy all on its own, combating infection and greatly improving blood circulation—which means immune activity—in the lungs. A simple steam with thyme or sage is very good for this problem.

Relevant tissue states: dampness, cold (depressed vitality)
Relevant herbal actions: antimicrobial, astringent, decongestant, diaphoretic, expectorant, pulmonary tonic.

Supportive Herbs

- Angelica
- Black Cohosh
- Black Elder
- Canadian fleabane
- Chamomile
- Coltsfoot
- Echinacea
- Elder
- Elecampane root
- Garlic
- Ginger
- Horehound
- Licorice
- Pearly Everlasting Flower
- Peppermint
- Pine
- Queen of the meadow
- Sage leaf
- Seneca snakeroot
- Slippery elm
- Thyme leaf

Fire cider

Makes about 1 quart

Traditional fire cider recipes are blends of pungent and aromatic stimulating expectorants that will heat you up and help you get the gunk out. In this version, we sneak in some immune stimulants and a good source of vitamin C. Do not consume this if you take pharmaceutical blood thinners.

1 whole head garlic, cloves peeled and chopped
1 (2-inch) piece fresh ginger, chopped
¼ cup dried pine needles
¼ cup dried sage leaf
¼ cup dried thyme leaf
¼ cup dried elderberry
¼ cup dried rose hips
2 tablespoons dried elecampane root
2 tablespoons dried angelica root
1 quart apple cider vinegar
Honey or water, for sweetening or diluting (optional)

1. In a quart-size mason jar, combine the garlic, ginger, and remaining herbs.
2. Fill the jar with the vinegar. Cover the jar with a plastic lid, or place a sheet of wax paper under the jar lid before you screw down the ring. (The coating on the bottom of metal mason jar lids corrodes when exposed to vinegar.)

3. Let the herbs macerate in the vinegar for 2 weeks or longer.
4. Strain, bottle, and label the finished fire cider. If the vinegar is too heating to be comfortable on your stomach, add some honey (up to one-fourth the total volume), or dilute your dose with water.
5. Take a shot (about ½ fluid ounce) at the first sign of mucus buildup in the lungs, and every couple hours thereafter until symptoms resolve.

Throat-soothing tea

2 teaspoons black cohosh root
2 teaspoons powdered Indian root
2 teaspoons chamomile flower
2 cups water
Honey, to taste

Combine the above herbs in a pan; cover with the water. Bring to a boil; reduce heat and simmer for 30 minutes; strain.
Add honey if desired. Take one tablespoon in two cups of water several times a day.

Sweet soothing tea

1 teaspoon marshmallow leaves or flowers
1 teaspoon coltsfoot leaves
1 teaspoon mullein leaves and flowers
½ cup boiling water
Honey

Combine the above herbs; steep one teaspoon of the mixture in the boiling water; strain. Sweeten with honey. Take one-half cup, three or four times a day, hot.
BRONCHITIS TEA #3
1 teaspoon elecampane root
2 tablespoons nettle leaves
1 cup boiling water

Combine the above herbs. Pour the boiling water over the herbs and steep for 30 minutes; strain. Sweeten with honey, if desired. Take up to two cups a day.
BRONCHITIS TEA # 4
1 to 2 slices of fresh ginger root
1 teaspoon pearly everlasting flowers or leaves
1 teaspoon redroot
1 cup boiling water

Combine the above herbs; steep in the boiling water for 30 thirty minutes; strain. Take one-half cup of the tea, three times daily.

Burns and Sunburns

A burn is an injury to the skin or other tissues caused by fire (or another form of heat), electricity, chemicals, or radiation. Burns are classified according to their severity as first-degree, second-degree, or third-degree. In a first-degree burn, the skin will turn red and swell but will not blister.

In a few days, there is complete healing, without scarring. The damage from a second-degree burn goes much deeper. The skin turns very red and there is blistering, although the skin heals without scarring. The most severe burn, third-degree, penetrates the skin, destroying both the epidermis and dermis (the segment of the skin beneath the epidermis).

A third-degree burn can result in scar tissue formation. Burn tissue can become necrotic and also develop into a serious infection. Skin elasticity can be destroyed. A third-degree burn may actually be less painful than a more superficial first- or second-degree burn because nerve endings in the skin are destroyed. Burns can also occur internally from swallowing very hot liquids or inhaling hot air (such as that from a fire).
A severe burn can cause dangerous systemic damage, such as respiratory tract injury, infection, and shock. Anyone suffering from a severe burn should seek immediate medical attention to counter these potentially life-threatening effects. Herbs, however, can help relieve the pain from a minor burn and encourage rapid healing.

Relevant tissue states: heat

Relevant herbal actions: anti-inflammatory, antimicrobial, antiseptic, vulnerary

Supportive Herbs
- Calendula flower
- Coneflower
- Echinacea
- Goldenrod
- Hyssop
- Linden leaf and flower
- Marshmallow
- Peppermint leaf
- Plantain leaf
- Rose petals
- Self-heal leaf and flower
- Sunflower
- Wild Indigo Root

Immediately following a burn, run cold water over the area—the skin retains heat for much longer than you'd expect. (If blisters form in the burned area, be very gentle with them and don't break them before they naturally slough off, if you can avoid it.) Then, gently clean the wound, removing any dirt or contaminant. Apply the herbs, combining antiseptics to prevent infection with cooling, wound-healing herbs to encourage tissue regeneration.
Apply any of the herbal allies in a wash, compress, poultice, or infused honey—don't use oily preparations (like salves) on burns, because they trap the heat in the tissue.
Do not underestimate the power of a marshmallow root poultice! Simply saturate a handful of marshmallow root with enough cold water to make a gloopy mass and apply it to the burn. Cover with gauze and leave in place for 20 minutes. Repeat frequently.

Burn~healing honey
Makes about 1 pint

Honey is the single best healing agent for burns: If you have nothing but plain honey, you're still in good shape. It gets even better, though, when you infuse these healing herbs into it ahead of time.

½ cup fresh calendula flower
½ cup fresh rose petals
1 pint honey, gently warmed

1. Put the calendula and rose petals in a pint-size mason jar.
2. Fill the jar with the warm honey. Seal the jar and place it in a warm area to infuse for 1 month.
3. In a double boiler, gently warm the closed jar until the honey has a liquid consistency. Strain the infused honey into a new jar, pressing the marc against the strainer to express as much honey as you can.
4. After cooling and cleaning a burn site, apply a layer of the infused honey and cover lightly with a gauze bandage. Refresh the application at least twice a day.

Sunburn spray
Makes 8 fluid ounces

A few spritzes cool the skin and begin to reduce inflammation.
1 tablespoon dried peppermint leaf
1 tablespoon dried plantain leaf
1 tablespoon dried self-heal leaf and flower
1 tablespoon dried linden leaf and flower
1 quart boiling water
4 fluid ounces rose water

1. Make a hot infusion: In a mason jar, combine the peppermint, plantain, self-heal, and linden. Pour in the boiling water, cover, and steep for 20 minutes.
2. Move the jar to the refrigerator until it's cold.
3. Strain out 4 fluid ounces of the infusion and transfer to an 8-ounce bottle with a fine-mist sprayer top. Use the remaining infusion for compresses or a cooling drink. It will keep, refrigerated, for 3 days.
4. Add the rose water to the spray bottle. Cap the bottle and label it.
5. Apply copiously and frequently. Keep the spray refrigerated when not in use.

Burn poultice

1 tablespoon dried coneflower flowers
1 tablespoon dried hyssop flowers
1 tablespoon dried goldenrod flowers
1 tablespoon dried sunflower petals

1. Combine the above ingredients; moisten with boiling water and place between two layers of cheesecloth; let cool and apply to the affected area.
2. When dry, remoisten. Use as often as necessary.

Immunity strengthener

30 drops echinacea tincture
20 drops wild indigo root tincture
1 cup warm water

1. Combine the above herbs in the warm water.
2. Take up to five times a day.

A burn can weaken the body, leaving you vulnerable to illness and infection. Use this tea to strengthen immunity.

Canker Sores

Canker sores are small sores usually found on the lining of the mouth, although they can also occur on the lips, on the tongue, or in the throat. Also called aphthous ulcers, they can be white or yellow and are surrounded by red, inflamed tissue. These small ulcers can be extremely painful for several days and may be accompanied by fever and swollen lymph glands. Canker sores can be brought on by stress, viral infections, poor dental hygiene, and nutrient deficiencies. Injuries (such as certain dental procedures) can also cause canker sores to develop.

Supportive Herbs
- Raspberries
- Black currants
- Big Sagebrush
- Echinacea
- Marigold

Anti-inflammatory mouthwash

½ cup barberry tea
½ cup white oak tea
½ cup echinacea tea
½ cup Oregon grape root tea

1. Combine the above ingredients in a glass container with a lid.
2. Use three times a day as a mouthwash. Be sure to swish the liquid around in your mouth for several minutes.

Cold Sores

Cold sores, those small yet painful blisters filled with fluid, emerge on the mouth due to the presence of the herpes simplex virus. Prior to their appearance, tingling, itching, and burning sensations may serve as early indicators of an impending cold sore eruption. The blisters typically develop a few hours or days after these initial warning signs. Over the course of a few days, they gradually dry out and form a crust. Generally, cold sores heal completely within one to two weeks.

Relevant tissue states: heat (inflammation)
Relevant herbal actions: immune stimulant, lymphatic, vulnerary

Supportive Herbs
- Burdock
- Echinacea
- Goldenseal
- White Oak
- Yerba Mansa
- Calendula flower
- Chamomile flower
- Linden leaf and flower
- Plantain leaf
- Self-heal leaf and flower
- St. John's wort leaf and flower
- Thyme leaf

Cold sore compress

This herbal recipe yields 5 cups of dried herb mix, providing approximately 50 applications. The direct application of this blend aims to enhance local immunity and promote tissue quality, allowing your body to better combat the virus. In the case of chickenpox or a full-body breakout, an herb-infused bath using the same formula can be beneficial. Adding a small amount of baking soda to the bathwater can help alleviate itching.

Ingredients:
- 1 cup dried calendula flower
- 1 cup dried plantain leaf
- 1 cup dried chamomile flower
- 1 cup dried linden leaf and flower
- ½ cup dried self-heal leaf and flower
- ½ cup dried St. John's wort leaf and flower

Instructions:
1. Combine all the dried herbs in a large bowl. Store the mixture in an airtight container.
2. To make a hot infusion, start by boiling water. Measure 2 to 3 tablespoons of the herb mix per quart of water. Place the desired amount in a mason jar or French press. Pour the boiling water over the herbs, cover, and steep for 20 minutes. (While the infusion is steeping, prepare a hot water bottle.)

3. Take a cloth and soak it in the warm herbal tea, ensuring you hold it by a dry spot and allow it to cool in the air until it reaches a comfortably warm temperature.
4. Lie down and place the moist cloth over the affected area. Cover it with a dry cloth, and then position the hot water bottle on top. Get into a comfortable position and allow the herbal infusion to soak into the skin for 10 to 20 minutes.
5. Repeat this process 2 to 3 times per day.

STEAM VARIATION: Another option is to perform a steam treatment using these herbs as they infuse. Create a blanket tent, position your face over a steaming pot containing the herbs, and steam your face for a few minutes before using the compress.

Cold sore balm

This gentle salve recipe creates approximately 5 ounces of product, providing a supply that can last around three months. The salve offers soothing relief for irritated cold sores, reducing inflammation and creating an unfavorable environment for the virus to thrive.

Ingredients:
- 1 fluid ounce of calendula-infused oil
- 1 fluid ounce of plantain-infused oil
- ½ fluid ounce of self-heal-infused oil
- ½ fluid ounce of chamomile-infused oil
- ½ fluid ounce of St. John's wort-infused oil
- ½ fluid ounce of thyme-infused oil
- 1 ounce of beeswax (additional beeswax may be needed)

Instructions:
1. Prepare the salve using the usual method (refer to specific instructions). If you plan to store the salve in small jars, create a softer consistency. For use in lip balm tubes, opt for a slightly firmer texture.
2. Apply the salve generously to the affected area, repeating the application 3 to 5 times per day.

Cold sore tea

Combine 1 teaspoon of burdock root and 1 teaspoon of dried and powdered goldenseal root in a glass container. Pour 1 cup of boiling water over the herbs and let them steep for 30 minutes. Allow the mixture to cool, then strain it to remove the herb particles. If desired, sweeten the herbal infusion with honey. Consume up to one cup of this herbal tea per day.

Cold sore mouthwash

In a glass container, combine 1 teaspoon of echinacea root, 1 teaspoon of yerba mansa root, and 1 tablespoon of white oak bark. Pour 1 cup of boiling water over the herbs. Allow the mixture to steep for 30 minutes, then cool and strain it. This herbal solution can be used as a wash to treat cold sores.

Constipation

Constipation refers to irregular or absent bowel movements. The frequency of bowel movements varies based on factors such as diet, physical constitution, and habits. While most people typically have one bowel movement per day, some individuals can go without one for two days or more without experiencing constipation. However, as waste products remain in the colon for a longer duration, more water is absorbed, resulting in drier and more compacted waste. Constipation can arise due to various reasons, including a poor diet, inadequate water intake, nervous tension, lack of exercise, drug use, inconsistent toilet habits, and excessive reliance on laxatives. Additionally, certain diseases such as thyroid problems, circulatory disorders, and colon disturbances (such as fistulas, inflammation, polyps, obstructions, and tumors) can also contribute to constipation.

Relevant tissue states: cold (stagnation), dryness, tension

Relevant herbal actions: bitter, carminative, demulcent, hepatic, laxative

Supportive Herbs

- Angelica
- Barberry
- Boneset
- Cascara Sagrada
- Cayenne
- Chicory
- Dandelion root
- Ginger
- Marshmallow
- Milk thistle seed
- Oregon Grape
- St. John's wort leaf and flower
- Sunflower

Sometimes, constipation is simply a sign of dehydration—drink some water! If it's a chronic issue, it may be an indication of a food allergy or simply a sign that you're not getting sufficient fiber in your diet. A good, thick, cold infusion of marshmallow solves both problems: It rehydrates better than water alone, and it includes a lot of polysaccharides and fibers that help move stool along. Constipation, especially when ongoing, can be traced back to sluggish liver function. Bile produced by the liver is a digestive fluid, but it also lubricates the intestines; when production is low, things can get stuck. Bitters and carminatives help spur digestive function, and liver-restorative herbs (hepatics) such as milk thistle can reestablish normal function.

Bowel-hydrating infusion

Makes 2½ cups of dried herb mix, which is sufficient for 14 to 18 quarts of tea. This delightful blend offers a tastier alternative to solo marshmallow, catering specifically to individuals with dry constitutions who often experience a specific type of constipation. If you find yourself struggling with hard-to-pass, dry, and compacted bowel movements resembling "rabbit pellets," this remedy is tailored for you. It is recommended to consume a quart or more of this tea daily.

Ingredients:
- 1 cup of dried linden leaf and flower
- 1 cup of dried marshmallow root
- ¼ cup of dried cinnamon bark
- ¼ cup of dried licorice root

Instructions:
1. In a medium bowl, thoroughly mix all the dried herbs. Store the mixture in an airtight container.
2. To prepare a cold infusion, measure 2 to 4 tablespoons of the herb mix per quart of water. Place the desired amount of herbs in a mason jar or French press. Pour cold or room-temperature water over the herbs, and allow them to steep for 4 to 8 hours before straining.

Bowel-motivating tincture

Makes 4 fluid ounces (30 to 60 doses). These bitters and carminatives will spur the bowels to movement by stimulating bile flow and intestinal peristalsis.

1½ fluid ounces tincture of dandelion root
1½ fluid ounces tincture of St. John's wort
½ fluid ounce tincture of angelica root
½ fluid ounce tincture of ginger

1. In a small bottle, combine the tinctures. Cap the bottle and label it.
2. Take 2 to 4 drops every 20 minutes until relief occurs.

Bowel-soothing tea

One large handful of boneset flowers
One large handful of dandelion flowers
4 ounces cascara bark
2 quarts water
Honey

Combine the above herbs in a pan and cover with two quarts of water; bring to a boil; boil until the mixture reduces to one quart; strain.
Take one cup before breakfast and one at bedtime. You may want to add honey to sweeten.

Purifying digestive tea

Combine 2 teaspoons of cascara sagrada, 3 to 4 slices of ginger root, 1 teaspoon of cayenne, and 1 teaspoon of Oregon grape root in a pan. Cover the herbs with 2 cups of boiling water, steep for 30 to 45 minutes, then cool and strain the mixture. Take one tablespoon at a time, up to two cups per day.

Cough and Cold

Cough and cold are common respiratory conditions that affect people of all ages. They are usually caused by viral infections, with the common cold being the most frequent culprit. Coughing and sneezing are the body's natural defense mechanisms to help clear the airways and expel irritants or infectious particles.

A cough is characterized by a repetitive, forceful expulsion of air from the lungs, often accompanied by a distinctive sound. It serves as a protective reflex to clear the throat and airways of mucus, irritants, or foreign substances. Coughs can be either dry (non-productive) or productive, where mucus or phlegm is coughed up.

The common cold typically presents with symptoms such as nasal congestion, runny nose, sneezing, sore throat, and a mild cough. These symptoms are often self-limiting and resolve within a week or two. However, in some cases, a cold may progress to a secondary bacterial infection or lead to more severe respiratory conditions, particularly in individuals with weakened immune systems.

Treatment for cough and cold primarily focuses on alleviating symptoms and supporting the body's natural healing process. This may include over-the-counter medications to relieve congestion, reduce coughing, or soothe a sore throat. Home remedies, such as drinking fluids, using saline nasal sprays, using a humidifier, and getting adequate rest, can also help manage symptoms and promote recovery.

It is important to note that antibiotics are ineffective against viral infections like the common cold and should only be used if a secondary bacterial infection is suspected.

Relevant tissue states: heat (irritation) or cold (depressed vitality), dryness or dampness
Relevant herbal actions: antitussive, astringent, decongestant, demulcent, diaphoretic, expectorant, pulmonary tonic

Supportive Herbs
- Agrimony
- Black currant
- Black Elder
- Blue Vervain
- Boneset
- Chamomile
- Coltsfoot
- Echinacea
- Elecampane
- Fennel seed
- Ginger
- Gingko Biloba
- Goldenrod
- Goldenseal
- Horehound
- Indian Root
- Licorice
- Mullein
- Osha
- Oxeye Daisy
- Peppermint
- Pine
- Pleurisy Root
- Queen of the Meadow
- Speedwell
- White cedar leaf tips
- Wild Cherry
- Wild Indigo
- Yarrow
- Yerba mansa
- Yerba sante
- Marshmallow
- Mullein leaf
- Sage leaf
- Thyme leaf

For herbs to work best, we need to differentiate between a hot, dry, irritated cough and one that is wet, but cold and unproductive.
When the lungs are dry, you'll have a racking, relentless cough; we use moistening herbs to correct this. Wet lungs rattle or gurgle and are most likely a response to infection. See Bronchitis/Chest Cold/Pneumonia or Cold and Flu.

Lung-lubricating tea

Makes 2¾ cups dried herb mix (enough for 18 to 22 quarts of tea)

For dry, hot lungs, these soothing and moistening herbs bring relief from a racking, unrelenting cough.

1 cup dried marshmallow root
1 cup dried mullein leaf
½ cup fennel seed
¼ cup dried licorice root, or to taste
Honey, for extra soothing (optional)

1. In a medium bowl, mix together all the herbs. Store in an airtight container.
2. Make a cold infusion: Measure 2 to 4 tablespoons of herbs per quart of water and place in a mason jar or French press. Pour in cold or room-temperature water and steep for 4 to 8 hours.
3. Strain the liquid and drink directly, or warm, if desired.
4. Add honey (if using) for extra soothing.

Antitussive oxymel

Makes about 1 quart (20 to 60 doses)

An oxymel is simply a blend of vinegar and honey, which combines the astringent and stimulating effects of the vinegar with the moistening and soothing aspects of the honey. Adding lung-specific herbs makes this a go-to for coughs of all kinds.

⅓ cup dried pine needles
⅓ cup dried sage leaf
⅓ cup dried thyme leaf
¼ cup dried ginger
1 quart apple cider vinegar
Honey, as needed for topping off the jar

1. In a quart-size mason jar, combine the herbs.
2. Fill the jar four-fifths full with vinegar; top off with honey.
3. Cover the jar and let macerate for 4 weeks.
4. Strain and bottle the oxymel. Cap the bottle and label it.
5. Take 1 to 3 tablespoons as needed.

Cough syrup

2 teaspoons coltsfoot leaves
1 tablespoon wild plum root
2 teaspoons mullein leaves
2 cups boiling water
1 pound honey

1. Combine the above herbs in the boiling water; in a nonmetallic container steep for 30 minutes and strain.
2. Add one pound of honey, heating and stirring until the honey is dissolved; cool and store in a glass container.
3. Take one tablespoon at a time, as needed.

Soothing cough and cold formula

30 drops echinacea tincture
20 drops wild indigo root tincture
2 cups white cedar leaf tips tea

1. Combine the above ingredients and take half a cup at a time, hot.
2. Take up to three times a day.

Lakota cough and cold formula

1 teaspoon goldenseal root
1 teaspoon mullein leaves
1 teaspoon osha root
1 teaspoon pleurisy root
1 teaspoon yerba mansa root
2 teaspoons yerba sante leaves
2 cups boiling water

1. Combine the above herbs and cover with the boiling water; steep for 30 minutes, cool, and strain.
2. Take two tablespoons at a time, as needed, up to two cups a day.

Lumbee cough and cold formula

3 teaspoons goldenrod leaves
4 teaspoons horehound leaves
2 teaspoons white pine inner bark
4 cups boiling water

1. Combine the above herbs in a cheesecloth; tie closed with a string.
2. Place the bag in the boiling water; boil for 15 minutes; cool; remove the bundle.
3. Take half a cup of the hot mixture at a time, as needed, up to two cups a day.

Quick-acting cough and cold formula

4 teaspoons agrimony leaves
2 teaspoons mullein leaves
2 teaspoons blue vervain leaves
1 teaspoon oxeye daisy
3 teaspoons horehound leaves
2 teaspoons speedwell
2 cups boiling water
1. Combine the above herbs in a nonmetallic container and cover with the boiling water; steep for 30 minutes, cool, and strain.
2. Take a tablespoonful every three hours, as needed, up to two cups a day.

Expectorating cough and cold tea

2 teaspoons boneset herb
2 teaspoons licorice root
2 to 3 slices ginger root
2 teaspoons wild cherry bark
2 cups boiling water

Combine the above herbs in a nonmetallic container and cover with the boiling water; steep for 30 minutes, cool, and strain. Take one to two tablespoons at a time, up to two cups a day, as needed, for a dry tickling cough.

Decongestant tea

2 slices fresh ginger
2 teaspoons pleurisy root
1 cup boiling water

1. Combine the herbs in a glass container; pour one cup of boiling water over the herbs; steep for 30 minutes, cool, and strain.
2. Take a tablespoon at a time, up to two cups a day. This tea is good for bronchial congestion.

Antitussive flower tea

1 teaspoon elderflowers
1 teaspoon yarrow flowers
1 cup boiling water

1. Combine the herbs in a nonmetallic container and cover with one cup of boiling water; steep for 20 minutes and strain.
2. Drink hot every two hours, as needed.

Quick-acting mullein cough syrup

1 cup of mullein tea
1 pound honey

1. Combine the above ingredients in a pan and heat until the honey is liquid.
2. Remove from heat, cool, and pour into a glass container. Take a tablespoon at a time, as needed.

Elecampane cough syrup

2 cups of elecampane tea
1 pound honey

1. Combine the tea with the honey and heat on low. Stir to dissolve the honey; when dissolved, remove the mixture from the heat.
2. When cool, pour into glass containers and seal.
3. Take two tablespoons at a time, as needed, up to one cup a day.

Horehound lozenges

1½ cups horehound leaves
1½ cups water
3 cups sugar
3 tablespoons corn syrup

1. Place the horehound leaves in a pan and cover with the water.
2. Bring the mixture to a boil and boil for 20 minutes.
3. Remove from the heat and cool. Strain the solution and add the sugar and corn syrup.
4. Place back on the heat, bring to a boil, then reduce heat to medium.
5. Cook until the mixture reaches 300°F (hard-crack stage).
6. Pour the syrup onto a large buttered baking sheet; cool, then break into one-inch pieces.
7. Use as you would any cough drop.

Cramps

Cramping muscles are characterized by involuntary muscle contractions that can be both painful and tight. They can occur due to various factors such as exposure to cold temperatures, dehydration, overexertion during exercise, imbalances in nutrients, and restricted blood flow to the muscles. Additionally, an imbalance in electrolytes, which include calcium, magnesium, potassium, and sodium, can contribute to muscle cramps. While muscle cramps commonly occur in the legs, often to a severity that hinders walking, they can also affect other areas of the body, including the arms, back, and virtually any muscle group.

Relevant tissue states: heat (inflammation), tension
Relevant herbal actions: anodyne, nervous tropho-restorative, relaxant, rubefacient

Supportive Herbs
- Black Cohosh
- Ginseng
- Wintergreen
- Yerba Mansa
- Cinnamon bark
- Ginger
- Goldenrod leaf and flower
- Meadowsweet flower
- Peppermint essential oil
- Wild lettuce
- Yarrow leaf and flower

A bit of delayed-onset muscle soreness after a hard day's work or an intense workout is normal. Rest well! Recovery time is when muscles grow stronger; if you don't give them time to recover fully, you'll confound your efforts. Eat well, too: providing the necessary nutrients speeds recovery. Bone broth with seaweed added is a great place to start.

Muscle-warming ointment

20 drops yerba mansa tincture
4 ounces wintergreen oil
1 pound petroleum jelly

1. Thoroughly mix the above herbs with the petroleum jelly.
2. Use as an ointment to relieve muscle cramps.

Muscle cramp tea

2 teaspoons black cohosh root
1 tablespoon ginseng root
2 cups water

1. Combine the above herbs in a pan and cover with two cups of water; bring to a boil; reduce heat and simmer for 30 minutes, cool, and strain.
2. Take two to three tablespoons up to six times a day.

Muscle rub

Makes 8 fluid ounces (100+ applications, 30-day supply)

These warming herbs increase local circulation, simultaneously reducing inflammation and soothing tension. If, after applications, you're still in a lot of pain when it's time to go to bed, take 1 to 2 drops of wild lettuce tincture for further relief.

2 fluid ounces ginger-infused oil
2 fluid ounces goldenrod-infused oil
2 fluid ounces tincture of ginger
2 fluid ounces tincture of meadowsweet
80 drops peppermint essential oil or cinnamon essential oil (or both!)

1. In a small bottle, combine the infused oils, tinctures, and essential oil(s). Cap the bottle and label it, including Shake well before each use.
2. Hold your palm over the bottle's mouth and tilt to deposit a small amount in your palm. Rub between your hands to warm the treatment, and apply to the painful joints.
3. Massage the liniment into the joints until your hands no longer feel oily. Really work the liniment into the tissue.
4. Repeat the application 3 to 5 times per day. More is better!

Diarrhea

Diarrhea is marked by frequent and excessive discharge of watery fecal material. Diarrhea can occur because of bacterial or viral infections or intestinal parasites. Certain chemicals and drugs can cause diarrhea, as can certain diseases, such as ulcerative colitis and cancer. Emotional stress can also bring on diarrhea. Food allergies, drinking caffeine or alcohol, or eating unripe fruit or spoiled food can also bring on an attack.
Excessive or prolonged diarrhea can cause dehydration, which can interfere with the absorption of nutrients. Diarrhea can be especially dangerous in children because they cannot tolerate much fluid loss.

Relevant tissue states: laxity (barrier compromise), dampness
Relevant herbal actions: astringent, demulcent

Supportive Herbs
- Agrimony
- Alumroot
- Angelica
- Barberry
- Blackberry
- Black Currant
- Canadian fleabane
- Catnip
- Cayenne

- Cinnamon bark
- Ginger Root
- Marshmallow
- Meadowsweet flower
- Mint
- Pine Bark
- Plantain leaf
- Raspberry
- Rose
- Self-heal leaf and flower
- Strawberry leaf
- Witch hazel
- Yarrow
- Yellow Dock

When the lining of the bowels loses integrity, excess fluid is lost. To counteract this directly, astringent herbs restore healthy tone to the mucous membranes, so water stays in the body where it belongs. Once this is accomplished, it's a good idea to follow up with some soothing demulcent herbs—especially if the diarrhea has been going on for a while, as that causes dehydration, which must be corrected.

Astringent tea

Makes 2¼ cups dried herb mix (enough for 14 to 18 quarts of tea)

The tannins in these herbs help bind lax tissues back together so fluids stay where they belong and barriers keep their integrity. Drink a quart of tea over the course of the day.

1½ cups dried self-heal leaf and flower
½ cup dried meadowsweet flower
¼ cup rose petals

1. In a medium bowl, mix together all the herbs. Store in an airtight container.
2. Make a hot infusion: Prepare a kettle of boiling water.
3. Measure 2 to 3 tablespoons of herbs per quart of water and place in a mason jar or French press.
4. Pour in the boiling water, cover, and steep for 20 minutes or until cool enough to drink.

TINCTURE VARIATION: If you prefer, make a tincture blend using the same proportions: Combine 1½ fluid ounces tincture of self-heal, ½ fluid ounce tincture of meadowsweet, and ¼ fluid ounce tincture of rose petal. Take 1 to 6 drops every 20 minutes until relief occurs.

Cinnamon powder capsules

Makes 20 to 24 capsules

When cinnamon is extracted into water—as an infusion or decoction—its demulcent quality is emphasized. However, if you swallow a capsule of the powder, the capsule dissolves in your GI tract and releases the dry powder, which then absorbs excess water and exerts an astringent effect on the intestinal lining.
This quells diarrhea quite nicely. The Capsule Machine, a handy manual capsule-filling device, helps with this recipe quite a lot.

20 to 24 empty gelatin capsules, size "00"
2 tablespoons powdered cinnamon

1. Fill the capsules with the cinnamon powder.
2. Take 1 to 3 capsules when you have diarrhea. If relief isn't obtained within an hour, take another dose.

Quick and easy diarrhea tea

Combine 3 tablespoons of agrimony leaves and 2 tablespoons of self-heal in a pan. Cover the herbs with 4 cups of water and bring the mixture to a boil. Reduce the heat and let it simmer for 30 minutes. Allow the infusion to cool and strain the liquid. Drink the herbal infusion as needed, up to one cup per day.

Soothing diarrhea tea

In a nonmetallic container, combine 2 teaspoons of alumroot, 2 teaspoons of blackberry leaves, 2 teaspoons of angelica seeds, and 1 teaspoon of Oregon grape root. Pour 2 cups of boiling water over the herbs and let them steep for 30 minutes. After steeping, strain the liquid. Consume the herbal infusion as needed, with a maximum of one cup per day.

Iroquois tea

Combine 2 teaspoons of raspberry leaves, 2 teaspoons of strawberry leaves, 2 tablespoons of yarrow, and 2 teaspoons of yellow dock root in a glass container. Pour 2 cups of boiling water over the herbs and let them steep for 30 minutes. After steeping, cool and strain the liquid. Consume up to one cup of the herbal tea per day. It's worth noting that the Iroquois utilized a similar tea for the treatment of bloody diarrhea.

Fatigue

Fatigue is more than just being tired. Instead, fatigue is a prolonged or excessive decrease in the ability to function, over and above what normal exertion would cause. Those who push themselves to the point of physical exhaustion are certainly familiar with fatigue. However, fatigue can be a symptom of more than overexertion; it is a symptom of a number of conditions including anemia, circulatory problems (such as angina pectoris, atherosclerosis, and high blood pressure), chronic fatigue syndrome, diabetes, hepatitis, inflammatory bowel disease, multiple sclerosis, and respiratory conditions including pneumonia and pleurisy.

Relevant tissue states: cold (depletion, depression, exhaustion)
Relevant herbal actions: adaptogen, exhilarant, stimulant
Supportive Herbs
- Angelica
- Ashwagandha root
- Blackberry
- Gingko Biloba
- Ginseng
- Gotu Kola
- Licorice root
- Mirabilis
- Pulsatilla
- Raspberry
- St. John's Wort
- Strawberry leaf
- Tulsi leaf

Fatigue is an indication that something is impairing recovery. Most of the time, it's simply a lack of sleep. (Believe it or not, healthy adults need 8 to 10 hours of sleep a night—every night—and most Americans only get 6 on weekdays, 8 on weekends!) Even if your fatigue is not immediately relieved by a good night's sleep, it's still important to prioritize sleep. While there can be other factors in play (malnutrition, chronic illness, stress, pharmaceutical side effects, etc.), sleep is irreplaceable. To counter fatigue, we should not underestimate the importance of movement for building energy. A little bit of motion can grow into greater kinetic energy if you cultivate it, gently and consistently. Tai chi and qigong are excellent for this. While you're working on that, we'll draw on the talents of our adaptogens and uplifting, stimulating herbs to help break through the fog and push forward.

Shake-it-off formula

Makes 3 fluid ounces (45 to 90 doses)

1 fluid ounce tincture of licorice
1 fluid ounce tincture of ashwagandha
1 fluid ounce tincture of tulsi

1. In a small bottle, combine the tinctures. Cap the bottle and label it.
2. Take 1 to 2 drops, at morning and noontime. Feel free to take additional doses whenever you need a boost.

Up-and-about morsels

Makes about 24 pieces

These tasty, restorative treats are a good way to get a substantial dose of beneficial herbs. This format is particularly useful because it provides the full complement of plant compounds instead of just those that are water soluble or alcohol soluble, as happens with a tea or tincture.

¼ cup powdered ashwagandha root
¼ cup powdered tulsi leaf
¼ cup powdered milk thistle seed
¼ cup powdered nettle leaf
3 tablespoons powdered licorice root
¾ cup nut butter
½ cup honey

Unsweetened shredded coconut, cocoa powder, powdered cinnamon, powdered ginger, cayenne, or whatever seems tasty to you, for coating

1. In a large bowl, blend the powders together.
2. Add the nut butter and honey. Stir to form a thick "dough."
3. Roll the dough into balls about the size of a walnut (1 inch).
4. Roll the balls in your coating of choice.
5. Eat 1 to 4 per day.

Pick-me-up tea

1 teaspoon Ginkgo biloba leaves
1 teaspoon dried mirabilis root
1 teaspoon dried ginseng root
1 teaspoon pulsatilla herb
1 teaspoon gotu kola leaves
1 teaspoon St. John's wort leaves
4 cups boiling water

1. Combine the above herbs in a glass container; cover with the boiling water; steep for 30 minutes; strain.
2. Take as needed.

Invigorating tea

1 teaspoon blackberry leaves
1 teaspoon strawberry leaves
1 teaspoon raspberry leaves
2 cups boiling water
Honey

1. Combine the above herbs in a glass container; cover with the boiling water; steep for 10 minutes; strain.
2. Sweeten with honey if desired. Drink as needed.

Fever

Fever is a temporary increase in body temperature, often indicating an underlying illness or infection. It is a common symptom experienced by individuals of all ages and is typically the body's natural response to help fight off infections and other health conditions.

A normal body temperature ranges between 97°F (36.1°C) and 99°F (37.2°C). A fever is generally defined as a body temperature above 100.4°F (38°C). It can be measured orally, rectally, or using a forehead or ear thermometer.

Fever is often a sign that the body's immune system is actively working to combat an infection. It can occur in response to various factors, including viral or bacterial infections, inflammation, certain medications, or underlying medical conditions. Common illnesses associated with fever include the flu, common cold, urinary tract infections, respiratory infections, and more. When the body detects an infection or other triggering factors, it releases chemicals that act on the hypothalamus, the part of the brain responsible for regulating body temperature. This causes the body to raise its temperature, resulting in a fever. As the body's temperature increases, it can lead to symptoms such as feeling hot, sweating, chills, body aches, fatigue, and changes in appetite or sleep patterns.

Fever itself is generally not harmful and can be a sign that the body is fighting an infection. However, it is important to monitor the severity and duration of the fever and seek medical attention when necessary, especially in cases of high or persistent fever, severe symptoms, or if there are underlying health conditions.

It is crucial to note that fever can be a symptom of serious infections or conditions, particularly in infants, young children, older adults, or individuals with weakened immune systems. Regular monitoring, proper hydration, and seeking medical advice when needed are key to managing fever and ensuring overall well-being.

Relevant tissue states: heat, dryness (dehydration)
Relevant herbal actions: diaphoretic, refrigerant

Supportive Herbs
- Angelica
- Boneset
- Cayenne
- Catnip leaf and flower
- Elderflower
- Garlic
- Ginger
- Juniper
- Marigold
- Osha Root
- Oxeye Daisy
- Peppermint leaf
- Sage leaf
- Skullcap
- Thyme leaf
- Tulsi leaf
- Wild Indigo Root
- Wild lettuce
- Yarrow leaf and flower

Fever is your friend: It's a vitally important immune response—and herbalists aren't the only ones saying so! The American Academy of Pediatrics released a clinical report in 2011 that stated: "It should be emphasized that fever is not an illness but is, in fact, a physiologic mechanism that has beneficial effects in fighting infection." So, don't give in to fever phobia—help your body do its work. Stay hydrated! Almost all serious problems associated with fever come not from the fever itself but from runaway dehydration. If a person is too nauseous to keep down fluids, sitting in a warm bath is a good way to rehydrate. Finally, remember that temperatures are relative to individuals. Children run hot, elders run cool, and constitution influences your baseline body temperature. A limp and unresponsive person at 99°F is in more trouble than an active, alert person at 101°F. So, always look at the person more closely than the thermometer.

Fever-inducing tea

Makes 3 cups of dried herb mix, which is ample for preparing 18 to 24 quarts of tea. This particular blend aims to promote a strong fever response by utilizing stimulating diaphoretics. These herbs not only assist in making the fever more productive but also facilitate sweating, thus aiding in making the fever more manageable. When a fever is low and lingering, and you desire to enhance its effectiveness, indulge in a generous mug of this tea.

Ingredients:
- 1 cup of dried tulsi leaf
- ½ cup of dried sage leaf
- ½ cup of dried thyme leaf
- ½ cup of dried yarrow leaf and flower
- ¼ cup of dried angelica root
- ¼ cup of dried ginger
- 1 garlic clove, sliced (optional, for added potency)

Instructions:
1. In a medium bowl, thoroughly mix all the dried herbs. Store the blend in an airtight container.
2. To prepare a hot infusion, start by boiling water. Measure 2 to 3 tablespoons of the herb mix (add the sliced garlic if desired) per quart of water. Place the herbs in a mason jar or French press. Pour the boiling water over the herbs, cover, and steep for 20 minutes.
For optimal results, reheat the infusion before consuming and drink it while it is piping hot.

For fevers that are low and persisting, this tea can help intensify the fever response and make it more effective. Remember to drink the tea while it is very hot to maximize its effects.

Fever-breaking tea

Makes 1¾ cups of dried herb mix, which is sufficient for preparing 14 to 24 pints of tea. This blend consists of relaxing diaphoretics and refrigerants that provide relief from excessive heat and tension during a fever, without further stimulating the fire within. The inclusion of wild lettuce in this mix can induce drowsiness, which is beneficial as sleep is a vital healing mechanism. Get yourself a cup and then go to sleep!

Ingredients:
- ½ cup of dried catnip leaf and flower
- ½ cup of dried elderflower
- ½ cup of dried peppermint leaf
- ¼ cup of dried wild lettuce leaf and stalk

Instructions:
1. In a medium bowl, thoroughly combine all the dried herbs. Store the mixture in an airtight container.
2. To prepare a hot infusion, measure 1 to 2 tablespoons of the herb mix and place it in a pint-size mason jar. Pour the boiling water over the herbs, cover, and steep for 20 minutes or until the infusion has cooled. It is recommended to drink this tea slightly cooler than usual.
3. Sip on a mugful of the tea whenever you wish to alleviate a fever.

Quick-acting fever tea

Combine 1 teaspoon of echinacea root and 1 teaspoon of white willow root in a pan. Cover the roots with 1 cup of water. Bring the mixture to a boil, then reduce the heat and let it simmer for 30 minutes. Allow the infusion to cool and strain the liquid. Take half a cup of the herbal infusion, up to four times a day.

Food Intolerances

Food sensitivities are extremely common and run the gamut from mild to life-threateningly severe. They cause all manner of gastrointestinal upsets—heartburn, IBS, bloating, and more—but can also contribute to systemic inflammation, neurological problems, and autoimmunity. In our opinion, everyone should periodically assess for sensitivity to a few common foods: Gluten, dairy, soy, corn, eggs, and nightshades (potatoes, tomatoes, peppers, eggplant, etc.) are all common culprits. A 30-day elimination period similar to what's described on Whole30.com, during which you avoid the suspect food entirely and track the severity of your symptoms, is the best way to identify if you have a sensitivity to a particular food.

Once your individual trigger foods are identified and eliminated from your diet, there's still some cleanup and reset work to do—that's where herbs really shine. A cup or two of herb-infused broth and a quart of gut-healing infusion in a day will have you feeling like a new person in no time.

Relevant tissue states: heat (inflammation), laxity (barrier compromise)

Relevant herbal actions: bitter, carminative, demulcent, hepatic, nervine, nutritive, relaxant, vulnerary

Supportive Herbs
- Angelica
- Barberry
- Bayberry
- Blue Cohosh
- Calendula flower
- Catnip leaf and flower
- Chamomile flower
- Coneflower
- Dandelion
- Echinacea
- Fennel seed
- Ginger
- Kelp
- Licorice root
- Marshmallow
- Meadowsweet flower
- Oregon grape
- Peppermint
- Plantain leaf
- Self-heal leaf and flower
- St. John's wort leaf and flower
- Tulsi leaf
- Yarrow leaf and flower

Flatulence, or gas, is commonly experienced as a symptom of indigestion. It often occurs when we eat too quickly or consume large quantities of food. Additionally, flatulence can be attributed to allergies or enzyme deficiencies, indicating difficulties in breaking down certain foods within our bodies. For instance, individuals who lack the enzyme lactase may struggle to digest the sugars present in dairy products, resulting in fermentation of milk sugars in the colon and the subsequent production of gas. Consuming high-fiber foods, beans, and cabbage can also contribute to the occurrence of flatulence.

Indigestion refers to any gastrointestinal disturbance, such as an upset stomach. Indigestion can occur if you eat too fast, eat too much, eat while emotionally upset, or, for some people, eat the wrong foods. Caffeine, high-fiber foods, alcohol, and carbonated drinks are often indigestion culprits. Sometimes allergies can cause indigestion. Indigestion can be a symptom of a number of diseases, including pancreatitis, ulcers, gastritis, and cholecystis. Often, however, there is no known cause for indigestion.

Gut-heal tea

Makes 4⅓ cups of dried herb mix, providing enough for approximately 20 to 40 quarts of tea. This well-rounded blend of digestive herbs encompasses a range of actions necessary for restoring healthy function to the stomach, intestines, and liver. It is a great blend, because it allows for easy customization. For instance, if you experience significant gut cramping, increasing the amounts of chamomile and fennel would be beneficial. If you tend to have a dry constitution, incorporating more marshmallow would be advantageous. If you are prone to excessive heat, omitting ginger would be advisable. Feel free to exclude any herbs you don't prefer and increase the quantities of your favorites. Aim to drink a quart or more of this tea each day.

Ingredients:
- ½ cup of dried calendula flower
- ½ cup of dried plantain leaf
- ½ cup of dried chamomile flower
- ½ cup of dried tulsi leaf
- ⅓ cup of dried catnip leaf and flower
- ⅓ cup of fennel seed
- ⅓ cup of dried peppermint leaf
- ⅓ cup of dried marshmallow leaf
- ¼ cup of dried ginger
- ¼ cup of dried licorice root
- ¼ cup of dried yarrow leaf and flower
- ¼ cup of dried St. John's wort leaf and flower (optional, see Tip)

Instructions:
1. In a large bowl, thoroughly mix all the dried herbs. Store the blend in an airtight container.
2. To prepare a hot infusion, prepare a kettle of boiling water. Measure 2 to 3 tablespoons of the herb mix per quart of water and place it in a mason jar or French press. Pour the boiling water over the herbs, cover, and steep for 20 minutes or until the infusion has cooled enough to drink.

Tip: If you are taking pharmaceutical medications, it is advisable to omit the St. John's wort from the blend.

Build-up broth

Makes about 3 quarts

Bone broth is very healing to the gut, especially when the bones have bits of collagen (gristle) attached. The amino acids in these parts help restore intestinal integrity, which is compromised by the food allergy reaction. Adding herbs enhances these healing and anti-inflammatory activities. If you feel particularly awful, forego solid food for a day and just have lots of broth!

One more reason to get in the bone broth habit: Broth made from bones with collagenous tissue still attached is rich in glucosamine and chondroitin. These nutrients are utilized by the body to rebuild healthy joints and connective tissues. You can buy glucosamine and chondroitin as supplements, but bone broth is a cheaper source and has so many other additional benefits!

1 cup dried calendula flower
¼ cup dried dandelion root
¼ cup fennel seed
¼ cup dried ginger
¼ cup dried kelp
Bones (such as from 1 rotisserie chicken; 6 pork chop bones; 1 lamb or beef shank; or the bones, head, and tail from 2 medium fish—really, any bones will do . . .)
3 quarts water, plus more as needed
1 tablespoon apple cider vinegar
Oyster, shiitake, or maitake mushrooms, for their nutritive and healing properties (optional)
Salt
Freshly ground black pepper

1. In a large pot over high heat, combine the herbs, bones, water, vinegar, and mushrooms (if using). Season with salt and pepper. Bring to a boil. Sustain boiling for 4 to 8 hours. Check often and add enough water to replace what has boiled away.
2. Strain the liquid and reserve. Compost the bones and herb marc, if desired.
3. Drink a mug of warm broth 2 to 3 times per day.

Stop-flatulence tea

Combine 1 teaspoon of dried angelica root, 2 teaspoons of peppermint leaves, and 1 teaspoon of bee balm leaves in a container. Take 1 tablespoon of the herb mixture and place it in a cup. Pour 1 cup of boiling water over the herbs, cover, and let it steep for 20 to 30 minutes. After steeping, strain the liquid. Take the herbal infusion as needed for relief.

Colon-soothing tea

Combine 2 teaspoons of bee balm leaves, 2 teaspoons of peppermint leaves, and 2 teaspoons of chamomile flowers in a container. Take 1 tablespoon of the herb mixture and place it in a cup. Pour 1 cup of boiling water over the herbs, cover, and let it steep for 30 minutes. After steeping, strain the liquid. Take the herbal infusion as needed for relief.

Quick-acting flatulence tea

Combine 1 teaspoon of catnip leaves, 1 teaspoon of grated ginger root, and 2 teaspoons of dandelion leaves. Place the herb mixture in a container and cover it with 2 cups of boiling water. Let the herbs steep in the water for 20 to 30 minutes. After steeping, strain the liquid. Take the herbal infusion as needed for relief.

Gut-clearing tea

Combine 1 teaspoon of blue cohosh root and 1 teaspoon of coneflower root in a glass container. Pour 1 cup of boiling water over the herbs, cover, and let them steep for 30 minutes. After steeping, allow the infusion to cool and strain the liquid. Take the herbal infusion as needed, up to one cup per day.

Daily digestive tea

Combine 1 teaspoon of angelica root, 1 teaspoon of grated ginger root, 2 teaspoons of chamomile flowers, and 2 teaspoons of peppermint leaves in a container. Take 1 tablespoon of the herb mixture and place it in 1 cup of boiling water. Let the mixture steep for 30 minutes. After steeping, cool and strain the liquid. Take the herbal infusion as needed, up to two cups per day.

Peppery indigestion tea

Combine 1 teaspoon of licorice root and 1 teaspoon of peppermint leaves in a nonmetallic container. Cover the herbs with 2 cups of boiling water and steep for 15 to 20 minutes. After steeping, strain the liquid. Take the herbal infusion as needed, up to one cup per day.

Hangover

A hangover is the unpleasant aftermath of consuming excessive amounts of alcohol. While enjoying a night of celebration or socializing can be fun, it's important to remember to drink responsibly to avoid the discomfort of a hangover the next day.

When you wake up with a hangover, you might experience a range of symptoms that can vary from person to person. These symptoms often include headache, fatigue, nausea, dizziness, sensitivity to light and sound, dry mouth, and overall feelings of malaise. A hangover can leave you feeling drained and less than your best self. Basically, it's your body telling you, "that's what you get for drinking too much!"

To alleviate the discomfort of a hangover, it's important to practice self-care. Stay hydrated by drinking plenty of water, as alcohol can dehydrate your body. Resting and getting some sleep can also help your body recover. Eating small, nutritious meals can provide your body with essential nutrients and help restore your energy levels. Time, rest, and taking care of yourself are usually the best remedies.

Take care of yourself and be mindful of your alcohol consumption to avoid the discomfort of a hangover. Remember, the best memories are made when we're feeling our best!

Relevant tissue states: heat (inflammation), dryness (dehydration), laxity (barrier compromise)
Relevant herbal actions: anodyne, antiemetic, anti-inflammatory, relaxant

Supportive Herbs
- Barberry
- Bayberry
- Betony leaf and flower
- Catnip
- Chaparral
- Chamomile flower
- Ginger
- Goldenseal
- Linden leaf and flower
- Licorice root
- Marshmallow
- Milk thistle seed
- Oregon Grape
- Plantain leaf
- Peppermint
- Self-heal leaf and flower
- St. John's wort leaf and flower

The number-one hangover preventive and simplest remedy is milk thistle capsules.
Milk thistle is one of the few herbs that are very effective in capsule form, and almost all commercially available brands are good quality. The best strategy is to take 2 capsules with a big glass of water before you start drinking, another 2 before bed, and 2 more in the morning. Sometimes this will prevent you from getting a hangover at all!

Take-it-easy next day infusion

This blend of dried herbs creates a soothing tea that effectively alleviates common hangover symptoms while aiding in rehydration. It is advisable to prepare the tea in advance, ensuring it is readily available when needed. Slowly consume a quart or more throughout the day for optimal relief.

Ingredients:
- ½ cup dried betony leaf and flower
- ½ cup dried plantain leaf
- ½ cup dried calendula flower
- ½ cup dried chamomile flower
- ⅓ cup dried linden leaf and flower
- ⅓ cup dried marshmallow leaf
- ⅓ cup dried self-heal leaf and flower
- 1 tablespoon dried licorice root
- 1 tablespoon dried ginger
- ¼ cup dried St. John's wort leaf and flower (optional, see Tip)

Instructions:
1. In a medium bowl, thoroughly mix all the dried herbs. Store the blend in an airtight container.
2. To prepare a hot infusion, prepare a kettle of boiling water. Measure 2 to 3 tablespoons of the herb mix per quart of water and place it in a mason jar or French press. Pour the boiling water over the herbs, cover, and steep for 20 minutes or until the infusion has cooled enough to drink.

Tip: If you are taking pharmaceutical medications, it is advisable to omit the St. John's wort from the blend.

No-fuss hangover tea

Combine 1 teaspoon of ripe barberry berries and 1 teaspoon of Oregon grape root in a nonmetallic container. Cover the herbs with 2 cups of boiling water, then steep for 30 minutes. After steeping, allow the infusion to cool and strain the liquid. Take up to one cup of the herbal infusion per day, diluting it in plenty of cool water.

Quick-acting hangover tea

Combine 1 teaspoon of bayberry root, 1 teaspoon of dried goldenseal root, and 1 teaspoon of Oregon grape root in a nonmetallic container. Cover the herbs with 2 cups of boiling water and steep for 30 minutes. After steeping, strain the liquid. Take 1 tablespoon of the herb mixture and add it to an 8-ounce glass of water. Throughout the day, drink several glasses of the herbal infusion.

Spicy hangover tea

Combine 1 teaspoon of catnip leaves, 1 teaspoon of peppermint leaves, and 1 teaspoon of dried chaparral leaves in a nonmetallic container. Cover the herbs with 2 cups of boiling water and steep for 20 to 30 minutes. After steeping, strain the liquid. Take half a cup of the herbal infusion at a time, up to two cups per day.

Headache

Headaches are very common and can be dull and steady, stabbing, gnawing, or throbbing. There are many kinds of headaches with many different causes. Sometimes tension, fatigue, or stress can cause a headache. Problems with the eyes, ears, nose, throat, or teeth can bring on a headache, as can allergies, injuries, infection, tumors, and any number of diseases. Headaches are also big business. In fact, Americans spend in excess of $1 billion each year buying medicines to help combat headaches. Most people take nonsteroidal anti-inflammatory drugs (NSAIDs) such as aspirin, ibuprofen, or indomethacin, or even stronger painkillers. But these drugs have unwanted, and sometimes serious, side effects, including ulcers and an increased tendency to bleeding. Herbs can offer a safer alternative.

Relevant tissue states: heat or cold, damp or dry, tense or lax
Relevant herbal actions: anodyne, anti-inflammatory, astringent, circulatory stimulant, relaxant

Supportive Herbs
- Betony leaf and flower
- Catnip
- Chamomile flower
- Feverfew
- Peppermint
- Pleurisy root
- White Willow
- Wintergreen
- Ginger
- Linden leaf and flower
- Marshmallow
- Meadowsweet flower
- Sage leaf
- Tulsi leaf
- Wild lettuce

Headaches arise from a variety of imbalances. Some are simple one-off causes—dehydration, sleep debt, dietary excesses, alcohol, caffeine, medications. For those, you want quick pain relief while you supply what's missing or simply wait for the body to recover. (When unsure of where to start, turn to betony.)

For long-term relief, it's important to identify your individual triggers, as well as the underlying patterns that contribute to your pain; this takes some experimentation. The following herbal remedies are designed to address the most common types of headaches we see, but try different combinations of herbs to refine the remedy and make it as personal as possible. If you have recurrent headaches and find this helps, drink a quart or more every day as a preventive.

Cooling headache tea

This blend of dried herbs is specifically formulated to alleviate headaches that are accompanied by a hot, sharp, and sensitive sensation. These types of headaches can be caused by tension, stress, anxiety, sinus congestion, or direct nerve pain. The herbs in this blend work to cool, relax, and promote drainage.

Ingredients:
- 1 cup dried betony leaf and flower
- 1 cup dried meadowsweet flower
- ½ cup dried linden leaf and flower
- ½ cup dried marshmallow leaf
- ¼ cup dried wild lettuce leaf and stalk

Instructions:
1. In a medium bowl, thoroughly mix together all the dried herbs. Store the blend in an airtight container.
2. To prepare a hot infusion, prepare a kettle of boiling water. Measure 2 to 3 tablespoons of the herb mix per quart of water and place it in a mason jar or French press. Pour the boiling water over the herbs, cover, and steep for 30 to 40 minutes. The tea can be consumed warm or cooled down to your preference. Drinking one cup of this tea should provide some relief from the headache.

Warming headache tea

This blend of dried herbs is specifically designed to address headaches characterized by a pale face and a cold, dull, and broad pain sensation. These types of headaches are often associated with conditions such as hypothyroidism, liver congestion, and circulatory stagnation. The herbs in this blend work to warm the body, gently constrict, and improve circulation. If you typically find relief from headaches with caffeine, this blend may be worth trying. For those experiencing recurrent headaches, consuming a quart or more of this tea daily can serve as a preventive measure.

Ingredients:
- 1 cup dried betony leaf and flower
- 1 cup dried tulsi leaf
- ½ cup dried chamomile flower
- ½ cup dried sage leaf
- ¼ cup dried ginger

Instructions:
1. In a medium bowl, thoroughly mix together all the dried herbs. Store the blend in an airtight container.
2. To prepare a hot infusion, prepare a kettle of boiling water. Measure 2 to 3 tablespoons of the herb mix per quart of water and place it in a mason jar or French press. Pour the boiling water over the herbs, cover, and steep for 30 to 40 minutes. The tea should be consumed warm to hot. Drinking one cup of this tea should begin to provide some relief from the headache.

Peppery headache tea

Combine 1 teaspoon each of feverfew leaves and peppermint leaves in a nonmetallic container. Pour 1 cup of boiling water over the herbs and steep for 30 minutes. Strain the infusion and add honey to taste. Take 1 tablespoon at a time, up to 1 cup per day.

Soothing headache tea

Combine 1 teaspoon of catnip leaves and 2 teaspoons of feverfew leaves in a glass container. Pour 1 to 2 cups of boiling water over the herbs and steep for 30 minutes. Strain the mixture and take up to 1 cup per day, a tablespoon at a time.

Heartburn/Reflux/GERD

Heartburn is burning stomach pain that can spread up into your throat. Heartburn occurs when hydrochloric acid from your stomach backs up into the esophagus. This condition can result if you gulp your food or drink too much caffeine or alcohol. It can also occur if you eat while stressed or eat certain foods (such as spicy or fatty foods). Antacids are commonly taken for heartburn, but herbs can be just as effective.

Note: If you suffer from heartburn, avoid peppermint. Although it is helpful in treating indigestion and other stomach problems, it can relax the esophageal sphincter and actually increase the tendency toward heartburn.

Relevant tissue states: heat (inflammation), laxity

Relevant herbal actions: bitter, carminative, demulcent, vulnerary

Supportive Herbs
- Barberry
- Bayberry
- Catnip leaf and flower
- Chamomile flower
- Chaparral
- Coriander
- Dandelion root
- Fennel seed
- Ginger
- Hops
- Kelp
- Licorice root
- Linden leaf and flower
- Marshmallow
- Meadowsweet flower
- Oregon grape
- Self-heal leaf and flower
- St. John's wort leaf and flower
- Yellow Dock

Contrary to what you might expect, heartburn is most often caused by low levels of stomach acid. When stomach acid is low, it causes a chain of problems in the digestive system that ultimately increase upward-moving pressure in the abdomen. This weakens the "trapdoor" between the stomach and the esophagus—when that's compromised, acid is more likely to splash up through and irritate the unprotected tissue there.

Reducing stomach acid production (with antacids or acid-blocking pharmaceuticals) temporarily relieves pain, but makes the underlying problem worse. To address heartburn, first we have to heal existing damage in the esophagus or stomach (inflammation and ulcers). Then we can work to restore normal acid levels to prevent recurrence.

That stomach-esophagus "trapdoor" (the lower esophageal sphincter, LES) can also be compromised by poor alignment and stress. When in a state of stress, saliva production decreases and digestive movement is inhibited. A rest-and-digest state of mind is required to retain the proper resting tone of the LES. This starts by being present with your food—slow down, chew thoroughly, take your time.

Marshmallow infusion
Makes 1 quart

If you have active heartburn, the first thing you need is a good cold infusion of marshmallow root. Keep this on hand for when there's an attack and to heal the damaged tissue in the esophagus. When heartburn happens, just sip on this slowly and you'll feel relief in no time.

2 to 4 tablespoons dried marshmallow root

In a quart-size mason jar, combine the marshmallow with enough cold or room-temperature water to fill the jar. Cover and steep for 4 to 8 hours. Keep refrigerated, where each batch will last for 2 to 3 days.

Preventive bitter tincture
Makes 3½ fluid ounces (30 to 60 doses)

This blend of tinctures is designed to restore normal stomach acid levels and reduce the conditions for heartburn. Take these drops before every meal to promote healthy digestion.

1 fluid ounce tincture of dandelion root
½ fluid ounce tincture of catnip
½ fluid ounce tincture of chamomile
⅓ fluid ounce tincture of fennel
⅓ fluid ounce tincture of meadowsweet
⅓ fluid ounce tincture of self-heal
½ fluid ounce tincture of St. John's wort (see Tip)

1. In a small bottle, combine the tinctures. Cap the bottle and label it.
2. Take ½ to 1 dropperful of the mixture 10 minutes before eating.

TIP: Omit the St. John's wort if you are concurrently taking pharmaceuticals.

Quick-acting heartburn tea

1 teaspoon dried angelica root
1 teaspoon crushed juniper berries
1 cup boiling water

1. Combine the herbs in a nonmetallic container and cover with the boiling water; steep for 20 to 30 minutes; strain.
2. Take a tablespoon at a time, as needed.

Soothing heartburn tea

Makes 1 cup of herbal infusion

To alleviate discomfort and promote relaxation, combine catnip leaves and oxeye daisy herb with boiling water. Steep for 30 minutes, then strain. Take a tablespoon of the herbal infusion at a time, as needed.

Hypertension

Hypertension can be classified into two primary types: essential hypertension and secondary hypertension. Essential hypertension, also known as primary hypertension, is the most common form, gradually developing over time without a specific identifiable cause. Secondary hypertension, on the other hand, arises as a result of underlying medical conditions or certain medications.

One of the striking aspects of hypertension is its tendency to remain silent in its early stages, often presenting no noticeable symptoms. However, if left uncontrolled, this silent companion can wreak havoc on the cardiovascular system and lead to serious health complications. Persistently elevated blood pressure places strain on the arteries and vital organs, including the heart, brain, kidneys, and eyes. This strain increases the risk of developing cardiovascular diseases such as heart attack, stroke, heart failure, and kidney disease.

Various factors contribute to the development of hypertension, encompassing a combination of genetic, environmental, and lifestyle influences. Risk factors for hypertension include a family history of high blood pressure, unhealthy dietary habits (such as consuming excessive sodium and inadequate potassium), physical inactivity, obesity, tobacco use, excessive alcohol consumption, stress, and the presence of certain underlying medical conditions like diabetes and kidney disease.

Diagnosis of hypertension typically involves measuring blood pressure levels using a sphygmomanometer. Blood pressure readings consist of two values: systolic pressure (the higher number) and diastolic pressure (the lower number). Normal blood pressure is generally considered to be around 120/80 mmHg. Hypertension is defined as blood pressure persistently equal to or greater than 130/80 mmHg.

Managing hypertension requires a comprehensive approach, combining lifestyle modifications and, in some cases, medication. Lifestyle changes may include adopting a balanced diet rich in fruits, vegetables, whole grains, and lean proteins, reducing sodium intake, engaging in regular physical activity, maintaining a healthy weight, moderating alcohol consumption, and quitting smoking. Medications, when prescribed by healthcare professionals, aim to lower blood pressure and minimize the risk of associated complications.

By embracing these evidence-based strategies and collaborating with healthcare professionals, individuals with hypertension can take proactive steps towards managing their blood pressure and reducing the risks associated with this intriguing condition.

Relevant tissue states: heat, tension

Relevant herbal actions: hypotensive, nervine, relaxant, sedative

Supportive Herbs
- Black Cohosh
- Black Currant
- Burdock
- Cayenne
- Dandelion
- Garlic
- Ginger
- Gingko Biloba
- Ginseng
- Goldenseal
- Gotu Kola
- Kelp
- Linden leaf and flower
- Marshmallow
- Raspberry
- Rose
- Slippery Elm
- Yarrow leaf and flower

Occasional high blood pressure is normal—it's a part of the natural response to stressful situations. Over time, though, high blood pressure can cause or worsen other cardiovascular problems. Herbs offer a nice suite of actions to reduce high blood pressure, often by addressing root causes rather than merely acting symptomatically.

It's worth noting that high blood pressure isn't always bad: New information indicates that hypertension that develops in the elder years may actually help reduce the risk of dementia.

Softhearted tea

Makes 2 cups dried herb mix (enough for 12 to 16 quarts of tea).

To promote relaxation and soothe both the mind and the physical heart, this herbal blend is highly beneficial. If you have a dry constitution, you can prepare it as a cold infusion. It is recommended to consume a quart or more of this tea daily.

1 cup dried linden leaf and flower
½ cup dried marshmallow leaf
½ cup dried rose petals

1. In a small bowl, combine all the herbs. Store the mixture in an airtight container.
2. Prepare a hot infusion: Boil a kettle of water. Take 2 to 3 tablespoons of the herb mixture per quart of water and place it in a mason jar or French press. Pour the boiling water over the herbs, cover, and steep for 20 minutes or until the tea is cool enough to drink.

Free-flowing circulation tea

1 teaspoon burdock root
1 teaspoon goldenseal root
1 teaspoon cayenne
2 teaspoons slippery elm bark
2 slices ginger root
3 cups boiling water

1. Combine the above herbs in a nonmetallic container, and pour the boiling water over them. Steep for 30 minutes, cool, and strain.
2. Take up to one cup a day, two tablespoons at a time.

Anti-congestive tea

2 teaspoons black cohosh root
4 teaspoons ginkgo biloba leaves
2 cups boiling water

1. Combine the herbs in a non-metallic container and pour the boiling water over them.
2. Let the mixture steep for 30 minutes, then cool and strain.
3. Take two to three tablespoons at a time, up to six times a day.

Arteriosclerosis preventive tea

to 3 ginger slices
2 teaspoons Ginkgo biloba leaves
1 teaspoon ginseng leaves
2 cups boiling water

1. Combine the herbs in a non-metallic container and cover with the boiling water.
2. Let the mixture steep for 30 minutes, then cool and strain.
3. Take up to half a cup per day.

Indigestion/Dyspepsia

Indigestion refers to any gastrointestinal disturbance, such as an upset stomach. Indigestion can occur if you eat too fast, eat too much, eat while emotionally upset, or, for some people, eat the wrong foods. Caffeine, high-fiber foods, alcohol, and carbonated drinks are often indigestion culprits. Sometimes allergies can cause indigestion. Indigestion can be a symptom of a number of diseases, including pancreatitis, ulcers, gastritis, and cholecystis. Often, however, there is no known cause for indigestion.

Relevant tissue states: cold (stagnation), tension
Relevant herbal actions: bitter, carminative, relaxant

Supportive Herbs
- Angelica
- Barberry
- Bayberry
- Blue Cohosh
- Catnip leaf and flower
- Chamomile flower
- Coneflower
- Dandelion root
- Echinacea
- Fennel seed
- Ginger
- Licorice root
- Oregon Grape
- Peppermint leaf
- Sage leaf

If you're having chronic digestive discomforts, take a hard look at your diet to see if you have any food sensitivities. Lucky for you, though, indigestion is a problem for which herbal quick fixes are ready at hand—read on for two simple, portable solutions.

Pre-emptive bitter tincture
Makes 4 fluid ounces (60 to 120 doses)

Indigestion often means just that—incomplete digestion. This formula stimulates all your digestive fluids—saliva, stomach acid, bile, and pancreatic enzymes—so digestion is as thorough and complete as possible.

1 fluid ounce tincture of dandelion root
1 fluid ounce tincture of sage
1 fluid ounce tincture of catnip
1 fluid ounce tincture of chamomile

1. In a small bottle, combine the tinctures. Cap the bottle and label it.
2. Take 1 to 2 drops 10 minutes before eating.

Carminative tincture
Makes 4 fluid ounces (60 to 120 doses)

This formula warms the body's core, stimulating your digestive organs and keeping the bowels from getting sluggish. If peppermint isn't your style, substitute angelica.

1½ fluid ounces tincture of ginger
1 fluid ounce tincture of fennel
1 fluid ounce tincture of peppermint (see headnote)
½ fluid ounce tincture of licorice

1. In a small bottle, combine the tinctures. Cap the bottle and label it.
2. Take 1 to 2 drops after each meal, or whenever your guts feel uncomfortably stuck.

Digestive tea
1 teaspoon blue cohosh root
1 teaspoon coneflower root
1 cup boiling water

1. Combine the above herbs in a glass container.
2. Pour the boiling water over the herbs; steep for 30 minutes; cool and strain.
3. Take as needed, up to one cup a day.

Strong digestive tea
1 teaspoon angelica root
1 teaspoon grated ginger root
2 teaspoons chamomile flowers
2 teaspoons peppermint leaves
1 cup boiling water

1. Combine the above ingredients in a container.
2. Take one tablespoon of the herb mixture and place in the boiling water; steep for 30 minutes; cool and strain.
3. Take as needed, up to two cups a day.

Quick-acting digestive tea
1 teaspoon licorice root
1 teaspoon peppermint leaves
2 cups boiling water

1. Combine the licorice root and peppermint leaves in a non-metallic container.
2. Pour the boiling water over the herbs and steep for 15 to 20 minutes.
3. Strain the mixture.
4. Take up to one cup per day, as needed.

Insomnia

Insomnia is any difficulty in sleeping. Some people find it difficult to fall asleep, while others can fall asleep easily but don't stay asleep. Nearly one-fourth of all Americans have an occasional problem sleeping, but some people (as much as 10 percent of the American population) suffer from chronic insomnia. Insomnia can occur for a number of reasons, including stress and nervous tension, excessive intake of caffeinated drinks, and irregular sleeping habits.

Insomnia can lead to fatigue and an inability to function at an optimal energy level during the day. Irritability, daytime drowsiness, and memory impairment often affect those suffering from insomnia.

Relevant tissue states: heat (agitation), tension
Relevant herbal actions: hypnotic, relaxant, sedative

Supportive Herbs

- Ashwagandha root
- Betony leaf and flower
- Catnip leaf and flower
- Chamomile flower
- Hops
- Linden leaf and flower
- Passionflower
- Rose
- Valerian
- Wild lettuce

Wild animals don't have insomnia. Hikers in the wilds don't either, actually. According to a 2013 study in the journal Current Biology, just a few days in an outdoor environment, with no artificial light exposure, is enough to reestablish normal circadian rhythms—even in people who are habitual "night owls" in their city lives. This tracks with a large and growing body of evidence that indicates that our electrically lit environments are directly responsible for most sleep disturbances we experience.

Reducing evening exposure to bright lights—including TV, computer, and smartphone screens—is one of the most important steps you can take to fight insomnia. Dimming lights and avoiding screens for at least an hour before bed, and taking the herbal remedies offered here, are sure ways to improve both the quantity and quality of your sleep.

End-of-the-day elixir

Makes 4 fluid ounces (60 to 120 doses)

This blend of relaxants and gentle sedatives doesn't force sleep but helps relieve the tension, anxiety, and distraction that make it difficult to transition into sleep. This formula (and any herbs taken to aid in sleep) is best taken in "pulse doses," which is much more effective than taking the total dose all at once right at bedtime. It gives the herbs time to start working in your system and emphasizes to the body that it's time to transition into sleep.

1 fluid ounce tincture of chamomile
1 fluid ounce tincture of betony
¾ fluid ounce tincture of ashwagandha
½ fluid ounce tincture of catnip
½ fluid ounce tincture of linden
¼ fluid ounce honey (plain or rose petal–infused)

1. In a small bottle, combine the tinctures and honey. Cap the bottle and label it.
2. One hour before bedtime, take 1 to 2 drops.
3. Thirty minutes before bedtime, take another 1 to 2 drops.
4. At bedtime, take the final 1 to 2 drops.

Sleep! Formula

Makes 4 fluid ounces (60 to 120 doses)

For this formula, we recruit wild lettuce, the strongest hypnotic (sleep-inducing) herb in this book. This is especially helpful if part of what's keeping you up at night is physical pain, as wild lettuce also has a pain-relieving effect. This formula, like End-of-the-Day Elixir, is best taken in "pulse doses."

2 fluid ounces tincture of wild lettuce
1 fluid ounce tincture of betony
½ fluid ounce tincture of chamomile
½ fluid ounce tincture of linden

1. In a small bottle, combine the tinctures. Cap the bottle and label it.
2. One hour before bedtime, take 1 to 2 drops.
3. Thirty minutes before bedtime, take another 1 to 2 drops.
4. At bedtime, take the final 1 to 2 drops.

Insomnia relief tea

1 teaspoon chamomile flowers
1 teaspoon hops
1 teaspoon valerian root
1 cup boiling water

1. Combine the chamomile flowers, hops, and valerian root.
2. Take one tablespoon of the herb mixture and place it in a cup.
3. Pour boiling water over the herbs and let them steep for 30 minutes.
4. Strain the mixture.
5. Drink the tea warm, as needed, in half-cup servings.

Sweet dreams tea

2 teaspoons catnip leaves
1 teaspoon hops
2 teaspoons chamomile flower
2 teaspoons passionflower
1 cup boiling water

1. Combine the catnip leaves, hops, chamomile flower, and passionflower in a glass container.
2. Pour the boiling water over the herbs, ensuring they are fully submerged.
3. Cover the container and let the herbs steep in the water for 30 minutes.
4. After steeping, allow the mixture to cool.
5. Strain the tea to remove the herb solids.
6. Drink the tea one hour before bedtime.

Menstrual cycle irregularities

The irregularities include various disruptions of the menstrual cycle. Each is addressed slightly differently, but a few overarching actions emerge that help with all of them: nourishing the body, improving circulation, and stimulating the liver and kidneys to clear away used-up hormones. Delayed or absent menses may be due to a lack of adequate nourishment, especially protein, or to disruptions in hormone levels. (Sometimes these share a cause. A high-sugar diet is nutrient-poor, and the havoc it wreaks on blood sugar levels has a cascade effect that disrupts hormone balance. Stress makes us tend to eat gratifying but poor-quality food, and excessive stress-response hormones interfere with the normal actions of estrogen and progesterone.)

Irregular cycles, with no predictable pattern, may also be due to poor nourishment, liver stagnation or strain, or an irregular lifestyle—especially erratic sleep habits. The daily cycle shapes the monthly cycle, like small and large gears interlocking in a watch. Overheavy bleeding generally comes from hormones not clearing efficiently at the liver, though it may also be connected with the development of fibroids or polyps. If heavy bleeding persists, seek medical attention.

Finally, let's talk about the most common menstrual ailment: dysmenorrhea, or menstrual pain, which usually begins just before menstruation, may occur in the lower abdomen or the lower back (and sometimes even into the thighs). Other accompanying symptoms may include nausea, vomiting, headache, and either constipation or diarrhea. This condition affects more than half of all women. There are two types of dysmenorrhea, primary and secondary.

In primary dysmenorrhea, there is no underlying pain causing the disorder. It is thought that the pain occurs when uterine contractions reduce blood supply to the uterus. This may occur if the uterus is in the wrong position, if the cervical opening is narrow, and due to lack of exercise.

Secondary dysmenorrhea is when the pain is caused by some gynecological disorder, such as endometriosis (when the endometrium, the tissue that lines the uterus, abnormally grows on surfaces of other structures in the abdominal cavity), adenomyosis (in-growth of the endometrium into the uterine musculature), lesions, inflammation of the fallopian tubes, or uterine fibroids. Uterine fibroids are tumors of the uterus that are not usually cancerous. Also known as myomas, these masses occur in nearly one-quarter of all women by the age of forty. Some women with uterine fibroids may have no symptoms. However, if symptoms are present, they include increased frequency of urination, a bloated feeling, pressure, pain, and abnormal bleeding.

Relevant tissue states: cold (stagnation), laxity

Relevant herbal actions: astringent, carminative, circulatory stimulant, emmenagogue, nutritive, rubefacient

Supportive Herbs

- Angelica
- Ashwagandha root
- Betony leaf and flower

- Black Cohosh
- Blue Vervain
- Chamomile flower
- Crampbark
- Dandelion leaf
- Elecampane
- Feverfew
- Ginger
- Goldenrod leaf and flower
- Kelp
- Marigold
- Milk thistle seed
- Nettle leaf
- Passionflower
- Peppermint
- Pulsatilla
- Raspberry
- Sage leaf
- Self-heal leaf and flower
- St. John's Wort
- Tulsi leaf

Steady cycle tea

Makes 3½ cups dried herb mix (enough for 20 to 28 quarts of tea)

This nourishing blend of herbs provides support for kidney, lymphatic, and endocrine systems, making it beneficial for menstrual irregularities. Customize the formula by adding ginger for warmth, betony for anxiety, and peppermint for taste. Drink a quart or more daily.

1 cup dried nettle leaf
1 cup dried dandelion leaf
½ cup dried goldenrod leaf and flower
½ cup dried self-heal leaf and flower
¼ cup dried tulsi leaf
¼ cup dried kelp

1. In a small bowl, combine all the herbs. Store in an airtight container.
2. Make a long infusion: Boil water in a kettle. Measure 2 to 3 tablespoons of the herb mixture per quart of water and place in a mason jar or French press. Pour the boiling water over the herbs, cover, and steep for 8 hours or overnight.

Bleed on! Tea

Makes 3 cups dried herb mix (enough for 20 to 26 quarts of tea)

To encourage menstruation, drink this tea for 3 days to 1 week before the expected start of your period. For best results, consume the tea hot and reheat as needed throughout the day. For a stronger effect, add a drop of angelica tincture to each cup of tea.

1 cup dried chamomile flower
1 cup dried tulsi leaf
⅓ cup dried goldenrod leaf and flower
⅓ cup dried ginger
⅓ cup dried angelica root

1. In a small bowl, mix together all the herbs. Store in an airtight container.
2. Make a hot infusion: Boil water in a kettle. Measure 2 to 3 tablespoons of the herb mixture per quart of water and place in a mason jar or French press. Pour the boiling water over the herbs, cover, and steep for 20 minutes or until cool enough to drink.

Daily soothing menstrual tea

To create a soothing and relaxing herbal infusion, combine 2 teaspoons of black haw root or bark with 2 teaspoons of passionflower in a pan. Cover the herbs with 2 cups of cold water and let it soak overnight. The next day, strain the mixture. Take half a cup of the infusion, up to four times daily, as needed for relief.

Dysmenorrhea tea

Combine black cohosh root, crampbark, black haw root or bark, and pulsatilla in a pan. Cover with water and bring to a boil. Boil for 10 minutes, then cool and strain. Take half a cup of the mixture, up to four times a day.

Cramp relief tea

Combine St. John's wort leaves and raspberry leaves in a glass container. Cover the herbs with boiling water and steep for 15 minutes. Strain the mixture and drink as needed to relieve cramps.

Nausea and Vomiting

Nausea and vomiting are common symptoms that can occur as a result of various underlying causes. They often go hand in hand, with nausea referring to the uncomfortable feeling of an urge to vomit, while vomiting is the act of expelling the contents of the stomach through the mouth. Nausea can manifest as a sensation of queasiness, discomfort, or an unsettled stomach. It is often accompanied by an aversion to food, increased salivation, and a general feeling of unease. Vomiting, on the other hand, is the forceful expulsion of stomach contents, which can provide temporary relief from the sensation of nausea.

Numerous factors can trigger nausea and vomiting. Common causes include gastrointestinal infections (such as viral gastroenteritis), food poisoning, motion sickness, pregnancy (morning sickness), certain medications, chemotherapy, pain, emotional stress, migraines, and various medical conditions.

Nausea and vomiting can be managed through various approaches depending on the underlying cause and severity of symptoms. These may include dietary modifications, such as consuming small, frequent meals and avoiding triggers or foods that exacerbate symptoms. Maintaining proper hydration is essential to prevent dehydration resulting from fluid loss during vomiting.

While nausea and vomiting are typically short-lived and self-limiting, they can sometimes indicate more serious underlying conditions that require medical attention. If vomiting persists for an extended period, is severe, or is accompanied by symptoms such as severe abdominal pain, high fever, blood in vomit, or signs of dehydration, it is advisable to seek medical evaluation.

Understanding and addressing the triggers of nausea and vomiting, seeking appropriate medical advice when needed, and prioritizing adequate hydration and nutrition are key to managing these symptoms and promoting overall well-being.

Relevant tissue states: heat (agitation), tension (spasm)
Relevant herbal actions: antiemetic, carminative, relaxant

Supportive Herbs
- Bayberry
- Bee Balm
- Catnip leaf and flower
- Chamomile flower
- Chaparral
- Fennel seed
- Ginger
- Horehound
- Oregon Grape
- Peppermint leaf
- Yerba mansa

One way or another, nausea almost always comes from food—a sensitivity, some indigestion, various potential infections. Especially if nausea happens frequently, look closely at your diet—keeping a journal can be helpful—to identify any patterns that occur around its appearance. Maybe when you eat on the run, or eat wheat products, or have really fiery spices—whatever it is for you, the only way to identify it is to pay attention in an organized way. After a bout of vomiting, some warm, slightly weak Calming Tea can be the easiest thing to drink for quite some time. Then slowly reintroduce broth, then soup, then stew . . . gradually progressing from food prepared to be very warm and moist to food that is more cool and dry, like salad.

Both of the following formulas are also excellent for morning sickness. If you feel you can't get anything down at all, just one drop of ginger tincture all by itself on the tongue can be helpful, or even just smelling strong ginger tea.

Calming tea

Combining the best herbal antiemetics, this mixture is effective in relieving nausea. Adjust the proportions of the ingredients based on your taste preferences. It can also be consumed preventively for those prone to nausea.

1 cup dried catnip leaf and flower
1 cup dried chamomile flower
½ cup dried peppermint leaf
½ cup fennel seed
¼ cup dried ginger

Mix the herbs in a medium bowl and store in an airtight container. To prepare, steep 2 to 3 tablespoons of the herb mixture per quart of boiling water. Cover and steep for 20 minutes or until cool enough to drink. Sip slowly and inhale the scent for relief from severe nausea.

Ginger emergency formula
Makes 5 fluid ounces (60 to 120 doses)

This mixture of tinctures is one to keep in your herbal first aid kit at all times. You never know when nausea will strike, and a quick herbal relief will be very welcome. Make this with ginger-infused honey if you have the time to prepare that in advance.

2 fluid ounces tincture of ginger
1 fluid ounce tincture of catnip
1 fluid ounce tincture of chamomile
1 fluid ounce honey

1.In a small bottle, combine all the ingredients. Cap the bottle and label it.
2.Take 1 to 2 droppersful every 20 minutes until relief occurs.

Antiemetic Tea:

Combine 1 teaspoon grated ginger root, 1 teaspoon yerba mansa root, and 1 teaspoon peppermint leaves in a nonmetallic container. Cover the herbs with 2 cups of boiling water, steep for 30 minutes, then cool and strain. Take a tablespoon at a time, up to two cups a day, as needed for relief from nausea.

Calming Tea:

Combine 1 teaspoon catnip leaves and 1 teaspoon chamomile flowers in a nonmetallic container. Cover with 1 cup of boiling water, steep for 20 to 30 minutes, then cool and strain. Take as needed for a nausea-soothing effect.

Rash

A skin rash is a temporary eruption on the skin that usually looks like small red or pink bumps. It may or may not itch. There may be scaly, round, or oval patches on the skin. A rash is usually a symptom of some other condition and can indicate a disease such as measles or chickenpox, an insect bite, an allergic reaction, a nutritional deficiency, or even dry skin.

Relevant tissue states: heat (inflammation), dryness or dampness, laxity
Relevant herbal actions: anti-inflammatory, astringent, demulcent

Supportive Herbs
- Burdock
- Calendula flower
- Comfrey
- Echinacea
- Evening Primrose
- Goldenseal
- Kelp
- Licorice root
- Marshmallow
- Oregon grape
- Plantain leaf
- Rose
- Self-heal leaf and flower
- Slippery Elm
- St. John's wort leaf and flower
- Strawberry
- Uva-ursi leaf
- White oak
- Yarrow leaf and flower
- Yellow Dock

A sudden appearance of a rash generally means you've come into contact with some kind of irritant—an irritating plant, a toxic chemical, or perhaps an insect bite or sting. Wash the area well with soap and water. Then apply insights from basic herbal energetics: If the rash is dry, use moistening herbs and preparations; if it's damp and oozy, use drying agents.

If there doesn't seem to have been any contact with an irritating plant, chemical, or other direct trigger, the rash may be an external reflection of an internal imbalance. Allergies can cause this, of course, as well as overworked internal detoxification systems.

Dry rash salve
Makes 9 ounces (60-day supply)

Salves are emollient due to their oil and wax content, especially when they have a moisturizing oil, like olive oil, as the base. In this simple formula, the herbs' healing and anti-inflammatory effects enhance the emollient effect.

3 fluid ounces calendula-infused oil
3 fluid ounces plantain-infused oil
2 fluid ounces licorice-infused oil
1 ounce beeswax, plus more as needed

1.Prepare a salve as usual (see here for complete instructions).
2.Gently apply a thin layer to the affected area at least twice a day.

Weepy rash poultice
Makes 4½ cups dried herb mix (enough for 12 to 18 poultices)

Contact with poison ivy and similar plants often produces a rash with fluid-filled blisters. These call for astringents, and those are best delivered in a water extract—a poultice or compress.
Learn to identify the plants that cause contact rash in your area! Poison ivy, poison oak, and poison sumac all grow in the US. Check out poison-ivy.org for great pictures and details about how to make a positive identification, as well as how to tell them apart from benign look-alike plants.

1 cup dried calendula flower
1 cup dried rose petals
1 cup dried self-heal leaf and flower

½ cup dried St. John's wort leaf and flower
½ cup dried uva-ursi leaf
½ cup dried yarrow leaf and flower
Boiling water, to make the poultice

1.In a large bowl, mix together all the herbs. Store in an airtight container.
2.Measure 4 to 6 tablespoons of the herb mixture and place in a heat-proof dish.
3.Pour just enough boiling water over the herbs to get them fully saturated—not so much that they're swimming. Let the herbs soak for 5 minutes.
4.Apply the mass of herbs, warm and wet, to the affected area. Cover with a cloth. Keep in place for 5 to 10 minutes, then gently pat dry.
5.Repeat 1 to 3 times per day.

TIP: If you don't have these herbs on hand, plain green or black tea bags will do the trick! Just get them warm and wet, apply them over the rash, and let them sit in place for 20 minutes.

Skin-soothing tea

1 teaspoon burdock root, 1 teaspoon Oregon grape root, 1 teaspoon echinacea root, and 1 teaspoon yellow dock root in a pan. Cover the herbs with 2 cups of water. Bring to a boil, then reduce heat and simmer for 10 to 15 minutes. Cool and strain the mixture. Take a tablespoon at a time, up to half a cup a day, as needed.

Rash wash

Combine 1 teaspoon comfrey root, 1 teaspoon white oak leaves or bark, and 1 teaspoon slippery elm bark in a container. Cover the herbs with 2 cups of water. Bring to a boil and let it boil for 20 to 30 minutes. Cool and strain the mixture. Use the resulting liquid as a topical wash, applying it as needed.

Sinusitis/Stuffy Nose

Sinusitis is an inflammation of the sinuses, marked by sinus congestion, headache, and pain around the eyes or cheeks. There may be a nasal discharge, fatigue, cough, fever, earache, and an increased susceptibility to nasal infections.

Sinusitis can be caused by allergies, bacterial or fungal infections, and viral infections (such as the common cold). However, nasal injury, a deviated septum (the separator between the two nasal passages), a swollen concha (the spiral air warmers in the nose), nasal polyps, or narrow sinuses can also cause sinusitis, as can cigarette smoke, dusty or dry air, or even infected tonsils or teeth.

Relevant tissue states: heat (inflammation), laxity (mucous membranes)
Relevant herbal actions: antifungal, anti-inflammatory, antimicrobial, astringent, decongestant, demulcent

Supportive Herbs
- Bayberry
- Black Elder
- Calendula flower
- Echinacea
- Garlic
- Ginger
- Gingko Biloba
- Ginseng
- Goldenrod leaf and flower
- Goldenseal
- Licorice
- Pau D'Arco
- Pine
- Rose
- Slippery Elm
- Valerian
- White Willow
- Wild Indigo
- Witch Hazel
- Marshmallow
- Sage leaf
- Thyme leaf
- Uva-ursi leaf
- Yerba mansa

Runny nose is a vital response to a cold or the flu! Believe it or not, mucus is full of antibodies. Drying it up with pharmaceutical decongestants makes the tissue more susceptible to infection. Keeping mucous membranes at a happy medium—not too dry, not too drippy—helps shorten the illness and prevent complications.

If not connected to a full respiratory infection, or if chronic or recurrent, the cause of symptoms is likely a complex of bacterial, fungal, and viral components. (This is why it can persist even after multiple rounds of antibiotics.) Antimicrobial herbs are less specific than antibiotic drugs, which is a benefit in this case, meaning that they can counteract a variety of pathogens and compromised states simultaneously.

Grating fresh horseradish and breathing its fumes, or eating prepared horseradish or wasabi, is a great way to clear the sinuses. If you've been blowing your nose a lot and the skin is irritated, some soft, simple salve or lanolin is very soothing.

Sinus~clearing steam bath

Makes 2 cups dried herb mix (enough for 4 to 8 steams)

Steaming is a universal treatment across cultures for any respiratory system troubles, including those related to the sinuses. The combination of hot steam and the evaporating volatile oils from the herbs makes it very difficult for pathogens to survive and stimulates immune response in the mucous membranes.

1 cup dried pine needles
½ cup dried sage leaf
½ cup dried thyme leaf
½ gallon water
5 garlic cloves, chopped, per steam (optional)

1. In a small bowl, mix the pine, sage, and thyme. Store in an airtight container.
2. Make and execute an herbal steam: In a medium pot over high heat, boil the water.
3. Place the pot on a heat-proof surface, someplace where you can sit near it, and make a tent with a blanket or towel.
4. Add ¼ to ½ cup of the herb mixture to the water, along with the garlic (if using).
5. Position your face over the steam and remain there for 5 to 20 minutes. (Bring a handkerchief, your nose will run as your sinuses clear!)
6. Repeat 2 to 3 times per day.

TIP: Similar microbe-clearing benefits can be gained by working with aromatic herbs as incense or a smudge stick (a tightly wrapped bundle of leaves, lit on one end to produce medicinal smoke). A study by Nautiyal et al. in the Journal of Ethnopharmacology found that "[when] using medicinal smoke[,] it is possible to completely eliminate diverse plant and human pathogenic bacteria of the air within confined space." Conifer trees like pine are particularly apt for this.

Sinus~relieving tea

Combine 1 teaspoon echinacea root, 1 teaspoon yerba mansa root, and 1 teaspoon goldenseal root. Take 2 teaspoons of the herb mixture and place them in a cup. Cover the herbs with boiling water and steep for 20 to 30 minutes. Strain the mixture and take it warm, up to 1 cup per day, as needed.

Mucus~freeing tea

Combine 1 teaspoon bayberry root and 1 teaspoon white willow bark. Cover the herbs with 2 cups of boiling water and steep for 15 minutes. Take the infusion warm, up to 2 cups a day.

Sore Throat

Usually, a sore throat is a minor problem that takes care of itself with time. Although we may not always be able to identify the cause of a sore throat, it most often occurs because of viral infections such as the flu or a common cold. It can also occur because of exposure to irritants such as dust or smoke, from allergies, or even from talking or yelling too loudly. A sore throat may make swallowing difficult and may lead to a hoarse voice.

Relevant tissue states: heat (inflammation), dryness or dampness
Relevant herbal actions: anti-inflammatory, antimicrobial, astringent, demulcent, mucous membrane tonic

Supportive Herbs

- Balsam Fir
- Bayberry
- Black Elder
- Blue Vervain
- Canadian Fleabane
- Cayenne
- Cinnamon bark
- Coltsfoot
- Comfrey
- Echinacea
- Ginger
- Goldenrod leaf and flower
- Indian Root
- Licorice root
- Marshmallow
- Osha Root
- Sage leaf
- Self-heal leaf and flower
- Seneca Snakeroot
- Slippery Elm
- Sumac
- Wild Cherry
- Witch Hazel
- Yerba sante

Sore throats are generally due to infection, whether that's a simple cold, the flu, or strep throat. When choosing remedies, it is helpful to differentiate between the hot, inflamed, dry sore throat and the cold, wet sore throat induced by post-nasal drip. Use extra demulcents for the former and astringent mucous membrane tonics for the latter. See also Cold and Flu and Immune Support.

Sore throat tea

Makes 2 cups dried herb mix (enough for 12 to 16 quarts of tea)

If you are prone to sore throat in the colder months, make a big batch of this every winter: as soon as you feel a tickle in your throat you can get yourself a hot steaming cup and avoid getting a full-on cold and raspy throat.

Add any spices you like, such as allspice, clove, or star anise. You can also include orange peel: simply chop the peel of your (organic!) oranges and let dry fully before adding.

Stir in some lemon and honey if you like the flavors. Lemon has some antimicrobial action, and the sour and sweet flavors both stimulate the flow of healthy mucus, which fights infection. You can also add a bit of butter, ghee, or coconut oil: less than ½ teaspoon per cup of hot tea. The medium-chain fatty acids (MCFAs) in these oils are topically antimicrobial and add a nice "coating" quality to the drink.

1 cup marshmallow root
½ cup dried ginger
¼ cup dried cinnamon bark
¼ cup dried licorice root

1. In a small bowl, mix together all the herbs. Store in an airtight container.
2. Make a decoction: Measure 2 to 4 tablespoons of herbs per quart of water and place in a lidded pot over high heat. Add the water and cover the pot. Bring to a boil, reduce the heat, and simmer for 1 hour.
3. To enhance the soothing effects of the mucilaginous herbs in this blend, cool the tea fully after decoction, then continue to cool for 1 to 2 more hours. Strain, and reheat before drinking.
4. Drink liberally throughout the day.

Herbal gargle

Makes 16 fluid ounces (enough for several gargles)

Sage is an aromatic astringent, and it specifically kills rhinovirus: a virus that causes many colds. Combining it with vinegar and salt enhances these properties. If you have a dry sore throat, you may want to follow this with a nice cup of marshmallow tea.

8 fluid ounces water
2 tablespoons dried sage leaf
8 fluid ounces apple cider vinegar
3 teaspoons salt

1. In a small pot over high heat, bring the water to a boil. Remove it from the heat and add the sage. Cover tightly and let infuse for 20 minutes.
2. Strain the liquid into a pint-size mason jar.
3. Add the vinegar and salt, cover the jar, and shake well.
4. Pour off 1 fluid ounce or so and gargle with it for 2 to 3 minutes. Rinse your mouth out with water afterward—the vinegar's acidity can wear down tooth enamel if left in place.
5. Repeat 3 to 5 times per day.

Throat-soothing tea

1 teaspoon Canadian fleabane leaves
1 teaspoon slippery elm bark
1 teaspoon echinacea root
2 cups boiling water

1. Combine the herbs in a nonmetallic container and cover with the boiling water; steep for 20 to 30 minutes; strain.
2. Take up to two cups per day, warm.

Fruity gargle

Combine 1 tablespoon elderberry fruit juice, 1 tablespoon sumac extract, and 1 teaspoon echinacea root extract. Gargle with the mixture as needed.

Sweet cough drops

1 teaspoon goldenrod leaves
1 teaspoon wild cherry bark
1 teaspoon licorice root
1 teaspoon yerba sante leaves
1 teaspoon slippery elm bark
2 cups water
3 cups sugar
3 tablespoons corn syrup

1. Place the above herbs in a pan and cover with the water. Bring the mixture to a boil and boil for 20 minutes.
2. Remove from the heat and cool. Strain the solution and add the sugar and the corn syrup.
3. Place back on the heat, bring to a boil, then reduce heat to medium. Cook until the mixture reaches 300°F (hard-crack stage).
4. Pour the syrup onto a large, buttered baking sheet; cool, then break into one-inch pieces.
5. Use as you would any cough drop.

Sprains and Strains

A sprain occurs when a ligament is severely wrenched, while a strain is a tearing and overstretching of muscle fibers. The same injuries that can cause a sprain can cause a strain as well. The difference is that a sprain involves ligaments and tendons, while a strain involves muscles. Sprains and strains are very common and can cause pain, swelling, bruising, and inflammation. Movement in the affected area is often limited because of the pain and/or swelling.

Most sprains and strains may heal without complications. But more severe injuries can become chronic, develop scar tissue, limit motion, and ultimately cause problems in surrounding tissues, nerves, vessels, and organs.

Relevant tissue states: heat (inflammation), tension and/or laxity

Relevant herbal actions: anti-inflammatory, circulatory stimulant, connective tissue lubricant, lymphatic, nerve tropho-restorative, vulnerary

Supportive Herbs

- Big Sagebrush
- Bilberry
- Black Cohosh
- Black Currant
- Cinnamon essential oil
- Gingko Biloba
- Ginger
- Ginseng
- Goldenrod leaf and flower
- Gotu Kola
- Horsetail
- Kelp
- Licorice
- Marshmallow
- Meadowsweet flower
- Peppermint essential oil
- Raspberry
- Self-heal leaf and flower
- Solomon's seal root
- St. John's wort leaf and flower
- Valerian
- White willow
- Wintergreen
- Yerba Mansa

The pain of an injured joint is your body speaking a warning to you. Heed it! Don't let a minor strain become a serious sprain. Rest the joint—but don't immobilize it; gentle movement allows blood to move through the injury site and speeds healing. Drink some bone broth (see Build-Up Broth), eat some seaweed, and work with herbs to reduce inflammation, improve blood exchange, and restore the connective tissues (tendons, ligaments, fascia).

One of the best methods for healing a sprain is alternating hot and cold compresses or baths. Heat exposure brings in fresh blood, while cold constricts the vessels and squeezes out stuck fluids. Alternate between 3 minutes of hot and 30 seconds of cold. Go back and forth a few times, and always finish with hot to bring fresh, healthy circulation to the area.

Sweet relief tea

Combine 1 tablespoon of raspberry leaves and 1 teaspoon of white willow bark. Pour 2 cups of boiling water over the herbs, cover, and steep for 30 minutes. Strain the mixture. Take the herbal infusion as needed.

Soft tissue injury liniment

Makes about 8 fluid ounces (100+ applications, 30-day supply)

3 fluid ounces ginger-infused oil
2 fluid ounces Solomon's seal-infused oil or tincture of Solomon's seal
1 fluid ounce tincture of St. John's wort
1 fluid ounce tincture of self-heal
1 fluid ounce tincture of meadowsweet
40 drops peppermint essential oil
40 drops cinnamon essential oil

1.In a small bottle, combine the infused oils, tinctures, and essential oils. Cap the bottle and label it, including Shake well before each use.
2.Hold your palm over the bottle's mouth and tilt to deposit a small amount in your palm. Rub between your hands to warm the treatment, then apply to the painful joints.
3.Massage the oil into the joints until your hands no longer feel oily. Really work the liniment into the tissue.
4.Repeat the application 3 to 5 times per day. More is better!

Topical pain relief

20 drops yerba mansa tincture
4 ounces wintergreen oil
1 pound petroleum jelly

1. Thoroughly mix the above herbs with the petroleum jelly.
2. Use as an ointment to relieve muscle pain.

Quick~acting pain relief tea

Combine 2 teaspoons of black cohosh root and 1 tablespoon of ginseng root in a pan. Cover with 2 cups of water and bring to a boil. Reduce the heat and simmer for 30 minutes. Cool and strain the mixture. Take 2 to 3 tablespoons of the herbal infusion, up to 6 times a day.

Stress

Experiencing an accelerated heart rate, elevated blood pressure, muscle tension, irritability, depression, stomachache, and indigestion are common indicators of stress. While many associate stress primarily with emotional strain, it can manifest in physical and biochemical forms as well. Physical stress may arise from injuries sustained in accidents or during surgical procedures, while biochemical stress can result from exposure to pollutants, pesticides, and inadequate nutrition. These various stressors trigger the body to produce higher levels of adrenaline as a coping mechanism. However, the release of adrenaline also leads to increased heart rate, elevated blood pressure, and muscle tension.

Sustained exposure to stress can give rise to a range of health conditions. These include accelerated aging, reduced immunity against infections, compromised immune function (which may contribute to conditions like chronic fatigue syndrome), and excessive hormone production (leading to adrenal fatigue). Counteracting the effects of stress requires adopting a well-rounded approach encompassing a balanced diet and a healthy lifestyle.

Relevant tissue states: heat (agitation), tension
Relevant herbal actions: adaptogen, nervine, relaxant, sedative

Supportive Herbs
- Ashwagandha root
- Betony leaf and flower
- Catnip leaf and flower
- Chamomile flower
- Elderflower
- Ginger
- Goldenrod leaf and flower
- Hops
- Kava Kava
- Linden leaf and flower
- Peppermint
- Pleurisy
- Rose
- Sage leaf
- Skullcap
- St. John's wort leaf and flower
- Tulsi leaf
- Valerian

Everyone's stress is the same, and everyone's stress is different. We all have the same physiological response to stress—racing heart, shallow breathing, narrowed focus, heightened cortisol and blood sugar. But we react to potential stressors differently—something that bothers one person might roll right off another's back. Whatever is stressing you, herbs can help both as a short-term rescue in the immediate moment and in the long-term to build more "nerve reserve" and poise in the face of difficulties.

Rescue elixir

Prepared in a compact 5 fluid ounces (40 to 80 doses), this remedy offers a quick respite from the chaos of a demanding day. For optimal results, it is recommended to find a moment of solitude in which to engage in a brief personal ritual. Begin by centering yourself and taking a few deep breaths, then administer the tincture. Take a few more calming breaths before reentering the bustling world. The power of this remedy is amplified by the inclusion of a mindful practice.

Makes 5 fluid ounces (40 to 80 doses)

Ingredients:
- 1 fluid ounce tincture of tulsi
- 1 fluid ounce tincture of betony
- ½ fluid ounce tincture of catnip
- ½ fluid ounce tincture of chamomile
- ½ fluid ounce tincture of elderflower
- ½ fluid ounce tincture of rose
- ¼ fluid ounce tincture of goldenrod
- ¼ fluid ounce tincture of sage
- ½ fluid ounce honey

Instructions:
1. In a small bottle, combine the tinctures of tulsi, betony, catnip, chamomile, elderflower, rose, goldenrod, and sage.
2. Add ½ fluid ounce of honey to enhance the taste and enjoyment.
3. Cap the bottle tightly and label it appropriately for future reference.

Soothe up! Tea

Makes 3¾ cups dried herb mix (enough for 22 to 30 quarts of tea)

This combination of herbs is perfect for those moments when it feels like everything is falling apart. Take a pause, prepare a cup of this tea, and savor it slowly to allow its warmth and relaxation to envelop you. Adjust the ingredients based on your specific stress symptoms. Include dried goldenrod and/or sage if you feel heavy and exhausted, or add dried chamomile and/or catnip for digestive upsets. Drink at least a quart of this tea daily.

Ingredients:
- 1 cup dried betony leaf and flower
- 1 cup dried tulsi leaf
- ½ cup dried linden leaf and flower
- ½ cup dried rose petals
- ½ cup dried elderflower
- ¼ cup dried St. John's wort leaf and flower (optional, see Tip)

Instructions:
1. In a medium-sized bowl, combine the herbs: betony leaf and flower, tulsi leaf, linden leaf and flower, rose petals, elderflower, and St. John's wort (if desired).
2. Store the herb mixture in an airtight container for future use.

Preparation:

1. Boil a kettle of water.
2. Take 2 to 3 tablespoons of the herb mixture per quart of water and place it in a mason jar or French press.
3. Pour the boiling water over the herbs, cover the container, and let the tea steep for approximately 20 minutes or until it reaches a suitable drinking temperature.

Tip: If you are currently taking pharmaceuticals, it is advisable to omit the St. John's wort.

Note: Embrace the therapeutic ritual of preparing and enjoying this tea blend mindfully, allowing it to restore balance and tranquility during challenging times.

Nerve-soothing tea

Combine 1 teaspoon of betony leaves, 1 teaspoon of kava kava root, 1 teaspoon of hops, and 1 teaspoon of dried skullcap in a nonmetallic container. Take 2 teaspoons of the herb mixture and place it in another container. Cover the herbs with 1 cup of boiling water, steep for 30 minutes, and then let it cool and strain. Take 1 tablespoon of the herbal infusion at a time, as needed, for relaxation and stress relief.

Calm down tea

Combine 1 teaspoon of powdered ginger, 1 teaspoon of powdered valerian root, and 1 teaspoon of powdered pleurisy root in a nonmetallic container. Cover the herbs with 2 cups of boiling water, steep for 30 minutes, then cool and strain the mixture. Take one tablespoon at a time, as needed, up to a maximum of two cups per day.

Shake-it-off tea

Combine 1 to 2 teaspoons of peppermint leaves and 1 teaspoon of valerian root. Cover the herbs with 1 cup of boiling water, steep for 20 to 30 minutes, then strain the mixture. Drink up to one cup per day, as needed.

Wounds

Most wounds are caused by cuts, abrasions, or other physical injuries. Wounds should always be cleaned thoroughly to avoid an infection. The bleeding that often accompanies a wound can usually be stopped by applying pressure to the wound. Excessive bleeding, or injury to major arteries, requires immediate emergency medical care. If a wound turns red, swells, throbs, or is hot to the touch and contains pus, it is a sign of infection: please contact a medical professional immediately in this case.

Relevant tissue states: heat (inflammation)
Relevant herbal actions: antimicrobial, astringent, emollient, lymphatic, vulnerary

Supportive Herbs
- Calendula flower
- Chamomile flower
- Goldenrod leaf and flower
- Kelp
- Marshmallow
- Pine
- Plantain leaf
- Rose
- Self-heal leaf and flower
- St. John's wort leaf and flower
- Yarrow leaf and flower

When working with a cut, scrape, abrasion, or other open wound, it's important to always follow the same order of operations:

Stop the bleeding. Direct application of pressure is usually the best way to accomplish this.

Clean the wound. Any particulate or foreign matter must be completely washed out of the wound or it will slow healing and allow infection to take root. A wound wash or soak with astringent, antimicrobial herbs is very effective for this stage.

Prevent or manage infection. Wound washes and soaks are also good here. Herb-infused honeys are extremely effective for this stage, serving both to disinfect and encourage healing. (Don't put tinctures directly into wounds unless you have no other option; even then, dilute them at 1 part tincture to 5 parts purified water, because alcohol inhibits cell growth.)

Encourage healing. Herb-infused honeys, poultices, compresses, and baths are all appropriate for open wounds. Once the wound closes (or if it was never very deep to begin with), you can transition to a salve. Choose herbs that are vulnerary, lymphatic (to drain blisters), and—especially in later stages—softening or emollient (to prevent scarring).

Wound wash

This recipe creates a blend of herbs for wound wash that can be used during the cleaning stage. It is recommended to start with a simple wash using rose water or nonalcoholic witch hazel extract if you're in a hurry. As the wound healing progresses, you can transition to using this formula for soaks and compresses. Adding ½ cup of dried marshmallow or kelp in the later stages of healing can provide emollient effects.

Ingredients:
- ½ cup dried calendula flower
- ½ cup dried plantain leaf
- ½ cup dried rose petals
- ½ cup dried goldenrod leaf and flower
- ¼ cup dried chamomile flower
- ¼ cup dried self-heal leaf and flower
- ¼ cup dried St. John's wort leaf and flower
- ¼ cup dried yarrow leaf and flower
- Salt (for the infusion)

Instructions:
1. In a medium bowl, mix together all the herbs. Store the blend in an airtight container.
2. Prepare a kettle of boiling water. Measure 4 to 6 tablespoons of the herb mixture per quart of water and place it in a mason jar or French press.
3. Pour the boiling water over the herbs, cover, and steep for 20 minutes or until cool.
4. Stir in 1 teaspoon of salt for each quart of infusion you've prepared.
5. Use the infusion to soak the wounded area or apply it as a compress over the affected area.
6. Repeat this process at least 3 times per day, or as frequently as possible.

Note: Adjust the frequency and duration of the soaks and compresses based on the progress of wound healing.

Pine resin salve

Makes 8 ounces (40-day supply)

Pine resin salve is the best choice for wounds that have closed or were never very deep. You can work with the resin of other conifers, too. Resin can be harvested directly from the trees—you'll find whitish globs of it along the trunk where branches were lost. Leave enough on the tree to keep the wound sealed—this resin is how the tree forms a scab!

It will probably have bits of bark, dirt, insect parts, etc., stuck in it—don't worry: you'll filter that out during processing.

After gathering resin, use a bit of oil to wash your hands—soap and water won't work. Just drop a bit of any liquid oil you have handy into your hands and scrub as if it were soap. The resin will soften and separate from your skin. Then you can use soap and hot water to wash it away.

You can use plain oil for infusing your resin but starting with an herb-infused oil means you get the good actions of all these herbs, instead of just those the resin contributes.

6 to 8 ounces pine resin or another conifer resin
8 fluid ounces total calendula-infused oil, goldenrod-infused oil, and/or plantain-infused oil
1 ounce beeswax, chopped or grated, plus more as needed

1. In a small pan over low heat, combine the resin and infused oil and heat gently, stirring frequently. The resin will soften and dissolve, infusing the oil with its virtues.
2. Pour this warm oil through a few layers of cheesecloth. Wrap the mass that remains and squeeze it to extract as much oil as possible.
3. Prepare a salve using this resin-infused oil (you will find the instructions in the second volume under salve)
4. Apply to the wound several times a day, using fresh, neat bandages each time.

Topical application for abrasions

Combine 1 teaspoon of white pine inner bark, 1 teaspoon of wild cherry bark, and 1 teaspoon of wild plum root in a pan. Cover the herbs with 2 cups of water. Bring the mixture to a boil and let it boil until the bark and roots become soft. Allow the mixture to cool, then strain it. To use, soak a clean cloth (preferably sterilized) in the solution and apply it to the affected area.

Topical wash for cuts

Combine 1 teaspoon of pleurisy root and 1 teaspoon of ginseng root in a pan. Cover the herbs with 2 cups of water. Bring the mixture to a boil and let it boil for 20 to 30 minutes. Strain the liquid. Apply the resulting infusion topically as needed.

Conclusion

I hope you have enjoyed reading this book as much as I've enjoyed writing it, and I hope it will accompany you in your ongoing journey to the discovery of Native American herbs and their medicinal uses.

If you found this book useful and are feeling generous, please take the time to leave a short review on Amazon so that other may enjoy this guide as well.

I leave you with good wishes and hopefully a better knowledge of the plants around us and their amazing powers. This volume is part of a seven-books series on Native American Herbalism from foraging and gardening native plants to making herbal remedies for adults and children. Check out the other volumes to gain a deeper understanding of the amazing wisdom and knowledge of our forefathers and to improve not only your health, but the health of our land as well.

The Native American Herbalist's Bible 4

The Gardener's Companion to Native Horticulture

Traditional Methods in Modern Practice to Grow Medicinal Herbs and Wildflowers

Linda Osceola Naranjo

Introduction

E ulu mau ka lewa, E ulu mau ka honua
Let the heavens continue to live,
Let the earth continue to live
E ho'opulu mau ka ua i ka 'aina
Let the rains continued to dampen the land
E ulu mau ka wao kele
Let the forest continue to grow
Alaila mohala a'e ka pua
Then, the flower (child) will bloom forth
Ho'ola hou ke kanaka.
And man will live again.
—Pule Ho'ola No Ka Honua
(Prayer of Healing for the Earth)

We live in a country where the cure for virtually any disease and ailment is within our grasp. In our forests, meadows, plains, and gardens grow small, seemingly insignificant flowers and herbs, plants that we don't look twice at, and trees of which we don't even bother to learn the name. Yet, they are the key to a better, healthier, and more sustainable way of life.

Our forefathers, more attuned with nature than we could ever imagine to be, understood that, and took carefully and sparingly the gifts that Nature offered to heal themselves and grow stronger.

We have lost that knowledge.

Only starting from the 1970s, a renewed interest in botanic medicine has uncovered the depth of the Native American knowledge of plants and their healing powers. The research has not only helped herbalists, but physicians and scientist as well that re-discovered substances that the Native Americans people knew about for hundreds of years.

This book is the extended edition of the best-selling The Native American Herbalist's Bible: 3-in-1 Companion to Herbal Medicine, offering four more volumes on gardening techniques, growing healing plants and wildflowers, and pediatric healthcare.

This is the unabridged companion to Native American herbs, their traditional and modern use, complete with appropriate doses and usage, gardening tips and techniques for both medicinal plants and wildflowers. The book is completed by a list of simple and effective recipes for the most common ailments for both adults and children.

You don't need to put at risk the delicate natural balance of your body and that of your loved ones by taking drugs and medications, if an easily available natural solution is just outside your door. Harvest carefully or grow your own herbs, learn to know your body and what works best for you, communicate with the nature surrounding you, and you will in a small way bring back a culture that for too long has been treated as inferior.

This book will teach how to find and treat the herbs the way the native American tribes did: from the forest to your herbalist table, but you will have to find your way to listen to your body and the plants around you.

To aid you in your holistic journey, we have decided to divide the book in seven handy volumes.

The first volume will give you a full theoretical approach to Native American medicine and the herbal medicines methods and preparations.

The second volume is a complete encyclopedia of all the most relevant herbs used in traditional Native American medicine, complete with modern examples, doses, and where to find them, making it a very effective field guide.

The third volume is a "recipe book" of sorts: it offers easy herbal solutions to the most common diseases a budding naturopath can encounter. It is meant as a jumping point to find your own way to treat yourself and your fellow man and will come in handy even to the most experienced herbalist.

This fourth volume provides a complete theoretical and practical approach to Native American traditional planting techniques and how they can be implemented in modern gardens.

The fifth volume is the native gardener's almanac for medicinal herbs. Foraging is not always an option and a lot of herbs are handy to have in your garden: this volume will guide you through the herbs that you can and (should) have in your garden.

The sixth volume continues the guide to the plants you can plant in your gardens focusing on healing wildflowers, which are not only good for your health, but for the planet as well, and they are not bad on the eyes either!

The seventh volume focuses on native pediatric healthcare. Treating children is a very delicate undertaking, their physiology is more sensitive to external agents, especially drugs. Natural herbalist treatments are effective and gentle in treating common, less severe, pathologies and they won't needlessly weaken your child's immune system. The herbs listed in this last volume have been carefully researched to specifically treat children and their ailments, avoiding any allergic reaction and boosting their immune system.

I am happy to guide through a life-changing journey in search of lost knowledge, amazing healing plants, and carefully crafted herbal remedies and I hope it will help you nurture a stronger relationship with the nature surrounding us and the many gifts it bestows upon us. To build a healthier relationship with nature we have to think in terms of biodiversity and how we may apply it to our own gardens and landscapes. To begin, what exactly is biodiversity At its core, biodiversity, short for biological diversity, encapsulates the variety and variability of life on Earth. This term is incredibly broad and can be viewed through multiple lenses. It not only involves the sheer number of distinct species in a particular area (species diversity), but also includes the genetic diversity within individual species and the variety of ecosystems (ecosystem diversity) that host these species. Biodiversity is essential for the stability of ecosystems and contributes to what we call 'ecosystem services'. These are the numerous benefits that humans derive from the environment, such as pollination of crops, purification of air and water, and the provision of food and medicinal resources.

In diverse ecosystems, species interactions form a web of compensatory mechanisms. In such vibrant ecosystems, if a certain species falters, another member of the ecological choir steps in to harmonize the rhythm of life, contributing to the overall system stability. Like a well-woven tapestry, ecosystems abundant in diversity demonstrate resilience against potentially destabilizing threats. They are better equipped to bounce back from challenges such as insect infestations, disease outbreaks, invasions by non-native flora or fauna, and climatic upheavals. Furthermore, plant diversity leads to the formation of a variety of micro and macro habitats, enhancing the overall biological productivity. The resultant increased photosynthetic activity aids in carbon sequestration, thereby improving air quality. Contrastingly, urban areas often exhibit low biodiversity with landscapes dominated by monocultures of grass or a limited selection of ornamental plants. However, we can infuse principles of ecology into our cityscapes and gardens.

To improve urban biodiversity, it's advisable to integrate a wide variety of plant species and forms, including trees, shrubs, herbs, and vines. This diversification creates numerous microhabitats that attract beneficial insects, facilitating biological pest control and reducing the need for chemical insecticides. Additionally, diverse plant communities are less susceptible to invasive species, curbing the prevalence of weeds and subsequently reducing herbicide use. Key indicators of successful biodiversity enhancement include the presence of birds, native bees, and butterflies. Measures such as planting native trees, creating a pollinator-friendly garden,

installing bird feeders, or incorporating a small water feature can stimulate wildlife diversity. Moreover, vegetation contributes to climate regulation via shade and evapotranspiration, thereby reducing energy costs.

The concept of biodiversity also extends beyond flora and fauna. Incorporating elements like deadwood logs and rocks into urban green spaces can attract decomposers, including fungi, lichens, and mosses (bryophytes), augmenting biodiversity while enhancing the aesthetic appeal of these spaces. From the macroscopic perspective, plant diversity facilitates an intricate network of micro and macro habitats, becoming inviting abodes for myriad creatures. Moreover, these variegated ecosystems possess an elevated productivity index. Augmented growth means heightened absorption of carbon dioxide, thereby contributing to air purification and fostering a healthier environment. Regrettably, our urban landscapes often showcase a stark contrast to this, becoming the epitome of monotony with homogenous expanses of lawns and a narrow palette of preferred ornamentals. Yet, it is within our grasp to integrate fundamental ecological concepts into our urban green spaces and backyard gardens.

Our journey towards a sustainable future commences by introducing a diverse array of plant life into our green spaces. Include an array of plant forms: towering trees, robust shrubs, delicate herbs, and climbing vines. Each additional species contributes to the creation of various microhabitats, serving as magnet for "beneficial" insects. These allies in disguise play a significant role in natural pest management, curbing our reliance on chemical insecticides. Moreover, biodiversity acts as a shield against invasive species, reducing the prevalence of unwanted weeds that typically flourish in monotonous turf landscapes, thus minimizing the use of herbicides. Look for signs of success in the fluttering wings of butterflies, the busy work of native bees, and the melodious twitter of birds - they are indeed the harbingers of healthy biodiversity. Attract these nature's marvels by planting native trees, cultivating a pollinator-friendly garden, setting up bird feeders, or introducing a small water feature. Plants also perform a remarkable job at modulating climate through shade and evapotranspiration, leading to lower energy consumption and expenditure. And remember, biodiversity is not confined solely to the realm of fauna and flora. Introducing elements such as deadwood logs and rocks can beckon a fascinating array of decomposers like captivating fungi, lichens, moss, and other captivating bryophytes. This not only boosts biodiversity but also adds a unique aesthetic appeal to your garden, ultimately creating a verdant landscape teeming with life and thriving in harmonious balance.

Ancient Methods

Many green-living enthusiasts are looking to Native American horticultural practices to learn how crops were cultivated in the past. For their existence, Native Americans had to rely on what they farmed as well as what was available in the wild. Some of the tactics they utilized in the past are still in use today with effectiveness.

Many of the practices that we use in our gardens today were developed by Native Americans. Corn, for example, was cultivated in rows to make pollination simpler. Beans that needed a trellis to grow were trained on poles or cornstalks. Fish from surrounding creeks or rivers were commonly used to fertilize gardens, and we still do so today with bone or fish meal.

Let's delve deeper.

A short history of Native American Gardening

The agricultural practices of Native American tribes in the Northeast left a profound impression on the early European settlers, who were astounded by their productivity and sustainability. The Native Americans had developed sophisticated techniques and systems that enabled them to cultivate the land effectively while maintaining its long-term fertility. The settlers witnessed the careful observation of nature, the efficient use of resources, and the deep understanding of the ecosystems in which they lived.

Today, as modern agriculture reveals its consequences such as soil compaction, erosion, fertilizer runoff, topsoil loss, and the high costs associated with petrochemicals for increased production, it has become imperative to revisit the techniques employed by Native Americans. Not only do these techniques offer a sustainable alternative, but they have also become a necessity.

The timeline of Native American settlement in the northeastern United States is a topic that continues to be studied and debated among researchers. While the exact dates are not conclusive, evidence from sites like the Meadowcroft Rock Shelter near Pittsburgh suggests human presence as early as 19,000 BP, although the accuracy of these dates is still subject to discussion.

By around 10,000 BP, it is widely accepted that Native American communities were well-established in the Northeast. These early inhabitants relied on foraging, hunting, and gathering as their primary means of subsistence. They developed a deep understanding of the local ecosystems and utilized the rich natural resources available to them.

The transition to agriculture in the region began to emerge during the Middle Woodland Period, which spanned from 1000 BC to AD 1000. This period marked a significant shift as Native Americans started engaging in deliberate cultivation of native grasses and other plants. This intentional cultivation was an important step toward the development of a more settled and agricultural lifestyle.

The Late Woodland Period, occurring from AD 1000 to 1500, brought further changes to the native subsistence patterns. During this time, a mixed economy emerged, where the cultivation of maize (corn), beans, and squash became dominant. This agricultural trio, known as the "Three Sisters," played a crucial role in the food security and cultural practices of many Native American tribes in the region. The intercropping system of corn, beans, and squash provided a sustainable and complementary approach to agriculture, enhancing yields and soil fertility.

The adoption of agriculture in the Northeast brought about social, economic, and cultural changes within Native American communities. It allowed for the development of more complex societies and the establishment of permanent settlements. The surplus food generated by agriculture supported population growth and facilitated the emergence of specialized crafts, trade networks, and social hierarchies.

The type of agriculture that emerged during the Late Woodland Period can be described as horticulture or extensive cultivation. Horticulture involves cultivating crops solely using handheld tools, as there were no domesticated farm animals in the Americas that could be used for plowing. Cultivated crops were combined with hunting, fishing, and gathering wild plant foods to ensure basic subsistence.

In the traditional horticulture practices of Native Americans in the Northeast, fields were prepared for planting through a systematic clearing process. Initially, saplings and underbrush beneath the largest trees were cleared, while the larger trees themselves were often left standing due to the effort required to fell them using stone axes. If removal was necessary, trees were killed by girdling, which involved removing a band of bark from the base to cut off moisture and nutrient flow. Controlled fires could also be set at the base of trees to weaken them until they fell. Once the underbrush and vegetation were cleared, they were allowed to dry and burned using fires created through friction drills. This burning process served the dual purpose of eliminating waste and providing ash, which acted as natural fertilizer for the soil. After the ash had cooled, women played a vital role, using stone celts, wooden dibbles, or tools made from turtle shells or deer scapulae to work it into the soil.

During the time of European contact, the Three Sisters crops were extensively cultivated by Native American communities in the Northeast, particularly among the Iroquois. This agricultural combination consisted of maize or corn, beans, and cucurbits such as squash and pumpkins. These crops were interplanted in a mutually beneficial manner, with the corn providing a structure for the beans to climb and the squash acting as ground cover to suppress weed growth and retain soil moisture.

The Three Sisters crops played a central role in the agricultural practices of the region during the Late Woodland Period, spreading through cultural contact and diffusion from Mesoamerica.

Before the adoption of horticulture, Native Americans in the Great Lakes region relied heavily on wild plants, utilizing over 130 species for food and 275 for medicinal purposes. Some of these native species were among the first intentionally cultivated, such as goosefoot and sunflowers, which emerged during the Middle Woodland Period in the Midwest and parts of the Northeast. However, the focus eventually shifted to the Three Sisters crops, which were introduced to agricultural production in Mesoamerica and spread throughout the region north of the Rio Grande through cultural exchange and diffusion.

In Native American communities, a complementary division of labor existed, with men engaging in hunting and land clearing for planting, while women took charge of planting, cultivating, and preparing the crops for consumption or storage. The growing season typically began in late March when women used hoes to create mounds, known as hills, several inches high and spaced about one to two feet apart. In April, when the soil had warmed and drained, maize seeds were planted in each mound. Once these seeds germinated and reached a height of three to four inches, bean and squash seeds were planted in the same mounds. The beans, being of the vining variety, used the growing corn stalks as support as they climbed, while squash plants spread across the ground, acting as natural ground cover. Alongside the staple crops, Native Americans in the Northeast also cultivated sunflowers and tobacco, with the latter primarily serving ceremonial purposes.

Problems of Modern Agriculture

With an annual population growth rate of 2%, the world is witnessing the addition of a staggering 130 million people each year. This exponential increase has led experts to project that by the mid-21st century, the global population will reach a jaw-dropping 9 billion, a significant leap from the estimated 6.7 billion in 2008. Such rapid growth presents an unprecedented challenge for agronomists, who are grappling with the urgent need to produce sufficient food to meet the demands of this expanding population.

In the 1960s, the advent of revolutionary crop hybrids, known as the Green Revolution crops, along with the widespread use of petrochemically-based fertilizers, herbicides, pesticides, and expanded irrigation, brought about remarkable surges in global food production. For several decades, food production outpaced the rate of population growth. However, by the late 1990s, this momentum began to wane. In 2008, the U.S. Department of Agriculture predicted a 2.6% increase in global food production, contingent upon favorable weather conditions in key agricultural regions. Unfortunately, the year proved challenging, with a 46% surge in food prices as demand caught up with supply.

Concurrently, agronomists have become increasingly aware of the detrimental repercussions stemming from intensive agricultural practices. Disturbing levels of topsoil erosion now afflict nearly one-third of the world's cropland. Geologist David Montgomery, in his enlightening book "Dirt: The Erosion of Civilization" (2008), highlights the alarming reality that agriculture is responsible for an annual loss of approximately 1% of topsoil. Shockingly, a single torrential downpour on exposed soil can wipe out a century's worth of productivity. The National Academy of Sciences has soberly determined that cropland in the United States erodes at a rate at least ten times faster than nature can replenish it. Sub-Saharan Africa, India, and China also face the adverse consequences of soil erosion, exacerbating the already reduced agricultural output in those regions.

Furthermore, the excessive application of chemical fertilizers poses an alarming ecological predicament. In a bid to maximize food production, modern farmers lavish around half a ton of petrochemically-based fertilizers per acre. Astonishingly, the Oregon State Agricultural Extension Service's recent study exposes that approximately half of the fertilizers applied in the United States merely serve to replenish the lost nutrients resulting from soil erosion. The repercussions are grave, as these fertilizers and other chemicals, propelled by runoff, contaminate streams and rivers. The subsequent ecological fallout manifests as the emergence of lifeless zones and rampant algae blooms, vividly exemplified by the devastating scenarios witnessed in the Chesapeake Bay and the Mississippi Delta. In fact, Science Daily's early 2008 report highlights the alarming expanse of the dead zone in the Mississippi Delta, stretching across a staggering 6,000 square miles, devoid of fish and shellfish.

Compounding the challenges faced by modern agriculture is the increasingly worrisome issue of soil compaction. According to the University of Minnesota Extension Service's 2008 report, the colossal weight exerted by a four-wheel-drive tractor equipped with a 325-horsepower engine compresses farmland to a depth of 24 inches, applying a staggering 13 tons of weight per axle. Such compaction restricts the crucial oxygen supply to crop roots, impeding their growth and development. Moreover, compacted soil exacerbates the impact of drought conditions as it struggles to retain adequate moisture. Modern agriculture's response to soil compaction entails resorting to additional chemical applications sprayed onto the soil before planting—an increasingly expensive recourse, particularly with oil prices soaring above the $100 per barrel threshold...

Benefits of Native American Agriculture

In recent years, researchers have gained a deeper appreciation for the incredible productivity and numerous advantages of native horticulture in the Northeast. Dr. Jane Mt. Pleasant, an agronomist at Cornell University and of Tuscarora descent, has played a pivotal role in this research. In the 1980s, Mt. Pleasant embarked on a journey to explore the cultivation methods employed by her ancestors. While the interrelationship among the Three Sisters crops had been recognized by scholars, it was often believed that native horticulture was primarily driven by technological necessity rather than being a highly efficient and advantageous system.

Dr. Pleasant emphasizes that the labor involved in native horticulture began in March, when the soil was cool and moist. Creating mounds of soil in fields served a dual purpose: draining excess moisture from the soil and raising its temperature, as cold air tends to sink. By mid-April, the soil would be perfectly prepared for planting and germination. The practice of mounding soil into hills also addressed the issue of soil compaction. By keeping the soil loose, the native system allowed for easy penetration of oxygen and moisture to the roots, resulting in stronger crop growth.

As Native Americans cultivated their fields and harvested their crops, they piled dead weeds, spent stalks, and vines onto the mounds. The decomposition of this plant material, combined with the ash from field burning, provided essential nitrogen, potassium, and phosphorus directly to the soil where plant growth occurred. Furthermore, as legumes, beans have the unique ability to transfer atmospheric nitrogen to the soil through the bacteria present on their root nodules. Although the quantity of soil nutrients added through this rough composting method may be relatively modest compared to manure or modern fertilizers, the effects are concentrated in the immediate vicinity of the crops, unlike the widespread application of fertilizers. Additionally, the practice of native horticulture, with its avoidance of large open fields, effectively minimized the erosive impacts of wind and rain. The use of ground covers and the accumulation of dead plant material on the mounds further contributed to erosion control.

Research also indicates that intercropping, or growing multiple crops in the same field, creates a diverse plant environment that exhibits enhanced resistance to drought, pests, and diseases. Nutritionists highlight the complementary nature of corn and beans. Both crops contain some of the essential amino acids required for cellular growth. However, corn lacks lysine and tryptophan, which are found in beans, while beans lack methionine and cystine, which are present in corn. The absence of any of these amino acids limits the body's ability to synthesize protein. Therefore, the combination of corn and beans in a single meal proves to be a successful nutritional strategy.

Following European contact, Native Americans in the Northeast demonstrated a willingness to adopt and adapt European farming methods as they interacted with European settlers. By the 1740s, some Native Americans began planting fruit trees and raising livestock as alternatives to traditional horticulture. Even today, in regions where Native Americans in the Northeast have access to land, these adaptations can still be observed. However, based on Mt. Pleasant's research and the support of agricultural extension offices, some Native Americans in the Northeast are now returning to the cultivation of the Three Sisters, not only to reaffirm their native heritage but also to enjoy the multitude of benefits that native horticulture provides.

Three sisters

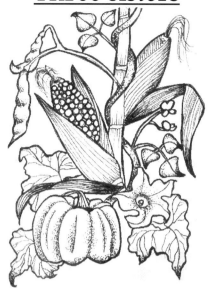

As you have discovered the three sister system was the most widely spread Native American horticultural systems.

Three separate seeds were sown in one enormous pile of dirt in this way. Corn, squash, and beans were among the seeds. As they matured, each of these seeds would contribute something that the others would require. The beans would add nitrogen to the soil, which would help the corn and squash grow well. The maize served as a trellis for the beans to climb. While the other two plants were growing, the squash offered cover and helped to keep pests away. Some Native Americans would first put a fish or eel in the hole, then scatter the seeds on top before covering it with earth. The soil received additional fertilizer as a result of this.

The Native Americans in the Northeast cultivated a variety of corn/maize that produced ears measuring around four to five inches long with eight rows of colorful kernels. The kernels came in a multitude of colors, including white, red, blue, yellow, brown, black, and spotted varieties, as reported by the Dutch in 1633. These kernels were consumed fresh during Green Corn Ceremonies, which are still celebrated by Native Americans in the region, or they were dried on the cob and stored. To dry the corn, the husks were peeled back, and the cobs were hung from house poles and roof supports. Once sufficiently dried, the corn was stored in pits dug into the ground, which were lined with bark or bluestem grass and reused year after year. Carefully dressed smooth walls, sometimes adorned with clam shells, can still be observed in archaeological sites.

Corn was commonly boiled in water or roasted in hot ashes. Dried corn could be transformed into hominy by boiling the kernels with wood ash, causing the hulls to soften, split, and swell in size. The ash and wood lye were then removed through repeated washings. Corn could be combined with beans to make succotash, a term derived from the Algonquin language, or ground into meal that could be mixed with animal fat or flesh. It could also be parched for use as travel food or made into cakes and baked in the ashes of a fire. Beans, on the other hand, were boiled at harvest and then dried for future use.

Squash was sliced into thin rings, strung on strings, and dehydrated in the sun.

Recent research has revealed that the traditional native farming methods, specifically the cultivation of corn, beans, and squash together (the Three Sisters), could yield over 4 million calories of food per acre. It's important to note that the cultivation techniques of the Three Sisters varied from east to west. In the western regions, the bean varieties were generally self-supporting, which meant they didn't need to be planted in the same hole as the maize and squash, unlike in other areas.

If you are interested in adding a three sister garden to your backyard, here is a list of heirloom varieties of beans and squash that were used by Native American tribes and survived to this day.

Corn

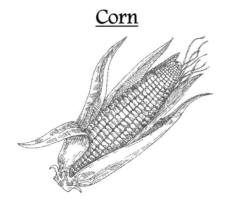

Corn, without a doubt, is one of the most extensively studied, manipulated, and, some argue, diminished vegetables from the New World. Its history is intricate and its literature vast. A great starting point to understand the evolution of corn from a sacred Native American food to the sugar-laden Coca-Cola corns of today is Betty Fussell's book "Story of Corn" (1992).

The industrialization of corn in America has brought about significant changes in agriculture, driven by genetic advancements that have transformed the once-sturdy corn varieties into a new generation of corns with remarkable differences. These transformations, however, contradict the principles of genetic diversity and seed preservation that are crucial for sustainable agriculture. It is ironic that corn, once a vital staple and cultural symbol for Native Americans, has now become one of the world's major cash crops. Unfortunately, this shift has led to its involvement in political corruption and the devastating destruction of the environment. Among proponents of seed saving and sustainable agriculture, there is a unanimous recognition of the importance of preserving corn as an heirloom vegetable.

Preserving corn as an heirloom presents unique challenges. As a mutated plant, corn relies on human intervention for pollination and seed production and cannot survive in the wild without assistance. Native Americans deeply understood this and held corn in religious reverence, unlike any other culture. Their attitude towards corn was not solely focused on maximizing productivity but on preserving its sacred essence. They believed corn possessed human qualities, and the purity of its seed color and types held profound metaphysical meanings in their spirituality. Native Americans excelled at seed saving, displaying remarkable skills as plant geneticists long before the concept was formally recognized.

Native American tribes categorized their corn varieties based on their intended uses, such as flour, hominy, porridge, and popping. Each type of corn was associated with specific ceremonies and festive recipes. While some corn varieties have been passed down to us from Native peoples, and we have adopted some of their dialect names, our usage and understanding of these corns have significantly changed over time. Porter A. Browne's "Essay on Indian Corn" (1837) documented thirty-five commonly grown varieties during that period, but only a few of them have survived to this day, with the rest likely extinct.

Horticulturists classify corn differently than Native Americans or early corn experts like Browne did. All cultivated corn varieties belong to the same species and can easily cross-pollinate with each other. Corn, relying on wind-blown pollen, is one of the easiest garden vegetables to cross-pollinate, even with a gentle breeze. This promiscuity in pollination has led to the emergence of numerous varieties that fall between the recognized types accepted by horticulturists. These garden varieties include popcorn, dent corn, flint corn, soft corn, and sweet corn.

Popcorn, one of the oldest and hardiest types of corn, thrives in areas where other varieties struggle. It can be planted earlier in the spring but easily crosses with neighboring corn varieties. To achieve the best results, popcorn kernels should age for over a year. They must ripen on the stalk and then be properly dried indoors before storage in insect-free and moisture-free containers. Freezing the corn immediately before popping can enhance its popping rate.

Dent corns, known as "she-corn" due to the dent or crease in the kernel, are starchy and commonly used for roasting, cornbread, and hominy. They are best suited for the South and Southwest regions, where various dent corn varieties have been developed. Flint corns, on the other hand, are the northern counterparts of dent corns. They contain a high percentage of opaline, a mineral that gives the ground corn a gritty or "flinty" texture. Flint corns are often used for grits and hominy, like many other field corn varieties.

Flour corns, also called soft corns, have predominantly starchy kernels when ripe, making them suitable for grinding into flour. Native American tribes cultivated these corns, which are believed to have originated in tropical regions. Corns with this genetic feature were among the first to be spread throughout the continent by Native Americans engaged in agriculture.

Native American tribes distinguished between two types of sweet corn. The first type is "green" or unripe corn, commonly found in most corn types during the "milky" stage. The second type is characterized by heavily wrinkled kernels and possesses natural sweetness due to its genotype. The sweet corn we are familiar with today belongs to this latter type. True sweet corn arrived in what is now the United States in the 1300s, originating from Peru, where it was used to make chichi, a fermented drink consumed in pre-Columbian times. Sweet corn's sweetness is derived from a recessive gene mutation that impairs the conversion of sugar to starch. Native Americans utilized this characteristic to store slow-ripening late-season varieties as "fresh" corn during the winter or to caramelize the corn while still in the husk over hot coals.

This slow drying process resulted in a sweet-tasting dry corn that could be eaten as a snack or incorporated into stews and vegetable mixtures. The Powhatans of Virginia, according to anthropologist Helen Rountree, made a corn-and-bean dish called pausarowmena, a staple dish during the winter. They harvested "green" corn or a variety of sweet corn in late summer and roasted it in the husk over hot coals until dry and slightly caramelized, resembling the present-day dry sweet corn of the Pennsylvania Dutch. This dry sweet corn was stored in middens and rehydrated with water as needed. It was often stewed with two types of beans, a large pole variety, and a small bush bean. This combination of dried sweet corn and two distinct types of beans constituted the true "succotash" of the Powhatans and related peoples in the Middle Atlantic region.

When planting open-pollinated corn varieties, a different approach is required compared to hybrids. For optimal results, plant the seeds in blocks or squares with five to six rows or, ideally, in rows 4 feet apart and hills 3 feet from one another, with four to six plants per hill. This method works well for heirloom varieties and ensures good pollination while providing space between the hills for squash. Pole beans can be planted among the clumps of corn and allowed to climb up the stalks, reviving the traditional three-sister system.

Among Native American tribes in the East, corn seeds were
typically treated in an herbal tea before planting. F. W. Waugh described some of these decoctions in his book "Iroquois Foods and Food Preparation." After soaking in the tea, the corn was left wet in a basket to sprout slightly before planting. This treatment was believed to protect the corn and may have produced an odor to mask it from birds and insects. Additionally, it helped separate viable seeds from weak ones and prevented seed from rotting in the ground.

To ensure effective seed-saving practices, it is necessary to have a minimum of 200 seed-producing ears in the garden. For genetic diversity, ripe and dry seed corn should be collected from twenty-five to fifty of the finest ears and mixed together. During this process, kernels must be meticulously sorted for color and the best characteristics of the variety. It is crucial to avoid inbreeding depression, as corn propagated from a limited gene pool can quickly and irreversibly decline in quality, similar to the consequences of close kin breeding in humans. The specified number of ears represents the critical mass required in the gene pool to maintain diversity and ensure the healthy survival of the corn variety. Saving seed for corn necessitates space, as 200 ears equate to at least 100 plants organized in twenty-five hills if following traditional planting methods.

Moreover, it is important to allow the seed corn to ripen on the plants and thoroughly dry before sorting it for storage. Sweet corn remains viable for up to three years, while other varieties can remain viable for five to ten years, or sometimes even longer. Animals can pose a significant threat to seed-saving endeavours, and it is prudent to overplant, considering potential losses. However, gardeners need not feel helpless in the face of corn thieves like raccoons, nature's expert pilferers.

A practical method to protect ears of corn from raccoons and squirrels is to wrap them with 3/4-inch-wide packing tape, preferably the kind reinforced with fiberglass or plastic webbing.
Start by encircling the ear with tape above its attachment to the stalk, then wrap it around the ear about 2 inches below the tip. Allow approximately 24 inches of tape per ear, ensuring it is not wrapped too tightly to allow proper expansion within the husk. The reinforced tape will prevent animals from pulling the ears off the stalks, and its resilient nature makes it difficult for raccoons and squirrels to chew through. This method also foils the efforts of crows.

Gourd Seed Corn

Native American communities cultivated gourd seed dent corn primarily for its use as flour corn, and its remarkable productivity still makes it an ideal choice for this purpose today. Historical records indicate that both white and yellow varieties of gourd seed corn were grown in regions of southern Virginia, the Carolinas, and the Upper South during the early settlements. Interestingly, the Iroquois people were also familiar with gourd seed varieties and cultivated them in the favorable microclimates along the Finger Lakes and Genesee Valley in western New York.

In Porter Browne's "Essay on Indian Corn," he mentioned yellow and white gourd seed corns, noting the existence of seven subvarieties of the yellow type. The white gourd seed corn likely had numerous subvarieties as well, although most of them have since become extinct. According to Browne, the true yellow type featured twenty-four rows of kernels on the cob, while the white variety could have as many as thirty-six rows. Through hybridization, a variety with sixteen rows was created by crossing the Sioux (a yellow flint type) with Yellow Gourd Seed.

The popular Maryland White Gourd Seed, prevalent in the late nineteenth century, also had sixteen rows, suggesting it may have been an early crossbreed. Many of the original gourd seed varieties were later crossed with northern corns to enable cultivation beyond the South.

Unfortunately, numerous old gourd seed corn varieties were lost between 1940 and the present. However, due to its disease resistance, there has been a renewed interest in its cultivation. The strain known as Texas Gourd Seed, formerly Maryland White Gourd Seed, was rediscovered in Texas and reintroduced commercially by Southern Exposure Seed Exchange in 1987. German farmers from the Upper South had brought this variety to Texas in the late nineteenth century, and it still retains many characteristics of the original white gourd seed corn. This particular strain is commonly grown among seed savers today.

Gourd seed dent corn plants can grow up to approximately 8 feet tall and typically produce two ears per stalk. The kernels, cream-colored and resembling thin "horse teeth" or gourd seeds, are densely arranged in rows ranging from eighteen to twenty-two. This distinctive kernel shape gives the corn its unique name. Gourd seed corn exhibits drought resistance, thrives in clay soils, and typically matures in approximately 120 days. When harvested while young and unripe, it can be consumed similarly to sweet corn. However, at this stage of ripeness, it is best grated for fritters, puddings, and pies. Additionally, it yields excellent flour, comparable to Mexican masa harina, and as a coarse meal, it produces delicious cornbread.

Ha-Go-Wa Corn (also known as Seneca Hominy or White Flint)

The Seneca people, like other Iroquoian tribes, have made it a priority to preserve numerous ancient corn varieties, driven by their religious and patriotic sentiments. Among these cherished varieties, Ha-Go-Wa holds a special place among the Senecas, being one of the oldest documented corn types associated with their tribal identity.

Seneca Hominy, as an heirloom corn, boasts a rich lineage and a storied culinary history. This resilient corn thrives in regions with short summers, making it suitable for cultivation throughout the country. It particularly excels in the South, especially when planted early. Seneca Hominy typically grows to a medium height of 6 to 8 feet, making it well-suited for small gardens. When planted in early May, it reaches the tassel stage in early July. Each stalk produces two 8-inch cobs positioned low on the plant, and its narrow leaves do not overshadow larger, leafy varieties of pumpkins or melons that may be grown alongside it. Compact watermelon varieties like Rattlesnake or King and Queen make excellent companion plants for Seneca Hominy. The kernels of Ha-Go-Wa corn are large, round, and predominantly white, often arranged in irregular patterns. A typical cob of Seneca Hominy should have twelve rows of kernels. Off-color kernels, such as yellow or red, which indicate cross-pollination, are best utilized for cooking rather than saved as seed.

The Seneca people exclusively use this corn variety to produce large hominy, small hominy (grits), and cornmeal, typically in the form of mush. The dry corn can be parched in the oven, resulting in various toasty flavors and a finer texture in the meal. The dry kernels can also be pounded to create cracked corn (samp), a versatile option for quick meals, particularly when cooked with beans. Additionally, the very young ears, known as "green" corn, can be consumed raw or boiled similarly to sweet corn.

Sehsapsing Corn (also known as Oklahoma Delaware Blue Corn)

In the vast cornucopia of Native American corn varieties, Sehsapsing stands as a hidden gem, cherished for its rich heritage and unique characteristics. This extraordinary corn, once cultivated by the Caney River Delawares in Oklahoma, has left its indelible mark on the corn collection at Iowa State University. However, its origins trace back to the lush fields of New Jersey, where the Siconese tribe referred to it as Sehapsink. With its intriguing story and remarkable attributes, Sehsapsing corn captivates the imagination of corn enthusiasts and gardeners alike.

Sehsapsing corn boasts a remarkable resilience and adaptability, thriving in diverse climates and soils. Its versatile nature makes it suitable for cultivation in various regions, from the sun-drenched plains to the fertile valleys. Standing tall and proud, Sehsapsing corn plants reach for the sky, reaching heights of up to 10 feet, a testament to their vigor and strength. Each sturdy stalk bears multiple cobs, generously providing an abundance of harvest. The cobs, adorned with a symphony of colors, showcase a tapestry of hues ranging from vibrant yellows to deep purples, a true feast for the eyes.

The kernels of Sehsapsing corn, with their distinctive shape and size, embody the essence of its uniqueness. Each cob bears rows of plump kernels, varying in color and texture. The velvety white kernels offer a delicate sweetness when enjoyed in their tender, immature state, reminiscent of the flavors of youth. As the corn matures, the kernels undergo a breathtaking transformation, transitioning to a kaleidoscope of shades, from royal purples to rich blues, capturing the essence of nature's artistry.

The versatility of Sehsapsing corn extends beyond its captivating appearance. This corn variety serves as a culinary canvas, inspiring culinary explorations and culinary creations. When harvested at its peak, Sehsapsing corn can be transformed into mouthwatering dishes that celebrate its natural flavors. Whether roasted to perfection, ground into nourishing flour, or incorporated into traditional recipes, Sehsapsing corn reveals its complex flavors, transporting taste buds on a journey of sensory delight.

Today, the legacy of Sehsapsing corn lives on, cherished by those who appreciate the stories woven into its kernels and the vibrant spirit it embodies. As gardeners and stewards of the land, we honor the traditions and wisdom of Native American cultures, keeping the flame of Sehsapsing corn burning bright, a living testament to the diversity and beauty of our agricultural heritage.

Tuscarora Corn

The Tuscarora flour corn variety weaves a tale of cultural migration and agricultural heritage. Its precise origins may be shrouded in mystery, but it is believed to have journeyed northward with the Tuscarora nation as they joined the esteemed Iroquois Confederacy in 1722. Hailing from the fertile lands of the Upper South, specifically present-day North Carolina, the Tuscarora people brought with them this cherished corn variety, also known as Turkey Wheat in early accounts from Virginia. It is quite possible that the Tuscarora corn shares ancestral ties with the ancient flour corn cultivated by the Powhatan and other tribes in the region.

Indeed, the whispers of history and the accounts of seed savers who have nurtured Tuscarora corn in the South lend credence to the belief that this corn variety flourished in those lands since time immemorial. While the Iroquois people have faithfully continued the cultivation of Tuscarora corn, it has remained relatively overlooked by non-Indigenous individuals. Perhaps its "heaviness" has led to its exclusion from the realm of commercial ventures, as it does not conform to the preferences of distilleries seeking corn for whiskey production or the demands of feed for pork. Nonetheless, the Tuscarora corn stands resolute in its primary purpose as a midseason flour corn, maturing gracefully over the course of approximately 120 days. These sturdy plants reach a height of 6 to 8 feet, bearing striking cobs that stretch up to 12 inches. Adorned with eight rows of substantial marble-white kernels, these cobs exude a sense of abundance and promise. Tapering in diameter from top to bottom, they hold within them the essence of the land and the traditions of the Tuscarora people.

In its young and vibrant state, Tuscarora corn can be savored and enjoyed akin to sweet corn, offering a tantalizing taste of its potential. However, it is when the kernels ripen and mature that the true splendor of this flour corn emerges. The resulting flour, delicately crafted from the snowy-white, velvety kernels of mature Tuscarora corn, possesses a texture that defies expectations. Soft and yielding, it serves as a testament to the resilience and resilience of this treasured variety. Unlike its counterparts, the mature Tuscarora kernels do not wither and shrink when dried, retaining their magnificence and allure.

As we celebrate the rich tapestry of our agricultural heritage, let us embrace the legacy of Tuscarora corn. It stands as a testament to the vibrant interplay between culture, land, and sustenance. Its journey from the sun-drenched fields of the Upper South to the lands of the Iroquois Confederacy is a testament to the resilience and adaptability of the crops that have nourished us throughout the ages. May the story of Tuscarora corn inspire us to honor and cherish the ancestral wisdom and the vibrant diversity of our agricultural tapestry.

Beans

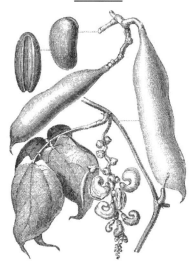

During early America, beans were not as abundant as they are today. Their functional uses took precedence over the characteristics sought after today. For instance, with certain pole beans, the focus was on drying the pods for long-term storage during winter rather than prioritizing tenderness when consumed fresh. Native Americans had a different perspective on categorizing beans compared to Europeans. They emphasized the usefulness of beans as a source of flour or their adaptability in dumplings and hearth breads.

Native Americans, before encountering Europeans, did not consume snap beans as we do today. Instead, they boiled the pods at the shelly stage and extracted the beans by pulling them between their teeth, discarding the pods.

An interesting trait found in old bean varieties is the presence of runners in bush beans. While the Pawnee Bush Bean, with its white seeds and brown speckles, lacks runners and exhibits uniform clusters of downward-hanging pods, it is not an ancient Indian bean. It has been modified by humans. A true pre-Columbian bush bean would have runners, possibly extending up to 3 feet. These old bush varieties had a weedy appearance and would entangle themselves by the end of summer. Native American women skillfully trained them around the base of sunflowers or other large-stemmed crops, providing support for the runners to wrap around. For Native Americans, beans held religious significance and the colors of the beans held sacred meanings.

Here are a few of the most notable native bean varieties.

Ohio Pole Bean

The Ohio Pole Bean is an incredibly significant Native American bean that has survived from the Midwest. It was cultivated during the 1790s by various tribes including the Delawares, Potawatomi, Shawnee, and Miamis who were encamped near Fort Wayne, Indiana. Early American farmers referred to it as the Golden Wax Bean. This remarkable bean variety produces large pods measuring 7 to 8 inches in length, growing on vines that reach 8 to 10 feet tall. Each pod contains 6 to 7 beans. The Ohio Pole Bean can be enjoyed as a snap bean when it reaches 4 inches in length, or it can be harvested as a dry bean for winter cooking. Its flavor has a delightful hint of walnuts and it serves as an excellent addition to potato salads.

Trail of Tears Bean

As per Cherokee tradition, the Trail of Tears Bean holds a poignant significance as it was carried from North Carolina to Oklahoma during the arduous forced march of the Cherokee Nation in the winter of 1838-1839, known as the Trail of Tears. During this devastating journey, thousands of Cherokees lost their lives, making the bean a powerful symbol of their struggle for survival and identity. It stands as one of the most evocative vegetables in the garden, embodying the resilience and endurance of the Cherokee people. The Trail of Tears Bean plants display lush olive-green leaves with brown veins, growing to a height of approximately 8 feet. They require sturdy support, often thriving when grown alongside tall corn. The 6-inch pods undergo a transformation, ripening from maroon brown to develop horizontal bands of black and tan as they dry. The seeds themselves are jet black, oblong, and possess a glossy appearance. While the young pods can be used as snap beans, the original purpose of the bean among Native Americans was for flour. It was commonly cooked in combination with blue and black corns. Interestingly, the indigenous people would add the ash of specific herbs to their stews instead of using salt. This alkaline reaction would release the vitamin B in the corn and cause the black beans to turn blue. A similar effect can be achieved by adding a small amount of baking soda.

Wild Pigeon Bean

Wild Pigeon is a traditional semi-pole bean that harkens back to the Eastern Woodland Native American heritage. It is characterized by its unique growth pattern, producing seeds in half-moon-shaped pods that grow close to the ground. The vines of Wild Pigeon typically reach a height of 2 to 3 feet, making them well-suited for cultivation alongside corn when planted in hills. Historically, the Iroquois people utilized this bean as a shelly bean, harvesting it at an immature stage. However, in modern times, it is more commonly enjoyed as a dry bean, often cooked together with corn and game.

The name "wild pigeon" draws its inspiration from the appearance of the now extinct passenger pigeon. Just like the gray and speckled feathers of the passenger pigeon, the coloration of the Wild Pigeon bean exhibits a similar gray hue with distinctive speckles. The timing of the bean's ripening and harvest coincided with the fall migrations of the passenger pigeon, further cementing the association between the two.

Amish Nuttle Bean or Corn Hill Bean

The journey of this unique bean variety unveils two captivating tales that intertwine to form its intriguing history. One narrative finds its roots among the Amish farmers of southeastern Pennsylvania, who affectionately named it Gnuddelbuhn, a whimsical term referring to its resemblance to rabbit droppings. Embraced by the Amish community, this dry bean holds a cherished place in their culinary traditions, enriching hearty soups and other traditional dishes that grace their Sunday gatherings. The light-hearted moniker adds a touch of humor to its identity, showcasing the warm spirit and creativity of the Amish culture. Yet, there is another chapter in the story of this remarkable bean, one that connects it to the corn-growing culture of the Seneca and other esteemed Iroquois peoples.

Known as the "Corn Hill Bean," this variety carries with it the weight of ancestral heritage and cultural significance. The Seneca of Oklahoma, in particular, have recognized it as one of their oldest bean varieties, treasuring its presence as a testament to their enduring traditions and ancestral ties. F. W. Waugh's seminal work, "Iroquois Food and Food Preparation," documents its inclusion under this name, capturing its place within the rich tapestry of Seneca history. True to its heritage, the Corn Hill Bean thrives when planted alongside corn hills, aligning harmoniously with the agricultural practices of the Seneca and echoing the traditions of generations past. It pairs beautifully with shorter corn varieties, reaching an average height of 5 to 6 feet, as it intertwines its tendrils amidst the sturdy corn stalks.

A late-season bean, it matures gracefully over a span of approximately 90 days, culminating in early September in the verdant landscapes of Pennsylvania. Delicate white flowers grace its vines, giving way to distinctive pods that bear the hallmark bumps and curves of the cutshort bean varieties. Each pod, measuring 3 to 4 inches in length, cradles the promise of abundance, containing 4 to 5 seeds within its embrace. As the season unfolds and the harvest approaches, the once vibrant pods surrender their colors to the passage of time. Transformed into drab purple-gray hues adorned with garnet speckles, the bean's outer coat becomes a canvas painted with nature's touch, a testament to the quiet beauty that emerges from the cycle of growth and maturation.

The Corn Hill Bean beckons us to embrace its duality, honoring the threads that bind together the Amish community and the Seneca people, each nurturing this bean with reverence and pride. It stands as a symbol of resilience, cultural exchange, and the timeless power of agriculture to connect us to our roots. As we savor its flavors and marvel at its history, let us celebrate the vibrant tapestry of human experience that finds expression through the simple yet profound act of cultivating and sharing the gifts of the land.

Squash

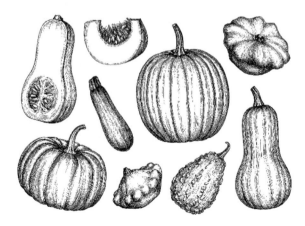

The term "squash" originates from the Algonquin word askutasquash, which refers to something that is eaten green or in an unripe state. While we commonly associate this with a specific category of squash grown during the summer, even field pumpkins can be consumed when they are young, and the Eastern Woodland Indians appeared to enjoy them in that stage. In the early 1800s, there was a variety known as the soft cymling or quash (Cucurbita pepo), which resembled a miniature sugar pumpkin and had an apple-like shape. It was harvested and eaten when still green, similar to how modern zucchinis are consumed. However, if left to ripen, it would develop a hard and woody rind, resembling a gourd.

In contemporary botanical classification, pumpkins and squash are divided into six species, with four encompassing the common varieties grown by American gardeners. Understanding these botanical classifications is crucial in preventing unwanted cross-pollination. It is possible to cultivate different types of squash within the same garden as long as they belong to different species. Squash varieties of the same species have the potential to cross-pollinate, so it is recommended to keep them separated by at least a quarter of a mile. Alternatively, hand pollination can be employed to ensure seed purity. Another method involves planting squash at three-week intervals, harvesting and removing plants of the same species to allow the next planting to flower and bear fruit. Additionally, removing the vines of early plantings creates space for other vegetables.

So, let's get to know the different species.

1. **Cucurbita maxima**: The family of Cucurbita maxima encompasses more than just impressively large field pumpkins. While size is certainly a notable feature of this group, it is not the sole defining characteristic. Maxima squash, as part of this family, exhibit their unique traits through long vines adorned with ample, hairy leaves that contribute to their distinct appearance. The stems of these squash are soft, rounded, and possess a spongy texture, adding to their intriguing nature. As we explore the diversity within Cucurbita maxima, we encounter a range of seed colors, from delicate white to earthy tan or brown, with creamy margins and a delicate membrane coating that envelops the seeds.

2. **Cucurbita mixta**: Cucurbita mixta is known for its spreading vines, large, hairy leaves, and seeds with crackable membranes.

3. **Cucurbita moschata**: Cucurbita moschata plants have spreading vines with hairy leaves. The fruit stems flare out at an angle and are hard, while the seeds have a dark tan margin.

4. **Cucurbita pepo**: Cucurbita pepo plants have prickly leaves and stems that can cause a rash. The fruit stem is angular with five sides, and the seeds are cream-colored with a white margin.

Seeds found in a Mexican cave indicate that the domesticated pepo species dates back approximately 10,000 years, making it the oldest and most widespread squash species in the New World.

There is a slight possibility of cross-pollination between Cucurbita moschata and Cucurbita mixta, but it is rare. To be safe, it is recommended to avoid planting these species close to each other. However, most heirloom varieties belong to different species, so this may not be a major concern. Keep in mind that squash plants have both male and female flowers on the same plant. In certain conditions, female flowers may drop without forming fruit, but the male flowers can be harvested for stuffed squash blossoms to avoid waste.

Planting pumpkins and squash follows similar techniques. Space hills 3 to 4 feet apart, adjusting as needed for larger-leafed varieties. Start seedlings indoors and transfer the strongest ones to large pots before moving them to the hills when the weather warms up. Well-established plants before late June are more resilient against squash beetles.
To save squash seeds, let the fruit fully ripen on the vine until the plants decline. Choose the best specimens with desired characteristics. Harvest the fruit and store it in a cool, dry place. Seeds become more viable with further aging in storage. Remove the seeds by scraping and washing them. Dry them on screens or paper towels for a few weeks, then store in airtight jars with dates in a cool, dark closet. Properly stored, squash seeds can remain viable for up to six years.

Appoquinimink
This ancient Native American winter pumpkin, believed to have originated in the vicinity of the Appoquinimink River in New Castle County, Delaware, can be traced back to a time before 1770. It was carefully preserved by Quaker farmers residing in the Odessa area and by the Nanticoke people who lived farther inland along the Delaware-Maryland border. What sets this winter storing pumpkin apart is its remarkable texture. Unlike mealy varieties, it boasts a dense and firm consistency, making it an excellent choice for hearth-baked breads. Its flavor is reminiscent of the renowned French heirloom squash, Muscade de Provence, but over the centuries, it has been specifically selected for its exceptional slow baking qualities. Notably, even the mottled skin of this pumpkin is edible. When fully mature, it typically weighs around 4.5 pounds and measures 7 to 8 inches in diameter and 6 inches in height. Furthermore, it excels in storage capability, remaining in good condition for at least six months.
Traditionally, Native Americans would bake these pumpkins by burying them whole in hot ashes for a minimum of one day. The local Quaker community, on the other hand, favored baking them in iron pots buried in ashes or hot coals. Regardless of the chosen cooking method, the addition of a touch of minced rosemary or herbs de Provence can greatly enhance the flavor profile of this pumpkin variety.

Summer Crookneck
The ancient heritage of the yellow Summer Crookneck squash is intertwined with the historical exchanges of Timothy Matlack and Thomas Jefferson in 1807. These correspondences, chronicled in Edwin Morris Betts' Jefferson's Garden Book, trace the origins of this unique squash variety to its indigenous roots in New Jersey.

Remarkably, it stands as a testament to the cultural legacy of the Lenape people who once thrived in the Delaware Valley. With its distinctive growth habit on a compact bush rather than a trailing vine, the Summer Crookneck squash showcases large, grayish-green leaves adorned with five lobes. At full maturity, the fruit grows to an impressive 8 to 9 inches in length, transitioning from a soft yellow hue to a vibrant yellow-orange shade. Notably, the skin surface bears prominent warts, a distinguishing feature that may manifest in subsequent generations due to potential cross-pollination with neighboring squash varieties. While the interior flesh typically displays a yellowish-white color, newer variants have emerged with a solid yellow hue, representing later developments. For culinary purposes, the squash is best enjoyed when harvested at a tender, very young stage. To obtain viable seeds for future cultivation, it is crucial to allow the Summer Crookneck squash to fully ripen. The skin should reach a pale orange, woody texture reminiscent of a gourd. Furthermore, leaving the fruit on the plant for an additional two weeks in this state facilitates the final aging process of the seeds, ensuring a higher proportion of viable seeds for the following season.

Mandan Squash

The Yellow Mandan Squash finds its origins in the Mandan Indians of the northern Great Plains, from which it derives its name. This variety is part of a group of similar North American squashes with ancient roots, making it a noteworthy heirloom. It is essential to distinguish the Yellow Mandan Squash from its close relative, the White Mandan Squash. The flesh of the Yellow Mandan Squash can range from pale orange to golden yellow, influenced by soil conditions, while its skin showcases a creamy yellow color. On the other hand, the White Mandan Squash is characterized by a distinct "sea foam white" skin, exhibiting a white shade tinged with green. Additionally, Yellow Mandan Squash fruits are smaller, weighing around 1 1/2 to 2 pounds, approximately half the size of true White Mandan Squash. When ripe, the Yellow Mandan Squash emits a pronounced fragrance and boasts better storage capabilities. It can be peeled, seeded, sliced like an apple, and dried for various culinary applications. It is important to note that among the available varieties, only Mandan and Yellow Mandan are currently offered through Seed Savers Exchange, as others have unfortunately vanished from seed lists. The compact nature of the Yellow Mandan Squash makes it well-suited for small gardens.

Its leaves resemble large grape leaves, and its low-lying growth habit allows the vines to coexist harmoniously with taller neighboring vegetables. This makes it an ideal companion plant for corn or when planted around the base of staked tomatoes. Furthermore, these plants exhibit abundant productivity. Personally, I dry this pumpkin to reconstitute it as paste or puree for my ongoing project building a Native American pantry. Dried pumpkin proves practical due to its easy storage and minimal space requirements. Alternatively, treat the mature fruit similarly to acorn squash. It's worth mentioning that when the young fruit reaches about 2 inches in diameter, it can be sliced and enjoyed raw with dips or cooked in a manner similar to zucchini.

Four sisters

In addition to corn, beans, and squash, certain southwest tribes grew a "fourth sister." They also planted the Rocky Mountain bee plant, which helped pollinate their gardens by attracting bees. One of the many common choices was the **Jerusalem artichoke**: a type of perennial sunflower with edible tubers, commercially known as the sunchoke (be careful though, these are most likely not heirloom varieties, but varieties bred to have knob-free tubers!).

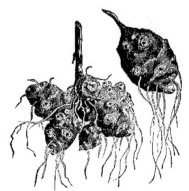

They were mashed like potatoes by Native Americans. It was also used in soups and stews as a thickening agent. They were cultivated in dried riverbeds and in fertile loam soils so that the tubers could be dug out easily once they were ripe. Jerusalem artichokes are highly suitable for cultivation due to their easy growth. The process begins by planting the tubers in well-prepared soil during the spring season. Throughout the summer, it is important to regularly weed the bed to prevent any competition that may arise with the emerging shoots of the artichoke plants. Once the fall season arrives and frost has caused the tops of the plants to wither, the roots can be harvested as needed. Gardeners have different methods for preserving the tubers: some choose to store them in damp sand, while others opt to leave them in the ground and cover them with straw over the winter. Either approach effectively preserves the Jerusalem artichokes.

Multiple varieties of artichoke can be grown within the same garden without issue, as long as they are propagated through their tubers. It is only when grown from seed that the potential for crosses arises. To maintain plant purity, it is advisable to cultivate the artichokes in contained beds. This precaution prevents them from spreading rapidly, interfering with hedges, impeding lawn mowers, or encroaching upon areas of the garden where they are not desired.

It was also rather common to train shooter beans using **sunflower** stems as we now use trellis.

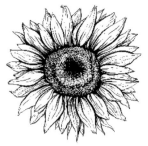

While trellis are useful, they are not pollinators and they don't look as nice, so consider using sunflowers as trellis not only for beans but for tomatoes, peas, or whatever you fancy growing.

Another plant that can be considered a "fourth sister" was **wild rice**.

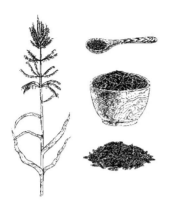

The American Indian diet included a lot of wild rice, making this fourth sister an obvious one. Wisconsin, Minnesota, and areas of the Great Lakes region grew it. Wild rice can only survive in three to eight feet of water. In order to live, the weather and water levels must be consistent.

Several weeks before the rice was ready to be harvested; women would enter the water. They tied the rice into little sheaves to prevent the rice kernels from falling into the water as they ripened. Rice is still gathered in boats now, as it was in the past.

While several people paddle a canoe, one person sits at the stern and knocks the rice grains into the canoe with long wooden rods before allowing the plants to spring back into place. Some grains are always left on the plants in order for them to re-seed the next year. Talk about mindful cultivation!

Dry land farming

For the natives of the American southwest, agriculture still played an integral part of their existence, despite the dry climate they called home, such as in the case of Anasazi agriculture, known as part of the Pueblo people today.

Evidence that they began to settle down in one spot for prolonged periods of time around 1200 B.C. and domesticate and produce crops from year to year helps to identify the historical boundary between hunter-gatherer civilization and the burgeoning Ancestral Puebloan civilization.

During the Basketmaker period, corn (maize) played a vital role as the primary crop. Its origins can be traced back to teosinte, a wild grass found in Mexico and Central America. The Ancestral Puebloan farmers, adapting to the colder and drier climate of the Southwest, likely engaged in cross-breeding various types of maize to select those best suited for challenging conditions. Alongside maize, squash was also cultivated, having been introduced from Mexico. Around 500 A.D., beans made their way into the North American diet, adding a new dietary component. The extended cooking time required for beans necessitated the use of pottery, which had replaced

baskets for food storage and cooking, enabling the successful incorporation of this nutritious legume into their cuisine.

The Cliff Dwellers of the Southwest region had a variety of food processing techniques. They commonly dried their crops by exposing them to the sun. Grinding stones, such as metate and mano, were used to stone-grind many types of food. Seeds were parched and crushed into meals over hot coals, while pine nuts were processed into a paste. Corn was ground to create cornmeal, an essential staple. To preserve their food, the Cliff Dwellers stored it in large pits, often protecting them from insects, animals, and dampness by wrapping them in baskets or ceramics.

The Ancestral Puebloans, unlike the Hohokam people to the south, did not construct massive irrigation canals. It was not irrigation in the traditional sense when they diverted and collected natural rain water. In general, they relied on the natural blessings of rain and runoff from melting snow for their dry-land cultivation. They often aided Mother Nature by constructing check dams, terracing hillsides, or situating farmland near arroyo and spring outlets. A 500,000-gallon reservoir at Mesa Verde was one of their major water conservation projects.

The Native Americans did not discard the cuisines of their nomadic forefathers, despite their reliance on domestic crops. Corn, squash, and beans, even in A.D. 1300, were insufficient to keep them alive. They continued to hunt deer, rabbits, and prairie dogs. And for food, they gathered wild plants. The pion pine nuts were roasted or crushed and eaten. They ate the banana yucca's ripe fruit and dried the prickly pear cactus' crimson fruit for later eating. Greens came from pigweed and amaranth.

Chinampas

Ancient farming practices continue to inspire innovative techniques in sustainable agriculture. One such technique is the chinampa system, which was the foundation of the Aztec Empire. Chinampas are highly productive farm plots surrounded by canals, and they played a crucial role in the Aztecs' rise to power. The Aztecs, once a small and impoverished tribe, settled in the area that would become modern-day Mexico City less than 200 years before their empire flourished. After initial conflicts with neighboring tribes, they were forced to retreat to two small islands in a lake. It was there that they adopted the chinampa system, a unique method of land reclamation and intensive agriculture. This system, which had been practiced on the lake's margins, proved to be one of the most productive and efficient farming methods ever devised. It not only provided the Aztecs with fertile land and surplus food but also enabled them to build a standing army that quickly expanded their empire across Mexico.

Although the Spanish conquistadors toppled the Aztecs and destroyed their magnificent pyramid temples, the chinampa system has persisted throughout history. However, after enduring for thousands of years, it now faces the threat of extinction. Chinampas are narrow strips of land surrounded by water were once vital to the region's agriculture. While many may not fully appreciate their significance today, the chinamperos, the caretakers of these gardens, and the tourists who visit the renowned chinampa center in Xochimilco, understand their importance.

The Valley of Mexico, a landlocked basin encompassed by volcanic mountains, is home to the extensive chinampa zone, covering around 3,000 square miles. In ancient times, the valley was filled with a large body of water known as the Lake of the Moon. Over time, it transformed into separate lakes due to evaporation, including Zumpango, Xaltocan, Texcoco, Xochimilco, and Chalco. The valley has been inhabited for centuries, with villages established as early as the late second millennium B.C. Teotihuacan, a significant city that emerged in the first or second century A.D., exerted its influence in the region. Since the Spanish conquest in 1521, the Valley of Mexico has undergone significant changes. Water was drained for agricultural purposes during the colonial era, and further depletion occurred when a tunnel was constructed in 1900. The demands of a growing Mexico City led to the tapping of springs and digging of wells, exacerbating the water scarcity. As a result, only isolated puddles of the Lake of the Moon remain, with parts of Lake Texcoco and Lake Xochimilco still existing. This drying has had a devastating impact on the chinampas, with most of the small urban centers disappearing over time.

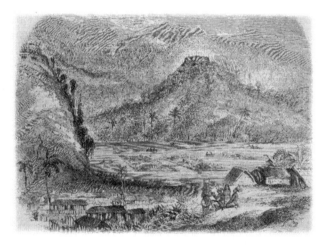

Each chinampa was a carefully crafted garden plot, typically around 300 feet long and 15 to 30 feet wide. Canals surrounded the chinampas, serving as transportation routes for farmers using flat-bottomed canoes. Before each planting season, the chinamperos would collect nutrient-rich mud from the canal's bottom and spread it onto the chinampa's surface. During the wet season, the water held within the chinampa provided moisture for the crops. However, additional watering was necessary as the dry season approached. Over time, the repeated application of mud elevated the surface of the chinampa, requiring excavation to lower it. The excess soil would be used to create new chinampas. An important technique in chinampa farming was the seed nursery. A layer of mud was spread over waterweeds, solidifying into blocks called chapines. Seeds were placed in holes in the chapines, covered with manure, and protected from frost and dry spells. The seedlings were then transplanted from the chapines to designated spots on the chinampa, covered with canal mud. Maize was the only crop that could be directly planted in the chinampa.

The industrious chinamperos skillfully cultivate a wide variety of crops, reaping the bounty of seven different types each year from their plots, including two dedicated to maize. In the flourishing fields of Xochimilco, ancient cultivation practices persist, nurturing the growth of five maize varieties, beans, chili peppers, tomatoes, and two delightful strains of grain amaranth, all cherished crops since pre-Spanish times. Alongside these native treasures, European vegetable introductions like carrots, lettuce, cabbages, radishes, beets, and onions thrive in harmony. Xochimilco, meaning "place of the flower gardens" in the Aztec Nahuatl language, resonates with the echoes of tradition as elders in the chinampa towns still converse in this ancestral tongue. The vibrant gardens burst with a myriad of blooms, with Nahuatl-named species like cempaxochitl ("twenty flower" or marigold), oceloxochitl ("jaguar flower"), and cacaloxochitl ("crow flower") adding a touch of enchantment. Dahlia, Mexico's esteemed national flower, adorns the landscape in countless captivating variations, while European imports such as carnations, roses, and lilies lend their exotic allure.

As the canals gracefully meander, their depths conceal a treasure trove of life. Carp and other fish species thrive in abundance, skillfully captured by the chinamperos using nets and spears. Among these aquatic marvels, the axolotl, a magnificent salamander, holds a special place. Revered by zoologists for its role as a laboratory animal and cherished by the people of Xochimilco for its tender flesh and absence of troublesome bones, the axolotl represents a unique delicacy. Regrettably, the once-teeming water birds that graced the canals have become a rare sight, their numbers diminished by the indiscriminate use of firearms, a sobering reminder of the delicate balance between human activities and the natural world. The island capital of the Aztecs, adorned by the marvels of chinampas, is a testament to their ingenuity and mastery of agriculture. The National Museum of Anthropology in Mexico City houses a precious Aztec map, meticulously crafted on native paper derived from the inner bark of a fig tree. This historical artifact provides a glimpse into the grandeur of the Aztec capital, encompassing the area that now lies beneath the railroad yards of Mexico City. Believed to be a tax record created by Aztec scribes, the map showcases the intricate network of canals arranged in a grid-like pattern, intersected by larger canals traversing diagonally. Alongside the canals, roads and footpaths can be seen, with wooden bridges connecting them as described by the Spanish conquerors. Within the heart of the capital, where the land was elevated and more solid, stood the substantial houses constructed from stone and mortar. This central area also housed prominent public edifices, including the majestic pyramid temples and the opulent palaces of the emperor and the high-ranking nobility. While these architectural marvels dominated the core, the majority of the population consisted of nonagricultural individuals, such as priests, politicians, craftsmen, traders, and soldiers.

Despite the diverse composition of its inhabitants, Tenochtitlan-Tlatelolco remained a city intertwined with chinampas, earning comparisons to the famed city of Venice by the Spanish conquerors. A bustling network of canals, vibrant with water vegetation, welcomed thousands of canoes laden with people and various goods on a daily basis. This lively aquatic transportation system facilitated the movement of both individuals and essential commodities throughout the city, adding to its vibrant atmosphere.

An Aztec poet has aptly described the astounding beauty of his native city:

The City is spread out in circles of jade,
Radiating flashes of light like quetzal plumes.
Beside it the lords are borne in boats:
Over them spreads a flowery mist.

It would not be an exaggeration to state that the existence of chinampas granted the ancient peoples of the Valley of Mexico intermittent dominance over a significant portion of the country for 1,500 years prior to the arrival of the Spanish. Consequently, a comprehensive examination of all facets of this exceptional system, as it presently operates, should be undertaken before the chinampas vanish entirely in the name of progress. In the face of our recent mistakes, which include the pollution stemming from the Industrial Revolution, oil spills from various industries, and human-induced climate change, scientists are diligently searching for methods to safeguard the planet. Interestingly, one of the most ingenious agricultural methods has been in practice for centuries. Sustainable agriculture is not solely a product of the twentieth century. Chinampas were constructed by forming small stationary islands through the accumulation of mud and decomposing plants. On top of these islands, maize, beans, chilies, squash, tomatoes, and various greens were cultivated. The vibrant flowers grown on the chinampas were also utilized for ceremonial purposes. Sturdy reeds were employed to enclose and anchor each chinampa, thereby providing stability to the islands. The process of mud dredging facilitated the creation of canals and naturally replenished the soil with nutrients necessary for crop growth. The resulting system of canals and gardens not only supported the cultivation of crops but also provided a habitat for fish and birds, contributing to the preservation of the ecosystem's health and offering additional food sources.

Contrary to degrading the ecosystem, the chinampas actually enhanced it. However, the development and maintenance of chinampas required substantial labor. These systems demanded various mechanisms and procedures to ensure the well-being of both the people and the soil. During the wet season, drainage systems were installed to prevent flooding. Waste collection systems were established to gather human excrement from settlements and utilize it as fertilizer for the crops. This not only prevented waste from contaminating the water supply but also aided in its enrichment. The transformation of unusable swampland into a flourishing garden by the Aztecs is a remarkable achievement in itself. Equally impressive is the coordinated effort, planning, and utilization of resources required to bring their vision to fruition. The concept of chinampas has transcended boundaries, finding application in other cities and nations, including examples along the Baltimore waterfront and efforts to clean up New York's polluted Gowanus Canal. Certain eco-businesses have even adapted the techniques of the Aztecs, developing innovative technologies reminiscent of the ancient floating gardens. Chinampas can facilitate plant growth, purify and conserve water, and do not necessitate vast expanses of land, thus appealing to modern-day gardeners seeking sustainability. The success of chinampas serves as a testament to the fact that the most inventive solutions do not always lie in the future but can be found in the past. This indigenous farming system's extraordinary efficacy reminds us that sustainability need not be expensive or reliant on cutting-edge technology. Sometimes, the best course of action is to look back and learn from those who got it right the first time.

Ahupua'a

Intensive rain-fed agricultural systems served as the cornerstone of the agricultural economies in Hawai'i and certain parts of Maui in the centuries preceding European contact. However, much of our knowledge regarding the functioning of these productive systems remains limited due to their abandonment in the nineteenth century. It is likely that Hawaiian farmers cultivated a winter crop called 'uala in the lower, warmer, and drier areas of the field system, while growing spring-summer crops in the upper, wetter regions. Management at the ahupua'a level in rain-fed agricultural systems potentially played a role in integrating environmental variability and sustaining yields throughout the year.

In ancient Hawai'i, prior to Western influence, the indigenous kanaka maoli people held a deep spiritual belief in the interconnectedness of all beings and the presence of mana, a spiritual power, in nature. They worshipped a multitude of gods, with four primary deities holding significant roles. Kane represented life, freshwater, and sunlight as the creator of mankind. Lono governed agriculture, clouds, and weather. Ku embodied leadership, medicine, and war as the god of the forest. Kanaloa presided over the wind and ocean. According to the kanaka maoli, they saw themselves as direct descendants of Wakea, the sky father, and Papa, the earth mother. This ancestral lineage emphasized their strong connection to the natural world.

The kanaka maoli believed in the concept of 'ohana, or family, extending beyond humans to include all living beings and even inanimate objects. They believed that everything possessed consciousness and the ability to communicate. By opening our receptiveness, we could perceive the aliveness and interconnectedness of everything around us, from the wind to the sounds and rocks. Wellness, characterized by harmony, arose from the constant interaction of all life forces. This harmony, known as pono, was maintained through the spiritual power of mana. Spiritual interrelationships were of utmost importance, and maintaining pono through right thoughts and actions was essential. Conversely, illness stemmed from the loss of pono and mana, affecting both humans and the environment. The kanaka maoli believed that plants and animals were their siblings, highlighting the interconnectedness of all life forms. It was the collective responsibility of everyone to malama 'aina, which means to care for the land and its natural resources. These relationships extended to all aspects of the cosmos. The kanaka maoli had a saying that reflected their worldview: "He ali'i no ka 'aina; he kauwa wale ke kanaka," which means "the land is chief; the human is but a servant." This saying underscores the reverence they held for the land and their recognition of humanity's role as caretakers rather than owners. The kanaka maoli had a unique land partition system that did not involve the concept of private property. Instead, the land was entrusted to the top chief or king, who held it on behalf of the entire community. The king appointed supervisors based on their status and rank to oversee different regions. The division of land started from the complete island (mokupuni) and continued down to individual family units.

In ancient Hawai'i, the kanaka maoli people recognized the mokupuni, or island, as divided into moku, the largest units that stretched from the mountains to the sea. Each moku was further divided into ahupua'a, narrower divisions that also extended from the mountains to the sea. The size of the ahupua'a was determined by the available resources, with larger ones in areas of lesser abundance. Each ahupua'a had an alii, or local chief, who was overseen by a konohiki.

Within the ahupua'a, there were smaller divisions called ili, typically consisting of two or three per ahupua'a, which made up the chief's estate. These ili could have noncontiguous pieces called lele. The mo'o referred to the arable areas within the ili that did not extend to the sea. Additionally, there were kuleana, small land parcels used by ordinary people for crop cultivation. The size of a kuleana, like that of an ahupua'a, depended on the land's natural fertility and abundance.

The ancient ahupua'a served as the basic self-sustaining unit, embodying the kanaka maoli's spiritual beliefs and interrelationships with the natural world. It followed the natural boundaries of the watershed, providing necessary resources such as fish, salt, fertile soil, and valuable trees. The ahupua'a fostered the sharing of specialized knowledge and resources specific to each local area. The self-sustaining environment of the ahupua'a relied on the interdependence of all life forms, from the mountains to the sea. The ahupua'a encompassed a wide range of products and resources, including trees for canoes, hardwood for tools, plants for medicine, and various materials for crafting. The kula plains and fields offered bamboo, grass for thatching, oil for lighting, and plants for medicine and decoration. The kai, the sea and shore area, provided fish, seaweed, and salt, along with resources from coconut trees and other coastal plants. The ahupua'a system operated as a self-sustainable ecosystem, with a core focus on the vital resource of wai, or freshwater. The people recognized the sacredness of water, utilizing it for agriculture and aquaculture. The konohiki oversaw the management of resources, while the maka'ainana enjoyed secure land tenure and participated in collective work. The kapu system regulated activities to maintain sustainable practices, ensuring the well-being of the community. Though the ahupua'a system has mostly vanished, its spirit and traditional knowledge persist through cultural practices and values. The importance of protecting Hawai'i's ecosystems and natural heritage remains crucial, as the health of the upland watershed influences the downstream environment and the livelihoods of the people. Preserving and learning from the wisdom of the past is vital in facing the challenges posed by the modern world. As the saying goes, "He ali'i no ka 'aina; he kauwa wale ke kanaka" — the land is chief; humans are but servants.

Agroforestry

Agroforestry, sometimes known as forest gardening, is the practice of planting trees, shrubs, herbs, and vegetables in a group to simulate a forest, or inside an existing forest, with each plant offering benefits such as shade, predator protection, life-giving humidity, and nutrients to the others. The prehistoric Eastern Woodlands were managed using silviculture, a practice aimed at enhancing tree growth and forest composition to improve hunting and boost wildlife populations. Native Americans also employed silvopasture, a method of grazing livestock among trees, to benefit forest health, sequester carbon in the soil, provide shade for animals, disperse seeds through cattle, and create more wildlife habitat. These strategies exemplified the deep understanding Indigenous peoples had of their environments and their ability to work harmoniously with nature. Controlled burning played a significant role in forest management across the Americas, with Indigenous peoples utilizing this technique to maintain and shape their forests. Through ecological succession, trees regrew over time, facilitating the movement of nutrients from the soil to an organic form, supporting the growth of diverse plant species, and promoting a healthy ecosystem.

Swidden agriculture, another practice employed by Indigenous communities, involved selective tree burning to utilize ash as a natural fertilizer for crops. This process not only enriched the soil but also stimulated regeneration and the growth of new vegetation. Over time, swidden agriculture contributed to the formation of grasslands in the Midwest and Southwest regions of the United States. Unfortunately, the displacement of Indigenous peoples from their ancestral lands through colonial tactics disrupted these traditional land management practices. As a result, forests have reclaimed territories that were once cultivated using swidden agriculture. Areas such as Wisconsin, Illinois, and the Texas Hill Country, which were previously characterized by grasslands, now boast thriving forests. The knowledge and practices of Indigenous peoples in silviculture, silvopasture, controlled burning, and swidden agriculture offer valuable lessons for modern forest and land management. By incorporating these principles into contemporary approaches, we can work towards sustainable forestry, improved biodiversity, and the preservation of our ecosystems. Nowadays, agroforestry is being considered as one of the most effective permaculture systems and the utopic idea of food forests has garnered mainstream interest. While a time-consuming and ambitious project, it can be easily implemented in our backyards and homesteads as well. Read on to the next chapter to discover how agroforestry and other traditional agricultural methods can be applied to today's gardening techniques.

...And Modern Practice

Taking a look back at history can do us a ton of good; that's true; however, we can also put these time-tested methods into use today.

Companion planting

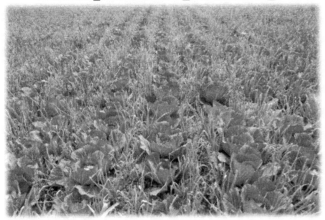

We all love having supportive friends, don't we? Like the three system taught us, plants like to be friends with one another!

Companion planting allows you to mimic nature in your garden and provide your crops with the greatest possible growing conditions, just like the three sisters system taught us. Companion planting is an excellent approach to boosting the health and productivity of your garden. Planting compatible plants close together allows them to benefit from each other's characteristics. Planting several types of plants close together can help your harvest develop faster, resist pests, and even improve the flavor.

Companion planting not only benefits your plants but also makes better use of your garden area, allowing you to gather more types in the same amount of space. Companion planting gives a lot of variety, which is great for pollinators, wildlife, and overall soil health. Understanding what plants go well together and how certain plants can help others can considerably boost your garden's production.

It helps to have a support network!

Conserves space
We all want to make the most of our available garden area. Plant a vining plant beneath a taller plant to save space in the garden that would otherwise be wasted. For more efficient gardening, plant fast-growing crops in between rows of slower-growing crops.

Provides protection and shade for other plants
Planting tall, strong plants with climbers in your garden can provide natural supports, removing the need for separate structures and staking. Lower-growing, climbing crops like beans, cucumbers, and peas can be supported by vertically tolerant plants like maize and sunflowers. Tall crops can also give shade to plants that don't need as much direct sunlight.

Useful for attracting beneficial insects
Many insects are helpful to gardens, and a wide variety of plants can improve the likelihood that they will visit frequently. Butterflies, bees, and birds are necessary pollinators for the healthiest growth in your garden. Also, for your prized plants, these cheerful insects are the best type of pest management. Beneficial insects will continue to visit your garden if you have a variety of plants and flowers with extended and different flowering periods.

Beneficial to the soil
Planting a variety of plants together might assist in keeping your soil moist and preventing erosion. It would be a waste of valuable garden areas to have open soil patches. Cucumber and squash plants provide excellent soil shade. In times of drought, shading the soil might be beneficial. Some vegetable plants help other plants by improving the soil quality. Beans, for example, assist in replenishing nitrogen in the soil as they grow.

Companion Planting Aids in the Control of Diseases and Pests
The Nasturtium is an excellent example of this. The aphid, a particularly damaging bug, adores the nasturtium plant. You can utilize the nasturtium plant as a host and sacrifice it to help safeguard surrounding plants that are affected by aphids by using clever companion planting.

Looking for beauty
Companion planting can benefit a variety of plants, not just vegetables. Companion planting might also provide purely aesthetic benefits. When you combine annuals and perennials, or plants with different bloom dates, you can create a garden that blooms continuously.

Plant	Beneficial Effects	Companion plants
Basil	Improves the flavor of neighboring herbs and repels flies and mosquitoes.	Tomatoes, Peppers, Asparagus, Oregano (avoid Sage or Common Rue)
Chamomile	Improves the flavor of any neighboring herb and attracts beneficial insects and pollinators	Cabbage, Onion, Cucumber
Garlic	Repels aphids, loopers, snails, and Japanese beetles.	Most Plants
Mint	Repels aphids, mosquitoes, and ants, and attracts bees.	Tomatoes, Most Plants (avoid combining Mint varieties)
Chives	Repels aphids.	Carrots, Tomatoes, Dill, and most herbs
Tarragon	Improves the flavor of any neighboring plant.	A great companion to Eggplant
Cilantro	Deters spider mites, aphids.	Spinach, Caraway, Anise, Dill
Sage	Repels some beetles and flies.	Rosemary (not Rue)
Dill	Discourages spider mites and aphids.	Onions, Corn, Lettuce, Cucumbers (not Carrots, Tomatoes, Fennel, Lavender, or Caraway)
Rosemary	Deters a variety of pests.	Beans, Peppers, Broccoli, Cabbage, Sage (not Carrots or Pumpkins)
Catnip	Repels harmful pests and attracts pollinators.	Pumpkins, Beets, Squash, Hyssop
Lavender	Repels harmful pests and attracts butterflies.	Cauliflower
Borage	Attracts bees and more than 100 beneficial insects, and repels tomato hornworms and cabbage worms.	Tomatoes, Squash, and Strawberries
Marjoram	Improves the flavor and increases the vigor of all vegetables.	Plant near any vegetables you want to boost
Thyme	Repels cabbage worms and carrot flies while attracting beneficial insects.	Chives, Onion, Parsley, Asparagus, Marigold, Nasturtium, Carrots and Lima Beans
Tansy	Makes an excellent herb near a compost heap. Attracts Honeybees to the garden.	Beans, Cucumbers, Squash, Corn, Roses, Raspberries, Peppers, Cabbage, and Potatoes
Summer Savory	Repels cabbage worms and carrot flies while attracting beneficial insects.	Beans and Onions
Lemon Balm	Repels mosquitoes and squash bugs.	Squash
Tarragon	Good companion to most plants. Repels Japanese beetles, striped cucumber beetle, squash bugs, sugar ants, mice, fleas & moths.	Other herbs. Chives, Sage, Etc.
Chervil	Radishes grow better and increase in flavor in the presence of chervil.	Radishes
Coriander	Enhances the flavor of many vegetables and repels aphids, spider mites, and potato beetles	Radishes, Peppers
Parsley	Attracts parasitic wasps, swallowtail butterflies, and repels asparagus beetles when gone to seed.	Tomatoes, Corn, and Asparagus
Mint	Repels cabbage moths.	Cabbage, Tomatoes

Terracing

If your home is on a hill or slope, you may believe that you won't be able to grow your own garden. But nothing could be further from the truth: the solution is a terrace garden design. You don't need quite an ambitious design like *Kanaki Maolo* with their *Ahapua'a*, but you can certainly take their lead!

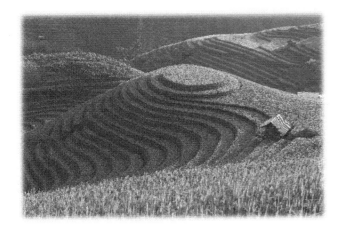

Terrace gardens allow you to cultivate a wide range of plants and vegetables without the danger of losing all of your hard work. This option allows any homeowner with steep slopes to build "mini-gardens" that minimize erosion by splitting hilly areas into smaller level parts, which would otherwise be impossible to cultivate. Water may be better distributed and absorbed into the ground this way.

Erosion prevention

Terrace gardening or farming has emerged as a practical solution to prevent erosion and transform steep hillsides into productive agricultural areas. Initially, farmers didn't prioritize aesthetics when contouring the hills, but the outcome turned out to be remarkably beautiful. A quick search for "rice terrace China" on Google showcases the stunning results achieved through hard work, love for the land, and the use of wood and stones. If you have stubborn hillside areas in your yard that are challenging to manage, terrace gardening can be a viable option. These areas are often difficult to mow and may have soil erosion issues due to steep slopes where grass or plants struggle to take root.

Moreover, steep hills can impede accessibility to certain parts of your yard. While you may desire a garden, unused space on a slope presents challenges. Garden terracing, inspired by the rice terraces in Asia, serves as a solution to prevent soil erosion and water runoff. If you have a sloping lawn that directs water and dirt into the street and drains, terracing can retain the water on leveled planes. This approach allows you to harness the benefits of the slope while preventing flooding in the drainage system.

This is particularly important because some towns are considering legislation that could exempt the government from liability for flood damage caused by sewage blockages in residential areas. As more new homes are built on green spaces, sewage backups are likely to become more prevalent. Terrace gardening can help mitigate these issues and promote sustainable land management practices.

Increases your potential garden area:

Using a sloped lawn for play or gardening can be challenging. However, terraces can provide additional square footage for these purposes by adding soil or compost to each level. Terracing creates flat platforms that can be utilized for play areas, seating, relaxation, or gardening. Each terrace level becomes a new space for planting flowers, vegetables, or herbs, improving both functionality and aesthetics.

More space for other features:

The options are limitless. What would you do if your yard had more level, open space? Would you consider starting a vegetable garden? Do you want to build a play structure for your children? Perhaps a koi pond with a small waterfall?

Wide variety of materials

Even in the absence of a steep hill, constructing a series of smaller terraces can still create varying levels and opportunities to experiment with different shapes, colors, and sizes of plants. These terraces provide the flexibility to arrange your garden in unique ways that wouldn't be feasible on a flat surface. Additionally, the choice of materials used to support the retaining wall can greatly enhance the overall aesthetic of your garden. Whether you opt for stone, cedar, brick, or other options, each material has its own distinct characteristics and can be adjusted to suit your preferences and style. The choice of materials adds another layer of customization and visual appeal to your terrace garden.

How to build your terraces

Choosing your materials

Terrace gardens can be made out of a variety of materials, such as bricks, rocks, and concrete blocks, although treated wood is the most popular. It has several advantages, including a lower cost than many other materials and the ability to mix in more seamlessly with natural surroundings. Landscape timbers, which may survive for many seasons in the garden, and cedarwood, which is great for vegetable gardens because it prevents chemicals from leaking into the soil, are two alternatives.

Preparing for slopes

Before you begin, keep in mind that whatever terrace garden design you choose must complement your surroundings. You'll need to consider a slope into your DIY terrace garden design plans if you're working with a slope. This necessitates determining the type of slope you're dealing with. The rise and run of the slope you're working with should be determined. The rise is the vertical distance from the bottom to the top of the slope, while the run is the horizontal distance from the top to the bottom. The height and width of each bed should be determined using these measurements.

Building the levels

If you're not hiring a professional to install your terrace garden, the first step is to dig a trench at the bottom of the slope for the first tier. Keep in mind that the deeper the trench will be, the more layers you have in your garden. It should, however, be kept level at all times, and the basic terrace layer should be placed within the trench.

The next stage is to dig a trench for the terrace garden's sides, making sure that the trench's bottom remains level with the first trench. Spikes can be used to hold your building materials together.

Finally, to verify that the terrace box is level, push up the soil in the back of the box towards the front. This may necessitate the addition of more soil. These processes should be performed for each of your garden's tiers.

Putting it together

The fun comes once the actual construction of your terrace garden is completed. It's now time to sketch out your landscape's botanical aspects. While maintaining your terrace garden will be necessary to protect its attractiveness, you can still make the most of your area by wisely selecting plants that will thrive in your hillside setting. In a hillside garden, you can cultivate a wide range of vegetables, fruits, herbs, and flowers. Radishes, various varieties of gourds, leeks, cucumbers, tomatoes, and limes are some of the easiest crops to cultivate in a terrace garden and are often quick to fruit. Ginger and mint, as well as thyme, Rosemary, lavender, and sage, are all beginner-friendly terrace garden herbs. And, of course, the flowers you select can enhance the attractiveness of your garden: avoid purely ornamental species such as hyacinths, primroses, pansies, and petunias, and opt instead for a native wildflower garden; you can have your pick amongst the 75+ native wildflowers carefully selected in the sixth volume of this series for their beauty, their effectiveness as pollinators, and their medicinal purposes. My personal favourites are marsh marigold, purple coneflowers, and trout lilies. Succulents, aloes, and various cacti are all low-maintenance plants that can be used year-round in a terrace garden. Just make sure that whatever you choose to grow in your garden, you've done your homework on what each plant requires to thrive, from ideal soil conditions to sun exposure.

"Catch the Rain" Irrigation

Although our planet is predominantly covered in water, not all of it is suitable for human use. Ocean and seawater cannot be consumed, and only a small portion of water is available for other purposes. This scarcity of usable water for drinking, domestic, and industrial needs persists globally. Water-stressed regions have addressed this issue by utilizing the limited rainfall they receive. This practice initially gained traction in areas with minimal rainfall and gradually spread to regions with more abundant precipitation, giving rise to modern rainwater harvesting systems. The concept behind rainwater harvesting is simple. Rainwater that falls on the ground is collected, stored, and later utilized. It can be purified for drinking, used for everyday tasks, and even employed in large-scale industries. In essence, rainwater harvesting involves the collection, purification, storage, and utilization of rainwater for irrigation and various other purposes. Rainwater harvesting techniques are employed by numerous individuals worldwide to reduce reliance on groundwater. This approach, which has been in practice

for thousands of years, is gaining popularity. In areas with ample rainfall, excess precipitation can be used to recharge groundwater through artificial recharge methods. Even today, rainwater remains a primary source of drinking water in many rural regions. One of its advantages is that it is free from pollutants, salts, minerals, and other natural or man-made impurities. In urban settings, rainwater collection is often facilitated through infrastructure, while the most basic approach to rainwater harvesting involves storage tanks. In this system, a catchment area such as rooftops is directly connected to cisterns, tanks, or reservoirs. Water can be stored in these containers until it is needed or utilized on a regular basis. If rooftops are sufficiently large to capture daily water requirements, they serve as excellent catchment areas. Alternatively, large bowls and tarps can also be used for rainwater collection.

Know your techniques

1. **Surface Runoff Harvesting:** Rainwater is collected in natural reservoirs, tanks, or infiltrated into underground aquifers before it becomes surface runoff.
2. **Rooftop Rainwater Harvesting (RRH):** Rainwater from rooftops is redirected and stored in a recharge pit, allowing it to slowly recharge the groundwater.
3. **Dams:** Barriers constructed to hold water, either by direct collection or through drainage systems. Dams are commonly used for irrigation and water treatment.
4. **Underground Tanks:** Excavated and cemented tanks placed below ground level to prevent water leakage. Rainwater is pumped into the tank through pipes, and pumps are used to extract the water.
5. **Rain Saucer:** A rain collection device resembling an upside-down umbrella or funnel, connected to a pipe to channel the collected water elsewhere.
6. **Rainwater Collection Reservoirs:** Rainwater is collected from roadways and pavements, although the water may be less pure and potentially polluted. It can be used for crop irrigation.
7. **Barrage:** A large dam with multiple apertures that can be opened or closed to control the water flow.
8. **Slopes:** Rainwater naturally collects at the bottom of slopes, providing an easy method of rainwater collection.
9. **Trenches:** Traditional trenches are used to direct rainwater to farms for irrigation purposes.
10. **Rain Barrels:** Specifically designed barrels for collecting rainwater from rooftops, typically available for purchase in retail stores.

So many options, right? Well, with so many options available, there are just as many pros to catching rain.

Simple to maintain

Rainwater harvesting systems offer several benefits to communities. Firstly, they enable efficient utilization of a valuable energy resource. By collecting and utilizing rainwater, we reduce the dependency on limited drinking water supplies and minimize wastage. Rainwater harvesting systems are built using simple technology, resulting in lower installation and operation costs compared to water purification or pumping systems. Additionally, these systems require minimal maintenance efforts and time. While rainwater may not be purified, it can be utilized for various purposes, further enhancing its versatility and usefulness within the community.

Self-sufficiency

Rainwater collection serves as a self-sustaining water source in regions where clean water is either expensive or scarce. It plays a crucial role in providing access to clean, potable water and enhances the overall availability of this vital resource. In developed countries, rainwater collection is often employed as an additional water supply rather than a primary source. By incorporating rainwater collection practices, overall water consumption can be reduced, promoting greater efficiency and sustainability in water usage.

Getting rid of water bills

Utilizing rainwater collected through a rainwater harvesting system offers numerous benefits for non-drinking purposes. By incorporating this alternative water source, homes and small businesses can experience substantial savings in their utility bills. On a larger scale, rainwater harvesting can provide ample water quantities to support various operations without placing excessive strain on local water supplies. Furthermore, rainwater harvesting contributes to the mitigation of soil erosion in diverse regions, allowing the land to restore its natural state. Rainwater can be stored in cisterns or other storage systems for use during periods of water scarcity, ensuring a reliable water supply.

It's irrigation-ready

The beauty of rainwater harvesting lies in its simplicity and minimal need for additional infrastructure. Most rooftops can be utilized as catchment areas, requiring minimal modifications to connect them to the harvesting system. This approach has the added benefit of reducing the environmental impact by minimizing the use of fuel-powered machinery and the need for extensive construction. Rainwater is naturally free from many of the toxins commonly found in groundwater, making it an ideal source for irrigation and watering plants. It provides a clean and chemical-free option to support healthy growth. Additionally, having large reservoirs of collected rainwater is particularly valuable in areas prone to forest and bush fires during the summer months, ensuring a readily available water supply for firefighting and prevention efforts.

Lessens the need for groundwater

The global demand for water is continuously rising due to population growth and increased water consumption. To meet these growing needs, many residential communities and businesses rely heavily on groundwater sources. However, overreliance on groundwater extraction has led to the depletion of aquifers in several regions, exacerbating water scarcity issues. Rainwater harvesting provides an effective solution to this problem by reducing the dependence on groundwater sources. By collecting and utilizing rainwater, communities and businesses can supplement their water needs without further depleting groundwater reserves. This helps to maintain stable groundwater levels and ensures the long-term sustainability of water resources. Rainwater harvesting systems enable the capture and storage of rainwater for various purposes such as irrigation, washing, and cleaning. By utilizing rainwater for non-potable uses, the demand for groundwater can be reduced, easing the burden on aquifers and allowing them to replenish naturally.

In times of drought, it's a good idea to have a backup plan

Rainwater harvesting is an economical and dependable method of obtaining clean water in regions with arid climates. It enables the collection and storage of rainwater for future use, particularly during drought periods. In dry climates, techniques like the construction of soil ridges help capture rainwater, preventing it from running off hills and slopes. This practice improves irrigation by providing water for crops even in low rainfall conditions. Roof surfaces can also be utilized to collect rainwater, which is then directed into storage tanks or reservoirs. The construction of dams and ponds further enhances water collection, ensuring a consistent water supply for irrigation, even during periods of limited rainfall.

It lowers the risk of flooding and soil erosion

During periods of heavy rainfall, rainwater is collected and stored in large-scale storage tanks, serving multiple purposes. One significant benefit is the mitigation of flooding in low-lying areas. By capturing and storing rainwater, excess water is removed from the immediate environment, reducing the risk of flooding. Additionally, rainwater harvesting plays a crucial role in minimizing soil erosion and preventing the pollution of surface water bodies. When it rains, pesticides and fertilizers applied to agricultural fields can be carried away by runoff, contaminating lakes and ponds. By collecting rainwater, these pollutants are intercepted and prevented from entering the water systems, promoting cleaner and healthier aquatic ecosystems.

Rainwater for drinking

Since rainwater is unaffected by groundwater salinity or contaminants, with the right catchment system it can be utilized for drinking.

...and non-drinking objectives

Rainwater that is collected for non-drinking purposes can be utilized in various everyday activities such as cooking, bathing, flushing toilets, cleaning clothes and utensils, watering the garden, washing cars, and more. By using rainwater for these purposes, there is no need to rely on purified drinking water, which can help conserve valuable drinking water resources. Rainwater is naturally soft and free from certain contaminants, making it suitable for many household tasks that do not require potable water. This not only helps reduce the demand for treated drinking water but also lowers water bills and promotes sustainability by utilizing a locally available resource.

Rainwater harvesting does come with certain challenges and considerations that should be taken into account:

Unpredictable rainfall

The availability of rainwater is dependent on the rainfall patterns in a particular area. In regions with inconsistent or limited rainfall, relying solely on rainwater may not be feasible for meeting all water needs.

Initial cost

Setting up a rainwater harvesting system can involve an initial investment, including the cost of equipment and installation. The expenses can vary depending on the system's size and complexity. Although the system can provide long-term cost savings, it may take several years to recoup the initial investment.

Maintenance requirements

Regular maintenance is essential for rainwater collection systems to ensure their proper functioning. This includes cleaning, inspecting for pests, preventing algae growth, and ensuring that the system is well-maintained. Neglecting maintenance can lead to issues such as clogging, contamination, or the creation of breeding grounds for pests.

Roofing considerations:

Some roof types, especially those made of certain materials, may leach chemicals, dirt, or animal droppings into the rainwater, potentially affecting its quality if used for watering plants or other purposes. It is important to consider the compatibility of the roofing material with rainwater collection.

Storage capacity limitations

The storage capacity of rainwater collection systems is determined by the size and design of the storage tanks or containers. In heavy rainfall events, the system may reach its storage limit, resulting in excess water flowing away if not properly managed.

Specific use limitations

Rainwater collected during the first rain event may not be suitable for watering plants due to potential contamination from roof materials or debris. However, it can still be utilized for non-potable household uses. Additionally, the availability of stored rainwater may be limited to the capacity of the storage system, which may not be sufficient for prolonged dry periods. Despite these challenges, rainwater harvesting remains an increasingly popular and environmentally beneficial method. It can be particularly advantageous in areas with abundant rainfall, providing a sustainable water source and reducing reliance on other water supplies.

"No-Till" Gardening

Plowing fields is one of the most significant contributors to land degradation. The primary goal of plowing is to bury agricultural leftovers, manure, and weeds while also aerating and warming the soil. This type of agriculture has been used for thousands of years, and many farmers are unable to imagine life without it. However, the tilled soil will deteriorate and become infertile over time.

Of course, there is another way to farm. No-till farming first gained popularity in the late 1970s and has steadily gained popularity since then. According to Roger Claassen, an agricultural economist with the USDA, only 5% of American farmers were no-till in 1988. In 2008, that percentage had risen to 25%. (and is likely higher now). However, there are disadvantages to the no-till method; it is not as straightforward as it appears. Here's a quick rundown of the benefits and drawbacks of no-till farming.

There are plenty of pros to this method.

It's cheaper

By eliminating the extra step of plowing each year, no-till can save a lot of money in labor and fuel over time.

Water comes easier

Crop leftovers on the surface from no-till farming absorb water and prevent runoff. Farmers in drought-stricken areas may benefit from this water retention.

Less runoff

Herbicides and other contaminants are kept out of adjacent water supplies due to the lack of runoff.

Higher yields

No-till farming can dramatically enhance crop yields, especially in locations with poor moisture levels. Lloyd, who farms wheat in Clay Center, Kansas, claims that since he quit plowing, his yields have increased by up to 50%.

There's plenty of literature available

The no-till movement is gaining traction, and there are numerous resources to assist you in making the switch. Many farmers had to wing it twenty years ago, learning the ins and outs by trial and error.

Of course, there are downsides.

Equipment can be expensive

Seeding equipment, such as a "no-till drill," can cost upwards of $100,000. This is a major expense, even if it is eventually incorporated into day-to-day operating savings.

Moisture can be an issue

Increased soil moisture levels can encourage the spread of previously controlled fungal infections.

Pesticides can be a crutch

Many no-till farmers report an increase in pesticide use, as weed disturbance was one of the plowing's key benefits. As a result, herbicide-resistant GM crops are becoming more popular.

It can be a long-haul

These improvements do not occur overnight. It can take years, if not decades, to reap the benefits of no-till farming (Lloyd made the switch 15 years ago.)

Seed Saving

In many parts of the world, genetically modified seeds have become the norm in order to increase yields and cut the cost of cultivating vegetables. Although modified seeds are ideal for large-scale agriculture, home gardeners can profit more from seed preservation, which results in a higher-quality product at a reduced cost.

For thousands of years, people have been preserving seeds for the following planting season. Because there were no garden centers where farmers and producers could buy seeds to sow, they saved their seeds from one season to start the next. Seed saving was one of the key reasons for the Neolithic revolution, laying the foundation for modern-day farming and transforming hunter-gatherers into self-sufficient settlements.

Rather than combing the countryside for what was naturally growing, people were able to manage and grow specific crops, which allowed them to thrive and eventually spread throughout the world.

Know your reasons

We can purchase seeds from agriculture and garden supply stores, but these aren't always the greatest varieties for where we live. Seeds that are kept from one season to the next have more time to adjust to your climate, resulting in a healthier vegetable or fruit that is less vulnerable to illness.

Seed saving offers not only a superior product, but it also saves money because you won't have to buy fresh seeds every year to begin your season. We are also helping to preserve susceptible strains by saving seeds and using them year after year, as many are being binned by seed sources for modified versions to save money. Seed saving saves money and provides a superior product while also benefiting the environment through diversity and providing you with seeds that are more tolerant of your climate and location.

Getting started

It's best to start by growing only one variety of each fruit or vegetable to avoid cross-pollination. Try to figure out how each plant is pollinated, and you'll be able to figure out which species are best for creating a seed-saving garden in no time. Check out what your neighbors are growing, and try to keep your plants as far away from theirs as possible to avoid cross-pollination issues.

You should only use the best seeds in our seed saving program, so start gathering seeds from the best quality plants you have at the end of the season. Never utilize plants that generated poor yields or struggled to thrive.

Various plants seeds must be processed in a number of ways, so look up how to harvest seeds for each plant species you want to use. After you've picked your seeds, make sure they're stored properly so they may be planted the next season. In Europe and the United States, there exist laws prohibiting copyright infringement on seeds, but these laws do not apply to the ambitious home grower. Start saving your seeds and encouraging your neighbors to do the same, and you'll be able to share and collaborate on the finest seeds to grow in your area that will produce the most delicious produce.

Food forest

Imagine the sensory delight of walking through a forest where nearly every tree, bush, and plant produce food, a forest that fertilizes itself and takes care of pests, and a forest that is built to last for years to come. Is this the state of nirvana? It's not a forest; it's a food forest.

A food forest is a permaculture gardening strategy that mimics nature's system of building self-sustaining, interconnected, and multi-layered ecosystems in which trees, bushes, plants, insects, and the area's terrain all work together to generate food indefinitely.

Does it seem too good to be true? The following are some of the advantages and disadvantages of creating a food forest garden.

Minimal work:

Nature takes over for the most part after the initial design and setup to fertilize, weed, and control pests in the forest garden in a sustainable manner. Other than harvesting, all that is necessary for years of delight is mulching, cutting back aggressive plants, and the occasional pruning.

Be ecologically sound:

Even a modest forest garden may be a transforming force that benefits the planet's health. It accomplishes this by allowing nature to do the work that chemical fertilizers, herbicides, and gas-burning machines would have done in traditional gardening, so avoiding pollution.

Be more self-sufficient:

Growing a food forest not only benefits the present but also leaves a lasting legacy for future generations. It provides an opportunity to pass down knowledge, values, and a connection to the natural world. Children who engage in the garden learn valuable lessons about the origins of food and the intricate relationships between all living beings.

In times of economic uncertainty, a food forest can provide a secure source of food for families. The diverse array of crops and plants grown in a food forest can offer sustenance and nutrition, reducing reliance on external food supplies. Additionally, surplus produce can be traded or shared within the community, fostering self-sufficiency and resilience. Food forests go beyond providing food alone. They can also serve as a source of medicinal plants and other materials that can be utilized for various purposes. This holistic approach to gardening expands the potential benefits and usefulness of the forest garden. One significant advantage of food forests is the quality of the produce they yield. Organic fruits and vegetables grown in a forest garden tend to contain more vitamins and nutrients compared to factory-farmed produce. Unlike mass-produced crops that prioritize long-distance transportation and pest resistance, food forests prioritize taste, quality, and nutrition. By eliminating the need for extensive transportation, forest gardens also reduce the environmental impact associated with long-distance food distribution. Overall, food forests offer a sustainable and regenerative approach to gardening. They provide a multitude of benefits, including food security, educational opportunities, cultural preservation, and a deeper connection to nature. By cultivating organic and diverse ecosystems, food forests contribute to a healthier environment and a more resilient and nourished community.

The downside is that they're a project:

While food forest gardens can yield food for years with little continuous labor, they do so at a cost. While there's nothing wrong with planting a food forest on the spur of the moment without forethought, the result is unlikely to be a self-sustaining garden. Before the gardener even plants the first plant in a hole, he or she must plan and build a successful food forest. Keep in mind that while it is feasible to plant everything at once, it is not necessary. The forest garden can expand and grow over time as time and money allow. If you don't have the time, space, or energy for a food forest there are some simpler options that still allow to incorporate the concept of agroforestry in our gardens and backyards. Let's take a look!

Permaculture

Permaculture gardens combine various elements of wildlife gardening, edible landscaping, and native plant cultivation to create a self-sustaining and productive ecosystem. These gardens serve multiple purposes, offering a diverse range of applications throughout the year. One key aspect of permaculture gardens is their ability to provide food and medicinal crops. They incorporate a variety of crops, herbs, fruits, and flowers, not only for consumption but also for their aesthetic value and potential use in crafts. Additionally, permaculture gardens attract wildlife, serving as habitats for birds, insects, and other beneficial creatures, contributing to a balanced and biodiverse environment. These gardens are often designed to provide peaceful retreats for meditation and exercise. A fundamental principle of permaculture gardening is the concept of minimizing waste. Garden waste is composted to create nutrient-rich soil supplements and fertilizers. Water management is also crucial, with water sources attracting wildlife and ensuring the moisture of the soil and plants. Permaculture gardens often incorporate water-saving techniques such as collecting rainwater using rain barrels, which not only conserves water but also provides nutrient-rich water for the garden. One notable advantage of permaculture gardens is the reduction or elimination of the need for pesticides. By attracting beneficial insects and wildlife that naturally control pests, permaculture gardens create a balanced ecosystem that minimizes pest problems. Companion planting is also utilized to further deter pests. Once a permaculture garden is established, it requires less maintenance, with watering, harvesting, and occasional mulching being the primary tasks.

Permaculture gardens are designed with intention, where each plant serves a specific purpose. Some plants are chosen for their food production, while others have medicinal properties or attract beneficial insects. Some plants improve soil quality, while others enhance the visual appeal of the garden. The overall goal is to create a harmonious and productive garden that takes full advantage of nature's offerings. In summary, permaculture gardens provide a holistic and sustainable approach to gardening, incorporating ecological principles, biodiversity, and multi-functional landscapes. They offer a wealth of benefits, including food production, wildlife habitat, natural pest control, water conservation, and aesthetic enjoyment. By emulating the patterns and resilience found in natural ecosystems, permaculture gardens create thriving and resilient environments that are both rewarding and profitable.

Alley Cropping

Alley cropping revolutionizes farming by employing a unique technique: planting trees in rows with ample spacing, allowing for the cultivation of various crops in the gaps between the rows. This innovative practice offers unparalleled versatility, accommodating both full-sun and partial-shade crops within the same system.

An effective approach to alley cropping involves a strategic crop sequence. In the initial stages, sun-loving crops thrive in the ample sunlight. As the trees mature and cast more shade, shade-tolerant crops gradually take their place in the alleys. Understanding the dynamics and competition between different plant species is pivotal to designing a successful alley cropping system that aligns with specific needs and objectives. Meticulous planning is the key to unlocking its full potential.

When implemented skillfully on a farm, alley cropping elevates overall productivity and diversifies the array of products that can be obtained. Simultaneously, it delivers remarkable environmental benefits. By effectively reducing soil erosion and optimizing the utilization of essential soil nutrients like nitrogen and phosphorus, alley cropping fosters sustainable land management practices. However, to achieve these outcomes, it is imperative to have a clear understanding of the short-term and long-term goals of the land, as well as a comprehensive knowledge of the intricate interactions between the selected trees, shrubs, and crops.

By incorporating alley cropping into farming practices, farmers can maximize land use efficiency, increase crop diversity, and promote sustainable agricultural practices. This approach allows for the integration of trees, shrubs, and crops in a mutually beneficial manner, leading to improved farm productivity and environmental stewardship.

Full-sun crops:
- Horticultural plants, such as tomatoes, corn and blackberries
- Forages, grains and oilseeds
- Tree crops, such as plums and nuts
- Seeds, such as wildflowers or select grasses
- Christmas trees
- Shrubs and other landscaping plants
- Trees for lumber and wood fiber products

Partial-shade crops:
- Herbal medicinal plants, such as ginseng, goldenseal and black cohosh
- Landscape plants like ferns, mayapples, and Jack in the pulpit
- Mushrooms such as shiitake

Silvopasture

Silvopasture, a dynamic land management system, harmoniously integrates trees, forage crops, and livestock to maximize the benefits of each component. Its adaptability allows for implementation in diverse settings, such as planted pine forests, fruit and nut orchards, and other types of woodlands, depending on the landowner's objectives and conditions. Silvopasture systems aim to generate high-value timber and potential fruit crops in the long term, while also reaping short-term economic advantages from livestock and forage. In the southeastern United States, a range of livestock species thrives in silvopasture systems. Large ruminants like bison and cattle, as well as small ruminants like goats and sheep, are commonly utilized. Interestingly, domestic geese have even been incorporated into fruit tree orchards to aid in weed and insect pest management, showcasing the versatility of silvopasture practices.

Establishing a successful silvopasture system requires thoughtful consideration of economic and management factors. In woodlands, except for pine plantations dealing with invasive woody shrubs, controlled browsing by goats and other small ruminants proves effective in reducing fuel loads and minimizing the risk of wildfires. By transforming such sites into permanent silvopasture systems, landowners can embrace a more sustainable land use approach. Landowners interested in implementing silvopasture have various options to explore. They can combine wood production with pasture for hay and silage, incorporate grazing livestock like cattle, bison, sheep, and llamas, introduce browsing livestock such as goats, or integrate weeder birds like geese, ducks, and turkeys with fruit and nut trees. Government agencies like the USDA-Natural Resources Conservation Service (NRCS) and the USDA-Forest Service (FS) offer specialized funding and technical assistance to support the establishment and management of silvopasture systems, empowering landowners to embark on this innovative and environmentally beneficial endeavor.

Crop rotation

Crop rotation is an ancient agricultural practice that involves shifting the planting locations of vegetables within a garden or field each season. This method has been utilized by farmers in civilizations such as ancient Rome, Greece, China, and the Middle East since as early as 6000 BC. Crop rotation is crucial for several reasons. First, vegetables belonging to the same plant family often share similar nutrient requirements and are susceptible to the same insect pests and diseases. When vegetables from the same family are continuously grown in the same area, it creates a favorable environment for pests and diseases to thrive. By rotating crops, the pests and diseases are disrupted in their life cycles, reducing their populations and the damage they cause to crops. Additionally, different vegetables extract different types and amounts of nutrients from the soil. When the same

crop is repeatedly grown in the same area, it depletes specific nutrients from the soil, leading to imbalances. Crop rotation helps to mitigate this by allowing different crops with varying nutrient needs to be planted in succession, giving the soil time to replenish and restore its nutrient levels naturally. Overall, crop rotation improves soil health, reduces pest and disease pressure, and maintains balanced nutrient levels in the garden or field. It is an effective and sustainable approach to maximize yields and minimize the reliance on synthetic fertilizers and pesticides.

Doing it yourself:

Crop rotation is indeed essential for reducing insect pests and pathogens, as well as maintaining soil fertility in specific areas of a garden. It is important to avoid planting vegetables from the same plant family in the same location year after year, as this can create a favorable environment for pests and diseases to persist. For example, if tomatoes are planted in a particular bed or area of the garden one year, it is advisable not to grow other Solanaceae family crops such as peppers, eggplants, and potatoes in the same bed or area the following year. Leaving an area fallow, without any planted crop, is not recommended as it can lead to soil erosion and weed growth. Instead, planting a cover crop or green manure can help maintain soil structure, prevent erosion, and provide beneficial organic matter when incorporated into the soil. Ideally, a successful crop rotation involves planting vegetables or cover crops from the same plant family in a specific area once every three to four years. In small gardens, this may be challenging to achieve, but shifting plant families planted in the same location from year to year can still help manage pests and diseases. Keeping a garden diary or map can be helpful for tracking the rotation of crops and planning for future plantings. This documentation can assist in ensuring a diverse rotation schedule and avoiding the buildup of pests and diseases in specific areas of the garden. By practicing effective crop rotation, gardeners can promote healthier plants, reduce reliance on pesticides, maintain soil fertility, and improve overall garden productivity.

Basic Gardening Tips

To make your plants thrive, you must locate the proper balance of sunlight, fertile soil, and water. It's also about pursuing your passion, so choose plants that you enjoy. No matter what degree of gardening knowledge you have, use the materials here as a starting point, and you'll have a lovely garden in no time.

Just as with everything else in life, gardening sounds easy at face value. It isn't until we receive our plants, as amateur gardeners, that we're reminded that plants are living beings that we are stewards of. There are a few basics to remember to help make the job a bit easier, though, no matter if you're dealing with herbs, vegetables, fruits, or flowers.

Know your Land

Enthusiastic advocates of native plants have widely promoted the idea that these plants are low-maintenance and well-suited to their native environments. While this holds true for many species, it is important to recognize that successful cultivation often requires replicating the specific conditions under which they naturally thrive. Each native plant has its own unique set of preferred habitats, and when cultivated in such conditions, they can indeed flourish with minimal intervention such as additional watering, fertilizers, and pesticides. Therefore, the key principle to bear in mind is selecting the right plant for the right place. By understanding the specific needs and habitat requirements of native plants, gardeners can create environments that mimic their natural homes and enjoy the benefits of low-input gardening with native species. To discover the plants that might grow in your backyard, check out the next two volumes of the series!

Water

The availability of water at a site is a fundamental factor that determines the suitability of plants. When selecting plants, it is crucial to consider the water needs of each species. Wetland plants, which thrive in water-rich environments, can still grow in good soil that is not consistently wet. However, if they are placed in dry conditions, they will struggle to survive. Similarly, plants adapted to dry conditions will suffer and potentially rot if they are exposed to excessive moisture. While there are exceptions to this general rule, such as floodplain trees that exhibit tolerance to both wet and dry conditions, this is rarely the case for the herbaceous plants growing beneath them. It is important to recognize these exceptions and account for them in plant selection. Understanding the water requirements of plants is essential for creating a thriving and sustainable landscape. By matching the water availability of a site with the specific water needs of chosen plants, gardeners can ensure optimal growth and avoid unnecessary struggles or failures. This approach promotes healthy plant establishment, reduces water consumption, and contributes to overall environmental sustainability.

Soil

The type of soil in which plants are grown plays a crucial role in determining their access to moisture and nutrients. To successfully cultivate native plants, it is important to replicate the soil conditions in which they naturally thrive. Different soil types, such as clay, sandy, silty, and loamy soils, have distinct characteristics that significantly impact water retention and drainage. Clay soils, composed of fine particles, tend to retain moisture and become wet during periods of heavy rainfall. Their compact nature makes them poorly drained. However, the small particle size allows clay soils to retain moisture for longer periods during droughts.

On the other hand, sandy soils have larger particles that do not retain moisture well. Excess water drains quickly through the large spaces between particles. Sandy soils are known for their fast drainage and lower water-holding capacity. Silty soils, with particles of medium size, strike a balance between clay and sandy soils. They hold moisture more effectively and are neither excessively wet nor excessively dry.

A loamy soil represents an ideal blend of clay, sand, and silt particles. It combines the water-holding capacity of clay, the good drainage of sand, and the balanced characteristics of silt. Loamy soils are generally considered the most favorable for plant growth. Organic matter, also known as humus, is a key component of healthy soils. It is responsible for the dark color often observed in fertile soils. Organic matter improves soil structure, enhances moisture retention, facilitates aeration, and provides essential nutrients. In addition, it supports a diverse community of beneficial soil microorganisms. Wetland soils, in particular, tend to have high organic matter content due to the slow decomposition of plant materials in constantly moist conditions. The presence of organic matter in soil is vital for sustaining plant life and supporting a healthy ecosystem. Without it, soil would lack crucial nutrients and the capacity to retain moisture, rendering the land barren and inhospitable. The preservation and enhancement of organic matter in soil are essential for maintaining the Earth's fertility and promoting sustainable agriculture and gardening practices.

Peat and muck are types of organic soils that form in continually saturated conditions. They can be found in wetland areas such as marshes, sedge meadows, and fens, where groundwater flows through bedrock or mineral soil. The high-water table in these areas keeps decomposing plant material saturated, leading to the accumulation of organic soils. The pH of peat and muck soils can vary depending on the specific environment. Organic soils in fens can range from acidic to alkaline, but commercially mined peat tends to be acidic. The pH level of soil is an important factor that influences nutrient availability and affects plant growth. Different plants have varying pH preferences. Some plants thrive in acidic soils with a low pH, while others prefer more alkaline soils with a high pH. When plants are grown in soils with pH levels that are outside their preferred range, they may exhibit signs of chlorosis, characterized by yellowing of the leaves instead of healthy green coloration.

Acidic soils are commonly found in regions with higher rainfall and where the bedrock substrate consists of materials like sandstone, metamorphic rock (such as chert), or igneous rock (such as granite). On the other hand, limestone is a basic rock that contributes to higher pH levels in soils. In urban areas, concrete, which contains lime, can also contribute to higher pH levels in the soil. Understanding the pH of the soil is crucial for selecting and growing plants that are well-suited to the specific soil conditions. By considering the pH requirements of plants and the natural pH of the soil, gardeners and farmers can make informed decisions about plant selection, soil amendments, and appropriate gardening practices. Adjusting the pH of the soil, if necessary, can be achieved through the application of amendments like sulfur or lime, depending on whether the goal is to make the soil more acidic or more alkaline.

Light

The exposure to sunlight is a crucial factor in the successful growth of plants. Different plants have varying degrees of tolerance to sunlight, ranging from those adapted to full sun to those designed for full shade. Understanding a plant's sunlight requirements is essential for ensuring its health and vigor. Plants that require full sun thrive when exposed to direct sunlight for a significant portion of the day. They need the intense light and warmth to carry out essential photosynthesis processes and promote robust growth. When these sun-loving plants are deprived of adequate sunlight, their growth becomes weak, and they may struggle to reach their full potential. On the other hand, there are plants that are adapted to varying degrees of shade. These shade-tolerant plants have evolved to thrive in the sheltered conditions where sunlight is filtered or limited. They are capable of photosynthesizing and growing with less direct sunlight.

In fact, exposing shade-demanding plants to prolonged periods of intense sunlight can lead to leaf scorch or damage. Gardeners should be aware that the timing of sunlight exposure also plays a role in plant health. Morning sun is generally cooler and less intense than afternoon sun, making it more suitable for plants that are sensitive to excessive heat or intense light. For sun-demanding plants, the morning shade may be tolerable because the midday and afternoon sun provide sufficient light and warmth to support their growth. However, for shade-demanding plants, exposure to the intense heat and harsh rays of the afternoon sun can be detrimental.

Furthermore, the intensity of sunlight can vary based on geographic location. Full sun in southern or western regions tends to be harsher compared to other areas. The increased heat and higher sun angle in these regions can have a more significant impact on plant growth and may require additional precautions or adaptations to provide the necessary shade or protection.

By understanding the sunlight requirements of plants and considering the timing and intensity of sunlight exposure, gardeners can make informed decisions about plant placement, providing suitable shade or sun exposure, and ensuring the optimal conditions for healthy plant growth.

Cold and heat

Hardiness, which refers to a plant's ability to tolerate cold temperatures during winter, is an important consideration in gardening. Plants have different levels of cold hardiness, and understanding their tolerance to winter temperatures is crucial for selecting suitable plants for a specific climate.

In addition to winter cold, summer heat also affects a plant's hardiness and overall health. High temperatures can place stress on plants, especially those that are adapted to cooler climates or have a preference for milder summers. The impact of summer heat is most pronounced in southern and western regions, where the intensity and duration of heat are greater. As you move towards northeast regions, the intensity of summer heat generally decreases. However, it's important to note that summer heat also plays a vital role in plant growth and the hardening off process, which prepares plants for winter. Adequate exposure to summer heat helps plants develop the necessary resilience and adaptability to withstand winter conditions. When describing a plant's heat tolerance or requirements, referencing resources like the American Horticultural Society's Plant Heat Zone Map can provide valuable information.

To summarize, selecting native plants that are suited to the specific soil, moisture, sunlight, and heat conditions of a particular location increases the likelihood of their overall health and survival. The principle of "right plant, right place" extends beyond temperature considerations and also applies to pest and disease resistance, as well as drought tolerance. By understanding the unique needs and adaptations of native plants, gardeners can create thriving and resilient landscapes.

Soil and pH

Compost has a pH of 6-8 when it's finished and ready to use. The pH of compost changes as it decomposes, therefore the range will shift at any moment during the process. The majority of plants like a pH of around 7, although some prefer a more acidic or alkaline environment. This is when knowing the pH of the compost comes in handy. Depending on the results, you have the option to fine-tune the compost and make it more alkaline or acidic. You may have observed that the temperature fluctuates while composting. The pH of the compost pile will fluctuate, just like the temperature, and not only at certain periods, but in different regions of the pile. This means that you should take a pH of compost from several different locations of the mound when testing it. You can test the pH of compost using a soil test kit and following the manufacturer's recommendations, or you can simply use a pH indicator strip if your compost is moist but not muddy. You can also use an electronic soil meter to determine the pH range of compost.

Lowering pH

The simplest method to achieve this is to add more acidic materials to the compost as it breaks down, such as pine needles or oak leaves. Ericaceous compost is the name given to this sort of compost, which essentially translates to "ideal for acid-loving plants." After the compost is ready to use, you can lower the pH of it. Add an amendment, such as aluminum sulfate, to the soil when you put it in. By encouraging anaerobic bacteria, you can make a very acidic compost. Composting is usually aerobic, which means the microorganisms that break down the materials require oxygen to function; this is why compost is turned. Anaerobic bacteria take over when oxygen is scarce. Composting in a trench, bag, or garbage can is an anaerobic process. Keep in mind that the final product is extremely acidic. The pH of anaerobic compost is too high for most plants, so it should be exposed to air for about a month to neutralize it.

Raising pH

The easiest technique to minimize acidity is to turn or aerate your compost to enhance air circulation and foster aerobic bacteria. Make sure there's enough of "brown" material in the compost as well. Some people believe that adding wood ash to compost will help to neutralize it. Every 18 inches, add a layer of ash. Finally, lime can be added to increase alkalinity, but only after the compost has been completed! It will release ammonium nitrogen gas if added directly to the processing compost. Instead, after the compost has been added, add lime to the soil.

Composting

First, what is compost?
Crop rotation is indeed essential for reducing insect pests and pathogens, as well as maintaining soil fertility in specific areas of a garden. It is important to avoid planting vegetables from the same plant family in the same location year after year, as this can create a favorable environment for pests and diseases to persist. For example, if tomatoes are planted in a particular bed or area of the garden one year, it is advisable not to grow other Solanaceae family crops such as peppers, eggplants, and potatoes in the same bed or area the following year. Leaving an area fallow, without any planted crop, is not recommended as it can lead to soil erosion and weed growth. Instead, planting a cover crop or green manure can help maintain soil structure, prevent erosion, and provide beneficial organic matter when incorporated into the soil. Ideally, a successful crop rotation involves planting vegetables or cover crops from the same plant family in a specific area once every three to four years. In small gardens, this may be challenging to achieve, but shifting plant families planted in the same location from year to year can still help manage pests and diseases.

Keeping a garden diary or map can be helpful for tracking the rotation of crops and planning for future plantings. This documentation can assist in ensuring a diverse rotation schedule and avoiding the buildup of pests and diseases in specific areas of the garden. By practicing effective crop rotation, gardeners can promote healthier plants, reduce reliance on pesticides, maintain soil fertility, and improve overall garden productivity.

Starting a compost pile

Composting can be a simple process of allowing plant materials to decompose on their own, but it can be slow and inconsistent. Active or hot composting involves supplying oxygen, adding moisture, and maintaining the proper carbon-to-nitrogen ratio to speed up decomposition. To ensure successful decomposition, it's important to have the right combination of ingredients. Carbon and nitrogen are essential components of composting. Carbon-rich materials include dead leaves, woody branches, bark dust, shredded paper, cardboard, straw, and wood ash. Nitrogen-rich materials include green plant trimmings, kitchen scraps, coffee grounds, and manures. A good compost pile should have more carbon than nitrogen. Too much carbon can slow down decomposition, while too much nitrogen can result in unpleasant odors. The ideal ratio, by volume, is typically 2 to 3 parts carbon (brown matter) to 1 part nitrogen (green matter). By following these guidelines and maintaining the proper balance of carbon and nitrogen, composting can be completed in a shorter timeframe, typically within 1 to 3 months. This active composting method allows microorganisms to work more efficiently, raising the temperature of the pile and speeding up decomposition.

Bin options

Before you begin "mixing your brew," it is a good idea to know what your options are!

Mass-produced bins or tumblers

Manufactured compost barrels or bins can be conveniently purchased online or from nurseries and garden retailers. These containers are designed to facilitate airflow and moisture while keeping pests out. They are typically made from materials such as wood, metal, wire mesh, or plastic.
Some compost bins are stationary and require manual turning of the compost to aerate it. On the other hand, compost tumblers feature a spinning mechanism that allows for easy turning of the material. Compost tumblers are particularly suitable for small urban yards, apartments with limited space, or balconies and patios.

DIYs:

A garbage can, plastic storage container, or milk carton can also be used to build a homemade compost bin. Come up with your own system using your imagination.

Multi-Bins:

If you have a large yard or property and anticipate generating a significant amount of compost, you can establish a compost pile or design a more complex composting system. This can involve the use of one or multiple bins made of materials such as wood, wire mesh, metal, or cinder blocks.
A popular option is the three-bin system, which allows for continuous production of compost. In this system, compost at various stages of decomposition is transferred from one bin to the next. The first bin is used for fresh plant waste and new additions to the compost pile. As the compost breaks down, it is moved to the second bin, where it continues to decompose further. Finally, the compost reaches the third bin, where it reaches its mature and fully decomposed state, ready to be used in the

garden. This three-bin system facilitates the management of composting materials and ensures a continuous supply of mature compost. It allows you to have different stages of composting in progress simultaneously, optimizing the decomposition process. By systematically transferring compost from one bin to another, you can maintain a steady production cycle and have a reliable supply of nutrient-rich compost for your garden.

The steps for creating compost

1. Break it down:
Enhance decomposition by cutting or shredding plant material into small pieces, facilitating microbial digestion.

2. Layer it up:
Create proper drainage and aeration by starting with a layer of twigs or straw at the bottom. Alternate layers of carbon-rich (brown) and nitrogen-rich (green) materials, resembling a lasagna, to ensure even distribution for microbial activity. End with a top layer of brown matter to control odors. Fill a composter or create a deep pile, ensuring sufficient volume.

3. Kick-start with a starter:
Although not essential, activators like chicken manure, comfrey leaves, grass clippings, or new weeds can accelerate decomposition. Commercial activators are also available.

4. Keep it moist:
If rainfall is scarce, lightly water the pile to maintain proper moisture. Excessive water will make the pile soggy and reduce temperature, hindering decomposition. Conversely, insufficient water will slow or halt the process. Aim for a consistency similar to a wrung-out wet sponge. Squeeze a handful of compost to assess moisture content; dripping indicates excess water, while no droplets suggest dryness. A few drops indicate the right moisture balance.

5. Cover it up:
Use tarps, plastic sheeting, or wood to cover open piles and retain heat and moisture.

6. Give it air:
Turn the compost every 1 to 3 weeks with a pitchfork or rotate a compost tumbler to provide aeration. Add water if needed to ensure moisture is evenly distributed.

7. Manage odors:
Use lime or calcium as necessary to discourage flies and neutralize odors. If a strong ammonia smell emerges, incorporate more carbon-rich materials like dry leaves or straw.

8. Prevent fires:
Monitor the internal temperature of the pile with a compost thermometer to prevent overheating.
Composting offers an excellent solution for reducing household waste and carbon footprint, particularly since kitchen and food waste constitute a significant portion of household garbage. When organic matter is sent to landfills without proper conditions for decomposition, it produces harmful methane gas, contributing to global warming and climate change. Kitchen countertop compost bins simplify the collection of scraps before transferring them to a compost bin or pile.

The Do's and Don't's of Composting

1. Carnivorous animal feces, like those from dogs and cats, should not be composted due to potential parasites and germs that are difficult to eliminate through standard composting methods.

2. Conduct a soil test to determine the specific needs of your soil. A soil test kit assesses pH and nutrient levels, providing valuable information to address any deficiencies. Private companies and local extension services often offer more comprehensive analyses. Repeat the test every 1 to 3 years.

3. Meat, bones, and fish leftovers decompose slowly, attract pests, and produce unpleasant odors.

4. Oil, fat, and kitchen grease take a long time to break down, attract pests, and contribute to strong odors.

5. Large wood chunks decompose slowly and may hinder the overall composting process.

6. Avoid using pressure-treated wood and railroad ties, as they contain hazardous compounds.

7. Maintain a healthy pH balance. Different plants have specific soil pH preferences. Some prefer acidic soil, like rhododendrons and azaleas, while others thrive in slightly alkaline or neutral pH. Soil pH can be adjusted by adding lime to increase alkalinity or sulfur to increase acidity.

8. Avoid composting plant matter treated with chemical pesticides or fertilizers, such as lawn clippings. It is crucial to create organic compost, especially for food crops, to prevent exposure to potentially harmful chemicals.

9. Exclude invasive plant seeds, such as pokeweed and butterfly bush, as well as weed seeds, from the compost. These seeds may sprout if the compost does not reach sufficient heat levels for an extended period. Most weed seeds require temperatures of 140 degrees F for at least 30 days to be destroyed.

10. Consider vermicomposting as an alternative method for producing organic materials. Red worms, or red wigglers, can be raised in enclosed bins to create nutrient-rich castings. Simply add kitchen scraps and damp bedding (shredded newspaper or cardboard) to the bin, and the worms will consume the material, resulting in valuable compost. Worms and bins can be purchased online.

11. Avoid adding unhealthy plant detritus to the compost, as pathogens can survive in finished compost and spread to healthy plants in the garden.

By being mindful of what not to compost, you can ensure the production of high-quality compost for a healthy and thriving garden.

Irrigation

All plants require frequent watering, although certain herbs require more than others. As a rule of thumb, when the soil is dry at the depth of a thumb, the plant needs water. However, take the time to learn about each herb's specific moisture requirements, and remember to plant like-minded plants together. Basil, for example, requires more water than lavender, which prefers perfectly dry soil between waterings, so do not combine the two herbs. Watering most herbs roughly once a week is a decent rule of thumb. During periods of high heat or drought, it may be necessary to water twice a week. Water in the mornings between 6 and 10 a.m. to avoid evaporation and to allow for deep root soaking.

Let's look a little further, though.
How much water is really needed?

It's difficult to know how much water the various herb varieties in your garden require. There are numerous variables that must be considered. Climate, solar exposure, and other factors are among them. Ideally in a self-sustaining system with properly selected plants according to your hardiness zone, hardly any watering should be required. However, most things in life are not perfect and our plants will most likely need a bit of help, unless you have opted for a permaculture garden (and successfully managed to build one!). The most sustainable option is rainwater irrigation, so you are not using water ex novo to irrigate your garden, but helping nature along. Check in the previous chapter the paragraph on "Catch the Rain" irrigation. Herbs need to be watered, but it is crucial to strike the right balance and avoid overwatering. The easiest way to avoid overwatering is to learn how to recognize it. You'll be able to figure out the best way to water herbs in your garden's specific setting over time. Many herbs are able to withstand the elements. They may survive in relatively dry soil. When the soil is damp, be on the lookout for wilting. Your herbs should, in theory, use the water you provide them quickly. You don't want to work with saturated soil.

Keep an eye out for the color of the leaves on your herbs. Too much water can cause yellow and black leaves to turn yellow. If you notice any mildew or fuzz on your herbs, it could be due to too much moisture. Observation is an important part of an effective herb watering strategy. You should spend daily time with your plants to see how water affects them. If required, take notes.

How often?
Understanding how often to water herbs becomes much easier once you've decided how much water your outdoor herb garden need, but you'll also need information about the local environment. Aim for a regimen that allows for consistent watering on a daily basis. Remember that underwatering is easier to correct than overwatering. Of course, depending on local rainfall and other conditions, you'll need to make adaptations.
This is the truth. It's possible that a daily watering plan won't be realistic. Many herb growers say that watering once or twice a week has yielded wonderful results. Just make sure the soil around the herb's base doesn't dry out too much.

What times?
Watering herbs is best done first thing in the morning. When you water when the weather is cooler, the water you apply will reach the root system of your plants more efficiently. When you water in the morning, say between the hours of 6 and 10, there is less risk of evaporation. This watering plan will also allow for a gradual drying of your herbs' leaves, eliminating mildew or disease caused by excess water.

Mulching

Mulching is an excellent time-saving practice in gardening, whether you're tending to flower beds, herb gardens, or vegetable gardens. When applied correctly, mulch reduces the need for watering, weeding, and pest control, resulting in healthier plants and more productive yields. To maximize the benefits of mulching, it's important to choose the right type of mulch for your specific garden needs. There are two main categories of mulch: organic and inorganic. Organic mulches include chopped leaves, straw, grass clippings, compost, wood chips, shredded bark, sawdust, pine needles, and even paper. In contrast, inorganic mulches consist of materials like black plastic and geotextiles (landscape fabrics). Both organic and inorganic mulches help to suppress weeds, but organic mulches have the added advantage of improving the soil as they break down over time. Inorganic mulches, although they don't enrich the soil, can still be a viable option for your garden.

For instance, black plastic, a commonly used inorganic mulch, warms the soil and retains heat, benefiting heat-loving plants such as chives and mint by providing them with optimal growing conditions. By selecting the appropriate mulch type and applying it correctly, you can enjoy the time-saving benefits of mulching while promoting the health and productivity of your garden.

Leaves and wood:
For mulching your flower beds and shrub borders, there are a few options to consider. You can visit a local garden center and purchase bags of attractive wood chips or shredded bark. Another cost-effective option is to contact your local tree-care or utility provider to inquire about any excess wood chips they may have available. Additionally, if you're environmentally conscious, you can chip your Christmas tree instead of discarding it. If you have trees on your property, you can create a nutrient-rich mulch by shredding the fallen leaves. Using a lawnmower with a bagger attachment, you can collect and cut the leaves into the ideal size for mulching. Wood chips or shredded leaf mulch can be applied anywhere on your property, but they particularly enhance the appearance of flower beds, shrub borders, and garden pathways. They blend well in woodland or shade gardens. However, it's important to note that wood chips are not suitable for vegetable and annual flower beds, as they can hinder digging and cultivation activities required in those areas.

Grass:
Grass clippings can be a convenient and easily accessible mulch option for your garden. However, it's also beneficial to save some of the clippings to use as a natural

fertilizer for your lawn. If you have excess grass clippings, you can utilize them as a nitrogen-rich mulch in your vegetable beds. This can help improve soil fertility and provide additional nutrients for your growing plants. Just make sure to apply a thin layer of grass clippings to avoid clumping and allow for proper air circulation.

Compost:
Extend the usefulness of your compost by repurposing it as mulch if you have any leftover. Applying compost as mulch not only enriches the soil but also promotes healthy plant growth. However, it's important to note that dry compost alone is not an ideal medium for plant roots to thrive in. To optimize its benefits, it is recommended to use a thin layer of compost around your plants and cover it with another type of mulch, such as chopped leaves. This combination helps retain moisture in the compost and keeps it biologically active, providing maximum benefits to your vegetables, fruits, and flowers.

Hay or straw:
For your vegetable garden, it is recommended to use straw, salt hay, or weed-free hay as mulch. These types of mulch not only give a clean and tidy appearance but also provide several benefits. They help retain soil moisture, suppress weed growth, and contribute organic matter to the soil as they decompose. However, it's important to take precautions to prevent slug and rat damage. Ensure that the hay you use is weed- and seed-free, and avoid placing it directly around the stems of vegetable plants or fruit tree trunks, as this can create hiding places for pests.

Plastic:
Using black plastic film sheets as mulch in a vegetable garden can offer several benefits. When tightly applied over the soil, black plastic conducts heat from the sun, creating a microclimate that is about three degrees warmer than an unmulched garden. This warmth helps to prevent the decay of fruits from vining crops like strawberries, melons, and cucumbers by keeping them dry and warm. Additionally, the mulch retains soil moisture and suppresses weed growth.

Infrared-transmitting (IRT) plastics, although more expensive, can further increase yields. These plastics not only warm the soil like clear plastic but also control weeds like black plastic. In raised bed gardens, the plastic sheet is placed over the entire bed, secured at the edges or weighed down with pebbles. Holes are then made in the plastic using a bulb planter, and plants or seeds are inserted. Since water cannot permeate the plastic, it's important to use soaker hoses or drip hoses on the soil surface to ensure proper hydration for the plants, as relying on rainwater alone may not be sufficient.

It's important to avoid using plastic mulch beneath bushes, as it can be detrimental to their long-term health. Shrub roots often grow near the soil surface, including directly beneath the plastic, in search of moisture and oxygen. Since water and air cannot penetrate the plastic, the shallow roots may suffer from lack of oxygen, moisture, and significant temperature variations. This can result in plant deterioration and eventual death.

Fabric:
Geotextiles, also known as landscape fabrics, provide a barrier that allows air and water to penetrate the soil while preventing weed growth. However, it is important to be aware of their limitations. Geotextiles can degrade over time when exposed to sunlight. To prolong their lifespan and improve their aesthetic appearance, it is recommended to cover them with an additional layer of mulch. Similar to plastic mulch, it is advisable to keep geotextiles away from shrubs. The roots of shrubs and weeds have the potential to grow through the landscape fabric, necessitating their removal when the fabric is taken out. Therefore, it is important to exercise caution and ensure that geotextiles are not placed in close proximity to shrubs to avoid any potential damage and the need for additional maintenance.

Do it the right way:
When using mulch for weed control, there are two important guidelines to keep in mind. Firstly, ensure that the soil is free of weeds before applying the mulch. Then, apply a thick enough layer of mulch to prevent new weeds from sprouting through. A four-inch layer of mulch is effective in discouraging weed growth, while shady areas may require a two-inch layer. If a garden bed contains a significant number of weed seeds or perennial roots, it is advisable to use a double-mulching technique. This involves placing the plants, watering them thoroughly, covering them with newspaper, and then applying mulch on top. Certain types of mulch, such as wood chips, can help retain soil moisture but may also contribute to soil warming. In the spring, it is recommended to pull the mulch away from perennials and bulbs to promote faster growth. It is important to avoid piling wet mulch against the stems of flowers and vegetables, as it can lead to plant decay. Maintain a one-inch gap between the mulch and the crowns and stems of plants.

When using mulch around shrubs and trees, it is essential to prevent the mulch from heaping against the woody stems. This can create a nesting area for rodents like voles and mice, which can cause rot. Deep mulch should be kept at least six to twelve inches away from the trunks to maintain the health of the plants.

How to Source Native Plants and Seeds

You may be wondering why there's so much buzz about gardening with native plants. Considering the increasing concern over global climate change and drought, you might suspect the main reason is to replace water-thirsty lawn with plants that only need a sip now and then. There are many nonnative plants that fill this need, however, so why should we choose native plants instead? Because native plants go beyond solving a single problem.

Native plants have adapted to the climate and soil conditions of the area where they grow naturally. Nectar, pollen, and seeds from these key plant species provide food for native butterflies, insects, birds, and other creatures. Common horticultural plants, unlike natives, do not give energetic incentives for pollinators and frequently require insect pest treatment to live.

Create a good habitat. Welcome native birds, insects, and butterflies to your yard by creating useful habitat. The best habitat is one with a variety of native plants appropriate to your locale. If you plant it, they will come. There will be no need to get in the car and drive for an hour to enjoy nature when it is right outside your door.

Save water. Many nonnative plants require supplemental water to thrive in our Mediterranean and desert climates. By planting natives, you will save water, and you can also enjoy longer periods of travel without worrying that your plants will be dead should the sprinkler system fail.

Say good-bye to toxic chemicals. Does walking through the aisle of garden chemicals at home improvement stores make your eyes itch and your nose run? Why would you want to have these toxic chemicals in your own yard? Native plants make it possible to enjoy a natural, toxin-free yard without worrying about health risks for adults, children, pets, and wildlife.

Treat your senses. Tickle your taste buds with sweet wild strawberries and piquant sage. Get a whiff of the spicy aroma of sagebrush. Stroke the smooth, sinuous bark of manzanita. Feast your eyes on the festive blues, pinks, and yellows of spring and the subtle, relaxing grays and tans of summer. Enjoy a symphony of birdsong year-round. Native plants can bring all this to you.

Enhance your sense of time. Although Californians have become accustomed to bright-green lawns and colorful flowers throughout the year, it is in observing the cycle of colors in the natural world that we can best appreciate each season and take note of time as months and years pass.

Feel at home. When returning from travels afar, the sweet, spicy, and earthy smells of a familiar environment help to settle you firmly in your own home, giving you an unmistakable sense of place and belonging.

End the tyranny of mow and blow. All gardens need maintenance. Lawn-dominated yards, though, require an endless repetition of mowing, blowing, watering, and applying chemicals. In contrast, native plants are easy to grow and call for minimal care once you understand the remarkable adaptations they have made to live in this unique climate. In a well-planned garden, once the plants get comfortable you won't need to do as much maintenance.

Feel good about being part of the solution. The environmental forecast is not good, but it feels great to know you can do something about it. One little garden may not matter much, but you can help the movement catch on so it spreads from yard to yard. When the news gets you down, a lizard sunning herself on a rock in your garden can lift you up.

Have fun in the garden. Gardening with native plants is a great adventure. If it isn't enjoyable, you are doing something wrong. Celebrate your successes and learn from your mistakes, but never stop having fun in the garden.

Now, to the hard part! Many native plants are quite difficult to grow from seed, so purchasing a plant is the only option. Most states have a state nursery that provides low-cost tree and shrub seedlings, and many local and midwestern regional nurseries sell native plants and seedlings, as well as seed. When acquiring plants, ask about provenance; make sure they are nursery-propagated or divisions from gardens—not pillaged from what's left of the wild. If a plant is inordinately cheap—especially if it is one of the more slow-to-propagate spring wildflowers—it may signal that it has been collected from the wild. Local plant societies and organizations occasionally salvage wildflowers from construction projects but always after obtaining permission from the landowner.

Many native plants do not conform to nursery mass production. They are programmed to grow roots with little top growth as an adaptation to the climate. Many upland oaks, shagbark hickory, pecan, Ohio buckeye, eastern hophornbeam, leadplant, New Jersey tea, prairie and large-flowered trilliums, and other spring wildflowers grow that way. This makes them more expensive than standard nursery items, but I guarantee they will be worth the wait and added expense in the long run. Dedicated native plant horticulturists and nursery professionals are slowly cracking the code to produce many of our more difficult native plants, including orchids.

Many other native plants are not grown in quantity because the demand for them is simply not there. Every native plant purchase you make helps the cause. I dream of a time when native bulbs are as easy to purchase as tulips and daffodils. I relish the thought of lawns filled with wild hyacinth and violet wood-sorrel rather than (or at least along with) Siberian squill and crocus. I also hope to see the day when drought-tolerant, difficult-to-transplant trees and shrubs will be as readily available as red maples and invasive Callery pears. Resist the temptation to buy cheap, easy-to-produce trees that usually are shorter lived. Many of our communities' native trees are mature and not being replaced—or if they are, the replacements are clones (mostly fruitless males). The rebirth of our priceless native flora can begin in our own backyards.

Here are your best option for sourcing native seeds and plants:

Seed swapping

Mark the last Saturday of January on your calendar, also known as Seed Swap Day. Even if this date has already passed when you read this, there are always opportunities to participate in local seed swaps or organize one in your area. Seed swaps can take various forms, ranging from casual gatherings among a small group of gardeners at someone's home to larger events held in public spaces. If you want to organize a larger event, consider hanging flyers and reaching out to your local town hall or Cooperative Extension to secure a suitable venue. The main objective is to exchange and acquire local seeds. These gatherings are not only practical but also enjoyable. Seeds of all types can be traded, allowing for a diverse exchange. You may want to specifically advertise the swap as a platform for trading wild-type native seeds, catering to those interested in indigenous and wildlife gardening. Vegetable farmers looking to share their open-pollinated heirloom varieties can also participate. Alternatively, you can keep the exchange open to any and all seeds gathered by participants. Seed swaps offer a wonderful opportunity to connect with other gardeners, diversify your seed collection, and contribute to the preservation of local plant varieties. Stay engaged and consider attending or organizing seed swaps in your area.

Sharing is caring

In the world of habitat gardening, we are all part of the same team! One of the greatest joys of this endeavor is the willingness of fellow gardeners to share their knowledge, ideas, inspiration, and even plants. To tap into this community spirit, explore your neighborhood and discover who has beautiful native gardens. Visit them on a day when they are not busy working outside, and you may find yourself leaving with a bounty of fresh plants or seeds.

Attending local plant seminars or events is another great way to connect with fellow gardeners. Take the opportunity to network and ask individuals if they have any plants or seeds they are willing to share. Some perennial plants can be divided by digging up a section of the root system, often referred to as a root ball or root clump. In such cases, having a bucket and shovel handy is beneficial. For other plants, seeds can suffice. If you are new to gardening, starting with root clumps can provide a sense of accomplishment as they establish and grow into robust plants without the need to worry about seed stratification, germination, or early weed management. However, be cautious as root clumps can sometimes come with unintentional "weed sharing," so it's important to be mindful of what you bring into your garden.

Embrace the camaraderie of fellow habitat gardeners, explore local resources, and be open to sharing and receiving plants and seeds. By engaging with the gardening community, you will expand your garden's diversity and foster a sense of connection with like-minded individuals.

A great use for social media

If you're looking to connect with fellow gardeners in your area, consider exploring gardening listservs. These online communities provide a platform for gardeners to share information, ask questions, and exchange plants and seeds. Additionally, you can check if there are any local groups on platforms like NextDoor, a free online service that connects people in the same neighborhood. Often, individuals within these communities are willing to share plants. Even if there isn't a specific gardening group, you can post a notice on a general wall expressing your interest in acquiring native seeds, plants, bulbs, and rootstocks.

Another option is to search for wildlife gardening groups on Facebook. For example, "Pitch in a Patch for Pollinators" is a new group formed by Habitat Network where people share photos of their gardens and engage in discussions about various topics, including where to acquire native seeds and plants. Since ecoregions tend to be large, there's a good chance you'll find someone within your ecoregion who is willing to share seeds or plants.

By actively participating in these online communities and platforms, you can connect with like-minded individuals, exchange gardening advice, and find valuable resources for your wildlife garden.

Seek out your AG office

During the spring season, many state and local agricultural extension agencies offer free seeds to the public for a limited time. These seeds are often provided by other gardeners and garden centers, allowing individuals who may not have access to seeds or find it challenging to purchase them to obtain them for free. To find out if there is a communal seed bank or seed distribution program in your area, contact your local Cooperative Extension office. You can use the HN Local Resources feature by entering your zip code and browsing through the results to find the link to your nearest Cooperative Extension office.

It's important to note that not all seeds available through these programs may be locally adapted to your area. It may require some research and effort to select the right seeds for your region. Additionally, since the seeds may have been collected and stored for some time, their viability may vary. Older seeds or those stored in less-than-ideal conditions may have lower germination rates. However, participating in these seed distribution programs can be a great way to access a variety of seeds and experiment with different plants in your garden.

Try local nurseries

Consider reaching out to smaller nurseries, particularly during their busy season, as they are often open to having volunteers help out. Smaller nurseries are also more likely to carry wild-type native plants compared to larger chain stores. When you visit a nursery, ask if you can volunteer for a few hours. While there's no guarantee of receiving free plants for volunteering, you'll likely gain valuable knowledge, meet like-minded individuals who share your interests in native gardens, and potentially receive discounts on plants, seeds, plugs, and rootstock. Spending time at a nursery is a great way to expand your plant collection as you immerse yourself in the gardening community.

Another approach you can try is networking and building connections. Nurseries typically go through different stages of plant development to produce the attractive quart-sized native plants they sell. They start with densely planted greenhouse cultivation and later divide the plants into plugs, which are then transplanted into larger containers. These plugs often have well-developed root systems and multiple leaves, enabling them to establish quickly when transplanted into larger containers.

Check with the nursery if they offer the option to purchase plugs instead of more established quart-sized plants. Plugs are smaller and generally less expensive, but they will require more care if you choose to directly plant them in your gardens. This can be a cost-effective way to acquire a larger quantity of plants and nurture them into thriving specimens.

Start yourself and draw others in

Consider becoming a seed saver and distributor to further enhance your gardening experience. Seed collection is a straightforward process, but proper storage is crucial. Create a well-ventilated room and use clearly labeled plastic or glass containers to store the seeds.

Ensure that the seeds are completely dry before placing them in containers. You can achieve this by leaving them on the plants until the first cold, dry days of the year or by physically harvesting them and drying them in a south-facing window. It's important to note that storing seeds in containers before they are fully dry can lead to mold formation.

Traditionally, harvesters left the seed heads in the fields to dry. The seeds or entire flower heads from individual plants were then collected and stored in different containers. To separate the seeds from the chaff or flower material, you can winnow the plants with flower heads. Once you have only seeds remaining, store them in individual containers for easy access when creating meadow mixtures or preparing species-specific seed packs.

Label your containers with the date of seed harvest, as well as the common and scientific names of the seeds. While many seeds can last for multiple seasons, their germination rate may decrease over time. As your seed collection grows, consider organizing a Seed Swap (Exchange) to share and trade seeds with other gardeners. This is an excellent way to keep your seed collection fresh and ensure successful germination opportunities are not missed.

Selecting Native Plants

It's time to remove invasive plants from your garden and replace them with fresh alternatives. Invasive exotics have a reputation for spreading beyond the boundaries of gardens and causing damage to natural areas. We've witnessed how English ivy suffocates wildflowers and weakens shade trees, and how Japanese honeysuckle strangles shrubs and small trees. Letting go of these old garden favorites is important for the future of our natural parks, forests, and fields.

Invasive species outcompete native plants by emerging earlier in the spring and retaining their leaves longer in the fall compared to native counterparts in the mid-Atlantic region. This extended growing period gives them a significant advantage. Additionally, invasive plants have no natural predators, such as insects or diseases, and they reproduce rapidly. In areas with high deer populations, many invasive plants are unpalatable to them, allowing invasives to quickly dominate.

When selecting a native plant replacement for an invasive species, consider the desirable qualities of the invasive plant you're removing. For example, if you appreciate the fragrant aroma or vining habit of Japanese honeysuckle,
replace it with native alternatives like the sweetbay magnolia (Magnolia virginiana), a tree with fragrant summer blooms, or the summer-blooming leatherflower vine (Clematis viorna) if you prefer a vining plant. By choosing these native options, you can enjoy the desired traits of honeysuckle without the negative impacts associated with invasiveness.

The next two books will focus on medicinal plants and wildflowers that were foraged and grown by the Native Americans and that can be a part of a beautiful gardens that serves both our medicinal purposes and the needs of pollinators, such as bees, butterflies, other insects, and even birds. Check out the next two volumes of the series to find the right plants for your garden!

The upcoming table shows the possible native substitutes to a series of common exotic ornamental plants that are invasive and not suitable for an eco-friendly garden.

Invasive ornamental plant	Characteristics	Better Alternative
Japanese Wisteria	Showy Flowers, Fragrance	Woodland Phlox, *Phlox Divaricatus* Sweet Azalea, *Rhododendron Canescens* Coast Azalea, *Rhododendron Atlanticum* American Wisteria, *Wisteria Frutescens*
Japanese Honeysuckle	Fragrant Flowers	Leatherflower, *Clematis Viorna* Carolina Jasmine, *Gelsemium Sempervirens* Trumpet Honeysuckle, *Lonicera Sempervirens* Sweetbay Magnolia, *Magnolia Virginiana* Purple Passionflower, *Passiflora Incarnata*
English Ivy	Drought Tolerant Evergreen	Plantain-Leaved Sedge, *Carex Plantaginea* Marginal Woodfern, *Dryopteris Marginalis* Woodland Aster, *Eurybia Divaricatus* Alumroot, *Heuchera Villosa* Creeping Mint, *Meehania Cordata* Allegheny Spurge, *Pachysandra Procumbens* Creeping Phlox, *Phlox Stolonifera* Solomon's Seal, *Polygonatum Biflorum* Christmas Fern, *Polystichum Acrostichoides*
Autumn Olive	Drought Tolerant	Strawberry Bush, *Euonymus Americanus* Wax-Myrtle, *Myrica Cerifera* Meadowsweet, *Spiraea Latifolia* Mapleleaf Viburnum, *Viburnum Acerifolium*

Barberry	Cheap/Nice Fruit	Strawberry Bush, *Euonymus Americanus* Shrubby St. Johnswort, *Hypericum Prolificum* Winterberry, *Ilex Ommissural* Deerberry, *Vaccinium Stamineum* Mapleleaf Viburnum, *Viburnum Acerifolium*
Purple Loosestrife	Long Bloom Season/Wet Tolerant	Swamp Milkweed, *Asclepias Incarnata* Sweet Pepperbush, *Clethra Alnifolia* Purple Coneflower, *Echinacea Purpurea* Gayfeather, *Liatris Spicata* Grass-Leaved Blazing Star, *Liatris Ommis* Green-Headed Coneflower, *Rudbeckia Laciniata* New York Ironweed, *Vernonia Novaboracensis*
Miscanthus Species	Strong Vertical and Fall/Winter Interest	Split-Beard Bluestem, *Andropogon Ternarius* Switchgrass, *Panicum Virgatum* Sugarcane Plumegrass, *Saccharum Giganteum* Little Bluestem, *Schizachyrium Scoparium* Indiangrass, *Sorghastrum Nutans*
Lesser Celandine	Early Color	Spring Beauty, *Claytonia Virginica* Yellow Ragwort, *Senecio Aureus* Other Spring Ephemerals, If Nursery Propagated
Asian Bittersweet	Showy Fruits	American Bittersweet, *Celastrus Scandens* Virginia Rose, *Rosa Virginiana*
Porcelainberry	Fast Grower/Colorful Fruits	Gray Dogwood, *Cornus Ommissu* Virginia Creeper, *Parthenocissus Quinquefolia* Swamp Haw Viburnum, *Viburnum Nudum*
Shrubby Honeysuckle	Replant After Removal	Spicebush, *Lindera Benzoin* Highbush Blueberry, *Vaccinium Corymbosum* Arrow-Wood Viburnum, *Viburnum Dentatum*
Burning Bush Euonymus	Fall Colors	Fringed Bluestar, *Amsonia Ommiss* Hubricht's Bluestar, *Amsonia Hubrichtii* Witch-Alder, *Fothergilla Ommissu* Oak-Leaf Hydrangea, *Hydrangea Quercifolia* Fetterbush, *Leucothoe Ommissu* Swamp Haw, *Viburnum Dentatum* Arrow-Wood Viburnum, *Viburnum Nudum*

Deciding what to grow

When it comes to selecting plants for your garden, several factors should be considered to ensure their success. First and foremost, you need to assess whether the plants are well-suited to your garden's specific growing conditions. This includes taking into account your local hardiness and heat zone, as well as the unique characteristics of your soils and the amount of sunlight or shade your garden receives. For example, while palm trees may evoke visions of tropical paradises, they are not suitable for Midwest climates due to their lack of winter hardiness. However, it's equally important to ensure that plants are compatible with your specific soil composition and lighting conditions, as these factors greatly influence their ability to thrive. Once you have a good understanding of your garden's growing conditions, you can move on to the next step: selecting plants based on their intended roles in the landscape. Each plant has unique qualities and functions that contribute to the overall composition of your garden. Some plants may serve as focal points or provide visual interest through their form, texture, or color. Others may be chosen for their ability to attract pollinators or provide habitat for wildlife. Consider the desired functions and benefits that you want your plants to offer, and select them accordingly. For instance, you might choose native flowering plants to support local pollinators or select shrubs that provide privacy or windbreaks. While aesthetics are often the starting point for many gardeners, it's crucial to remember that beauty alone is not enough. The plants you choose should not only be visually appealing but also capable of thriving in your specific growing conditions and fulfilling the intended functions in your landscape. A successful garden requires plants that can withstand the challenges of the growing season and winter. Selecting plants solely for their beauty without considering their suitability to your garden's conditions may result in disappointment and unsuccessful plantings. Therefore, aesthetics should be the final consideration, adding the finishing touch to a well-designed and functional landscape. Here are a few factors that will help you determine the right plants based on the environmental condition. Use the next two books to determine the plants you can grown based not only on the conditions of your garden, but on your medical needs and on the pollinators you want to attract.

Using the Hardiness Map:
The USDA Plant Hardiness Zone Map, last updated in 2012, is widely recognized as the authoritative resource for determining the suitability of plants in specific regions. Developed by the Agricultural Research Service (ARS) of the United States Department of Agriculture (USDA), this map can be accessed on their official website. The map divides regions into distinct zones, each spanning a range of 10-degree Fahrenheit intervals, based on the average minimum winter temperature experienced in that area. By referencing this map, gardeners can make informed decisions about which plants are most likely to thrive in their particular zone.

Environmental conditions:
When planning a garden or selecting plants, several factors should be taken into consideration.

These include:

1. Soil: Understanding the type and quality of your soil is crucial. Factors such as texture, fertility, pH level, and drainage capacity can significantly impact plant growth.
2. Climate: Consider the climate of your region, including the average temperatures, seasonal variations, and length of growing season. This information helps determine which plants are suitable for your area.
3. Elevation: Higher elevations can influence temperature and weather patterns, so it's essential to know your specific elevation and its impact on gardening conditions.
4. Drainage: Good drainage is important for plant health. Assess the natural drainage patterns of your garden to avoid issues like waterlogging and root rot.
5. Aspect: The orientation of your garden (north, south, east, west) affects sunlight exposure. Different plants have varying sunlight requirements, so consider the aspect when choosing plant locations.

6. Sun/ Shade: Determine the amount of sunlight your garden receives throughout the day. Some plants thrive in full sun, while others prefer partial shade or full shade.
7. Precipitation: Understand the average rainfall in your area to ensure plants receive adequate water. This helps guide irrigation practices and plant selection.
8. Microclimates: Microclimates refer to localized variations in climate within a given area. Factors like proximity to buildings, wind patterns, and vegetation cover can create microclimates that affect plant growth.
9. Frost dates: Know the average dates of the first and last frosts in your region. This information is crucial for timing planting and protecting sensitive plants from frost damage.
10. Other environmental factors: Consider any other environmental factors specific to your location, such as strong winds, salt spray near the coast, or pollution levels.

Available sources:
When selecting plant material for your garden, it is generally recommended to choose species that originate from and are native to your specific geographic region. These regions are defined by ecological boundaries rather than political ones and are often referred to as ecoregions. The Nature Conservancy in the U.S. and the Conservation Data Centers in Canada provide reliable delineations of these ecoregions. Using native plant material that closely matches the environmental conditions of your planting site can lead to better development and performance of the plants.

This is because native species have often become genetically adapted to local environments to varying degrees. However, it is important to note that species-specific knowledge may be limited, so a cautious approach is advised to ensure the success of plantings in both the short and long term. It is crucial to obtain native plant material from reputable nurseries rather than digging them from natural areas. This helps prevent the local extinction of native plants and supports conservation efforts. While it can sometimes be challenging to find native plants in nurseries, it is worth the effort to seek them out. If it becomes necessary to transplant from the wild, it is essential to follow proper foraging guidelines and exercise caution to minimize any negative impacts on natural plant populations.

Amount of work to prepare your site:
Having the right planting tools is important for successful planting. When purchasing prairie seeds, you may inquire about a Truax drill for large sites or hand-operated seeders for small sites. Hand-sowing prairie seeds is a common option that can result in more natural planting patterns, providing a closer resemblance to the way seeds would be dispersed naturally. Before planting, it is essential to ensure that the current vegetation is free of weeds. If you are dealing with thin lawns or thinly vegetated areas, inter-seeding (no-till) or plugging plants into the existing vegetation can be considered. This approach can help minimize the emergence of new weeds and encourage the growth of native plants.

Know what's regionally appropriate:
There are a number of plants that you should not buy or plant in your area. These plants may not be native to your area, despite their beauty. Natural controls keep these plants in check in their natural habitat. Some species, however, become invasive when introduced into a new habitat without natural predators or competitors. Invasive plant species have the potential to spread and suffocate native plants and animals. To avoid bringing invasive species into your yard, check to see if a plant is appropriate for your area. Consult resources such as Invasive.org and the USDA Natural Resources Conservation Service PLANTS Database for advice.

Manageable need for ongoing maintenance:
Is there anything that will compete with natural species, such as noxious weeds or problem species? Before planting indigenous, seek professional assistance on control tactics and elimination. Herbicides, hand pulling, weed wrenches, cultivation, and mowing are some of the possibilities. Make a weed-control strategy. Weed control can be done in a variety of ways. Choose the one that best fits your needs. Mulch can assist in choking weeds and nourish seedlings in early plantings. Mow before weeds grow 6-12 inches in prairie/savanna plantings. When there is enough fuel to complete a thorough burn, execute safe controlled burns in plant communities that are naturally maintained by fire, such as prairies, savannas, and many pine woods. Plan to mow and remove clippings if burning isn't an option. Weed control and wildlife protection are frequently required for tiny seedlings in tree and forest plantings.

No matter what, keep records:
Keep track of where the plant material you utilize came from. This is especially critical for large-scale restorations, such as those at nature centers or other educational facilities. Detailed information on the plants utilized and their suppliers will help us analyze their success or failure and adjust our plant selection tactics as appropriate. Given the projected climate changes as a result of global warming, this may become increasingly relevant.

Planning your garden
A well-thought-out strategy is crucial for establishing a successful home garden. Here are some important considerations to keep in mind during the planning process:
1. Select a location with loose, fertile, level, and well-drained soil. Avoid areas where water collects or the soil remains consistently damp, as most vegetables do not thrive in poorly drained soil.
2. Choose a planting location where weeds are less likely to grow. This will help ensure that your vegetables have a better chance of growing well without competing with invasive plants.
3. Adequate sunlight is essential for the growth and productivity of most plants. Avoid planting in areas that will be shaded by buildings, trees, or shrubs. Reserve shaded areas for plants that prefer less sunlight, such as ferns or shade-loving plants. Most vegetables require a minimum of 6 hours of sunlight per day.

4. Be mindful of planting vegetables beneath the branches of large trees or in close proximity to other plants. This can deprive them of essential nutrients and water. While a food forest can be a great option, it should be well-designed and carefully planned, as discussed in the chapter on agroforestry.
5. Whenever possible, place your garden near a water source. While some regions may receive enough natural rainfall to sustain a garden, regular watering can greatly enhance its success. This is especially important during prolonged periods of drought or when growing seedlings.
6. Remember that very few people have the perfect garden setting, so do your best to find the most suitable location available to you. With proper planning and care, you can create a thriving and productive garden anywhere.

Calculating the size:
One common mistake made by enthusiastic first-time gardeners is creating a garden that is too large to manage effectively.

It's important to consider the following factors when determining the size of your garden:
1. Consider the available space: If you live in an apartment or flat, a planter box or container garden may be suitable. However, if you have a suburban or rural setting with ample space, you can consider a larger garden.
2. Time commitment: Assess how much time you can dedicate to gardening. If you have limited time due to work or school, it may be challenging to maintain a large garden. Start with a smaller garden that you can manage within your available time.
3. Involvement of family: If gardening is a family activity and there are multiple members involved in its maintenance, a larger garden may be feasible. Additionally, a larger family can consume more vegetables, justifying a larger garden size.
4. Purpose of the garden: If your garden is primarily for pleasure and aesthetics, a container garden or flower bed may be sufficient. However, if you intend to grow vegetables for canning or freezing, you will require a larger space to accommodate a higher yield.
5. Consider spacing requirements: Some vegetables require ample space to grow. Adequate spacing between rows is crucial, with a minimum of 3 feet between rows recommended. If you plan to grow multiple rows of vegetables, calculate the necessary width accordingly. For example, if you want to have ten rows of vegetables, your garden should be at least 30 feet wide.

Considerations for planting:
1. What is the size of your available space? Mint should not be grown in a tiny garden. They take up an excessive amount of space. Other herbs that do not claim and climb, such as Rosemary, can be planted anywhere.
2. The more productive each row is, the more vital it is in a tiny garden. Basil, parsley, chives, and other fast-growing plants are the ones to grow if you want to harvest soon and get the most out of your space.

3. What is the nutritional value of your food? Although all herbs are beneficial, some are more nutrient-dense than others. Grow a variety of plants to add diversity to your diet.
4. It is a personal choice. This is especially crucial if the garden is solely for personal enjoyment or recreation. Grow plants that your family enjoys.

Lighting:
Remember, herbs needing more light will need open space facing the north; those needing shade will need to have coverage by fences or sheds – some shade-providing source!

Timing:
We're lucky in that herbs are very forgiving; however, keep in mind that it is best to plant herbs in spring; if that isn't an option, any time that the ground isn't frozen will do.

Are you considering wildlife?
If you have a love for observing and experiencing the beauty of nature, such as listening to bird songs, watching hummingbirds feed, or witnessing the grace of butterflies, you may be interested in increasing the wildlife presence on your property. The term "wildlife" can mean different things to different individuals, ranging from birds like cardinals, nuthatches, or hummingbirds for bird enthusiasts, to rare species for avid birders, or even butterflies for passionate gardeners. However, attracting wildlife to a specific location is not a random occurrence. It is a result of creating a suitable environment. To encourage more wildlife, certain wildlife management strategies need to be employed.

These strategies involve modifying the habitat, managing animal populations, or implementing measures to accommodate the needs of both wildlife and people, particularly landowners. By adopting wildlife management practices and creating a hospitable habitat, you can increase the presence of various wildlife species on your property. This may involve providing food sources, creating shelter or nesting areas, offering water sources, and minimizing disturbances that could disrupt wildlife populations. Ultimately, by taking steps to enhance the habitat and manage the environment, you can create a welcoming space for wildlife, allowing you to enjoy and appreciate the diverse array of animals that may visit or reside on your property. Take a look at the last chapter of this volume for more information.

Know the four elements:
In a wildlife habitat, there are four essential components that contribute to the survival of wildlife: food, water, shelter, and space for raising their young. When planning your wildlife habitat strategy, keeping these requirements in mind will increase your chances of success in attracting and supporting a diverse range of wildlife species. Different species have specific nutritional needs that can vary with age and season. Some species may rely on berries, while others prefer nuts, acorns, grasses, grains, seeds, or floral nectar. By providing a variety of food sources in your habitat, you can cater to the dietary needs of different wildlife species. Water is equally crucial for wildlife survival. Installing a pond or birdbath can quickly attract wildlife to your habitat. Allowing your pond to overflow may even create wetland areas, which can further enhance the habitat for certain species.

Cover is essential for wildlife as it provides protection from the elements and predators, as well as nesting and resting areas. Shrubs, grasses, trees (including dead trees), rock and brush piles, nesting boxes, and abandoned structures can all serve as valuable sources of cover for wildlife. Finally, wildlife requires adequate space to raise their young. Many animals establish and defend their territories. For example, if you provide nesting boxes for bluebirds, they should be placed at least 300 feet apart to avoid territorial conflicts. However, some species like purple martins and wood ducks do not defend territories. Additionally, certain species have specific space requirements, such as ruffed grouse needing 10 acres of lake or wetlands, or loons requiring 100 acres of suitable habitat. By incorporating these elements into your wildlife habitat, you can create an environment that supports the needs of various species, enabling them to thrive and reproduce successfully.

Cover the basics:
An understanding of the basic tenets concerning habitat and how these habitats correlate with various wildlife species is critical before engaging in a comprehensive analysis of a wildlife habitat. The concept of 'niche' frequently comes up in wildlife habitat discussions. This term encapsulates the notion that every species within a community carries out a distinct role within that collective. Take woodpeckers, for instance, who feast on insects tucked under tree barks and burrow holes into tree trunks, or beavers, which are renowned for felling trees and constructing dams, exemplifying highly specialized species.
Certain organisms are referred to as generalists, often seen in competition with each other. Medium-sized omnivores like raccoons and foxes all feed on the same fruits and small mammals, however, the diversity of their food sources equips them for robust competition. All species possess a distinctive role in the ecosystem that aids other organisms, including humans.

Consider squirrels, who inadvertently aid the ongoing propagation of forests. They stash away acorns as food reserves, yet fail to retrieve all, resulting in new oak trees springing from the forgotten acorns. Other animals and birds also play a part in dispersing seeds across the landscape. Acorns and beechnuts heavily depend on blue jays for their long-distance dispersal. These birds transport the nuts to far-off locations and bury them in soft soil or under leaves. As per a study, 50 blue jays in Virginia relocated 150,000 acorns within a month. While some of these acorns were retrieved and consumed later, a significant portion remained and helped in forest regeneration. In a forest habitat, plants grow across various vertical layers. Some wildlife species depend on the ground layer, which comprises herbaceous plants, for sustenance, but also seek shelter from the tree canopy, the highest layer.

The middle layer consists of shrubs. By emulating nature and planting in layers, different species can have diverse feeding and nesting habits. Although it's not mandatory to eliminate lawns, maintaining them within manageable proportions can support wildlife and save both time and money. The costs associated with mowing, applying chemicals, weeding, and watering can be hefty, both financially and temporally. The term 'edge' represents the juncture where two or more differing plant communities or successional stages converge, like where a forest adjoins an open area. The transition between plant communities can sometimes be abrupt or defined, other times it can be a gradual shift from one plant community to another. The latter tends to be more wildlife-friendly.

Diverse ecosystems signify stability and the capacity to adjust to change. Landscaping with a broad variety of plants tends to foster thriving wildlife. Certain plants will be evergreen or form dense thickets for cover, while others will be valued for their blooms and fruits. It's essential to understand the requirements of the wildlife species inhabiting your region. In gardens, ornate double-petaled, frilly blooms are visually appealing, but they are inaccessible to butterflies for nectar, so it's better to provide flat, more open blossoms that butterflies prefer. The planting of invasive foreign species, like the multiflora rose and Japanese honeysuckle, which can outcompete native plants and are nearly impossible to eradicate, should always be refrained from.

Planting a mixture of trees, shrubs, and flowers that bloom or bear fruit at different times throughout the year can cater to the needs of wildlife year-round. For example, crabapple trees yield fruit in the fall and winter, cherry trees in the summer, and hickory trees produce nuts in the fall. For optimal results, food, water, and cover should be positioned closely. This lessens predator mortality when animal species move from one habitat element to another.

Above all else, remember your responsibility:
A field of wildflowers is one of the most beautiful things we may see in nature for many of us. We have a deep desire to reach out and select a flower in a gorgeous butterfly-filled meadow or along a public forest route lined with spring beauties, irises, or wake-robins from childhood into maturity. We've dedicated an entire book to Wildflowers because we all have such fond recollections of them. Millions of people visit public lands each year, and if just a small percentage of them individually selected a few flowers, there would soon be none left for the rest of us to enjoy.

Almost all wildflowers are delicate, and many quickly wilt and die after being harvested. The long-term consequences of uninformed individuals harvesting wildflowers go far beyond the loss of the flowers themselves. When wildflowers are gone, a key chain of events is set in motion that will last for years. On a micro-scale, wildflowers support entire ecosystems for pollinators, birds, and small creatures, which humans don't frequently notice. Butterflies and other insects, as well as small birds and animals, rely on seeds, nectar, and pollen for sustenance and survival.

Furthermore, some pollinators are not particularly mobile, have restricted home ranges, or are dependent on a single plant species, and perish when their habitat is eliminated.

1. All living organisms must reproduce in order to survive. Digging up wildflowers, picking them, or collecting their seed reduces a plant's ability to reproduce and has a negative impact on its long-term survival in that place.
2. Taking wildflowers out of the wild can have a negative impact on pollinators and other creatures who rely on them for food and shelter.
3. The majority of wildflowers that are dug from their original habitat do not survive transplantation.

So, unless it is absolutely necessary, find your seeds for wildflowers through seed swapping, local nurseries, or even through websites, rather than robbing a delicate, and ever fragile biosystem.

Designing a Native Garden
The design process described here will ensure that you select plants workable for your site without added inputs—which means that whatever your garden style, you will be gardening sustainably. When the right plant is put in the right place, its need for fertilizer, watering, and pesticides is greatly reduced. A happy plant is more vigorous and resistant to weather calamities and pests.

Inventory
To create a successful planting design that utilizes native plants to their optimum, you must begin by doing an inventory of your planned garden's site. Foremost is to identify the soils on the site. Are they wet, moist, or dry? Composed of sand, loam, clay, or gravel? Is there bedrock and, if so, what kind of stone is it? It's ridiculous to amend a site for your desired plants. Instead, pick plants that will thrive under the existing soil conditions. When in doubt, check your local soil survey and/or get a soil test. Next, know your site's orientation. It is critical to know north from south, east from west, because of the angle of the sun and where it casts cooler shadows, where it beats down most intensely (from the southwest), and how the sun changes through the seasons. The sun rises directly in the east on the vernal and autumnal equinoxes, but rises in the northeast in summer, southeast in winter. Winds are also a factor, almost universally southwesterly in summer and from the northwest in winter. You even have to think about the aspect of the land. Is it flat? Is it sloping, and if so which direction? Note these variations if you have topography. Those who garden on the east sides of bluffs never see the sunset and have a much more sheltered site; those on the west sides of a hill may never see the sunrise and may get baked by the afternoon sun. The inventory should note all existing plants. This is a great clue in interpreting the site's conditions and an indicator of what plants will do well in there. Gardeners with a bare, blank slate can look nearby for such plant clues. Trees are your best indicator because they have been there a long time. A good inventory must also map all utilities, including overhead and underground wires, gas lines, water and sewer lines, and septic fields, so that plantings are compatible with and allow access to such infrastructure, thus preventing future headaches. You also want to call 811 and get underground utilities flagged, a service provided in all regions to prevent homeowners and contractors from accidentally digging into them.

Analysis

Once you've identified existing plants on or near your site, look into the conditions under which they thrive. It is not enough to determine your hardiness zone, you have to take into consideration the particular microclimate of your location. What are you doing with that research? You are analyzing the situation. Do the same for the soils: analyze the conditions and note any anomalies. It is often best not to fix them but to work with them. Don't forget compass directions and the sun and wind changes through each season. Think of where sunny and shady sites are, how to screen the southwestern sun from your home or outdoor seating space in summer. Note to block the cold northwesterly winds in winter. Here is an example based on my own gardening experience. When I started growing in my backyard, I looked at the county's soil survey and learned that I had a uniform droughty clay soil, shallow to limestone bedrock in places. I inventoried where there were exposed rocks. The ridgetop property sloped eastward, draining into a ravine to the southeast. I noted the directions and existing large trees to the southwest that cool the house in afternoon; to the northwest, shingle oaks with marcescent (held through winter) leaves made a nice windbreak. The north and east sides of the house reflected a more cool and moist microclimate, the west side of the house was hotter and drier.

The existing trees were all second-growth species (shingle oak, honeylocust, black cherry, elms, hackberry) that are known to be very drought tolerant. Under the trees grew roundleaf groundsel, so I knew I would be able to grow woodland wildflowers that thrived in dry upland woods. An open meadow area to the south had milkweeds and a few other prairie plants—indicators of well-drained, dry soils. That demonstrated that upland, dry prairie species would do well in that site. No trees or wildflowers indicated moist or wet conditions.

Scheme

Putting together a basic scheme is the final step in the design process. Everyone wants a beautiful garden that is easily cared for and a sound investment. But since you're reading this book, you're probably also interested in a landscape that celebrates spirit of place; a garden that is ecologically balanced and sustainable; a yard that includes edible and medicinal plants; plantings that attract birds and other wildlife; insect-friendly borders that support bees, pollinators, butterflies, moths—and so on. So what is your style? Do you embrace traditional landscapes of order, or do you like natural landscapes? If you want a more natural look, be sure to research the regulations or landscape ordinances of your neighborhood or community first. Be prepared to get a variance and discuss what you are doing with your neighbors. Think about what you are capable of maintaining or how you plan to maintain your landscape. Landscape maintenance is a critical part of your scheme, so you must consider a plant's behavior and suitability for a particular landscape, be it formal or natural.

Yes, there are Midwest native plants that can be used traditionally; already most of our trees and some shrubs are embraced and readily utilized in landscaping, as are some ornamental grasses. But most native evergreen shrubs, vines, perennials, groundcovers, bulbs, and annuals are much less understood and cultivated. Some examples of those that have made the jump to "popular" include our native wisteria as a vine and prairie dropseed as a perennial. Traditional styles where plants are grown in an orderly fashion show the hand of humans over nature. Plants usually must stay put and be segregated; only groundcovers are allowed to spread, and then only uniformly. Plants must be well behaved and under control. This is the typical style of suburbia, where shade trees, select ornamental trees, foundation plantings, hedges, and a few perennials prevail, adorning a lush, turf grass lawn. Natural styles embrace the hands of Mother Nature and allow plants to naturalize freely and behave as they would in the wild. This allows for complex relationships and mixes of species that can look unkempt or untidy to many people. To the trained ecologist's eye, however, the pattern here is best described as "disordered hyperuniformity"—order at large distances, disorder at shorter distances. It's how plants are arranged in a native prairie.

There are in-between styles, the average perennial border being a good example, where relatively well-behaved plants are planted in groupings that create compositions that are usually synchronized for bloom through the seasons and in such a way so that the ornamental characters of the plant create artistic compositions based on color and texture. Follow your own choice of aesthetic schemes to make your landscape fit your needs and help give it some parameters, so that it is not all hodgepodge. The color palettes of our native plants through the season have their own splendor, whatever their original habitat. Clean, defined edges to natural landscaping along with signage are helpful for neighbors accepting of only a formal landscape. I certified my landscape with the National Wildlife Federation, North American Butterfly Association, and Monarch Watch and have posted the signs they provided. Other local and national groups will do the same, including Wild Ones and the Xerces Society. You can also post your own signs—the idea is to communicate, somehow, what you are doing and what your natural landscape reflects.

Always embrace problematic site conditions. If you can't beat 'em, join 'em. A wet spot can become a wetland garden; a dry locale should embrace what does well in that habitat. Dense shade can usually support moss and ferns or other woodland wildflowers. Sandy sites have a whole suite of plants that thrive under those conditions. Make peace with what you are given, and a better, more sustainable design, unique to you and your site, will ensue. Capture your spirit of place and bloom where you're planted. There are native plants that thrive in every niche.

Garden Styles

Several garden styles lend themselves to incorporating native plants. Here we will look at prairie, woodland, water, and rock gardens, as well as edible landscapes.

PRAIRIE GARDENS

No other garden style provides more appropriate, beautiful, and productive biomass to a landscape than a prairie garden, especially in the Midwest, whether you are starting from scratch or adding to a remnant prairie, meadow, or grassland with existing natives. The most meaningful prairie gardens include only native plants found in the local area. Prairie gardens provide exceptional food and cover for beneficial insects and wildlife. Virtually all are composed mainly of midsummer- to fall-blooming wildflowers, as the spring-blooming wildflowers are most costly to plant and challenging to establish. Prairie plantings also usually favor the larger warm-season grasses that are easier to establish. Smaller grasses like prairie dropseed and cool-season grasses like river oats get ignored, along with the many wonderful sedges. A prairie planting is the epitome of a natural landscape, so must be planned and well thought out, particularly with regard to how it works with local landscape ordinances. Its long-term maintenance must be carefully considered along with its flammability. In urban contexts, a landscape variance, clean edges, and signage are usually necessities. Burning is often not allowed, so an annual or occasional cut will be necessary. A flail mower is an ideal tool for cutting a prairie and chopping it into lovely mulch.

Almost all prairie gardens begin with a clean, weed-free plot in full sun. Plantings are most economical when started from seed, but using plant plugs can speed up the project. Select species for the planting mix that fit the site's soils whether sand, clay, or loam; wet, moist, or dry. Be careful with certain exuberant species: some may be integral but better added after more conservative species are established, so there is competition to keep them in check.

Your local native plant nursery will be able to recommend methods best suited to establishing a prairie garden in your particular area. I strongly suggest a mix of plugs and seed for smaller projects, starting with plugs or plants of some of the neglected spring wildflowers, smaller grasses, and sedges. Keeping weeds out through mowing high the first season or two also will help, while the long-lived prairie plants develop their roots. Black-eyed Susan and other short-lived, disturbance-dependent annual or biennial plants provide early color and suppress weeds; they will fade out as long-lived species become established. They will also prove to the uninformed that you aren't just tending a patch of weeds.

WOODLAND GARDENS
Beloved spring ephemeral wildflowers, spring-flowering trees, dazzling fall color, the promise of cool—all these are the inspiration for our common love of woodland gardens. They are a no-brainer for wooded landscapes. Just be sure to pick plants compatible with the types of trees and the environment you have. Some gardeners in new, treeless landscapes want woodland gardens and that is not a problem either: start on the shaded north or east side of your home and plant trees that will eventually allow you to expand your woodland plantings. Most trees grow surprisingly fast when well sited and cared for, so refrain from choosing short-term, quick trees. I always recommend oaks and hickories. Oaks are more readily available at nurseries, but hickories can be grown from nuts that you collect, and they grow well in the shade, taking their time and being quite beautiful from seedling to sapling stage, with attractive buds and tropicalesque foliage. Some highly desirable small woodland trees, such

as eastern redbud and pagoda dogwood, grow really fast and jumpstart your woodland garden.

One of the beauties of a woodland garden is that every type of plant is used to create the most complete, layered picture: canopy trees, understory trees, woodland shrubs, perennials, and so on. Vines must be carefully matched with young trees; you don't want them to smother their host, and they are best added to existing, more mature trees or against buildings or structures. Use fallen leaves for natural mulch, but don't let it get too thick until perennials are established. Surprisingly, most woodland wildflowers need bare earth to germinate, so you can rake away select spots or let foraging songbirds scratch through the leaf litter to open up new seedbeds. Woodland gardens always have a focus on spring, but the other seasons must be included as well. Ferns have striking foliage that replaces spring ephemerals after they go dormant, and there are also some wonderful, if subtle, summer-blooming wildflowers, such as Culver's root and alumroot.

Fall in the woodland garden is often exuberant: various shade-loving asters and goldenrods create an outstandingly colorful display, with abundant nectar, pollen, and seeds for winter songbirds. Solomon's seal, false Solomon's seal, Jack-in-the-pulpit, and many other woodland plants have exquisite berries in late summer and autumn too. Winter in the woodland garden should highlight some of our fine native evergreens, including Christmas fern and the stunningly patterned leaves of hepaticas.

WATER GARDENS
Claude Monet and his limpid paintings of water lilies popularized the water garden for eternity—not so surprising, given the beautiful subject. Water gardens are inherently intriguing. The sound of water, its exquisite reflective properties, its cooling nature, and the special suite of creatures it attracts make it a very popular garden type. Water plants are the showiest Midwest wildflowers, and many other lovely grasses and even more of our gorgeous wildflowers require wet feet. Water gardens are not rain gardens; they must be sited out of major rainwater drainage, or they will quickly fill in with silt and debris. Obviously, they must be lined with soils that hold water or with a waterproof liner to be effective. Circulating water is needed for aeration, and filters are required to maintain water clarity, so gardens do not become cesspools. New construction styles pump water from below the pool so that it filters through gravel for purification and does not get clogged with leaves or other debris.

Design a water garden with various water depths for all sorts of plants, from those marginal plants that like wet feet to those that require a water depth of at least 18 inches. Water plants can be containerized and moved about, or even overwintered in the deepest parts of unheated pools, where the water doesn't freeze. Water gardens with waterfalls, bubblers, and heaters that provide fresh water to wildlife and birds through all seasons are a naturalist's delight. There is no finer way to observe many of our colorful migrant songbirds, especially warblers, which relish drinking and bathing in such features. Water is also a requirement for the life cycle of garden frogs and toads, whose peeps and trills are so welcome after a long winter; pools without fish or with shelves or nooks that fish cannot get to are best for these amphibians. Dragonflies and damselflies, a group of increasingly popular and dynamic insects, also require water for their eggs and juvenile life stages. Adult dragonflies and damselflies are wonderful predators of mosquitos and other nuisance insects, eating many of them on the wing.

ROCK GARDENS

Rock gardens, a garden fad of the 1920s, have lately seen a resurgence in popularity. They are ideal places to cultivate drought-tolerant native plants that grow wild on rock outcrops, cliffs, glades, talus slopes, and glacial deposits. Any landscape site with natural rock outcroppings is a likely place to try one. Rock gardens are also a good choice where steep changes of grade occur, and they can actually be living walls, where stones are dry stacked with a soil mix between them. Sharp drainage is essential for all rock gardens, though some rock garden plants thrive in wet scree or gravel. When constructing a rock garden, use local stones and—crucially for aesthetics—set them in such a manner that they appear to be naturally occurring. Soil mixes between the rocks should be equal parts local topsoil, gravel, and compost. A gravel mulch can be applied to give a clean, neat look and to keep plants from rotting in wet weather. Rock gardens that also function as retaining walls must have a sturdy footing and good drainage—that is, be backed by coarse gravel and drainage tile; this allows excess moisture to drain away and prevents frost heaving in winter. Each layer of stone on a living wall should be stepped back about ½ inch for buttressed support. The same soil mix should be placed between stone layers as recommended for any rock garden. An engineer should approve any wall taller than 4 feet to ensure that it is stable in the long term. Plant living walls in spring; this gives the plants a chance to root in before summer's heat

and, ideally, to be so well rooted by winter that frost heaving is not a concern. A mix of clay and sphagnum moss can be pressed around new plants to hold them in place as they establish.

EDIBLE LANDSCAPES

Edible landscaping, a concept first popularized by landscape designer Rosalind Creasy, simply means using food plants in the garden in a functional and aesthetically pleasing way, just as one would ornamentals. Gardeners and nongardeners alike have embraced both edible plants and edible landscapes, and these two trends have only gained momentum with the sustainability and foodie movements. The benefits of this garden style are the delicious treats produced by the plantings. Yes, there are native plants of all types, from shade trees to groundcovers, that are edible and should be valued for that reason. Pecans and highbush and lowbush blueberries are commercial successes. Other edible species are just as tasty but don't meet shipping or shelf-life criteria, so are rarely found beyond local growers' and farmers' markets.

Incorporating native edibles into the home landscape definitely adds value to a sustainable garden, allowing one to celebrate and savor the bounty of the seasons. A collection of native food-yielding plants grown in a natural woodland manner is termed a food forest. Such a garden is both productive and ecologically sound. It's a good way to use many of the native edible plants that don't conform well to recommended planting and care for prime production; wild black raspberry plants, for instance, are too disease-prone to be cultivated in a formal, trained bed, but when allowed to run through open woodlands or woodland edges, there are always some that produce fruit to enjoy. Take a look back at the chapters on agroforestry and food forests for more information.

Methods of Propagation

In the modern world of commercial nurseries, cultivars and hybrids have taken center stage. These are carefully cultivated plant varieties that have been selectively bred to exhibit specific traits such as compact size, vibrant bloom colors, double flowers, and consistent growth patterns. While these characteristics may be visually appealing to some, they often come at the cost of reduced reproductive capacity and genetic diversity, which are essential for adapting to diverse environmental conditions. To maintain these desired traits, nurseries rely on asexual reproduction methods, bypassing the natural process of sexual reproduction. In contrast, the natural environment thrives on the sexual reproduction of plants through the production of seeds. This natural propagation method leads to a wide range of variations among individual plants, as each seed carries unique genetic traits that influence how a plant responds to environmental stressors such as heat, drought, flooding, and other disturbances. The diversity preserved through seed propagation is intrinsic to the survival and adaptability of wild native plants, representing their optimal strategy for navigating future environmental challenges

It is important to recognize the value of preserving the genetic diversity found in wild native plants. By prioritizing seed propagation and embracing the inherent variations among individuals, we can ensure the resilience and long-term sustainability of plant populations in the face of changing environmental conditions. While cultivars and hybrids may offer certain aesthetic benefits, we must not overlook the importance of genetic diversity and the role it plays in the continued adaptation and evolution of plant species.

Germinating from seeds

Propagating indigenous plants is a truly fascinating process that doesn't necessitate any fancy equipment. In fact, native seeds are naturally adapted for germination in outdoor settings, whether it be in beds or pots. Interestingly, many native species tend to germinate more successfully outdoors compared to the controlled environment of a greenhouse. This is because the stable temperature and high humidity inside a greenhouse can create an ideal breeding ground for rot and other issues. When practicing outdoor propagation, the seeds of native plants exhibit a remarkable responsiveness to their environment. Each species has its own unique set of requirements for germination, which may align with the cool temperatures of early spring for some, while others may require the warmth of summer. The seeds patiently await the perfect conditions to emerge and start their journey of growth and development.

This natural process of outdoor germination allows for a harmonious synchronization between the native plants and the environment they inhabit. It ensures that each species has the opportunity to germinate and establish itself when the conditions are most favorable for its specific needs. By embracing the innate timing and preferences of indigenous seeds, we can enhance the success of propagation efforts and foster the diversity and resilience of native plant populations. Seeds can be sown in seed flats or plastic pots that have a diameter ranging between 4 to 10 inches and a depth of at least 3 inches. These can be placed in a spot with plenty of shade. A modest nursery, with 10–20 pots, can easily be established beneath a garden bench for hobby gardeners. It's conveniently located away from pets and children, provides shade, and is easy to maintain. An open-air cold frame also serves as a suitable location for a nursery area for seed flats and pots. Tending to a dozen pots is as simple as caring for a single one, and if you try cultivating a variety of species, you'll enjoy great success. If you end up with surplus plants, they can be gifted to someone else.

Sowing the seeds:

Native seeds can be planted in high density (in close proximity to each other). The label should include the name of the plant and the date of sowing. A good guideline to follow is to plant the seeds 1/8 to ¼ inches apart and to a depth equivalent to the thickness of the seed. Seeds that are as fine as dust are barely covered. After sowing, the seeds should be topped with coarse sand, which is more suitable than potting soil as it helps prevent the seeds from being washed away by rain. If nearby weeds pose a threat, cover the flats with a spun poly material like Reemay. Maintain the hydration of the seeds by watering them every few days or once a week.

Wait for full germination

The germination process of native seeds is a fascinating journey that unfolds at its own pace. Unlike cultivated plants, such as vegetables and annual flowers, native plants have not been selectively bred for rapid germination. As a result, the germination timeline of wild seeds can vary significantly. Some seeds may sprout immediately after planting, while others exhibit a sporadic germination pattern that can span weeks, months, or even years. This diverse germination strategy allows wild plants to disperse their offspring gradually, providing them with a greater capacity to adapt to changing environmental conditions. For seeds that do not require any pretreatment, germination can occur within a timeframe ranging from a week to several months after planting.

On the other hand, certain species may have specific dormancy requirements, such as winter stratification, before they can germinate. These seeds remain dormant until the right conditions occur, breaking their dormancy and triggering germination. It's worth noting that flats or pots that fail to germinate in the first year should not be discarded. Instead, patience is key, as some seeds may take longer to germinate and may surprise you with their emergence in subsequent years. One practical approach to sowing native seeds is to plant them outdoors during the fall or winter seasons. This eliminates the need for artificial cold stratification, which involves refrigerating the seeds, that some species require when planted in the spring. By taking advantage of the natural cycles and conditions of the seasons, we can simplify the propagation process and align it with the innate tendencies of native seeds. Embracing the unique germination patterns of native seeds allows us to appreciate the resilience and adaptability of these plants. It encourages us to be patient, observant, and attuned to the natural rhythms of nature, as we witness the beauty of new life emerging from the soil.

Root cuttings

Understanding the seasonal dynamics and their impact on the propagation of plants through root cuttings is crucial for successful gardening practices. For a long time, the significance of "on" and "off" seasons in root cuttings' ability to generate stem buds was overlooked. However, recent research has shed light on the variations in root potential and the futility of propagation attempts during unfavorable seasonal conditions. The lack of awareness regarding these fluctuations may have contributed to the underutilization of root cuttings as a propagation method among gardeners.

Therefore, it is essential to assess whether the plant of interest exhibits distinct seasonal responses and determine the most opportune time to acquire root cuttings. While it may seem logical to take cuttings during the growing season, experience has shown that this approach often yields unsatisfactory results. However, there has been some improvement when cuttings were obtained very early or late in the season. While a few plant species can be successfully propagated at any time of the year, they are relatively rare. Horseradish serves as a notable example, as it can readily regenerate from each root piece, often becoming a tenacious weed.

In contrast, most other plants exhibit a seasonal response. While initial observations suggested that winter was the most favorable time for propagation, it is now understood that the crucial factor is not winter itself, but rather the dormant season. It is important to note that not all herbaceous plants go dormant during winter. For plants that initiate growth in the new year, root cuttings taken after this period may not respond effectively. Successful propagation is typically achieved during the plant's dormant season, which could occur in late summer or early autumn. Although root cutting propagation can generally be attempted throughout a plant's dormant season, it is advisable to focus on the mid-section of that season for maximum response. Attempting propagation while dormancy is still being established or as it begins to wane may not yield optimal results.

Preparing the plant

Before embarking on the propagation of root cuttings, it is crucial to properly prepare the parent plant. This preparation will promote the growth of roots that are more inclined to generate stem buds and give rise to new plants.

To enhance the regenerative potential, lift a healthy plant prior to the onset of the growing season and trim back any top growth. Using a knife, carefully sever the roots near the base of the plant. Then, reinsert the plant into the ground. This act of trimming disrupts the balance between the plant's roots and shoots, stimulating rapid growth in the following season as the plant strives to restore equilibrium. Consequently, the vigorously growing roots will exhibit greater capacity for developing stem buds.

Root growth is most vigorous at the beginning of the season, gradually slowing down as the season progresses. By the time the dormant season arrives, root growth comes to a complete halt. The section of a root that experienced the most rapid growth during the spring season will possess the highest potential for bud production. In other words, the faster a root grows, the better its capacity to generate stem buds. Therefore, if you have an ample supply of root material, it is advisable to take root cuttings solely from the upper portion of the root that initiated growth in early spring. To obtain cutting material, lift the parent plant and trim away any top growth. Rinse off the soil by immersing the plant in a bucket of water or using a hose.

This will allow you to identify the young roots that are suitable for propagation. Cut these roots near the base of the plant, ensuring a clean, perpendicular cut. Replant the parent plant in the garden. Trim off the thinner end of the root by making an angled slice. Remove any small side roots from the cutting to facilitate ease of handling and subsequent planting. It is important to note that taking roots from the parent plant for propagation also functions as a form of root pruning, stimulating the growth of more roots that can be utilized for propagation in the following season.

Size of a root cutting

The size of a root cutting can significantly impact its success, especially when a single root provides multiple cuttings. It is crucial to determine the smallest feasible size for a root cutting to optimize the utilization of the available root material. The size of a root cutting is influenced by two key factors. Firstly, the cutting must possess enough stored nutrients to initiate and sustain the development of a stem bud until it produces green leaves and becomes self-sustaining. Secondly, the cutting requires adequate food reserves to support itself during the process of regrowth. Therefore, the size of the cutting consists of two components: the regrowth part and the survival part. The size of the survival part depends on the duration it takes for the cutting to regenerate.

This is influenced by the temperature in which the cutting is propagated. Warmer environments promote faster stem growth. For instance, a root cutting planted outdoors during winter might not sprout a shoot until May, whereas the same cutting placed in a propagator with a temperature range of 65-75°F (18-24°C) could regenerate in approximately four weeks. The food reserves necessary for survival in these two temperature conditions differ significantly. However, the size of the regrowth part remains consistent irrespective of the propagation temperature. Therefore, a general guideline for determining the size of a root cutting is based on the variable factor of temperature.

If the roots of the parent plant were pruned one year prior to taking the cuttings, all roots will exhibit one year's growth and have a relatively uniform thickness. Consequently, the cutting length remains the same. For outdoor plantings, a cutting should be at least 4 inches long, as it will need to survive for approximately 16 weeks. In slightly warmer environments, such as a cold frame or unheated greenhouse, regeneration occurs in approximately eight weeks. Thus, a smaller survival portion is required, and the cuttings only need to be slightly over 2 inches long. In a warm greenhouse or propagator with a temperature range of 65-75°F (18-24°C), the regeneration time is reduced to four weeks. This further decreases the required survival time and food reserves. In such an environment, root cuttings need only be about 1 inch long.

Recognizing the top of a root cutting

Recognizing the "polarity" of a root cutting—that it has a top and bottom, or in other words, a "right way up"—is key when propagating plants. Many guides recommend planting root cuttings horizontally, primarily because it's difficult to identify the top and bottom due to the absence of leaves or buds. However, this isn't the case with stem cuttings; they are not planted sideways. Therefore, it's not logical to expect root cuttings to be planted that way, regardless of the direction their roots eventually grow. Root cuttings planted upright and correctly usually perform best, given they were taken from a healthy plant and placed under appropriate conditions.

In contrast, cuttings planted on their side seldom exceed a 40 percent success rate. To properly identify the top and bottom of a root cutting and ensure it is planted in the correct orientation, there is a simple technique you can follow. Begin by making a flat cut perpendicular to the root at the point where it was separated from the parent plant. This flat cut will serve as a reference point. Then, at the bottom end of the root cutting, make a diagonal cut to remove the thin section. It is important to consistently use this method when cutting roots. By employing this technique, regardless of any changes or handling the root cutting may undergo later, you will always be able to recognize its correct polarity and ensure it is planted with the right side up. This ensures proper growth and development of the root cutting in its new location.

Planting

To ensure successful growth, root cuttings require a supportive medium that prevents drying out, allows for proper air circulation, and provides essential nutrients during the regeneration process. While outdoor soil can suffice, it is often more convenient to initially plant root cuttings in a container before moving them outdoors once they have established. Select a container that can accommodate the number of root cuttings you intend to propagate, allocating about 1-1.5 inches of space for each cutting. For instance, a 3.5 inch pot can accommodate seven cuttings. Fill the container with a peat-based compost that contains loam, as this helps maintain adequate moisture levels and supplies nutrients consistently. Use a flat board to level the compost with the rim of the container and press it down until it sits about half an inch below the rim.

Create a hole in the compost using a dibber or similar tool, and carefully plant the root cutting, ensuring that the top of the cutting aligns with the top of the compost. Gently press the compost back around the cutting, and evenly distribute the remaining root cuttings throughout the container. Cover the cuttings with grit, and again use the flat board to level the grit with the rim of the container. The weight of the grit slightly compresses the compost, causing the tops of the cuttings to rise into the grit layer, creating optimal air circulation for the bud that will develop at the top of the root cutting. Avoid watering at this stage. Label the container for identification and place it in a suitable environment, such as a propagator or cold frame, depending on the size and specific needs of the root cuttings. Monitor their progress and provide appropriate care until they are ready to be transplanted outdoors.

Aftercare

To maintain proper aeration in the compost during the propagation of plants from root cuttings, it is important to minimize watering. This not only helps prevent the cuttings from rotting but also promotes air circulation within the compost. In some cases, if the root cuttings were initially planted in adequately moist compost and the environment remains humid, additional watering may not be necessary.

It is common for the first growth to be in the form of a stem and green leaves, without the development of roots. The roots typically emerge later from the base of the new stem.

Even if the roots do develop from the cutting, they usually appear after the growth of the stem and leaves. It is important to avoid watering until the roots become visible, as excess moisture can lead to rotting. Once the stem and leaves have emerged, it is advisable to move the plant to a well-lit area. If the plants were propagated in a warm environment (around 70°F or 21°C), it is recommended to gradually acclimate them to normal outdoor conditions. This process, known as "hardening off," allows the plants to adapt to the changing environmental conditions before being planted outside or transferred to larger pots. Hardening off helps reduce the risk of transplant shock and ensures a smoother transition for the plants.

Spores

Ferns are indeed ancient plants that have been on Earth for almost 300 million years. They're a part of the Pteridophytes group, which also includes other prehistoric plants like club mosses and horsetails. During the era of the dinosaurs, these plants grew to substantial sizes, some even reaching over 100 feet. The warm and humid climate during that period was ideal for the growth of these plants.

When growing ferns indoors from spores, here's a simplified step-by-step guide:

1. Prepare the environment
You'll need a fresh, clear plastic container, sterile peat-based potting soil that has been soaked with boiling water and cooled, and water in a misting bottle (that has also been boiled and cooled).

2. Prevent contamination
Make sure your container is thoroughly cleaned to avoid the growth of mold or algae after you've sowed the spores. In nature, ferns usually germinate in moss, rotting wood, or damp soil in shaded areas, like along a stream.

3. Sow the spores
Fill the container halfway with moistened potting soil. Open the lid, hold the fern spores in your hand and sprinkle a light dusting of spores over the soil surface, just as you would season food with a pinch of salt.

4. Maintain the right conditions
Lightly spray the inside of the container with the misting bottle and place it in a warm area with good light but away from direct sun or strong artificial light. Monitor the container over the next weeks for signs of germination. Unless the soil appears dry, keep the container closed; if it does appear dry, lightly spray the soil.

5. Watch for germination
Initially, germination will appear as a green layer on the soil surface. After that, little flat green prothallia will appear, indicating sexual reproduction. If you see small fern fronds after a month or more, you'll know you've successfully moved from the reproductive to the juvenile fern stage.

6. Continue care
At this point, you can remove the cover of the container. Keep watering your plants regularly, but not too much to avoid rotting. It may be necessary to start using a very dilute seaweed fertilizer.

7. Repot and acclimate
When the small ferns reach about an inch in height, repot them in a good organic compost-based potting soil. Start acclimating them to the outdoors by moving the pots to a shaded area outside in early summer. This will help them adjust to the natural growing season.
Remember, growing ferns from spores is a delicate and slow process. Patience is key, and with good care, you'll see the efforts pay off!

Troubleshooting

Even seasoned horticulturists encounter difficulties while trying to cultivate a flourishing garden of local plants and wildlife. Here's some advice to navigate through the most frequent challenges.

Some like it cold
If you're dealing with seeds that demand a period of cold and it's already progressing into late spring, you still have the option to plant them by fabricating a winter scenario. Envelop the seed tray in plastic film or sow your seeds in pre-moistened sand or vermiculite, then refrigerate them in a sealed plastic bag for about two months. Following this mock winter, bring them out and place the tray in the open air.

Too big for your tray
During the initial growth season, many seedlings of native species can continue in their original seed tray. If the seedlings seem excessively crammed during the first summer, they can be carefully pulled apart and placed in individual pots. However, avoid moving the seedlings to their ultimate location until the subsequent spring. Ensure the plants are always labeled. When repotting, unless the species is a tree, group 3-10 seedlings together per pot. This guarantees the presence of multiple individuals, leading to genetic diversity and the ability to produce viable seeds in the new planting. Bi-weekly, feed the seedlings with a weak solution of seaweed-based fertilizer to ensure their health and strength.

Winter is coming
Like a garden needing a steady snow blanket, germinated pots and flats demand protection during winter. It's ideal to shield them using several layers of winter-grade Reemay wrapped in white plastic. Be aware that rodents might find your covered nursery appealing for nesting if the plants aren't frozen before being covered. To err on the side of caution, set up mouse traps under the covering.

Still got troubles? Put them to bed!
A germination bed can enable seedlings to grow larger before repotting, which also helps reduce the frequency of watering compared to flats or pots. Pick a spot that offers full to partial shade for forest species and partial shade for most other varieties, except for plants demanding full sun. Construct a frame using 2" x 10" or 2" x 12" raw-cut lumber (avoid pressure treated, as it releases harmful chemicals). A four-foot-wide by ten-foot-long bed can accommodate a substantial number of seedlings for several years. Alternatively, logs of 6 to 10 inches in diameter can be used. Affix sturdy screening to the bottom, flip it, and secure it. Fill it with a weed-free compost-based potting mix. You can make your own growing medium by mixing 3 parts weed-free compost or leaf mold, 1 part vermiculite, and 1 part coarse builders' sand. Unlike potting soil based on peat moss, which is sterile and nutrient-poor, compost and leaf mold teem with beneficial microorganisms and release nutrients slowly over time. Seeds can be sown in 4' rows across this bed, marked with durable plastic labels for identification. If the bed is situated near a weed source, like an old field or lawn full of dandelions, cover it with Reemay.

Phenology Tips and Tricks

Have you ever heard the "When cherry trees bloom, a robin makes a nest"? That is phenology, nature's calendar! Phenology is an essential facet of our planet's existence. Many birds lay eggs to coincide with insect availability, ensuring their hatchlings have ample food. Similarly, insects often emerge concurrently with the appearance of leaves on their host plants. Earlier blossoming translates to an earlier onset of allergies for people. For farmers and gardeners, understanding plant and insect growth cycles is crucial to timing the application of fertilizers and pesticides and for scheduling plantings to evade frost periods. The phenomenon of phenology impacts species numbers and distributions, ecosystem functions, food chains, and even global water and carbon cycles. Temperature and precipitation shifts can also influence phenology. Clearly, phenology can provide valuable insights into the health of our ecosystems.

Many gardening enthusiasts start planning their forthcoming garden virtually as the first leaves start changing colors, definitely before the first frost. However, a stroll through the garden offers the most relevant information regarding the timing of different plants. Climate, weather, and temperature cues interact with the environment, affecting the dynamics of plants, animals, and insects – this is phenology. So, what exactly is phenology, and how can it assist us in appropriately timing planting and fertilizing in our gardens? Using Phenology as a Chronometer Gardeners, being outdoorsy people, are typically astute observers of natural cycles. Even on overcast days expecting rain, the bustling activities of birds and insects herald the arrival of spring. Birds intuitively know when it's time to commence nest-building. Like overwintering insects, early spring bulbs intuitively know when it's time to break through the surface.

Noticing these repeating natural cycles can offer gardeners valuable insights. Even before the term phenology was coined, farmers have traditionally used these cycles as cues to sow and fertilize their crops. The lifespan of a lilac, for instance, is now commonly used as a guide for landscape planning and planting. Phenology-focused gardeners might interpret signs such as leaf emergence and the progress of blossoms from bud to decay. For example, in the world of phenology, it's deemed safe to plant frost-sensitive crops like beans, cucumbers, and squash when lilacs are in full bloom. However, it's important to remember that phenological events progress from west to east and south to north when using lilacs as a gardening reference. This is known as the "Hopkins' Rule," suggesting that events are delayed four days for every degree of latitude northward and 14 days for every degree of longitude eastward. This rule isn't rigid; it's merely a guide. The natural events predicted by this rule can be affected by the altitude and topography of your location.

Common Phenology checkboxes

- Timing of the first bud (of various plants)
- Timing of the first flowering (of various plants)
- The first migration of animals
- The first appearance of insects
- The appearance of hibernating animals and insects

Temperature and day length are important to trees, shrubs, herbs, and flowers alike; they develop on a predictable schedule dependent on local conditions. Other natural events, such as bird migrations and the appearance of insects and amphibians, herald the arrival of spring.

It's only natural to utilize these occurrences as predictors of when the weather is suitable for planting.

1. Crocus blooming means it's time to plant radishes, parsnips, and spinach.
2. It is okay to plant peas, onion sets, and lettuce when the forsythia is in bloom.
3. When the daffodils bloom, half-hardy crops like beets, carrots, and chard can be sown.
4. Before planting potatoes, wait for dandelions to bloom.
5. When the maple trees begin to leaf out, perennial flowers can be planted.
6. Transplant cabbage and broccoli when the quince blossoms.
7. Before planting bush beans, wait for apple trees to bloom.
8. Plant pole beans and cucumbers once the apple flowers have fallen.
9. It will be okay to sow fragile annual flowers and squashes once the lilacs are fully bloomed.
10. When the lily-of-the-valley is in full bloom, transplant tomato transplants to the garden.
11. It's time to plant morning glory seeds when the maple leaves have grown to full size.
12. When the bearded irises are in flower, peppers, and eggplant can be transplanted.
13. It's okay to plant heat-loving melons like cantaloupe while peonies bloom.

For everything there is a season

The following rules are a good overall scheme for the tasks you will have for each season, of course there are plants that have different needs, but these are good rule of thumbs nevertheless, modelled after the most common kitchen herbs.

Spring

As the spring season unfolds in full bloom, it brings with the joy of stepping outside, breathing in the fresh air, and brushing off winter's remnants from the garden. Now is the moment for nurturing new life, seeding and planting, and prepping for the upcoming season. This period or autumn is the perfect time for redesigning your herb garden or starting a new one. At the beginning of this phase, you'll be able to harvest only the herbs that have made it through the winter. Among the first ones to sprout are chives, angelica, fennel, mint, sorrel, and lemon balm. However, by late spring, the entire herb garden is teeming and ready for harvesting.

GROW:
• Start sowing seeds of annual herbs either indoors from early spring or directly outside when late spring arrives, following the guidelines given on the seed packet.
• Sow seeds of herbaceous perennials and shrubs according to the season recommended on the packet. Check seeds sown in autumn and left outside during winter.
• As the seedlings begin to sprout, thin them out and transfer the healthiest ones to pots for planting outdoors in late spring and early summer.
• Segment herbaceous perennials and replant the divisions or pot them up.
• Plant new herbs outside and ensure they receive ample water during establishment if the weather is dry.

MAINTAIN:
• Prune old stems of herbaceous perennials back to the ground level.
• Clear out old growth, leaves, and winter debris (which can be composted) to reveal self-seeded plants. Transplant or pot up desired plants such as fennel or borage or let them stay.
• Meticulously weed the garden to eliminate perennial weed roots, and aerate compacted soil with a garden fork.
• If the soil is excessively dry, water it thoroughly before spreading mulch. If required, blend in an organic, slow-release granular fertilizer, ensuring the mulch doesn't touch plant bases or trunks.
• Water the garden as necessary during dry periods.
• Neaten up pots by weeding and mulching, repotting where necessary.
• Begin feeding pots with organic liquid fertilizer from early spring.
• Once the threat of frost is minimal, remove winter protection like cloches during the daytime initially, and gradually relocate potted plants that overwintered indoors once it's warm enough.

PRUNE:
• To manage their growth, decisively prune shrubs like elder and rosemary in early spring, if required.
• Once the threat of severe frost is past in mid- or late spring, shape shrubs and subshrubs like bay, sage, thyme, and hyssop neatly.
• Guide new growth of climbers and replace or loosen old ties as necessary.

Summer

Herbs truly shine in summer, exhibiting their most vibrant and succulent growth in the early to mid-season. Moreover, they provide a continuous yield over the growing season as they flower and seed.

During summer, all herbs are ready to be harvested in one form or another. Gather leaves as required and snip bundles for drying before they flower to use when fresh foliage is not at hand. Harvest the flowers for culinary use or decoration, and collect the seeds for cooking or sowing the following year.

GROW:
• By early summer, plant any herbs sown in spring that have not yet been moved outdoors, either in the ground or large pots.
• Continue sowing annuals outside in early summer and once more in late summer for overwintering, following the instructions on the packet.
• Take cuttings of perennials and shrubs.

MAINTAIN
• Regular deadheading will help sustain repeat-flowering plants like marigolds.
• After herbaceous perennials have bloomed, trim them back to stimulate new foliage growth before fall.
• Prune back completely to the ground (ideal for herbs like chives) or to a lower stem point (for herbs like mints and lemon balm).
• Continue watering as necessary, particularly for potted plants, and apply a liquid fertilizer to pots every couple of weeks.
• Remove weeds as needed, ideally before they can bloom and seed.

PRUNE:
• After flowering, prune shrubs like lavender and thyme to prevent them from growing leggy. Trim back to a leaf, discarding the flowered stem part.
• Trim hedges in midsummer to maintain their shape.
• Prevent mints from spreading by cutting off the stolons as they grow over the edges of pots or along the ground.

Autumn

As the growing season winds down, it's time to preserve the remaining harvest and reflect on the triumphs and trials of your garden. An 'evaluation' is an extremely helpful exercise - jot down potential changes, plants to relocate, or strategies to adopt for the coming year. If a redesign or new bed has been in the works since the summer, this is the ideal time to prep the soil and plant.

Many plants continue to yield harvestable seeds and sometimes fruit into the fall. Even annuals such as basil can linger a while if the initial frosts are tardy. However, as the days become chillier and darker, basil leaves harden and become coarse, so collect any soft ones and use or preserve them early in the fall. Evergreen herbs will survive and allow picking into the winter.

GROW:

• Dig up a small portion of herbs like mint and chives, including an ample amount of roots, and pot for indoor growth. This way, they can provide fresh leaves all winter long.
• Sow seeds that need the winter cold ('stratification') to sprout, or of any herbs to start growing now for bigger, earlier plants to transplant in the spring. Check each seed packet for additional details.
• If still suitable, propagate herbs from cuttings.
• Split herbaceous perennials in early autumn. Replant the sections to increase stock or pot up to share.

MAINTAIN:

• Ensure new plantings are adequately watered until they are established, particularly if the season is dry.
• Thoroughly weed the garden.
• Apply a layer of mulch now if it wasn't added in the spring; nevertheless, an autumn mulch can be added in addition to the spring layer where the soil needs improvement.
• Keep an eye on the garden and remove any fallen stems that land on other plants.
• If frost is predicted, move potted plants needing winter protection under cover and erect cloches or similar over ground plants.

PRUNE:

• Secure any long, flailing stems of climbers before winter winds lash and snap them.
• Prune back herbaceous perennials where their dead growth is damp (such as angelica and lovage); where the stems could damage other plants if they fall (like fennel); or where self-seeding is unwanted. Other stems can be left - the seed heads can be appealing and provide sustenance and shelter for birds and invertebrates.

Winter

Contrary to popular beliefs, winter is not be a period of inactivity at least for the astute gardener. Considering potential new plantings, sketching ideas, and perusing books and catalogs (but remember the size of your garden when ordering!) are all valuable tasks. Outdoors, keep an eye out to prevent any damage.

Aside from overwintered and indoor herbs, winter harvests are mainly limited to evergreen shrubs like rosemary and thyme, and resilient plants like parsley. Be careful not to harvest too heavily.

GROW:

• Sow chili seeds in late winter, following the instructions on the packet.
• Sow other leafy annuals for microgreen harvest, provided there is sufficient light and some basal heat, such as from a heated propagator.

MAINTAIN:

• To enhance winter harvests, keep parsley under the protection of a cloche or similar.
• Ensure the soil in pots doesn't dry out completely.
• Particularly in windy weather, check that winter protections are still effective.
• Cut back any stems or other growth from herbaceous perennials that have fallen onto lower plants.
• To prevent splitting and to allow light to penetrate, brush or shake off heavy snow from the tops of plants and from cloches and fleece coverings.
• Prepare for the upcoming growing season by cleaning pots and tools.

Medicinal Herb Garden

Herbalists have a broad definition of "herb," encompassing any plant or plant part used for promoting health, including mushrooms. However, from a botanical perspective, an "herb" refers specifically to leafy plants that die back in winter and lack woody stems. Garden centers and horticulturists may also limit the term "herbs" to culinary plants with leafy mounds of growth. Chefs often refer to "herbs" as the leaves of culinary plants, distinguishing them from spices like seeds, roots, and barks. While there are already excellent herbal products available in the market, there are compelling reasons to grow your own plants and create your own remedies. Working directly with plants and making personal remedies enhances your skills as an herbalist, improves your well-being, increases your effectiveness as a practitioner, and contributes to your overall growth as a person.

Here are six reasons why growing your own herbs is worthwhile:

1. **Freshness**: Creating remedies with fresh herbs allows you to customize them according to your preferences, resulting in stronger and more potent remedies compared to store-bought alternatives.
2. **Cost-effectiveness**: Making your own herbal remedies can be much more affordable, as you can produce potent remedies at a fraction of the retail cost. This becomes especially evident when compared to purchasing small quantities of commercial products.
3. **Customization**: Instead of amassing a wide range of remedies, carefully consider the best plants for your specific needs. Start with small quantities, gradually building an herbal medicine cabinet tailored to you and your family. Crafting your own blends can be more effective than pre-made formulas, and it's an enjoyable process.
4. **Self-sufficiency and empowerment**: Growing your own herbs allows you to access remedies directly from your backyard or medicine cabinet, providing a sense of self-sufficiency. You don't need to rely on running to the store for every ailment. The more you learn about plants and gain confidence in your skills as a home herbalist, the stronger and more empowered you'll feel in taking care of yourself, your family, your community, and the environment.
5. **Sustainability, stewardship, and confidence**: By growing your own herbs, you ensure access to high-quality plants. You develop a connection with the plants, ensuring their authenticity and promoting sustainability by avoiding unethically harvested herbs in commerce. Becoming a steward of your land and the plant kingdom, you contribute to a deeper ecological balance that benefits not only the plants but also the diverse organisms that rely on them.
6. **Connection**: Growing, harvesting, and making medicine with plants allows you to establish a deeper connection with your remedies. It goes beyond a simple powder or pill—it involves communing with individual plants and immersing yourself in the broader ecosystem. Nature has healing qualities, whether through nibbling on a leaf or appreciating the beauty of flowers and their pollinators.

When selecting herbs to grow, consider the following:
- Choose herbs that address your specific health needs and align with the benefits you desire.
- Consider the plants that thrive in your growing conditions and environment, including native species.
- Trust your intuition and listen to how your body responds to different herbs. Experiment with small quantities to determine which plants resonate with you and produce the desired effects.

Remember, your herb garden doesn't need to start with an extensive collection. Begin with a few plants that genuinely attract your interest and get to know them intimately before expanding your herbal garden.

Remember the basics

Observation is indeed a crucial first step in creating a successful garden, as highlighted in the chapter on designing a native garden. By closely observing your property throughout the seasons, you can gather valuable insights that will guide your gardening decisions. Here are some key aspects to observe:

1. **Plant Growth and Placement**: Pay attention to the natural distribution of plants on your property. Notice which plants thrive in specific areas, as this can indicate their preferred growing conditions. For example, the presence of horsetail and jewelweed suggests a damp spot. Identify areas with different light conditions, such as full sun, shade, or partial shade.
2. **Soil Characteristics**: Observe variations in soil composition across your property. Hills or slopes may have drier, sandier, or rockier soil at the top, while the bottom might be moister and more fertile. While some plants have specific soil preferences, most plants will do well in well-drained soil rich in organic matter. Conducting a soil test can provide you with important information about the soil's pH and nutrient levels, helping you determine if any amendments are necessary.

3. **Microclimates:** Take note of microclimates created by buildings, fences, or stone walls. These structures can create areas of shade, reflect heat and sunlight, and offer protection from wind, light frosts, and animal activity. Identify north-facing areas that receive minimal sunlight, south-facing areas that are sunny, and east/west-facing spots that receive varying levels of shade throughout the day. Planting the same type of plant in different microclimates can help you identify the optimal location for its growth.

By observing these factors, you can make informed decisions about plant selection and placement, optimizing the growing conditions for each species. Additionally, consulting your local extension office or organic land care organization can provide valuable tips and information about soil testing companies, further enhancing your understanding of your garden's unique characteristics.

Building a Bed

When it comes to building garden beds, the lazy lasagna gardening method is a simple approach that works well regardless of your soil type. Begin by selecting the location and size of your garden bed and deciding whether you want to frame it with materials like wood, brick, stones, or simply edge it with a lawn edging tool. For formal beds, such as those for culinary herbs that require regular harvesting and tending, it's best to avoid making the bed too wide to ensure easy access without stepping on the soil. A width of three to four feet is typically suitable. If possible, construct the bed in the fall so you can plant in the spring. This allows the soil to settle and gives beneficial microbes time to thrive. However, if you're short on time, you can build and plant your beds on the same day.

Here's a step-by-step breakdown:

1. **Optional Soil Loosening:** To improve the quality of your soil and promote deeper penetration, you can use a broad fork to break up compacted soil. This step is not essential but can be beneficial.
2. **Cardboard or Newspaper Base:** Lay flattened cardboard boxes (although not technically organic due to glue, they are effective and readily available) or several layers of wet black-and-white newspaper over the designated area. This technique helps smother grass and most weeds, and over time, the base will break down into the soil as the bed becomes established.
3. **Edging or Framing:** Use an edger tool to create a perimeter around the bed or construct a bed frame. If stone is not within your budget, untreated pine boards are a convenient and relatively affordable option, lasting 5 to 10 years in our yard. Opt for boards that are 2 inches thick and 6 to 8 inches wide. Cedar is more expensive but offers increased durability. Avoid pressure-treated wood, as it can release toxic chemicals into the soil.

4. **Filling the Bed:** Begin by layering twigs and small branches at the bottom of the bed for drainage, followed by a thick layer of leaves or straw. Then add a mixture of loam and compost. If you have sufficient space and materials, continue layering in this manner until the bed is full. Use compost covered with leaf mulch for the top layer. Over time, the soil will naturally settle.
5. **Planting:** When you're ready to plant your seedlings, gently pull back the mulch and dig a hole slightly larger than the plant's root system. Carefully remove the plant from its pot and untangle any bound roots. Place the plant flush with the soil line in the hole, fill in with soil, and gently tamp down the soil around it. If desired, create a small indentation in the soil to help retain water or slightly raise the plant in waterlogged areas. Water the plant thoroughly and surround it with mulch.

After planting, keep a close eye on the newly planted seedlings and water them periodically until they become established. If possible, choose a day with light rain in the forecast to plant, rather than during hot sun. Avoid planting most annuals and tender perennials until the threat of frost has passed. Tender perennials are herbs that can only survive year-round in warm climates and are prone to perishing if exposed to frost. If possible, gradually acclimate new seedlings to the outdoors by placing them outside for increasing periods, or at least wait for a week of mild weather before planting.

Getting Supplies

To obtain organic compost and loam, consider purchasing them from landscape supply companies that offer delivery services. They typically deliver by the truckload or square yard. Alternatively, you can gather loam from other areas of your yard, such as a spot where you have been depositing grass clippings and leaves over the years. If you have access to well-aged manure, either from your own livestock or local farms, it can be a valuable addition to your soil. Keep in mind that horse manure may contain more weed seeds, but it is often readily available.

In our own soil improvement project, we introduced a small flock of chickens to our property, and they have been incredibly beneficial. We apply their coop shavings to the beds during fall and winter, covering them with leaf mulch. However, it's important to note that crops in these beds should not be harvested until 90 to 120 days after the application of chicken coop shavings for safety reasons. Additionally, composting grass clippings, garden waste, and kitchen waste can provide valuable organic matter for your garden. Using chopped leaf mulch saved from the previous fall can help retain moisture, reduce weed pressure, and gradually enhance the soil ecology. It serves as an excellent option for enriching your garden beds. Lastly, building a medicine wheel garden is another exciting option that you can explore in the next volume of this series. You will gain in-depth knowledge about this type of garden and its unique benefits. But here is a snippet to get you interested.

The Medicine Wheel Garden

The circle represents infinity since it has neither beginning nor end and is all-encompassing. For ages, Native Americans have used this emblem in medicine wheel garden designs. What is the purpose of a medicine wheel garden?

There are various different medicine wheel garden designs, but they all have one thing in common: a circle that is divided into four unique garden regions and filled with medicine wheel garden plants.

Traditionally, it symbolized the connection to the cosmos and the Creator. Refer to the first volume for an in-depth examination of medicine and spirituality in Native Americans cultures. Modern medicine wheel garden design are an attempt to recreate this kinship with the land and a higher power, or it may just be a technique to include medicinal herbs and plants into the garden in a meaningful way. Refer to the next volume of the series to find out which plants suit best your personal medicine wheel garden and for a more in-depth examination of the meaning of the medicine wheel garden.

Building your garden

There are a few main types of medicine wheel gardens you could undertake.

1. The first is to draw a little circular rock outline in a location that holds significance for you. Additional stones can be used to divide the circle into quadrants. Then wait for natural plants to take root. Traditional herbalists think that the plants that self-sow in this sacred garden are the ones you most require.
2. Another medicine wheel garden idea has the same circular and quadrant pattern, but you get to choose which plants will be in each quadrant. Different plants can be planted in each segment. For example, one or two quadrants could be dedicated to culinary herbs, another to medicinal herbs, and yet another to native plants — or you could mix it up and include all three, as well as some annual blossoms and veggies.

Tools required:

The preparation for a medicine wheel garden is the same in each circumstance. For marking, gather five marker stakes, a hammer, measuring tape, compass, and rope or line.

The process:

1. Make a hole in the ground with a stake. This will serve as the garden's focal point. Use the compass to determine the four cardinal directions (N, W, E, and S) and mark them with a stake. The perimeter of the garden will be determined by the distance between the central stake and the cardinal stakes, which is entirely up to you.
2. Remove any sod or rocks from the interior of the circular garden. Smooth it out. If necessary, add compost to the soil. The medicine wheel garden plants you choose will determine what else the soil need. The soil should be well-draining and slightly alkaline in general.
3. To make trails, lay plastic or landscape fabric from each outer stake to the center, then cover them with gravel, rocks, or other material. Replace the stakes

with pebbles if desired, and then outline the rest of the garden area in the same way.

Your medicine wheel garden should be unique and tailored to your preferences. You can even build triangular beds to fit in the circle of the medicine wheel garden. The only criterion that must be followed is a circle with four sections fenced off. The circle's outline and bisections can be created using large, medium, or little stones or bricks, pavers, wood, or even seashells — whatever you choose, as long as it's natural. A medicine wheel garden can be further personalized by adding other features. Statuary, orbs, crystals, and other garden art will transform the garden into your own personal sanctuary.

Mulch

Embrace the power of mulch! As you discovered in the previous chapter, it offers numerous benefits for your garden, including weed prevention, moisture retention, organic matter enrichment, improved drainage, earthworm nourishment, and enhanced microbial and fungal diversity in the soil. Despite the potential drawbacks of using mulch, such as attracting slugs and ticks and reducing self-seeding activity, the benefits of mulching outweigh the risks. There are various materials available for mulching, including pine needles, wood chips, newspaper, straw, grass clippings, sawdust, wool, and leaves. Among these options, leaves are a personal favorite.

If feasible, it is recommended to shred or mow over the leaves before using them as mulch. This helps prevent them from smothering the soil, aids in their faster breakdown to enrich the soil, and allows perennials to emerge. During the fall season, leaves can be collected in a bag using a lawn mower and then deposited in a pile or directly onto the garden beds. It's important to ensure that the leaves come from yards without pesticide use and invasive seeds, such as bittersweet berries. Excessive amounts of oak, hemlock, or chestnut leaves should be avoided.

Wood chips are suitable for woodland plants and trees, but they take longer to decompose and may temporarily deplete nitrogen from the soil. To counteract this, organic fertilizer or blood meal can be sprinkled onto the area. Additionally, acquiring free wood chips from road crews trimming around power lines every few years can be a great resource for mulching shrub and tree beds along the forest's edge, as well as creating garden walkway paths.

Soil amendments and fertilizers

Aged manure and compost are excellent natural fertilizers that can provide ample nourishment for your garden, often eliminating the need for additional amendments. North Country Organics Pro-Gro is a recommended all-purpose fertilizer that can be sprinkled in with new plants or used in spring to give your plants a boost. Neptune's Harvest fish and seaweed emulsion is also popular, although it may attract raccoons and skunks due to its fish content. Biochar is a beneficial amendment that enhances nutrient and water retention in the soil. Depending on the specific needs of your soil, organic amendments like blood meal, fish emulsion, seaweed, greensand, lime, wood ash, and other nutrient-rich materials can be considered. Local non-profit organic associations can provide guidance on where to obtain a soil test and purchase these items. They may offer bulk orders, and well-stocked feed and farm stores might carry organic fertilizers as well.

However, it's important to note that compost, manure, and mulch often don't suffice in balancing and improving various soil types over time. But, if you opt for native plants and carefully plan your garden design, you may not need any additional soil amendments. Native plants have the remarkable ability to thrive without external assistance, making them a sustainable choice for your garden.

The Lifespan of a Plant

Herbs can vary in their life cycles, with some needing to be replanted each year, others living on a specific two-year cycle, and some being long-lived perennials. The specific life cycle of an herb depends on factors such as the planting zone and freezing temperatures.

Annual herbs complete their life cycle within a year, dying after the first frost or once they have set seed. They can be replanted each year or allowed to self-seed for the next growing season. Examples of annual herbs include calendula and dill.

Perennial herbs, on the other hand, return each year, continuing to grow and thrive. The majority of herbs fall into this category, such as lemon and bee balm.

Biennial herbs have a two-year life cycle. During the first year, they focus on herbaceous growth, and in the second year, they produce flowers and fruits or seeds before dying. Examples of biennial herbs include burdock, mullein, and foxglove.

Tender perennials are herbs that can survive winter only in warm climates. In colder regions, they are typically treated as annuals or brought indoors for protection. Examples of tender perennials are lemongrass, lemon verbena, gotu kola, bacopa, ashwagandha, and rosemary.

Short-lived perennials are herbs that have a relatively short lifespan, easily dying off or lasting around three years. Examples include artichoke (in warm climates), St. John's wort, and certain mallows. When growing herbs, it's important to consider the time it takes for them to establish themselves. Some plants may require more time before they can be harvested for medicinal purposes. In such cases, you may opt for wild trees like cherry bark and birch, which can often be found in established form for pruning. Additionally, it may take several years for shrubs and trees to produce flowers and berries. The age of the plant, species, and growing conditions all play a role in determining when they will reach maturity. Providing full sun, good soil, and regular moisture can promote faster growth and increased flower and fruit production.

Follow these guidelines for the plants that can be harvested for medicinal purpose only after they have established themselves.

Garlic: plant in the fall, harvest the following summer

Biennial roots: in the fall of the first year or spring of the second (before it flowers)
Examples: mullein, burdock

Most perennial roots: 2–3+ years (but when you weed them, use all that good stuff!)
Examples: yellow dock, marshmallow, valerian, elecampane
Echinacea roots: 3–4 years

Black cohosh roots: 3+ years

Mimosa bark/flowers: 2+ years

Roses/hips: 3–5 years

Elderflowers/berries: 3–5 years

Hawthorn flowers/berries: 3–10 years

Linden flowers: 5–10 years

Most bark: 2–5 years (or as a rule of thumb when they are big enough to prune)
Examples: cramp bark, wild cherry, mimosa, birch

Common garden herbs

Let's take a look at the most common plants for a medical herb garden that can be used in the kitchen as well.
The following plants are not native to the United States and therefore were integrated only later or not at all in Native American medicine.
Even if they are helpful and yummy added to savory and sweet dishes (which is why I have included them), I really encourage you to choose native plants with the help of the next volume, tailored to your medical needs and your environment.

Garlic

Habitat: The Garlic plant (Allium sativum) is native to Central Asia, specifically in the region that includes present-day Kazakhstan, Uzbekistan, and Tajikistan. However, it has been widely cultivated and naturalized in many parts of the world, including Italy and southern France. In these regions, garlic has become a staple ingredient in the local cuisine and is used in a variety of national dishes. Its distinct flavor and aroma add depth and character to numerous recipes, making it a popular and beloved ingredient in Mediterranean and French cooking traditions.

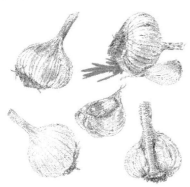

Identification: Garlic plants typically have a height of around 60 cm (2 feet). They have long leaves that emerge either from a short, hard stem above the bulb or from a softer pseudostem composed of overlapping leaf sheaths, depending on the specific cultivar. The bulb of the garlic plant is covered in a protective membrane skin and contains multiple cloves, which are edible bulblets. When the garlic plant flowers, the bracts surrounding the flowers split apart, revealing a spherical flower cluster enclosed by papery, tapering bracts. Occasionally, flower stalks may produce sterile blossoms and small bulbils, which are secondary bulbs that grow in place of flowers. Garlic is typically cultivated as an annual crop, with cloves or top bulbils used for reproduction and propagation.

Taste: The bulbs have a strong onion-like scent and a harsh flavor, therefore they are rarely eaten fresh.

Medicinal parts: The plant's bulbs contain the most medicinal properties, however, the green stems of the plant offer some benefits as well.

Medicinal Uses: Garlic is a vital plant for managing respiratory tract infections, including cold, flu, pneumonia, bronchitis, tonsillitis, strep throat, and sinus infections. This is because some of the most antimicrobial aspects of garlic you've ingested exit the body through the lungs as you exhale—that's how you get garlic breath. On the way out, they directly destroy fungi and bacteria while stimulating an immune response against viruses in the mucous membranes. This makes garlic a remedy specific to microbial infections of the lungs. These antimicrobial agents function anywhere they can reach, so topical application of garlic—to a wound on the skin, in the digestive tract, or at the site of other infections—will also be antibacterial and antifungal. However, raw garlic can also cause damage to skin and digestive tract tissue, so it's important to buffer garlic's heating action with oil when applying it to the skin and to be conscious of your body's reaction when consuming raw garlic. If raw garlic is too intense, consider "pickling" it—combine peeled garlic cloves in a jar with half apple cider vinegar and half honey and let soak for a month. Garlic pickles retain all the benefits but are gentler on the digestive system. By improving the quality of the blood and stimulating circulation while lowering blood pressure, garlic can have beneficial effects on the cardiovascular system. Plus, garlic is packed with antioxidants, which help lower cholesterol levels.

Gardening Tips: To grow garlic, you can plant bulbs "in the green" or sow seeds in a location that receives dappled shade and has rich, moist soil. When planting bulbs, choose a spot with suitable conditions and gently press them into the soil at the appropriate depth. If sowing seeds, follow the instructions on the seed packet for proper planting depth and spacing. Garlic plants prefer soil that is well-drained and rich in organic matter. In early summer, after the leaves have died back, you can cut them back to keep the garden tidy. This will also allow the energy to focus on bulb development below ground. Removing seed heads is recommended to prevent the plants from spreading extensively, as garlic can self-propagate through both bulbs and seeds. By preventing seed production, you can control the spread of garlic and ensure that its multiplication remains more contained within the planting area.

Rosemary

Habitat: Rosemary (Rosmarinus officinalis) is a herb that is native to the dry and rocky regions of the Mediterranean, especially along the coast. The name "Rosmarinus" is derived from the Latin words "ros" and "marinus," which translate to "dew" and "sea," respectively. This name reflects the herb's ability to thrive in coastal areas where it can capture the moisture from the sea air. Rosemary has a long history of use by the Greeks and Romans, dating back to ancient times. It was highly valued for its aromatic fragrance, culinary uses, and medicinal properties. The ancient Greeks believed that rosemary improved memory and mental clarity, and it was often used in religious ceremonies and as a symbol of remembrance.

Due to its resilience and adaptability, rosemary has spread beyond its native Mediterranean range and is now cultivated and enjoyed in many parts of the world.

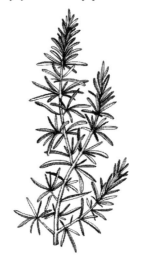

Identification: The plant can reach a height of 2-6 feet and a width of 2-4 feet, and it blooms from June to July. It is preferable to cultivate Rosemary indoors for the first winter and then put them outside in late spring. From stiff, tall kinds to rounded bushes and squat, thick tufts to rock-hugging creepers, Rosemary comes in a variety of forms. Height might range from 1 foot to 6 feet or more. Plants are densely covered in slender, resinous, aromatic leaves that are normally 1 to 1 inch long and lustrous dark green above, grayish white beneath. Throughout the winter and spring, little clusters of – to inches blooms in various colors of blue (rarely pink or white) emerge; the bloom occasionally returns in the fall.

Taste: The leaves are floral, nearly pine-like in taste.

Medicinal parts: The leaves are the part of the plant generally used, however Rosemary flowers are also edible.

Medicinal Uses: Rosemary has a rich history in traditional medicine and has been associated with several potential health benefits. It is believed to have properties that can help relieve muscle pain, improve blood circulation, strengthen the immune system, enhance memory, promote hair growth, aid in digestion, and protect brain health and eye health. The antioxidants and anti-inflammatory compounds found in rosemary are thought to contribute to these effects. However, further research is needed to fully understand the mechanisms and effectiveness of rosemary in treating specific health conditions. As always, it is advisable to consult with a healthcare professional before using rosemary for medicinal purposes, particularly if you have any existing medical conditions or are taking medications.

Gardening Tips: For optimal growth, rosemary prefers well-drained soil and full sun exposure. It is important to avoid consistently wet soil, especially during the winter months, as rosemary does not tolerate excessive moisture. Pruning rosemary after it flowers is recommended as it helps stimulate bushier growth and allows for maintaining its desired shape. By trimming back the plant, you can encourage new growth and keep the rosemary plant healthy and attractive.

Basil

Habitat: Basil is a tropical and subtropical Asian annual herb that is so easy to grow that even inexperienced gardeners can plant it with confidence. It grows well in hot, humid environments and blooms from spring until frost throughout the South.

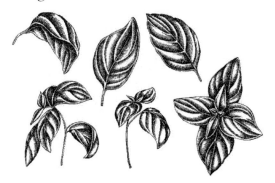

Identification: The 2 foot-tall, bushy plant produces spikes of little white or pinkish flowers, but it's renowned for its shining green leaves, which are oval in shape and 12 inches long, with a clovelike scent and spicy-sweet flavor that make them necessary in the kitchen. There are countless variations on the subject, such as purple or variegated foliage, dwarf globe or columnar habits, huge or tiny leaves, and white, pink, or purple flowers.

Taste: Herbal and pungent, Basil is a frequently topping sought out for slices of pizza and making fresh pesto.

Medicinal parts: While the leaves are the most sought-after part of the plant, Basil flowers are potent and fresh as well, offering a sharper flavor as compared to the mild leaves.

Medicinal Uses: Basil offers numerous health benefits when consumed in the diet, used as herbal medicine, or as an essential oil. Traditionally, basil has been used for treating snakebites, colds, and nasal inflammation associated with colds. It contains macronutrients like calcium and vitamin K, as well as various antioxidants that contribute to its health-promoting properties. Different basil varieties contain specific chemical compounds that give them unique scents and additional health benefits. For instance, sweet basil contains a high concentration of eugenol, which gives it a clove-like aroma and possesses antioxidant properties. Lime and lemon basils contain high levels of limonene, providing a citrusy scent and additional antioxidant benefits.

Tulsi, also known as Holy Basil, is a specific basil species with notable therapeutic properties. It has traditionally been used for addressing "stuck emotions" such as depression, PTSD, and general moodiness. Recent research has revealed that tulsi can help restore the brain's ability to convert short-term memory into long-term memory, assisting individuals in moving past difficult experiences and emotions. Tulsi also uplifts the spirit and acts as an adaptogen, promoting hormone balance and offering support for various issues like sleep troubles, blood sugar regulation, and menopause. Additionally, tulsi can aid in moderating cravings, making it beneficial for those aiming to reduce sugar intake, overcome food allergies, or quit smoking or drinking. Tulsi is known for its diaphoretic properties, meaning it helps induce sweating and is useful for managing fevers and flu symptoms. In Hindu cultures, basil holds religious significance and is grown extensively for its protective influence on temples and homes. Furthermore, basil branches can be hung to repel insects, including mosquitoes. Overall, basil, particularly tulsi, provides a wide range of health benefits and is valued both for its culinary use and its role in traditional medicine and cultural practices.

Gardening Tips: Basil plants thrive in warm conditions and require ample sunlight to flourish. In cool-temperate climates, it is best to grow them under cover or on a sunny windowsill to provide the necessary warmth. Basil prefers well-draining soil that is light in texture. Most culinary basil varieties are annuals, meaning they need to be re-sown each year. It is advisable to discard old plants after their growing season. However, there are tender perennial varieties such as 'African Blue' that can be overwintered in a heated greenhouse or propagated through cuttings to ensure their survival for multiple seasons. To promote bushier growth in basil plants, it is recommended to regularly pinch out the growing tips. This practice encourages lateral branching and results in a fuller and more compact plant.

Spearmint

Habitat: The mentha spicata grows in damp areas, such as along stream banks and along shorelines. This herb may grow from low elevations in the mountains to higher elevations. The Juncas and Veronicas are two species that are closely related. Although it is native to Europe, it is widely distributed throughout temperate North America.

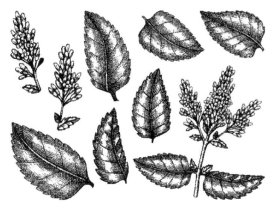

Identification: Looking like a small bush that spreads quickly, the opposite leaves are 2-8cm long, 6-40mm broad, narrow-oval to elliptic-oval, gradually tapering to a pointy tip, and strongly serrated along the margins, and attach directly to the stem. The lavender flowers have a 5-lobed tube-shaped calyx and a 4-lobed tube-shaped corolla and are 3-5mm long. From June through August, this plant blooms, in other parts of the year, the bush will be magnificently green.

Taste: Sweet with a cooling, prickly sensation.

Medicinal parts: The leaves

Medicinal Uses: Spearmint is known for its medicinal properties and has been used to treat various ailments including flu, colds, headaches, skin conditions, nausea, and irritable bowel syndrome (IBS). It is also valued for its calming effects. Traditional uses of spearmint include the treatment of flatulence, menstrual pain, diarrhea, nerve and muscle pain, and indigestion. One of the key benefits of spearmint is its ability to soothe the muscles in the stomach and enhance bile flow, which makes it an effective remedy for indigestion. The menthol compound present in spearmint improves blood circulation and provides a cooling sensation that helps alleviate pain. This quality makes it particularly helpful in relieving menstrual cramps.

In addition, spearmint possesses anti-inflammatory, antiviral, and antibacterial properties. These attributes make it a suitable choice for relieving sinus congestion caused by allergies, infections, or the common cold. The menthol content in spearmint contributes to improving airflow in the nasal cavity, providing relief from nasal congestion.

Gardening tips: When planting spearmint, it is recommended to choose a location with moist and nutrient-rich soil. It can thrive in both partial shade and full sun. However, it's important to note that spearmint has a tendency to spread rapidly through its creeping stolons, which are overground roots. Without proper monitoring, it can become invasive and overtake other plants in the area. To control its growth, planting spearmint in a large pot, container, or a dedicated raised bed is a good solution.

After spearmint flowers, it is advisable to cut it back to the ground. This promotes the growth of fresh leaves, ensuring a continuous supply. In autumn, once the stems have died back, it is recommended to cut the plant down to the ground for maintenance and to prepare it for the following season. By following these practices, you can keep your spearmint plant healthy and prevent it from spreading uncontrollably.

Lemon Balm

Habitat: Lemon Balm, Melissa Officinalis, is widely grown in Europe, but it is primarily grown in the United States. It can be seen growing wild in sunny fields and along highways. It's a perennial that can be grown from seed or by root division in rich, sandy, or loamy soil

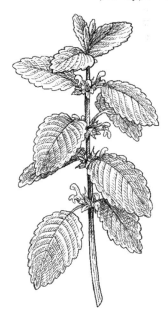

Identification: The square, branching erect stem grows to about 3 feet in height. The leaves are brilliant green, oval, and serrate, and grow in opposing pairs. When crushed, the entire plant has fine hairs and a citrus smell. The blooms are two-lipped, bilabiate, yellow-white to rose-colored or even bluish, and occur in clusters at the joints or on little branches at the joints. From July to August, it blooms.

Taste: Citrusy with a slight pang.

Medicinal parts: The leaves

Medicinal Uses: Lemon balm optimizes digestive and immune health and helps balance the nervous system. It effectively calms bloating, gas, and indigestion. Lemon balm promotes relaxation and aids in managing stress. It supports cognitive function, improving focus and maintaining a calm state. Lemon balm has a positive impact on sleep, making it helpful for insomnia. Its mild sedative properties promote relaxation and restful sleep. Drinking a cup of chamomile and lemon balm tea a few hours before bedtime can contribute to better sleep. Incorporating lemon balm into your daily routine, for example enjoying a nightlylemon balm tea, can enhance overall well-being. It supports digestive health, boosts the immune system, balances the nervous system, promotes relaxation, and improves sleep quality.

Gardening Tips: To grow lemon balm, choose a location with moist, rich soil and provide it with full sun or partial shade. After the plant has finished flowering, trim it back to the ground. This will encourage the growth of fresh leaves and prevent the plant from self-sowing too widely. In autumn, when the stems have died back, cut the plant down to the ground. Following these maintenance steps will help you keep your lemon balm healthy and thriving.

Fennel

Habitat: Fennel (Foeniculum vulgare) is a perennial herb belonging to the Apiaceae family. It is renowned for its edible shoots, leaves, and seeds. Native to southern Europe and Asia Minor, fennel is widely cultivated. However, it should be noted that it is considered an invasive species in certain regions, such as Australia and parts of the United States.

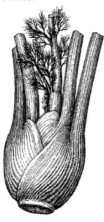

Identification: Cultivated fennel typically reaches a height of approximately 3 feet. Its stalks are adorned with finely divided leaves consisting of several linear or awl-shaped segments. The plant produces small yellow flowers arranged in grayish complex umbels. The fruits of fennel are greenish brown to yellowish brown oblong ovals, measuring about ¼ inch in length. These fruits have five noticeable longitudinal dorsal ridges and are dry in nature.

Taste: A distinctly licorice taste with a floral aftertaste.

Medicinal parts: Shoots, leaves, and seeds.

Medicinal Uses: Fennel is a warming herb known for its ability to improve digestion and liver function. It is particularly beneficial in counteracting the cold and stagnant conditions commonly seen in our population today. This herb is effective in relieving gas and bloating in both adults and children, as well as colic in babies. Fennel can be added directly to foods that may cause gas or bloating, or consumed as a tea after meals. For babies,

a small amount of fennel tea given on a spoon or through a dropper can be quite effective. Additionally, fennel has antispasmodic properties, making it a valuable remedy for intestinal cramping, whether it is due to temporary indigestion or a chronic condition such as irritable bowel syndrome (IBS). Its antispasmodic action is also beneficial in soothing menstrual cramps and relieving the constriction and spasms associated with asthma.

Gardening Tips: Fennel is a versatile plant that can grow in various soil types and positions, but it thrives best in full sun and well-drained soil. It has a tendency to self-sow, spreading around the garden, unless the flowers are deadheaded to prevent seed production. In autumn or winter, it is recommended to cut back any dead stems to maintain the plant's health and appearance.

Oregano

Habitat: Origanum vulgare, commonly known as oregano or wild marjoram, is a fragrant perennial herb from the mint family (Lamiaceae) that is highly valued for its aromatic dried leaves and flowering tops. Originally hailing from the hills of Europe and western Asia, oregano has adapted and become naturalized in certain regions of Mexico and the United States.

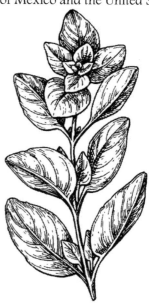

Identification: In regions with mild climates, oregano is typically cultivated as a small evergreen subshrub. Its compact oval leaves are arranged in pairs on opposite sides of the stem and are covered with glandular trichomes, giving them a slightly fuzzy texture. The young stems are typically square-shaped and covered in fine hairs, while older stems become woody. Oregano produces small clustered flowers that can vary in color from white to pink to pale purple.

Taste: Peppery and earthy bite.

Medicinal parts: The leaves.

Medicinal Uses: Oregano possesses digestive and antifungal properties that make it beneficial for various conditions. It can be used to address chronic candidiasis due to its antifungal properties. To ensure its effectiveness in the stomach and intestines, oregano capsules are recommended for this ailment. Supplementing with oregano can also aid in treating low stomach acidity, heartburn, and indigestion. Oregano helps alleviate gas and soothe an upset stomach. Its antifungal and antimicrobial properties, derived from compounds like carvacrol and thymol, make it effective against Candida Albicans and various bacteria such as staphylococcus aureus, salmonella enteric, klebsiella pneumonia, and Escherichia coli. Oregano contains beneficial components such as vitamin C, vitamin A, sterols, oleanolic acid, ursolic acid, triterpenoids, rosmarinic acid, borneol, thymol, and carvacrol. For treating infections, oregano tea can be consumed or the oil can be topically applied to the skin. It's important to dilute the oil with a carrier oil to prevent skin irritation, as it can cause burns if applied directly. However, it should never be ingested internally. Oregano tea is prepared using dried leaves of the oregano plant.

Gardening Tips: Oregano can be grown from seeds, which are typically planted in the garden after the last frost has passed. Alternatively, you can propagate it from cuttings or use established plants. It is important to ensure that the soil temperature is around 70 degrees Fahrenheit before initiating any planting. When planting oregano, spacing them approximately ten inches apart is recommended. This herb thrives in warm, sunny locations with well-drained to dry soil conditions. To encourage the growth of fresh leaves, it is advisable to trim back the stems once flowering has concluded.

Lovage

Habitat: Lovage comes from the Mediterranean region of Europe/Asia, however, the plant grows well in many climate zones that have temperate months.

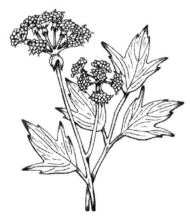

Identification: Divided, glossy, deep green leaves grow to be 2 feet long on this ornamental herb. In the summer, hollow stems emerge from the leaves clumps, crowned by flat-topped, greenish yellow flower clusters. In ideal conditions, flowering plants can grow to be 6 feet tall and wide, although the average height is 3 feet tall and spread.

Taste: Celery-like flavor profile. The leaves of the plant carry an herbaceous quality like a floral licorice.

Medicinal parts: Leaves when green and fully grown are the most beneficial. Lovage seeds are excellent for cooking.

Medicinal Uses: Lovage, a plant with origins in the Mediterranean, has been used for centuries in herbal remedies. It has found its way into alcoholic beverages and various recipes worldwide. Its medicinal properties include anti-inflammatory effects, skin conditioning, menstrual support, and gastric relief. One of its well-known uses is as a digestive aid, providing relief from flatulence and stomach discomfort. Lovage has also been valued for its ability to strengthen the heart, aid in respiratory health, act as a diuretic, treat kidney stones, and purify the blood. In medieval times, it was employed as a treatment for gout, rheumatism, and skin issues. Lovage remedies have a long history dating back to the 12th century and were significant in the teachings of the medieval School of Salerno. Nutritionally, lovage is rich in various nutrients and minerals, including abundant amounts of vitamin C and B complex. It contains quercetin, which helps inhibit histamine and alleviate allergy symptoms. Many women have reported finding relief from menstrual symptoms by using lovage supplements. Extracts of lovage in cosmetics can aid in reducing acne, promoting clear skin, and treating dermatitis. Additionally, lovage's diuretic properties make it useful in body cleansing routines without causing electrolyte loss. This attribute also contributes to its potential to support kidney health. The herb shows promise in easing arthritis sensitivity, improving respiratory processes, and possessing antibacterial properties.

Gardening Tips: Plant lovage in well-drained, fertile soil that receives full sun or partial shade. Ensure the soil remains consistently moist for optimal growth. If you do not plan to harvest the seeds, it is recommended to cut down the stems after flowering. This will encourage the development of fresh, leafy growth. In autumn, when the stems have died back, cut them down again to prepare the plant for the dormant season. By following these pruning practices, you can maintain the health and vitality of your lovage plant.

Coriander (Cilantro)

Habitat: Coriander, scientifically known as Coriandrum sativum, is an annual herb in the Apiaceae family, also referred to as cilantro or Chinese parsley. It is widely recognized as a popular herb and spice used in various cuisines. Although native to the Mediterranean and Middle East regions, coriander is cultivated worldwide for its culinary applications.

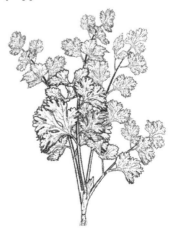

Identification: The coriander plant features a slender hollow stem and delicate bipinnate leaves, growing to a height of 1 to 2.5 inches. It produces small flowers in clusters known as umbels, which can be pink or whitish in color. The fruit of the coriander plant is a dry schizocarp, consisting of two semiglobular fruits fused together along their inner edges. This creates a single smooth and nearly spherical fruit, measuring approximately 0.2 inches in diameter. The fruits are yellowish brown, emitting a mild fragrance and offering a flavor that combines hints of lemon peel and sage.

Taste: Savory and peppery; traditionally used in many meat dishes.

Medicinal parts: Both the leaves and seeds have medicinal and culinary uses

Medicinal Uses: Cilantro, also known as coriander, has been used for its digestive properties, aiding in stimulating appetite, treating dyspepsia, and relieving gastrointestinal spasms. It has also been traditionally employed to alleviate chest pains and coughs, both when applied topically and taken internally. Cilantro has demonstrated effectiveness in managing conditions such as dysentery, diarrhea, vomiting, and indigestion. It possesses antispasmodic and expectorant qualities, making it useful for bronchitis and coughs. Additionally, cilantro can be applied topically to reduce inflammation associated with rheumatism and arthritis. The seeds of cilantro have been utilized to address insomnia and anxiety, as well as to alleviate flatulence. Research suggests that cilantro can contribute to reducing insulin resistance and lowering blood sugar levels. The seeds are also known to have cholesterol-lowering properties, making them beneficial for cardiovascular health. When cultivating cilantro, it is important to choose the appropriate variety based on whether you desire the leaves or seeds. Sow the seeds in well-drained soil under full sun, unless you intend to harvest the leaves and roots, in which case dappled shade is preferred to prevent premature bolting. Adequate watering is necessary to keep the plants healthy. Remove dead plants in autumn to maintain the garden's cleanliness.

Artichoke

Habitat: This formidable Mediterranean native thrives in well-prepared heavily mulched, compost-rich, mildly acidic soil with plenty of room to grow. One plant can reach 4 to 6 feet in height and width! It can be challenging in cooler climates; start it indoors. In subtropical climates, it will produce for several years. Cardoon (*C. cardunculus*) has similar properties.

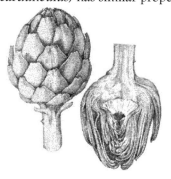

Identification: Artichoke grows into a tall plant, reaching heights of 4-6 feet. It features arching, deeply lobed, silvery, glaucous-green leaves that can measure 19-32 inches in length. The flowers of the artichoke form a large head, producing an edible bud that measures 3-6 inches in diameter. The bud is composed of interlacing triangular scales, with purple florets in the case of the globe artichoke variety. The edible portion of the artichoke primarily consists of the fleshy lower parts of the involucral bracts and the base, referred to as the heart. In the center of the bud, there is a mass of immature florets known as the choke or beard. However, these become inedible as the flower matures and grows larger..

Taste: The bitterness — and potency — mellows with cooking. Take it with meals in a small dose — sip, spray — it works better if you taste it. It's too bitter as tea, but enjoy a splash of a bitter blend (with aromatic carminatives and a hint of sweetness) in seltzer.

Medicinal parts: leaves

Medicinal Uses: The Arabs, Greeks, and Romans cultivated artichoke and cardoon for food and medicine for millennia, and from those populations it spread to the world. The leaves act as a simple bitter to promote digestion and liver detoxification, much like the more famous gentian root, yet far easier and more sustainable to grow and harvest in abundance. We use bitters to increase gastric juice and enzyme production, ease many cases of reflux and heartburn, improve peristalsis (the muscle action that moves food through the GI tract), encourage the liver to detoxify more efficiently, improve bile production and excretion, increase our ability to digest fats, indirectly move the bowels, reduce blood sugar, regulate appetite, control sugar cravings, and more. Human studies support its benefits in dyspepsia, gastric motility, cholesterol, hypertension, and appetite control.

Gardening Tips: Of all the heirloom varieties, the globe artichoke is by far the easiest to cultivate. Artichoke seed should be started indoors in the early spring and the seedlings transplanted to pots, then moved to the garden after all threat of frost has passed. The plants should be set out on hills 4 feet apart with one or two plants per hill. The artichoke produces huge silvery gray leaves that are quite striking as garden ornaments in their own right, but they cannot be crowded. Artichokes need good air circulation during humid weather; otherwise, they will develop mildews, molds, and other fungus diseases. Do not expect an artichoke crop the first year, for it is usually the second-year plants that begin to produce. They will yield crops for five to seven years, but regardless, new beds should be started every year. When the plants send up flower heads, only one or two buds should be left on the stem in order to increase their size. These are harvested right before the flower head opens to bloom. Artichokes that bloom will produce seed, but the seed is not usually true. Not only do artichoke varieties cross with one another, but artichokes also cross with cardoons. It is therefore common practice to propagate the plants from suckers, choosing the best that appear over the course of the growing season.

Ashwagandha

Habitat: Ashwagandha (Withania somnifera) is a plant that is widely distributed throughout India, ranging from the northern tropics to southern regions. It is also cultivated extensively due to its use as a natural health supplement. In addition to India, ashwagandha is native to other countries such as Nepal, Yemen, and China.

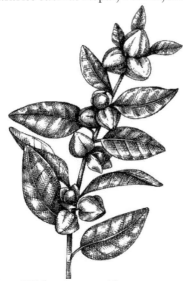

Identification: *Withania somnifera,* commonly known as ashwagandha, is a relatively short and tender perennial shrub that typically grows between 14 to 30 inches in height. It has branches covered in a downy or woolly texture that radiate from a central stem. The leaves are elliptical in shape, dull green in color, and typically measure around 4 to 5 inches in length. The flowers of ashwagandha are small, bell-shaped, and green in color. As the fruit ripens, it turns into a reddish-orange hue.

Taste: Ashwagandha's name means "smells like horse" because of the strong scent of the roots. Don't dry ashwagandha near other herbs as it can flavor them.

Medicinal parts: roots fresh or dried

Medicinal Uses: Ayurvedic practitioners revere ashwagandha as one of the most effective, multipurpose, safe medicinal plants for vitality. According to ancient ayurvedic wisdom, taking ashwagandha regularly for a year will give you the strength of a stallion for the next 10 years. This includes deep energy, physical strength, calm mind, better sleep, perky and stable mood, cognitive prowess, more muscle, nourished nerves, less pain, reduced cancer risk, healthy immune and respiratory systems, stronger thyroid function, improved libido, enhanced hormones and fertility, and more. Ashwagandha is one of my favorite herbs for myself and clients. You often see results within a few days, with further improvement over time. Ayurvedic practitioners often stir the powder into hot milk (cow, coconut, or almond), ghee, or other warm, fatty substance based on the belief that this would better send ashwagandha to the fat-lined nervous system. It's a great addition to "golden milk," which is traditionally made with turmeric, honey, hot milk, and a pinch of black pepper. I add a pinch each cardamom and nutmeg and sometimes blend in egg and vanilla extract (eggnog!). Ashwagandha is extremely safe, but avoid it if you react to other nightshade-family plants like tomatoes and potatoes. To avoid overstimulating the thyroid, seek an herbalist's or naturopathic doctor's guidance if you have hyperthyroid disease or are on thyroid medications and want to use herbs (always keep your medical doctor in the loop, too).

Gardening Tips: Start seeds indoors (easy to germinate) and/or plant seedlings outdoors after the threat of frost. Treat it like an annual in cool climates and grow it like tomatoes: ashwagandha loves heat, sun, and well-drained soil (rich to sandy) without competition from nearby plants. Dig up the root in the fall before frost in its first year in cool climates or, in warmer zones, the second fall when the berries are ripe red-orange.

Chamomile

Habitat: You'll find German chamomile tea on the shelf in almost every country in the world. Although many different types of chamomile exist and can be used somewhat interchangeably — including the perennial Roman chamomile (*Chamaemelum nobile,* formerly Anthemis nobilis) and petal-less pineapple weed (*Matricaria discoidea*) — German remains the most popular. German chamomile has gone through several Latin name changes, including *Matricaria recutita* and *Chamomilla recutita.* English camomile is a perennial herb, while German camomile is an annual herb.

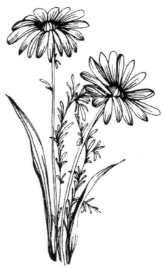

Identification: German chamomile (Matricaria chamomilla) has thin and feathery bipinnate leaves that are somewhat hairy. It typically grows to a height of approximately 20 inches. On the other hand, English chamomile (Chamaemelum nobile) has larger and thicker leaves that are not bipinnate, and its stems are not hairy. English chamomile plants are shorter and wider compared to German chamomile plants.

When it comes to the flowers, German chamomile has tiny flowers that are approximately one inch in diameter. The center of the flowers is yellow, while the petals are white, resembling a daisy. In contrast, English chamomile flowers have larger centers, and the petals that surround the blossom are sparse and sometimes even absent. In some varieties of English chamomile, the plant may not flower at all. Additionally, the receptacle of German chamomile has a hollow interior, while the receptacle of English chamomile has a solid interior.

Taste: Mellow, apple-like sweetness. Faintly fruity scent.

Medicinal parts: flower heads

Medicinal Uses: Chamomile gently calms the nerves; improves digestive juices; functions as a mild bitter and carminative; decreases gastric inflammation; eases spasms, pain, gas, and colic; and discourages pathogenic gut bacteria. These properties make it a superb, well-rounded herb for digestion and the gastrointestinal tract for both babies and adults. Its calming effects also quell anxiety, teething pain, insomnia, and fussy behavior. In fact, chamomile is specifically indicated not just for babies but also for adults who act like fussy babies. It's also fantastic where emotional tension brings digestive discomfort. Chamomile's anti-inflammatory and calming effects also help with skin irritation, making it popular in skin care as a toner, bath, or cream. For this, it also offers vulnerary healing and light antiseptic properties. As a flower essence, chamomile soothes the solar plexus belly area, quelling anxiety and digestive distress. Chamomile has a fantastic safety record for all ages; however, some people with daisy-family allergies may react to chamomile. (For those folks, catnip offers similar nerve-digestive benefits.)

Gardening Tips: Direct sow seeds or plugs in well-drained soil and harvest or deadhead regularly to keep it producing more flowers. We harvest only the small flower heads of chamomile, which means you'll need a lot of plants and time to harvest a sufficient amount. That's why good chamomile costs so much. Allow some seeds to self-sow for the next year.

Sage

Habitat: Sage, a member of the mint family Lamiaceae, is native to the Mediterranean region. However, it has successfully naturalized in various locations around the world.

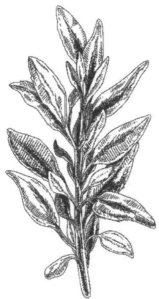

Identification: The Old World cultivar of sage, scientifically known as S. officinalis, is a recommended choice. It typically grows to a height and width of up to 2 feet. The plant produces purple flowers, although white, pink, or purple variations can also occur. The oblong leaves of this cultivar can reach up to 2 inches in length and 1.5 inches in width. They have a grey-green color, with a rugose texture on the upper side and a nearly white underside, thanks to the presence of short, soft hairs.

Taste: Potent earthy-herbaceous-aromatic flavor. Perfect for autumn cuisine!

Medicinal parts: leaves fresh or dried

Medicinal Uses: Sage shares medicinal benefits with close relatives lavender, rosemary, oregano, and thyme, yet it has its own special affinities. It's profoundly drying and helps with conditions of excess secretions: heavy perspiration from stress, daytime hot flashes, or overactive sweat glands; night sweats; and postlactation leaking. It affects hormones by providing plant estrogen and inhibiting prolactin. As an antimicrobial, it's useful in a variety of forms: a gargle for sore throats, a foot powder for sweaty feet and fungus, an antiseptic vinegar spray for countertops. As an aromatic, whether you take it internally or inhale its aroma, sage provides wisdom by perking up cognitive function and helping to fight the effects of aging on the brain. Anti-inflammatory aromatic properties also make it useful for cold, achy joint pain and arthritis, especially with lemon and ginger. Sage, a bitter carminative, improves digestion, fights intestinal pathogens, and makes it easier to digest fat.

Gardening Tips: Native to the Mediterranean, sage likes it warm and dry and will do well near "like-minded" herbs including lavender, horehound, thyme, and rosemary. It may die off after a few years, especially if it gets too cold or damp. Older happy plants produce beautiful purple flowers throughout most of the growing season. Several other species of sage have similar properties but are rarely winter-hardy.

It's Time to Harvest!

Harvesting herbs can be a straightforward process once you understand the general guidelines. While specific plant profiles may provide more detailed instructions, the key is to harvest when the plant appears vibrant, fragrant, and flavorful - essentially when it's thriving and "happy." For aromatic herbs, it's best to harvest them earlier in the day when their flavors are more concentrated. If you plan to dry the herbs, wait until the dew has evaporated and consider the weather forecast if you rely on warm, sunny conditions for dehydration. Flowers should be harvested just as they begin to open. Roots and barks are typically harvested in spring or fall, but you can adjust the schedule to fit your needs. Whether it means venturing out at night with a headlamp to beat frost or digging up a root in mid-June, adapt the process to your schedule and circumstances.

Aerial parts and leaves

When it comes to harvesting herbs with leaves and branching stems, there are a few approaches you can take. One method involves harvesting the top portion of the plant, typically around one-quarter to two-thirds of its height. It's important to leave a few sets of leaves behind and trim just above a leaf node. This technique encourages new growth and ensures the plant's vitality. However, if time is limited or you have a substantial amount of material to harvest, you can opt for a more expedient method known as giving the plant a "bad haircut." This involves cutting across the top portion of the plant in a straight line. Although the plant may initially appear somewhat untidy, it will regrow and rejuvenate itself. For herbs such as chives, parsley, and lemongrass that lack branching or leafy growth, a different approach is required. In these cases, you can cut the plants down to the ground, leaving about one-third to two-thirds of the plant untouched. This helps stimulate new growth and ensures a continuous supply of fresh herbs. Additionally, with chives and lemongrass, you can also trim the grassy tops (excluding the tightly rolled stalks) from the upper portion of the plant. Always remember to harvest in a manner that promotes future growth while providing enough material for your desired remedies or culinary needs. This ensures a sustainable harvest and the continued health of your herb garden.

Flowers and Buds

To preserve the quality of harvested flowers, it's important to follow proper techniques. Start by pinching off newly opened blossoms, including any green sepals or bracts at the base of the flower. In most cases, it's recommended to leave the whole flower head intact, as is the case with calendula, red clover, and chamomile. However, for certain flowers like roses and dandelions, you may choose to remove only the petals. When it comes to drying the flowers, ensure they are laid out in a single layer to allow for proper airflow. This will help prevent moisture build-up and minimize the risk of fermentation and mold during storage. One option for drying is to use a dehydrator, which provides controlled temperature and airflow to expedite the drying process. Make sure to monitor the flowers closely and remove them from the dehydrator once they are completely dried. Properly dried flowers can be stored in airtight containers, such as glass jars or resealable bags, in a cool and dark place. Regularly check for any signs of moisture or mold, and discard any flowers that show these issues. By following these guidelines, you can ensure the long-lasting quality of your dried flowers for various purposes, such as herbal remedies or decorative arrangements.

Bark

Timing is crucial when harvesting bark for its medicinal properties. For optimal results, it's recommended to harvest bark in early spring when the tree's sap is rising but before it has fully leafed out. Another suitable time is in the fall when the leaves have started changing color and dropping. However, in certain situations, such as when pruning the tree for maintenance, bark can be harvested at any time of the year. When identifying the medicinal part of the bark, focus on the inner bark, which is typically juicy, green, and aromatic. This inner bark should be separated from the outer bark and the inner woody pith to ensure you're obtaining the desired medicinal properties. When pruning branches specifically for bark harvesting, target twigs and branches with a diameter of approximately 1 1/2 inches or smaller. For smaller branches, there's no need to remove the outer bark. It's worth noting that the pruning technique employed will impact the tree's growth. A "heading cut" made above a strong node encourages bushy growth, while a "thinning cut" involves removing the branch entirely. In the case of harvesting bark from wider branches or the trunk, the outer bark needs to be removed. After pruning, remove any leaves from the branches and use a knife or peeler to scrape off the bark. For the twigs, clippers can be used to trim them, as they will be utilized for making medicine. Depending on the bark's characteristics, it may easily peel off, allowing you to slice it down the length or strip it by hand. If you intend to create a tincture with the harvested bark, consider adding 10 percent glycerine or honey. This addition helps stabilize the tincture and prevents the astringent tannins present in the bark from precipitating out over time, ensuring the tincture retains its potency.

Roots

Harvesting roots is typically recommended in spring or fall when plants are not primarily focused on leafy growth and flowering. However, it's important to consider specific plant requirements and individual circumstances, as there may be exceptions to this general guideline. To extract the roots from the ground, a garden fork can be utilized to loosen the soil around the plant. Depending on the plant and soil conditions, tools such as a sharp spade, hori hori (Japanese gardening knife), or digging stick may be used to slice or pry the roots out. For plants with spreading roots like burdock and nettle, or those with easily removable roots like mullein and valerian, a digging stick, hori hori, or CobraHead weeder can be employed to work the roots out effectively.

Once the roots are out of the ground, gently tapping them against the ground or a rock helps loosen and remove excess dirt. Rinse the roots with a garden hose sprayer on the power-wash setting or immerse them in cold water, swishing them vigorously to further clean them. If any dirt remains clinging to the roots, a potato scrubber and cold water can be used to remove it. After harvesting, it is advisable to process the roots promptly. Chop them into smaller pieces using tools such as a hatchet, loppers, clippers, or a wood chipper, depending on the size and hardness of the roots. There are two main options for further handling: dehydration or immediate use of the fresh roots in preparations. If you choose to dehydrate the roots, they can be dried in a single layer in the oven at a low temperature of around 100 to 120°F (38 to 49°C). Alternatively, you can incorporate the fresh roots directly into your preparations.

Garden Design for Pollinators and Wildlife

Pollination is not just an intriguing aspect of nature, but a vital ecological function for the survival of the human race and terrestrial ecosystems. Without pollinators, we would face the perilous loss of almost all the 1,400 crop species that provide our food and plant-based products. Bees and other pollinators play a crucial role in bringing us larger, more flavorful fruits and increasing crop yields. In the United States alone, the value of pollination services for agricultural crops is estimated at ten billion dollars, and globally, it exceeds three trillion dollars.

Flowering plants, through the process of photosynthesis, use carbon dioxide produced by plants and animals during respiration to produce oxygen, making the air breathable. With rising carbon dioxide levels in the atmosphere due to increased fossil fuel usage and deforestation, which destroys vital forests often referred to as the "earth's lungs," pollinators become even more essential for the reproduction of wild plants. Even if soil, air, nutrients, and other life-sustaining factors are present, existing plant populations would decline without the assistance of pollinators.

Additionally, flowering plants contribute to the well-being of our environment in various ways. Their roots help hold the soil in place, preventing erosion, while their foliage acts as a natural cushion, reducing the impact of rainfall on the earth's surface. By cleansing water and facilitating moisture return to the atmosphere through pollination, flowering plants contribute to the overall health and balance of ecosystems.

Even if you don't want to embark on the challenging yet rewarding task of building a wildflower garden there are still a few ways to make your garden pollinator-friendly.

1. Utilize a diverse selection of blooming plants throughout the seasons, ranging from early spring to late fall. Plant them in clumps rather than solitary to facilitate the discovery and utilization of these plants by pollinators. Opt for flora that naturally occurs in your region, as native plants have adapted to the local temperature, soil conditions, and pollinator populations. Remember that nocturnal creatures like moths and bats are attracted to flowers that bloom at night.

2. It is advisable to avoid modern hybrid flowers, especially those with "doubled" blossoms. Plant breeders often unintentionally removed essential elements like pollen, nectar, and fragrance while striving to create aesthetically pleasing blooms for human enjoyment.

3. Whenever possible, minimize the use of pesticides in your garden. If pesticide use becomes necessary, opt for the least hazardous options available. Before purchasing any products, carefully read and follow the labels, as many chemicals can be particularly harmful to bees. Make sure to use the pesticide product responsibly, spraying it when bees and other pollinators are not active, preferably during the nighttime.

4. Integrate larval host plants into your garden to support caterpillars and attract beautiful butterflies. Embrace the fact that these caterpillars will consume the plants, so it's best to place them where leaf damage is acceptable. Remember that not all host plants may be visually appealing, as some may even resemble weeds. Utilize a butterfly guide to identify the most suitable plants to include and create a butterfly habitat in your garden.

5. Create a moist salt lick to attract butterflies and bees. You can achieve this by using a dripping hose, drip irrigation line, or by placing your birdbath directly on bare soil. Add a pinch of salt (preferably sea salt) or wood ashes to the damp area.

6. Provide additional nesting locations for native bees by leaving dead trees or branches intact, ensuring they do not pose any safety hazards to people below. To create artificial nesting sites, drill holes of various diameters approximately 3 to 5 inches deep in a scrap piece of lumber attached to a pole or beneath eaves, forming a bee condo.

7. Consider using a hummingbird feeder to supplement nectar supplies. Prepare artificial nectar by combining four parts water with one part table sugar. Avoid using artificial sweeteners, honey, or fruit juices. Place a red object near the feeder to attract hummingbirds. To prevent mold growth, make sure to clean the feeder with hot soapy water at least twice a week.

8. Understand that butterflies require more than just nectar to survive. They are also attracted to unpalatable food sources such as moist animal droppings, urine, and decaying fruits. To observe and attract different butterfly species, place slices of overripe bananas, oranges, and other fruits, or a sponge, in a dish of lightly salted water. Sea salt is preferred over regular table salt, as it contains a wider range of micronutrients.

In the sixth volume of this series you'll find a comprehensive guide on growing native wildflowers that attract pollinators and native wildlife. Discover all the possibilities to create a vibrant and captivating meadow in your garden.

Key design elements

Native plants and indigenous animals have a mutually beneficial relationship in which animals rely on plants for food, shelter, and breeding, while plants benefit from animals through pollination, seed dispersal, pest control, waste decomposition, and soil maintenance. For more suggestions on designing a native garden, refer back to the earlier chapter.

Layers. To create a habitat garden, it is important to incorporate structural diversity by including a variety of plants and different layers such as trees, shrubs, grasses, and groundcovers. Woodland gardens are well-suited for achieving this diversity. When considering the replacement of non-indigenous plants, a strategic approach is recommended to prevent wildlife from being disturbed or abandoning the garden. Instead of completely removing intact vegetation, gradually replace sections with new indigenous plants. Dead trees, shrubs, logs, rocks, sticks, mulch, and fallen leaves can provide valuable habitats for insects and reptiles. It is important to avoid collecting logs and rocks from bushland areas where they are already serving as habitats. Nesting hollows play a vital role in the breeding and nesting of various bird and mammal species, as the decline of old trees has led to a scarcity of natural hollows. Consider installing nest boxes in your garden to help address this issue.

Food. Many native animals rely on a variety of plants that offer nectar, pollen, seeds, fruit, leaves, and roots as a source of food. Additionally, dead plant material can serve as a valuable food resource. Insects that inhabit the plants, mulch, and soil play a crucial role in providing food for birds, lizards, frogs, and mammals.

Host Plants. Certain insects, including butterflies, have specific host plants on which they lay their eggs. These host plants are crucial for the survival and reproduction of native caterpillars, which are often small, nocturnal, and discreet in their presence within your garden. If you want to attract and retain butterflies in your garden, it is important to include these host plants. The volume on wildflowers provides detailed information on which plants are known to attract butterflies.

Water. To attract wildlife to your garden, especially during the summer months, it is essential to provide a reliable water source. Placing a shallow birdbath on a pedestal near a dense or prickly shrub can offer protection to birds while they bathe and drink. Additionally, frogs require a permanent or semi-permanent water source to keep their skin moist and create suitable breeding conditions. Creating a space with a small puddle in the soil or a wide dish of damp sand will attract butterflies, as they gather to take in water and obtain essential salts and minerals from the soil.

Shelter. Native wildlife requires suitable shelter to protect themselves from adverse weather conditions, predators, and competition from other species. They rely on finding safe havens where they can establish their nests and raise their offspring. Providing adequate refuge is essential for their survival and reproductive success.

Creating habitats with diverse vegetation, including trees, shrubs, and dense plantings, offers hiding spots and secure nesting sites for wildlife. Dead trees and shrubs can also serve as important habitats for a variety of native species.

Responsible pet ownership. To safeguard the native wildlife in your yard, it's important to take measures to prevent pets, particularly cats and dogs, from disrupting their habitat. Keep your pets indoors during the night to minimize the risk of them preying on wildlife. While collar bells on cats can offer some assistance, their effectiveness in deterring hunting behavior is limited. It is crucial to actively manage and supervise your pets to ensure the safety and well-being of the local wildlife population.

Natural pest control. A diverse range of wildlife in your garden can greatly enhance its natural pest control capabilities. Birds, bats, frogs, lizards, spiders, and insects like praying mantises all play a role in keeping insect populations in check. It is important to regularly monitor your garden for pests, and it's generally advisable to tolerate a minor infestation as it can attract natural predators. For certain pests like snails, you can manually remove them by hand. Additionally, you may consider using home remedies like linseed oil traps to control pests such as earwigs.

Encourage others. Encourage your neighbors to join in creating habitat gardens as well. By doing so, you can collectively attract and support a greater diversity of wildlife throughout the entire area. A network of interconnected habitat gardens provides a larger and more interconnected habitat for birds, butterflies, pollinators, and other wildlife to thrive. Consider organizing community events or sharing resources and knowledge with your neighbors to inspire and guide them in creating their own habitat gardens. Together, you can create a thriving ecosystem that benefits both the local wildlife and the community as a whole.

Gardening for Birds

Creating a bird-rich landscape in your garden involves considering their basic needs: water, cover, and food. While a birdbath and native screening hedges provide water and cover, the key to attracting a variety of birds lies in providing the right food sources. Although bird food can be purchased in bags, observing a songbird's nest reveals that they predominantly feed their young with protein-rich invertebrates like spiders, caterpillars, and moths. While marketed plants with berries are beneficial, it's the plants that host a multitude of caterpillars that truly enhance a bird-rich garden. Doug Tallamy has emphasized this concept, and his website, bringingnaturehome.net, offers a valuable list of plants and the number of butterflies and moths they support. Native trees excel in this regard, as they provide ample food for caterpillars and young birds. In contrast, non-native trees like Norway maple (Acer platanoides) and London plane (Platanus ×acerifolia) do not support any caterpillars, thus limiting their value to bird populations.

Once nesting season is over, fruits, berries, and seeds become important food sources for birds. Acorns, native cherries, dogwood berries, eastern red cedar cones, and the seeds within pinecones and birch fruits are highly sought after. By incorporating a diverse selection of plants that bear fruits ripening throughout the season, from early summer to fall, and those that persist into winter, you can transform your garden into a haven for birds. By providing the necessary elements of water, cover, and a variety of food sources, your garden can become the most bird-friendly place in your neighborhood, attracting and supporting a thriving bird population.

Gardening for Butterflies

Native invertebrates, including butterflies, bees, ladybirds, ants, gnats, beetles, spiders, dragonflies, and lacewings, play vital roles in the environment. They serve as plant pollinators, help recycle waste, control pests, and provide a crucial food source for native birds, frogs, reptiles, and mammals. Butterflies are a delightful addition to any garden. To attract butterflies, provide a dish of damp sand to satisfy their need for moisture and salts. Place a flat rock where they can bask in the morning sun and offer a sheltered spot for them to rest during the midday heat. Planting flat flowers like daisies that are easily accessible for feeding on nectar will also attract butterflies. They are particularly drawn to flowers in colors such as blue, yellow, and red. Creating large clusters of flowering plants increases the chances of attracting butterflies to your garden. To encourage them to stay, include host plants where butterflies can lay their eggs and support their life cycle.

Where do butterflies go in winter? It's surprising how few gardeners think about that, but it's the cornerstone of sound gardening for these beautiful creatures.
Each butterfly has a particular way of surviving winter, beginning with several that overwinter as adult butterflies. Yes, even in the frigid north, several species survive sheltered in cracks and crevices of wood and in outbuildings—but probably not in your butterfly house purchased for garden décor. Many survive the winter as a chrysalis hanging from a stalk, branch, fence, or just about any obscure support or, as with the skippers, as a pupa snuggled in a nest of dead vegetation. Others survive the winter as a caterpillar: a couple create little sleeping bags of remnant leaves, tethered to the plant with their silk; most simply overwinter in fallen leaves. Finally, some butterflies (hairstreaks in particular) overwinter as eggs, poised to emerge and feed on young growth. Surprisingly, almost a third of midwestern butterfly species are colonists and migrants and do not survive the winter here.

All this means that a certain level of garden maintenance is crucial to a butterfly-friendly landscape. Rake up all the leaves, cart off all the dead stems, clean up every brush pile, and you will inadvertently kill a lot of butterflies. It also highlights that all three stages of a butterfly's metamorphosis are needed and should be accommodated. You may apply pesticides thinking you are not hitting a butterfly, but are you impacting its unseen eggs, caterpillar, or chrysalis?

Most butterflies need a specific set of related host plants for their caterpillars to eat and grow and make more butterflies. Provide the host plants, and the butterflies will find you and colonize. Adult butterflies need nectar or other sustenance to survive, so planting nectar-rich flowers or putting up a butterfly feeder, filled with spoiled fruit, does the trick. If you plant and maintain properly, butterflies will come and certainly enrich your backyard gardening experience.

Moths are even more important to a healthy garden's web of life, but they don't get the respect they deserve. They require the same gardening plant selection, care, and maintenance considerations as butterflies, as they too have a complete metamorphosis, from egg to adult.

Conclusion

I hope you have enjoyed reading this book as much as I've enjoyed writing it, and I hope it will accompany you in your ongoing journey to the discovery of Native American herbs and their medicinal uses.

If you found this book useful and are feeling generous, please take the time to leave a short review on Amazon so that other may enjoy this guide as well.

I leave you with good wishes and hopefully a better knowledge of the plants around us and their amazing powers. This volume is part of a seven-books series on Native American Herbalism from foraging and gardening native plants to making herbal remedies for adults and children. Check out the other volumes to gain a deeper understanding of the amazing wisdom and knowledge of our forefathers and to improve not only your health, but the health of our land as well.

The Native American Herbalist's Bible 5

The Gardener's Companion to Native Medicinal Herbs

Everything you need to know to Select and Grow Native Plants for your Home Apothecary

Linda Osceola Naranjo

Introduction

*You have noticed
that everything an Indian does is
in a circle; everything the power of the world
does is done in a circle. The sky is round, and I have
heard that the earth is round like a ball and so are all
the stars. The wind, in its greatest power, whirls. Birds make
their nests in circles, for theirs is the same religion as ours.
The sun comes forth and goes down again in a circle. The
moon does the same, and both are round. Even the seasons
form a great circle in their changing, and always come
back again to where they were. The life of a man is a
circle from childhood to childhood, and so it is
in everything where power moves*
Black Elk, Oglala Sioux medicine man (1863–1950)

We live in a country where the cure for virtually any disease and ailment is within our grasp. In our forests, meadows, plains, and gardens grow small, seemingly insignificant flowers and herbs, plants that we don't look twice at, and trees of which we don't even bother to learn the name. Yet, they are the key to a better, healthier, and more sustainable way of life. Our forefathers, more attuned with nature than we could ever imagine to be, understood that, and took carefully and sparingly the gifts that Nature offered to heal themselves and grow stronger. We have lost that knowledge. Only starting from the 1970s, a renewed interest in botanic medicine has uncovered the depth of the Native American knowledge of plants and their healing powers. The research has not only helped herbalists, but physicians and scientist as well that re-discovered substances that the Native Americans people knew about for hundreds of years. This book is the extended edition of the best-selling The Native American Herbalist's Bible: 3-in-1 Companion to Herbal Medicine, offering four more volumes on gardening techniques, growing healing plants and wildflowers, and pediatric healthcare. This is the unabridged companion to Native American herbs, their traditional and modern use, complete with appropriate doses and usage, gardening tips and techniques for both medicinal plants and wildflowers. The book is completed by a list of simple and effective recipes for the most common ailments for both adults and children. You don't need to put at risk the delicate natural balance of your body and that of your loved ones by taking drugs and medications, if an easily available natural solution is just outside your door. Harvest carefully or grow your own herbs, learn to know your body and what works best for you, communicate with the nature surrounding you, and you will in a small way bring back a culture that for too long has been treated as inferior. This book will teach how to find and treat the herbs the way the native American tribes did: from the forest to your herbalist table, but you will have to find your way to listen to your body and the plants around you. To aid you in your holistic journey, we have decided to divide the book in seven handy volumes.

The first volume will give you a full theoretical approach to Native American medicine and the herbal medicines methods and preparations.

The second volume is a complete encyclopedia of all the most relevant herbs used in traditional Native American medicine, complete with modern examples, doses, and where to find them, making it a very effective field guide.

The third volume is a "recipe book" of sorts: it offers easy herbal solutions to the most common diseases a budding naturopath can encounter. It is meant as a jumping point to find your own way to treat yourself and your fellow man and will come in handy even to the most experienced herbalist.

The fourth volume provides a complete theoretical and practical approach to Native American traditional planting techniques and how they can be implemented in modern gardens.

This fifth volume is the native gardener's almanac for medicinal herbs. Foraging is not always an option and a lot of herbs are handy to have in your garden: this volume will guide you through the herbs that you can and (should) have in your garden.

The sixth volume continues the guide to the plants you can plant in your gardens focusing on healing wildflowers, which are not only good for your health, but for the planet as well, and they are not bad on the eyes either!

The seventh volume focuses on native pediatric healthcare. Treating children is a very delicate undertaking, their physiology is more sensitive to external agents, especially drugs. Natural herbalist treatments are effective and gentle in treating common, less severe, pathologies and they won't needlessly weaken your child's immune system. The herbs listed in this last volume have been carefully researched to specifically treat children and their ailments, avoiding any allergic reaction and boosting their immune system.

I am happy to guide through a life-changing journey in search of lost knowledge, amazing healing plants, and carefully crafted herbal remedies and I hope it will help you nurture a stronger relationship with the nature surrounding us and the many gifts it bestows upon us.

Spiritual Gardening

The previous volumes focused on the exceptional methods that our forefathers had to live off the land and thrive in nature without exploiting it. However, a practical approach often neglects the spiritual aspect, which is why I would like to take this chapter to explore the sacred space we create when we garden consciously. No one is a better teacher than our forefathers and the most visual expression of their connection to nature is certainly the medicine wheel garden. I have already extensively covered the subject in the first book of the series, but as we approach gardening the herbs for our health rather than foraging in these new volumes of the series, I think it is important that we recollect the importance of a sacred space within us and on the grounds we care for.

There exists a dimension of human experience where communication between plants and humans is possible. Throughout history, humans have engaged with this dimension, seeking a deep connection with the sacred and listening to the wisdom shared by plants. However, in modern times, this way of life has been marginalized and dismissed as primitive and superstitious.

The knowledge acquired through this intimate relationship with plants predates the emergence of what we now call science. In this realm of human experience, people sought closeness with the divine, aiming to understand the Creator's desires and manifest the spiritual visions bestowed upon them. Remarkably, the knowledge gained through this process proved effective, as scientific study has revealed. It is astonishing to observe this knowledge from the perspective of our scientific world, as we struggle to comprehend the information gathered in that other realm. Unfortunately, in the industrialized nations, we have largely abandoned this form of knowledge gathering, and as a result, we have become impoverished in many ways.

For Earth-centered peoples like Native American tribes, the sacred is immediate and pervasive throughout the world. By cultivating a willingness to engage with the deeper aspects of the Earth, individuals can establish a closer relationship with the spiritual realm. This profound connection can provide guidance and purpose to their lives and communities. Over time, this deepened relationship empowers individuals to invoke the sacred through ceremonies, shaping its influence in human affairs for the betterment of the community, healing, instruction, and upliftment.

When humans embark on sacred journeys, they possess the innate ability to recognize the sacred and discern patterns of sacred expression. Sacred travelers often focus on specific aspects or patterns of the sacred world, dedicating their lives to understanding Spirit through those particular expressions. One such example is the manifestation of the sacred through plants. This sacred expression through plants has always been regarded by Earth-centered peoples as a pathway to becoming holy, a means of attaining knowledge, wisdom, and harnessing the immense power of the sacred for the benefit of the community.

While the names of most of these holy individuals may remain unknown, they have left traces of their wisdom in human DNA and within the sacred landscape. Traveling through sacred territories may seem formidable, but knowing that our ancestors have traversed these paths before us brings comfort. It is possible to discover the remnants of their presence and follow in their footsteps. Heed the wise words of Crashing Thunder's father:

If you wish to obtain real blessings, so that you can cure even more people, you will have to fast a long time and sincerely for these blessings. If four or perhaps ten of the powerful spirits bless you, then someday when you have children and anything happens to one of them, you will not have to go and look for a medicine man, but all you will have to do will be to look into your own medicine bundle. Look therein and you will be able, with the medicine you find, to cure your children of whatever ailments they have. Not only that, but after a while you will be called to treat your fellow men. Then you can open your medicine bundle and not be embarrassed, for you will know how to treat an individual who is ill and needs medicines since you will possess those that are good for him. You will know where the seat of his trouble exists, and since you will have obtained these blessings only after the greatest effort on your part, whatever you say and do will be efficacious. If you declare that he will live, then he will live. If you make proper offerings to your medicine, and if you speak of your medicine in the way you are accustomed to do, and if you ask your medicine to put forth its strength in your patient's behalf, the medicine will do it for you. If, in truth, you make good offerings of tobacco to your plants, if you give many feasts in their honor, and if you then ask your medicines to put forth their strength, and if, in addition, you talk to them like human beings, then most certainly will these plants do for you what you ask. You can then accept the offerings patients make to you without any embarrassment and your children will wear these offerings and will gain strength from them. They will be well and happy. So be extremely diligent in the care you take of your medicines. Medicines are good for all purposes. That is why they were given to us. We are to use them to cure ourselves. Earthmaker gave them to us for that purpose.

There exists a way of relating to the natural world that fosters ecological sustainability. When we recognize the sacredness and interconnectedness of all life, it becomes difficult to exploit or harm species that are seen as relatives or sacred expressions of Spirit. Unfortunately, in industrialized societies, many people have lost touch with this perspective, reducing the Earth and its components to mere resources or subjects of study. This devaluation of life has had serious consequences for our planet and our own well-being. By devaluing other members of the ecosystem, we have devalued ourselves. The restoration of the Earth and our lives necessitates a capacity to revere and establish connections with all forms of life.

Establishing a sacred relationship with plants begins by experiencing and treating each plant as if it were a person, just as you would wish to be treated. All beings possess awareness and are woven from the fabric of Spirit, enabling communication among us. With nonhuman inhabitants of the Earth, this communication takes the form of ceremony. Ceremony may or may not involve words, but the crucial aspect is the communication of meaning, which should embody a genuine feeling of reverence for plants and life. Without this deep reverence, the form itself holds little significance, as plants can perceive and sense our true intentions.

To initiate your connection with plants, it is essential to genuinely appreciate and like them. A simple way to begin is by finding a plant in the wild that moves you or to which you feel drawn. Sit by the plant, admire its beauty, and allow yourself to fall in love with it. In this process, as you would with a beloved person, observe how the plant appears and feels to you in the present moment. Offer a prayer or engage in a brief conversation with the plant, seeking its permission to sit with it and appreciate its presence. Observe how you feel in response and contemplate the plant's potential response to your interaction.

Many individuals in Western culture have lost touch with this way of relating to plants and may struggle to differentiate between projection and the plant's genuine response. Unlearning what we have been taught takes practice and effort. It is akin to the story of the raven that spent years attempting to imitate a dove, only to realize that it had forgotten how to be a raven. Similarly, we have been conditioned to be something we are not, disconnecting us from our innate feelings, intuitions, and spiritual experiences. Our culture has prioritized rational processes and skepticism toward other forms of knowledge gathering, severing our roots to the Earth. Reconnecting with the sacred realm of plants requires "unlearning" our overdependence on rational thought and reawakening our other faculties. We must learn to "think like a mountain," where the well-being of all life is considered, and human beings assume their rightful place within this perspective.

It is indeed possible to see the world in this manner. As we embark on the journey of unlearning, the old knowledge and ways of perceiving the world gradually resurface of their own accord. John Seed, an Australian rainforest activist, shares a story of two sisters reclaiming their land by focusing on a small corner of a field where native plants still thrived. They diligently removed the seedlings of introduced plants each spring, allowing native grasses and plants to flourish and even bringing back species thought to be extinct in the area. The reclamation project gained momentum, overcoming challenges as it encountered an erosion gully. Seed emphasizes that a similar situation exists within ourselves, where the removal of introduced beliefs leads to the resurgence of native knowledge within us.

In this process of unlearning, of reconnecting with plants and hearing their wisdom, profound realizations begin to unfold. Among these, the pain of the Earth becomes acutely apparent and impossible to escape. To harness the power of plant medicine, trustworthiness is crucial, and our word to plant relations must be inviolate. Trust, like in any relationship, is built on honoring commitments. The more trustworthy we are, the more the plants will reveal to us, thereby increasing our power and responsibility.

When first learning about plants, it is helpful to have someone introduce you to them, focusing on three or four different species. Spend time with these plants daily if possible. Learn about their medicinal properties and incorporate them into your own life. By regularly contemplating and deepening your emotional relationship with plants, they will naturally become an integral part of your being. Observe them in the wild, noticing their growth patterns in each season. These questions and reflections serve as a starting point for building your relationship with the plants in your garden, and additional insights will arise as you embark on this spiritual journey.

- How does the plant taste?
- Do all parts taste the same?
- How does it feel to your touch?
- How does it smell?
- What other plants and animals gain benefit from them?
- How does their coloration vary from ecosystem to ecosystem?
- How does it feel to you to pick a plant and make medicine out of it and be healed by it?
- Are their roots different from season to season? From year to year?
- Do they taste different as medicine from season to season, from year to year? How do they feel in your body?
- What effects do they have?

Attentiveness to detail is fundamental in the Earth-centered peoples' relationship with plants, leading to a profound understanding of their uses, their connection to humans, and their role within the ecosystem. This knowledge combines meticulous analytical information with deep emotional and spiritual experiences, forming the reservoir of power carried by practitioners of sacred plant medicine.

Indigenous communities have long recognized the dual nature of knowledge about sacred plant medicine. They possess a far greater understanding of the plants in their environment compared to Western botanists. Their training and observations are meticulous, often surpassing the complexity of Western identification systems. They can identify and name each plant in their territory at any stage of growth, from seedling to withered leaf.

For instance, the Barasana Indians in Colombia can identify all their tree species without relying on fruits or flowers, a feat that eludes many botanists with academic training. Some indigenous cultures even employ classification systems more intricate than those currently utilized by Western botanists. Harold Conklin's research demonstrated the significance of comprehending folk classifications in ethnobotany, emphasizing that "there are important distinctions between any two systems of classification." The Hanunoo people, for example, name a greater number of plants compared to Western scientists, highlighting the necessity of recognizing this fundamental difference. Similar intricate classifications and naming practices have been observed in various other cultures, such as the Zapotec, who seek to establish connections among plants through multiple dimensions.

In the development of this comprehensive body of knowledge, one's senses, particularly one's feelings, become gateways to establishing a relationship with the natural world and plants. The body recognizes plants in ways that are inaccessible through pharmaceuticals, and thus, it becomes a reliable source of information. Understanding how the body responds to plants fosters self-trust and confidence in the knowledge received.

To foster a deep connection with plants, it is often beneficial for individuals to carry a plant they feel drawn to in a medicine pouch around their neck, positioned at heart level, for an extended period, perhaps up to a year. This practice allows the body to acclimate to the plant's presence, and thoughts of the plant become frequent and natural.

During sleep, placing the root of a plant one is working with under the pillow can facilitate access to dream medicine associated with that particular plant, deepening the personal relationship.

When gathering plants for personal use, it is essential to offer prayers and tobacco as a means of honoring and acknowledging their intrinsic nature and character. Prayer and offerings are integral to establishing a relationship with plants and recognizing the reciprocal nature of taking from the natural world. Placing a small amount of tobacco into the hole from which the plant was taken is an offering to Nono'mis, the Earth, the grandmother of mankind, expressing gratitude for the benefits derived from her body as ordained by Ki'tshi Man'ido.

While making offerings and prayers to plants and the Earth is important, it is crucial that these actions go beyond mere routine behavior. They should be rooted in genuine reverence and gratitude. Many individuals who offer tobacco may do so mechanically, lacking inherent reverence for the plant and failing to grasp its living essence and equality with the picker. They do not know how to treat plants as fellow beings. However, as you deepen your understanding of how the Earth and plants feel and think, you will realize that they value sincerity of intent and emotional connection more than the specific form of the offering. For us today, this genuine offering of ourselves is the most significant gesture we can make to our plant relatives and the Earth.

Despite occasional disagreements among indigenous cultures, medicine people, and their students regarding the correct form of offering or prayer, these debates usually stem from cultural differences rather than disrespect. As you develop your relationship with plants, allow your forms of offering and prayer to emerge naturally from your personal connection with them, without feeling obligated to adhere to rigid rituals.

However, regardless of the form you develop, seek the deeper truth underlying the offering of tobacco and prayers. There is a profound reality beneath these practices. Regardless of cultural variations, the act of prayer and offering is always present, albeit in different ways and at different times for each individual and culture.

Another essential aspect of offering prayers in a way that establishes a deep connection is the understanding of Earth medicine. The power of the Earth flows into everything that is born from it. When a plant is harvested, this vital flow of life force is disrupted, and specific intention is required to ensure that the power of Earth medicine remains within the plant and does not dissipate.

This knowledge is crucial for preserving the life force and Earth medicine within a plant intended for medicinal use. However, actualizing this requires sensitivity to the existence of this force and the ability to interact with it knowingly. The act of praying and conversing with the plant initiates this process, but the primary action that anchors this power within the plant originates from the herbalist. The Seminole people, for example, use their breath, but this act is symbolic. It is the life force carried by the breath and directed through it that activates the medicine. Similarly, in the case of maintaining the strong life force of the Earth within the plant, it is the conscious interweaving of the herbalist's life force with that of the plant and the Earth that accomplishes this.

The Medicine Wheel Garden

The Medicine Wheel embodies the core elements of a sacred relationship with the Earth, reflecting the indigenous understanding of life as a circle where all elements of the web of life coexist and human beings progress through life on a great wheel. It holds particular significance as a profound expression of the Earth-centered experience, encompassing the belief in distinct stages of human development that transcend psychology and environment, with plants playing specific roles at different points along the wheel.

The Medicine Wheel has been and continues to be utilized in religious ceremonies, with its various segments representing complex aspects and intersections of the life cycles of plants and the humans who care for them, spiritual growth, the seasons of the year and of an individual's life, and the circularity of the universe. These aspects will be explored further in the next subchapter.

The name "Medicine Wheel" originates from the well-known wheel located atop Medicine Mountain in Wyoming's Bighorn range. Constructed between 300 and 800 years ago, this wheel resembles a bicycle wheel when seen from above. It consists of a central hub made of cairn-like rocks with 28 "spokes" extending outward. Additional cairns are erected at regular intervals around the wheel. During the Summer Solstice, the cairns and spokes align with the rising and setting sun, as well as the rising of specific stars. These alignments are specifically designed for that location, which is accessible for visits only during the summer months (I encourage you to visit if possible).

Native perspectives on healthcare place a strong emphasis on community. Individual well-being is intricately connected to the harmony of family and community, as well as pride in one's ancestry, and medicine gardens are integral to this cycle. Each medicinal plant holds spiritual medicine, and during the healing process, gratitude is expressed for the insight received in selecting the appropriate plant medicine, understanding its proper use, and finding ways to reciprocate and contribute to the plant's survival.

The Native American medicine wheel symbolizes the cycles of life, honoring each stage with reverence and allowing us to appreciate the significance of every step in our journey, gaining new perspectives on our growth patterns. It serves as a circle of learning that each person must complete to fulfill their life's journey.

In sustainable gardening, an objective is to highlight the interconnectedness of all life and celebrate circles by incorporating circular designs or structures throughout the landscape.

Our ancestors possessed a profound knowledge of the natural world. They could navigate the wilderness with ease, recognizing the abundance of food and medicinal plants that surrounded them. Their lives were intricately intertwined with the Earth, fostering deep relationships and a profound understanding of the interconnectedness of all living beings.

In those days, the Earth was viewed as a self-contained ecosystem, capable of sustaining itself and providing for all its inhabitants. This understanding was not just intellectual but rooted in a deep spiritual connection to the natural world. Our ancestors recognized their role as caretakers of the Earth, understanding that it was their responsibility to preserve and nurture this sacred bond.

Modern spiritual gardening aims to recapture this innate connection and revive our relationship with the Earth and its bountiful gifts. It is a conscious effort to align ourselves with the wisdom of our ancestors, embracing their reverence for nature and their deep respect for the Earth's intricate balance.

In spiritual gardening, we seek to cultivate not only plants but also a sense of reverence, mindfulness, and gratitude for the Earth's abundance. It is a practice that goes beyond the mere act of planting and harvesting; it is a way of life that honors and celebrates the interconnectedness of all beings and recognizes our role as stewards of the Earth.

Through spiritual gardening, we strive to reclaim our inherent bond with the Earth, fostering a harmonious relationship where we give back as much as we receive. It is an invitation to embark on a journey of self-discovery, mindfulness, and healing through our interactions with nature.

The physical journey of life begins at birth, symbolized by the southern direction of the hoop in the Medicine Wheel. We all travel in a circle from the South to the North until we reach the home of the elders in the North. Just as the seasons change, we too evolve and progress, passing through different stages of the cycle and learning from each. The medicine wheel serves as an analogy for life, constructed from the earth beneath our feet.

- Birth, childhood, adolescence, adulthood (or old age), and death are the stages of life.
- Spring, summer, winter, and fall are the four seasons of the year.
- Spiritual, emotional, intellectual, and bodily affairs are the aspects of life.
- Fire (or sun), air, water, and earth are the natural elements.

We'll be seeing all of these elements represented.

The "Creator Pole" holds a significant place within the Medicine Wheel, and its shadow plays a role in marking the passage of time throughout the year. Positioned at the center of the circle, the Creator Pole represents the focal point from which the circle's outline is drawn, much like the center of a compass.

For Native Americans, observing the sun's position in the sky, tracking the rising and setting of stars, and noting the emergence of bears from hibernation were all important indicators of time. The cycles of the moon were also named based on the events or natural phenomena occurring during those periods. Different tribes assigned unique names to lunar cycles, such as "laying geese" or "coming caribou." Counting the number of full moons that had passed served as a way to mark the passing of a year for many Native American nations.

The original Medicine Wheels, which date back thousands of years, exhibit peculiar arrangements of pebbles. It is speculated that these arrangements were used to chart the lunar and solar cycles. Knowing the precise location of a shadow at a specific time each year may have signaled the beginning of significant events or important transitions. The space between the two curving lines in the image represents the areas where the shadow of the pole would fall throughout the year. The top line, marking the winter solstice, indicates the onset of winter, which usually occurs around December 21 or 22, the shortest day of the year with the longest shadow. Some Indian tribes view this day as the start of a new cycle of rebirth and renewal.

The Medicine Wheel and its connection to celestial cycles and natural phenomena demonstrate the deep understanding and reverence that Native Americans had for the passage of time and the interconnectedness of all things. It reflects their profound spiritual connection to the Earth and the cosmic forces that shape our world.

Each tribe or nation had their own description, unfortunately I couldn't include them all, so I opted for the one used by the Sioux of the American southwest:

Month	Description
January	The moon of strong cold and frost in the teepee
February	Bone moon (very little food left in reserve from the summer, so people gnaw on bones and eat bone marrow soup)
March	The moon of the buffalo cows that drops their calves
April	The moon of the greening grass
May	The moon when the ponies shed
June	The moon of creating fat
July	The moon when the wild cherries are ripe
August	The moon when the geese shed their feathers

Practical Tips for a Spiritual Approach

These ritual aspects are part of our cultural background; but even if you lack that cultural background, you can still find within you and your deeper roots a relationship with the plants you decide to grow. Designing a Medicine Wheel Garden is just one, albeit very powerful, way to honor the earth and support the Circle of Life.

But what are the other ways in which you can restore the connection with the Earth and be an active, positive force in the Circle of Life.

1. Show reverence and remember the interconnectedness of all life forms, honoring the Earth and its sacredness.
2. Grow endangered and at-risk plants to contribute to their conservation and restoration.
3. Create habitats that attract and support birds, butterflies, bees, and other beneficial creatures.
4. Plant native and historical trees, plants, vegetables, herbs, and wildflowers to preserve biodiversity.
5. Choose heirloom seeds, save and share them, or let them naturally disperse for continued growth.
6. Express joy, gratitude, and compassion for the Circle of Life, appreciating the interconnected web of relationships.
7. Designate a sacred space for ceremonies and rituals, fostering a deeper connection with nature.
8. Arrange seating areas strategically to immerse oneself in the beauty of the garden, from different perspectives and times of day.
9. Enhance soil fertility and health to support the growth of vibrant and resilient plants.
10. Foster thoughts, actions, and words that promote peace and harmony with the Earth and its ecosystems.
11. Embrace organic and flowing forms in the garden design, incorporating curves and natural shapes.
12. Create a special area in the garden to honor and remember ancestors, using plants as symbols of remembrance.
13. Design enchanted spaces for children to explore and connect with nature, fostering their sense of wonder and imagination.
14. Regularly reflect on how to reduce the ecological footprint and minimize harm to wildlife and the environment.
15. Cultivate a mindful partnership with the Earth, actively working towards its well-being and sustainability.
16. Repurpose and recycle natural materials, finding creative uses for shells, stones, branches, and other organic elements.
17. Embrace the sensory richness of diverse plant species, engaging all senses in the garden experience.
18. Preserve untouched wild areas within the landscape, creating sanctuaries for native flora and fauna to thrive undisturbed..

Planning a Medicine Wheel Garden

T he notion of the circle, representing profound unity and harmony, holds sacred significance. It symbolizes the interconnection and interdependence of all life on Earth, a belief deeply ingrained in ancient cultures for millennia. This reverence for planetary health served as a steadfast foundation, nurturing physical and mental well-being while fostering the perpetuation of the Circle of Life.

Recognizing the Earth's vitality and the opportunity for attunement with its consciousness, we acknowledge that all life forms constitute an Earth community. A garden offers a tangible space to experience and embrace this truth. Whether it be a Medicine Wheel Garden, a humble home apothecary garden, a flourishing food forest adorned with heirloom vegetables, a permaculture sanctuary, or a native woodland or prairie garden, each sustainable option we explored in the previous volume provides a model for growth rooted in conscience.

The circle embodies the sacred essence of Harmony, Truth, wholeness, unity, perfection, and infinite existence. Its natural presence pervades the world, serving as a fundamental form of life. Just as wheels smoothly propel vehicles forward, circles facilitate the graceful movement of all things through space, embodying synchronized harmony.

Life, in its diverse forms, is bound by a common thread. Indigenous peoples eloquently refer to life's myriad expressions as "People." Trees are known as Tree People, flowers as Flower People, and creatures of the air as Butterfly People or Winged People. Those who inhabit water are Water People, while humans are the Two-Legged People, and those who walk on four legs are the Bear People or Wolf People. In this journey, we shall acquaint ourselves with the Herb People and the Wildflower People, natives of our Land.

To visually embody this Circle, we can create a Medicine Wheel by drawing an equal-armed cross within a encompassing circle. This simple act results in four distinct wedges, each facing a cardinal direction. These Sacred Directions serve as focal points, each representing a season, an element, an animal, and carrying symbolic significance within Native cultures.

Guided by spirit beings from each direction since birth, we are bestowed wisdom from various perspectives. These experiences throughout our lives cultivate an awareness of the Earth, enabling profound connections within the Circle of Life.North is represented by the top wedge, which is white in hue and signifies winter, Eldership, Reflection, Deep Spirituality, and Life Understanding.

East is represented by the right-hand wedge, which is yellow in color and represents spring, planting, birth, new beginnings, second chances, and a connection to the physical world.

South is represented by the bottom wedge, which is red in color and signifies summer, growth, the teen years, mental development, and intellectual understanding.

West is represented by the left-hand wedge, which is dark or blue in color and denotes fall, harvest, adulthood, and deep emotional knowledge.

The circle's center represents you or your community. Of course, depending on which are your cultural roots and what resonates with you, there are numerous ways to imagine a Medicine Wheel.

The key thing is to focus on the four parts of life that are portrayed and the contemplative discoveries that can be made within each of them.

You'll need a compass and a permanent mean to identify the four cardinal directions if you want to make a Medicine Wheel Garden.

The obvious choice is rocks, but sculptures, bricks, or even large letters may suffice as long as they are weatherproof. Because you'll be walking on the spokes, flat stones or some form of paving would be ideal. Perhaps a large flat rock or a smaller circle packed with gravel for the circle's center.

Then you get to choose which colors represent the four qualities to you and plant various plants of that hue in each wedge. You might find that you have spirit guides for each element when you meditate in the garden, in which case you'll want to include items that remind you of them.

You can also choose to honor the four elements in your garden design. Here are a few ideas:

Earth: Choose a serene location in nature to create a sacred circle. Place twelve stones, representing the cardinal directions of East, South, West, and North. In the center, position five smaller stones symbolizing Above, Below, Within, Love, and Peace. Let this be a space of balance, reflection, and connection.

Fire Element: Consider the soothing practice of burning sage incense as you stroll through your garden. The gentle wafts of sacred smoke has a calming effect and also benefits your plants, particularly those troubled by insect pests. Embrace this mindful act of smudging to create an atmosphere of tranquility and support the well-being of your cherished green companions.

Air Element: Enhance the ambiance of your garden by adorning a tree with a delicate wind chime. Let its melodious tones dance on the breeze, capturing the essence of the wind and carrying your heartfelt prayers and intentions into the garden. As the chimes resonate, they infuse the space with healing vibrations and positive energies, nurturing a sense of tranquility and harmony. Allow this harmonious interplay between nature, sound, and intention to create a sacred atmosphere within your garden sanctuary.

Water Element: Enhance the natural allure of your garden by carefully selecting a serene spot to install a delightful birdbath. Nestle it next to a flourishing shrub, creating a harmonious and inviting space for birds to gather, drink, and bathe. Remember to change the water in the birdbath daily, providing a clean and refreshing oasis for your feathered friends.

As you explore your landscape, take a mindful stroll to identify areas where water can be collected and utilized. Observe the contours of the land and seek opportunities to capture rainwater or repurpose runoff for irrigation purposes. Consider incorporating a small pond, a rain barrel, or other innovative water management systems to harness and maximize the natural resources available.

By embracing water conservation and wise utilization, you not only nurture the health and vibrancy of your garden but also contribute to the sustainability of the ecosystem. Let the presence of water in your landscape serve as a reminder of our interconnectedness with nature and the responsibility we have to be mindful stewards of the environment.

A Medicine Wheel, like any garden, will be a work in progress.

Your garden will also teach you to honor the season and the everlasting cycle of life, to mark the seasons be sure to celebrate and reflect upon the aims you wish to achieve in the piece of land that is under your care on each solstice and equinox.

Winter Solstice

The winter solstice, marking the beginning of an important cycle of life in late December, invites reflection and planning. As landscapes lie dormant and growth pauses, it is an opportune time to envision and set goals for the upcoming year. Similar to planting a garden, choices must be made regarding the seeds we wish to sow and the changes we aspire to make. Let these questions guide your contemplation:

1. What do I want to achieve in the next year?
2. What seeds do I wish to plant for my life during the upcoming year?
3. What new plants can I introduce to my landscape to bring joy and nourishment?
4. What changes do I desire to make in my life? How can I transform my landscape?

Embrace this moment of stillness and introspection to shape your intentions, envisioning the possibilities that lie ahead. Just as a well-tended garden requires thoughtful planning and deliberate action, so too does the cultivation of a fulfilling life and a vibrant landscape. Let these questions ignite your imagination and inspire your journey towards growth, abundance, and harmony.

Spring Equinox

The spring equinox, arriving in late March, heralds a season of growth and opportunity. It is a time to lay the foundation for realizing your goals and dreams. Embrace this moment of renewal and take proactive steps towards success. As you embark on this journey, consider the following questions:

1. What steps do I need to take to achieve my goals?
2. Am I facing any resistance or obstacles along the way? How can I address them?
3. What actions, words, thoughts, or emotions will nurture the growth of my seeds?
4. What changes do I want to make in my life to align with my goals and aspirations?

By identifying the necessary actions and addressing any barriers, you empower yourself to move forward with confidence and determination. Share your goals with others, engaging in networking and seeking support from like-minded individuals. Embrace new ideas, stretching your mind and exploring uncharted territories. Plant the seeds of intention, and nurture them with focused efforts, positivity, and a mindset primed for growth.

Summer Solstice

As the summer solstice approaches in late June, a season of celebration and abundance comes into view. It is a time for garden parties, where friends and family gather to enjoy the bountiful rewards of the seeds sown earlier in the year. As you revel in the beauty and abundance surrounding you, reflect on the following questions:

1. What is blooming or growing well in my landscape?
2. Where do I see abundance in my life and surroundings?
3. What is my favorite bloom or most cherished aspect of my landscape? Conversely, what challenges or obstacles have arisen?
4. What issues or aspects of my life have I become more aware of during this season?
5. What valuable lessons have I learned along the way?
6. How can I transform these lessons into opportunities for personal growth?
7. How can I celebrate the achievements I have made or am currently making?
8. How can I acknowledge or celebrate the earth, wind, water, or any element of the Circle of Life in my festivities?

As you bask in the warmth of summer, let joy and gratitude fill your heart. Embrace the season of abundance and take time to appreciate the gifts that have bloomed in your life.

Autumn Equinox

As the autumn equinox arrives in late September, it marks the magnificent conclusion of the cosmic cycle of seasons. Now is the time to reap the fruits of your labor and reflect on the abundance that has been bestowed upon you. Take stock of the blessings you have received and express gratitude. Share your experiences with others, celebrating your journey thus far. As you prepare to enter the season of the West, characterized by introspection and slowing down, consider the following questions leading up to the winter solstice:

1. What are the fruits of the seeds I planted at last year's winter solstice?
2. What have I achieved and accomplished this year?
3. What valuable lessons have I learned and what experiences have I enjoyed since the beginning of the year?
4. Who am I today, in this moment of reflection and self-discovery?
5. Where would I like to steer my life's path from here onwards?
6. What seeds do I want to plant at the upcoming winter solstice, setting intentions for the next year's journey?

By reflecting on the outcomes of your previous seeds, acknowledging your achievements, and embracing the lessons and joys of the year, you gain clarity about your current identity and aspirations. Contemplate the path you wish to embark upon, envisioning the directions you desire to explore and the goals you wish to set. As the winter solstice approaches, you will have the opportunity to plant new seeds, birthing fresh intentions for the year ahead.

Understanding the Meaning

Infinity, perfection, and the everlasting are all represented by the circle, which has neither beginning nor end.

The circle is articulated in many symbolic ways in our lives and in our varied cultures:

- **The wedding band:** Universally regarded as a symbol of protection and bonding, the wedding band takes the form of a circle, representing the eternal nature of love and commitment between partners.
- **Hindu depiction of the Wheel of Existence:** Hindus symbolize the vastness of existence as a circle, illustrating the continuous cycle of birth, life, death, and rebirth. This circular representation captures the essence of the eternal nature of the soul's journey.
- **Yin Yang symbol:** Derived from Eastern philosophies, the Yin Yang symbol exemplifies the interdependence and balance of opposing energies. The circle within the symbol signifies the harmony and equilibrium achieved when these energies coexist in a state of dynamic balance.
- **Tibetan Buddhist mandalas:** Tibetan Buddhism utilizes mandalas as symbolic artwork and sand paintings to represent paths to enlightenment. These intricate circular designs serve as visual aids for meditation, guiding practitioners towards spiritual awakening and a deeper understanding of reality.
- **Ancient labyrinths:** Labyrinths, constructed in circular form, have held significant spiritual meaning across cultures. In Christian labyrinths, the center represents the Universe or the venerated "Creator-God," while the winding trails leading to the center symbolize a metaphorical pilgrimage towards divine connection and spiritual enlightenment.

These examples highlight the diverse and profound symbolism attributed to the circle across different cultures and belief systems. The circle's encompassing and unbroken nature speaks to concepts of unity, eternity, balance, and spiritual significance, making it a powerful symbol that transcends time and borders.

The sacred hoop and circle were important to Native American culture in describing their link with the universe and the Creator.

The Native Americans and Lower Canadian tribes held the circle of the Universe in utmost reverence, considering it a spiritual blueprint for all human actions. By incorporating the circle into their everyday duties and conduct, they infused ritual meaning into every aspect of existence. The Plains Indians, for instance, conducted circular gatherings for ceremonies, meals, dances, and even in the structure of their dwellings, such as the tipi.

To the Native Americans, the circle symbolized not only the vastness of the universe but also the cycles of growth, death, and rebirth. They observed these cycles in the rising and setting of the sun and moon, the planting and harvesting of crops, and the birth and passing of each individual. Thus, the medicine wheel became a powerful tool for honoring and celebrating nature's cyclical patterns through ritual, song, dance, and offerings.

Ceremonial practices permeated every facet of Native American culture, going beyond mere symbolism. Ceremonies provided a means to communicate with Nature in a way that transcended the limitations of human language. Even ordinary daily activities were performed in a ritualized manner to honor the natural cycles that governed their lives.

For the Native Americans, every moment of life held sacred significance as they deeply valued the abundance of food, crops, water, and their harmonious coexistence with Mother Earth. Their relationship with the Earth was one of spiritual encounter, transforming everywhere they walked, ate, and slept into hallowed ground where ceremonies and rituals were established to honor and revere the interconnectedness of all things.

The sacred circle served as a stylized framework to depict the vastness of the universe and the interconnectedness of its components. The four cardinal directions held special significance, each guarded by an animal totem. Archaeologists and historians have extensively theorized about the ritualistic and ceremonial purposes of the ancient medicine wheels, particularly the specific placement of animal totems, as their true intention was not explicitly recorded.

Different civilizations devised their own unique rituals and methods to depict their relationship with the cosmos or their Creator. Medicine wheels, mandalas, sacred circle teachings, labyrinths, stone megaliths, and other tools were employed as expressions of this profound connection and to explore their place within the greater cosmic order. Each of these practices served as a means to deepen their understanding and express their reverence for the Universe and its intricate web of life.

Beyond the physical shape, gardening is linked to the sacred circle notion. A life cycle is represented by a circle. Plants and flowers go through the same life cycle as humans, including birth, adolescence, adulthood, and death.

The life cycle of plants follows a natural progression from seed germination to growth, blooming, seed development, and eventually plant death. While some plants have long lifespans, the cycle is particularly evident in annual blooms that last for a single season.

Without the inclusion of traditional rituals and ceremonies, the concept of the Medicine Wheel can be adapted for use in the garden. By labeling your garden as a "Medicine Wheel Garden," you honor ancient traditions and add depth to the design and implementation process.

A garden designed in the shape of a strong circle, paying homage to the cardinal directions, can incorporate animal totems represented by stones or boulders resembling animals. Four basic spokes intersecting through the center reinforce the movement of the spirit and the embodiment of your chosen focus within the garden. This personalized sacred garden space becomes truly unique.

To infuse your garden with sacredness, customize it according to your own preferences and belief systems. Begin with the fundamental structure of the circle and the four quadrants, and then add elements that resonate with you, such as crystals, feathers, flowers, spheres, garden art, or other symbolic items. Tailor the size of the sacred circle to fit your garden, ensuring that you create a space where you can move around without disrupting its sacredness. Trust your intuition and follow what feels right, allowing the creation of a space where you are spiritually connected to each plant you grow. This connection enables you to honor and express gratitude for the medicinal and nutritional benefits they provide.

The goal is to cultivate a sacred environment where you feel a deep spiritual connection with the plants, fostering a sense of reverence and appreciation. By honoring the plants and expressing gratitude, you establish a harmonious relationship that extends beyond their utilitarian value.

Picking Your Spot
The type of plants that can grow in the area will depend on whether it is sunny or shady. Then decide on the size of the bed; for a beginner, five to ten feet across would suffice, while a garden with a diameter of 20 to 30 feet will be enough for an expert gardener. Place a stake in the ground and attach a half-diameter string to it. Walk around a circle while keeping the string taut and marking points throughout the circumference with little sticks.

Mark the Directions
With larger sticks, indicate north, south, east, and west. Determine the directions with a compass. If possible, go out on a starry night, identify the Big Dipper, and picture a line extending from the dipper's bowl's last two stars. The bright North Star, which denotes true north, is indicated by that line.

Clean Up the Site
Within the circle, dig up grass or other plant matter. It is advisable to go against using pesticides or other chemicals, as this would negate the objective of planting medicinal plants.

Work in organic compost or composted manure at approximately 50 pounds for a small garden and two or three times that for a large one, using a pitchfork or shovel.

Clean Up the Guideposts
Remove the stick markers from the picture. Mark the circle and quadrants with cobble-sized rocks. Cover walkways with gravel or river stones if the garden is large enough.

Continue Upkeep
Seeds or transplants should be sown by placing straw or bark around the bases of the plants to conserve soil moisture and keep weeds at bay. Try distributing rocks throughout the quadrants as well. The rocks operate as heat sinks, absorbing heat during the day and releasing it at night, maintaining a consistent temperature for the plants. During dry spells, water is essential.

Native Medicinal Herbs for your Garden

This is a carefully chosen selection of Native plants that you can grow in your herbal garden. It covers herbs, shrubs, and groundcover plants, wildflowers warrant a volume of their own, the next volume of this series For each plant are indicated its medical uses, solvents, hardiness zone, sourcing and habitat, gardening techniques, and consumption methods. However, for more information on their identification, their traditional and modern uses please refer to the second volume of the series. Whereas in the second volume the plants were chosen for their health benefits, in this volume the plants were also chosen for the benefits they can provide in a garden either because they are endangered species which warrant replication in a native garden, or because they are excellent pollinators. Several plants are only present in this volume: for these plants the traditional and modern uses, as well as the identification have been reported in this volume. Happy reading!

Aloe Vera

Medicinal Aloe, Barbados Aloe.

Liliacee.

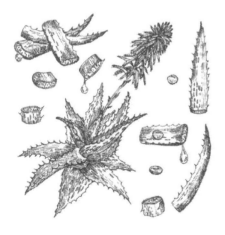

Medical Uses: Aloe Vera was utilized by Native Americans to soothe and treat their skin, as well as nourish and protect it from harsh climates such as dry deserts. It was also used to make soap and to heal sunburn. Today, the component may be found in a variety of skin-soothing products, including after-sun creams, face masks, and moisturizers. Check the second volume for more information on all the amazing uses this plant

Solvents: Water.

Hardiness Zones: Zones 8-11.

Sourcing: You can find Aloe Vera plants at any big box store or garden center. Even if you don't have a garden or you can't grow it, you can keep a potted aloe vera at home, it's extremely useful and forgives forgetfulness and infrequent waterings.

Gardening Tips: Begin by placing your aloe vera in a location that receives ample bright, indirect sunlight. A south-facing window or a well-lit spot outdoors with partial shade is ideal. Ensure you use a well-draining soil specifically formulated for succulents or cacti. This type of soil allows excess water to flow through, preventing root rot and promoting optimal growth.

When it comes to watering your aloe vera, it's essential to strike the right balance. Aloe vera is a drought-tolerant plant, so it's important not to overwater it. Water deeply, allowing the soil to completely dry out between waterings. This mimics the plant's natural habitat and helps prevent the onset of root rot. As a general rule, during the warmer months, water your aloe vera approximately every two to three weeks. In the colder months, when growth slows down, reduce watering to once a month or when the soil is completely dry.

Choosing the right container is also crucial for aloe vera's well-being. Opt for a pot that provides proper drainage with sufficient drainage holes. This allows excess water to escape and prevents the plant's roots from sitting in stagnant water, which can lead to root rot. Additionally, select a pot size that provides ample room for the plant's growth, ensuring it isn't cramped.

Temperature plays a significant role in the health of your aloe vera plant. Aim for temperatures between 55-80°F (13-27°C) to maintain optimal growth. Avoid exposing your plant to extreme temperature fluctuations, as it may result in stress or damage.

Lastly, consider occasional fertilization. While aloe vera plants can survive without fertilizer, a light application of a balanced, water-soluble fertilizer diluted to half strength can promote healthy growth. Apply the fertilizer sparingly during the active growing season, typically in spring and summer, following the package instructions.

Consumption Methods: While many herbs in this book are commonly used in tea, this won't be the case for Aloe Vera. Aloe Vera is typically used in lotions and salves or raw as the gel-like contents of the plant can be directly rubbed onto the skin or made into juice.

Warnings: It is important to exercise caution when consuming aloe vera. While aloe vera gel and products derived from it are widely used in skincare and cosmetics, the internal consumption of aloe vera should be approached with care. Aloe vera contains compounds called anthraquinones, specifically aloin, which can have laxative effects and may cause abdominal discomfort, cramping, and diarrhea, particularly when consumed in excessive amounts.

Moreover, aloe vera plants may also contain other compounds that could be harmful if ingested in large quantities. It is crucial to ensure that any aloe vera product intended for consumption is specifically formulated and labeled as food-grade or intended for internal use.

If you are considering incorporating aloe vera into your diet or using it for its potential health benefits, it is recommended to consult with a healthcare professional or a qualified herbalist.

Alumroot

Jill-of-the-Rocks, Coral Bells.

Heuchera.

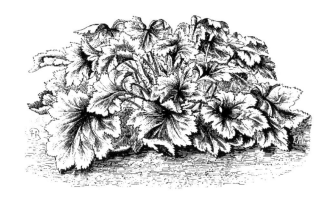

Identification: The evergreen leaves are handsome from spring through winter, sometimes with purplish undersides; they seldom reach 12 inches in height. The airy stems of flowers rise 24–30 inches. The flowers themselves reward close inspection; they are light green and asymmetrical, with a longer top side, and sport cute orange protruding stamens—they may not be pink, but hummingbirds appreciate them and nectar from them all the same. Alumroot grows in almost any well-drained soil. It is hands down the hardiest heuchera species, growing on prairies throughout the northern Great Plains.

Traditional Uses: Alumroots were essential medicinal herbs for both indigenous peoples and herbalists in North America. In the 18th century, a powerful astringent derived from the roots was reputedly used to treat cancer. The roots were used to treat wounds, sores, and liver diseases by Native Americans in the interior, and the Secwepemc created a solution of the leaves to treat diarrhea. Plants of this genus are also employed as a mordant to attach dyes by craftspeople.

Medicinal parts: roots and leaves

Solvents: Boiling water, alcohol.

Hardiness Zones: Zones 4-9.

Sourcing: From low to mid-elevations, Alumroot can be found on damp, grassy bluffs, rocky slopes, and forest edges. It can be found from British Columbia to just beyond the border of northwestern California, passing through western Washington and Oregon. In eastern Oregon and Idaho, there are a few isolated clusters. You can carefully forage it or easily find it at a reputable local nursery

Gardening Tips: For successful cultivation of alumroot (Heuchera spp.), selecting the ideal planting location is crucial. Choose a shaded area in your garden that offers protection from intense sunlight, particularly during the hottest parts of the day. Alumroot thrives in partial shade to full shade conditions, as excessive sunlight can scorch its delicate foliage.

Before planting, it is important to prepare the soil properly. Start by clearing the planting area of any weeds or debris. Alumroot prefers well-draining soil, so ensure that the soil has good drainage to prevent waterlogging and root rot. If your soil is heavy or clay-like, consider amending it with organic matter such as compost or well-rotted manure. This will improve soil structure, enhance moisture retention, and provide essential nutrients for healthy growth. When it's time to plant, dig a hole that is slightly larger than the root ball of the alumroot plant. Gently remove the plant from its container, being careful not to damage the roots. Place the plant in the hole, making sure that the crown (where the roots meet the stem) is level with or slightly above the soil surface. Backfill the hole with soil, gently firming it around the roots to eliminate air pockets. Water the plant thoroughly after planting to settle the soil and provide initial hydration. Proper watering is essential for alumroot's health. While alumroot prefers consistently moist soil, it is important to avoid overwatering, as this can lead to root rot. Monitor the soil moisture regularly by checking the top inch of soil. Water the plant when the soil feels slightly dry to the touch, aiming for a deep watering that reaches the root zone. Mulching around the base of the plant with organic material, such as wood chips or straw, can help retain soil moisture and suppress weed growth.

In terms of fertilization, alumroot generally doesn't require heavy feeding. However, you can apply a balanced slow-release fertilizer in early spring to provide a nutrient boost. Follow the package instructions for proper dosage and application method, ensuring you don't overfertilize, as this can lead to excessive foliage growth at the expense of flowering. Regular maintenance is important for alumroot's longevity and appearance. Remove any faded flower stalks promptly to encourage new blooms and prevent seed formation. Trim damaged or diseased leaves as needed to maintain the plant's overall health and aesthetics. Division can be done every few years in early spring to rejuvenate the plant and control its size. Dig up the plant, separate the clumps, and replant them in suitable locations. By following these detailed instructions, you can create an optimal growing environment for alumroot, resulting in healthy plants that enhance the beauty of your garden year after year.

Consumption Methods: Alumroot has long been esteemed for its astringent and styptic properties. The root of the plant contains high levels of tannins, which contribute to its potent therapeutic effects. Alumroot can be utilized both internally and externally to address various ailments.

When taken internally, alumroot is commonly used as a mild astringent to help alleviate conditions such as diarrhea and dysentery. It can also be used as a gargle or mouthwash to relieve sore throat or mouth ulcers. Externally, alumroot is a valuable ingredient in topical preparations. Its astringent properties make it particularly effective for reducing bleeding and promoting the healing of minor cuts, wounds, and bruises. A decoction or infusion of alumroot can be applied as a compress or used in a bath to help soothe skin irritations, such as rashes or insect bites. It is important to note that individuals with sensitive skin may experience mild irritation, so a patch test is advisable before using alumroot topically. The combined application of a poultice made from the mashed root of alumroot (Heuchera spp.) and the resinous pitch extracted from Douglas fir (Pseudotsuga menziesii) has demonstrated efficacy in wound treatment. To utilize this remedy, the poultice should be carefully prepared, ensuring that the mashed root and pitch are thoroughly mixed. Once prepared, the poultice ought to be covered with a clean cloth and gently applied to the open wound. This application helps promote healing and provides a protective barrier. Moreover, the chewed leaves or roots of alumroot can serve as effective dressings for wounds when used independently. By directly applying the chewed plant material to the affected area, it aids in the healing process and provides a natural barrier against potential contaminants. In addition to wound care, alumroot offers a traditional application to promote hair growth. To harness this benefit, the plant can be crushed, creating a paste that is then rubbed onto the scalp as a tonic. This botanical treatment stimulates the hair follicles, potentially enhancing hair growth. The dose of alumroot can vary depending on the intended application. For internal use, a standardized extract or infusion is typically recommended. A common dosage range is approximately 1-2 grams of dried alumroot root or leaf per cup of boiling water, steeped for 10-15 minutes. This infusion can be consumed up to three times daily. It is advisable to consult a qualified herbalist or healthcare professional to determine the appropriate dosage and duration for specific health concerns.

Warning: Overdosing can cause gastric upset.

American Ginseng

Man-root, Ginseng.

Panax quinquefolius.

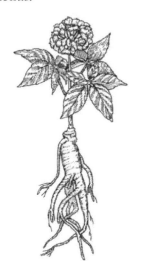

Medical Uses: The Ojibwe has a long-standing tradition of using American ginseng (Panax quinquefolius) for its medicinal properties. They have employed it as a tonic for boosting vitality and stamina, as well as for its adaptogenic effects, assisting the body in adapting to physical and mental stressors. The Seneca tribe has also recognized the medicinal value of American ginseng (Panax quinquefolius). They have traditionally used it as a natural remedy for various ailments, including enhancing cognitive function, improving digestion, and supporting overall immune health. Check the second volume for more information on its uses and consumption.

Solvents: Boiling water, alcohol.

Hardiness Zones: Zones 3-7.

Sourcing: American Ginseng can be found in deciduous forests throughout the United States, mainly in the Appalachian and Ozark regions, as well as eastern Canada. If the soil is rich and moist, it is a candidate for supporting American Ginseng. Do not forage it, acquire seeds from a reputable source

Gardening Tips: Ginseng, known as "man root" due to its leg-like appearance, has been revered by the Chinese for centuries, valued for its cognitive enhancement, stress reduction, energy restoration, and anti-inflammatory properties. The popularity of Ginseng reached North America in the 1700s, where American Ginseng (Panax quinquefolius) emerged as a sought-after herbal remedy alongside the original Red Ginseng (Panax ginseng). However, the demand for American Ginseng led to near extinction in the 1970s, resulting in strict regulations on wild harvesting. Today, wild Ginseng remains superior, but cultivating it on private property is a viable option to avoid legal complications.

To steward a ginseng population, the first step is locating a wild population, often found in shaded areas under certain tree species like tulip-poplars, jack-in-the-pulpit, rattlesnake fern, sugar maple, and wild ginger. Timing is crucial for planting Ginseng seeds, as they germinate better after the berries turn red, typically in late August. Stewardship should occur after the berries are red but before the harvest season begins, respecting the natural life cycle of the plant.

Growing Ginseng at home requires patience and careful attention. Stratified seeds or purchased seedlings are recommended to ensure successful germination and growth. Choose a well-shaded location with proper drainage and limited weed competition. Raised beds with netting or containers with drainage reservoirs can mimic the ideal forest-like conditions Ginseng thrives in. Plant seeds in the fall at a depth of 12 inches or place roots in early spring under 3 inches of soil, following the natural rhythm of the plant.

Ginseng thrives in shady, forest-like environments with rich, well-draining soil that is slightly acidic. When selecting a location for your ginseng patch, choose an area under the canopy of deciduous trees, where the plants can receive filtered sunlight.

Begin by preparing the soil. Clear away any debris or competing vegetation, ensuring that the area is free from weeds and grass. Ginseng seeds have a dormancy period and require a stratification process to improve germination rates. To simulate this natural process, place the seeds in a moist medium, such as peat moss or sand, and store them in a cool location (around 40°F or 4°C) for several months. This stratification period breaks the seed's dormancy and prepares it for germination.

Once the stratification period is complete, it's time to sow the ginseng seeds. Gently press the seeds into the prepared soil, ensuring they are spaced at least a few inches apart to allow sufficient room for growth. Cover the seeds lightly with a thin layer of leaf litter or compost to mimic the natural forest floor. This layer helps maintain moisture levels and provides insulation for the seeds.

Water the newly planted seeds regularly, ensuring the soil remains consistently moist but not waterlogged. Mulching around the plants with a layer of organic matter, such as leaf compost or wood chips, can help retain moisture and suppress weed growth. Ginseng requires patience, as it takes several years for the plants to reach maturity and develop their characteristic root.

As your ginseng plants grow, keep an eye out for pests and diseases. Slugs and deer can pose a threat to young ginseng plants, so implementing protective measures like slug traps and fencing can be beneficial. Proper ventilation and spacing between plants are also crucial for preventing fungal diseases.

In autumn, ginseng enters a dormant phase, and the foliage will begin to turn yellow. This is an indication that the plants are preparing for winter. It is important to resist the temptation to harvest the roots too soon. Ginseng typically requires a minimum of five to six years of growth before the roots can be harvested for their medicinal properties. Waiting for the roots to reach their full potential ensures a higher concentration of beneficial compounds.

Harvesting ginseng roots requires careful attention to prevent damage. Gently loosen the soil around the base of the plant and slowly extract the root system. Take care not to break or damage the roots, as this can diminish their value. Once harvested, the roots can be cleaned, dried, and stored in a cool, dry place for future use.

Harvesting mature Ginseng roots in the fall requires careful handling to preserve their value. The roots can be consumed raw or used fresh in teas, soups, and stir-fries. Alternatively, they can be dried and sliced or grated for future use. Steaming or making tea by steeping freshly sliced Ginseng in boiling water are also popular consumption methods. For those who prefer not to consume the plant directly, alternative forms such as pills, salves, lotions, and soaps are available.

Warnings: While American ginseng offers numerous potential health benefits, it is essential to be aware of certain precautions and potential risks associated with its use. Firstly, ginseng can interact with certain medications, such as blood thinners, anticoagulants, and immunosuppressants, so it is crucial to consult with a healthcare professional before incorporating it into your routine, particularly if you have underlying health conditions or are taking prescription medications. Additionally, some individuals may experience allergic reactions or side effects, including headaches, digestive issues, and changes in blood pressure. Pregnant and breastfeeding women, as well as children, should exercise caution and consult a healthcare professional before using ginseng. Lastly, wild harvesting of American ginseng is strictly regulated to protect the plant's population and preserve its natural habitat. Engaging in legal and sustainable sourcing practices is of utmost importance to ensure the long-term availability of this valuable herb.

Anise Hyssop

Blue Giant Hyssop, Fragrant Giant Hyssop, Lavender Giant Hyssop.

Agastache foeniculum.

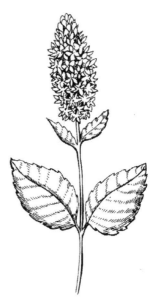

Identification: Both the flowers and leaves of this popular aromatic perennial herb are edible; they taste just like licorice, and you have only to rub the foliage when passing by to release the anise scent. The violet-blue florets stand out from the more-purply calyxes for a strikingly showy flower that produces a seed head that holds well into winter. The plant is in flower over a long period, from early summer into autumn, and grows 3–4 feet tall.

We rarely design a landscape with the late-season hole created by dormant perennials in mind, but that's when yellow giant hyssop is at its showiest, bringing interest to the garden. The late-summer flowers are inconspicuous but very rich in nectar, with hummingbirds and other pollinators vying for position. When in bloom, the plant dances with swallowtails and hummingbirds and, later, goldfinches vie for position on its seed heads. The fruiting heads are marvelous atop exuberantly tall, sturdy stems, like torches in winter. Yellow giant hyssop grows 5–7 feet tall in well-drained moist soils in full sun to light shade. Plant it at the back of a perennial border with a woodland backdrop. It's best in a natural landscape, insectaries garden, or bird garden, as it brings in creatures, including deer (unusual for a mint), exceedingly well. Individual plants are short-lived but self-sow readily.

Purple giant hyssop is quite similar to yellow giant hyssop, only with pale bluish or purplish florets. Its common name overstates the reality of its light-colored flowers, as the photo shows, but they are as rich in nectar as both anise hyssop and yellow giant hyssop and appreciated by an equal cloud of pollinators. Purple giant hyssop grows as large as yellow giant hyssop, 2–5 feet tall, and has similarly simple cultural requirements: just give it well-drained garden soil. Its showy fruiting heads look great at the back of a perennial border or in the winter landscape.

Traditional Uses: Anise hyssop has been utilized in traditional herbal medicine for a long time, particularly by Native Americans. Anise hyssop, when infused in tea, can help to reduce congestion by acting as an expectorant (clearing mucus from lungs and airways). A cold infusion can be used to ease chest discomfort produced by coughing too much, and it can also be used to treat respiratory infections and bronchitis when combined with licorice. Because a hot infusion produces sweating, it can be used to treat fevers; the Cheyenne were known to utilize anise hyssop in sweat lodges as a result of this property.

Solvents: Boiling water, alcohol.

Hardiness Zones: Zones 4-8.

Sourcing: Anise hyssop, a native of North America, grows wild in grasslands, dry woodlands, and plains.

Gardening Tips: To begin, choose a suitable time for planting Anise Hyssop. Wait until after the last frost and aim for the spring season. Seedlings can be planted anytime between spring and early summer. Consider incorporating this herb into various garden settings, such as borders, wildflower gardens, herb gardens, or butterfly gardens. Allow sufficient spacing of 18 to 24 inches between plants, or use them as specimens in containers. With a height ranging from 2 to 5 feet and a width of 1 to 3 feet, Anise Hyssop makes an excellent addition to the middle or rear of perennial borders. Enhance its presence by companion planting it with Japanese anemones, native biennial brown-eyed Susan (Rudbeckia triloba), goldenrods like Solidago rugosa 'Fireworks,' or fragrant herbs such as garlic, chives, oregano, and thyme.

Anise Hyssop thrives when exposed to direct sunlight. While it can tolerate partial shade, inadequate sunlight may result in leggy growth. Ensure your plants receive healthy, well-drained soil composed of sand, loam, chalk, or clay. Avoid heavy clay soils as they may hinder drainage, leading to potential root rot issues. Aim for a neutral pH level, and if your soil is acidic, consider adding lime. Ideally, the soil should be dry to moderately moist, although established plants can generally tolerate dry conditions. Effective drainage and overall dryness of the soil are crucial factors for winter survival.

During the initial four weeks after planting, provide water to newly planted Anise Hyssop if there is no rainfall. Water deeply and slowly to encourage the development of deep and spreading roots. Once the plants have established themselves, they are remarkably drought-tolerant, requiring minimal watering.

To maintain the vigor and health of your Anise Hyssop, incorporate compost into the soil every other year during early spring. Apply a shovelful of compost around the base of each plant, leaving a couple of inches of space between the compost and the main stem.

Once Anise Hyssop is established, it generally requires minimal upkeep. To encourage continuous flowering and prevent the formation of seed heads, it is advisable to deadhead any spent flowers. Additionally, periodic trimming will help the plant maintain its best appearance. Pruning in early spring, cutting back up to one-third of the woody material, will promote a bushier growth habit. Use sterilized pruning shears or loppers with sharp edges. Make angled cuts to prevent moisture from accumulating near the stem. In most parts of North America, Anise Hyssop will brown and die back during the winter. Cut back the plant in late winter, removing any dead plant material just above a promising bud node. Alternatively, if you prefer, you can leave the plant alone and add a little extra mulch around the root region. If rejuvenation is necessary, cut back Anise Hyssop stems to within 6 to 12 inches from the ground.

Dividing Anise Hyssop every 3 to 5 years is beneficial for maintaining the vitality of the plant and invigorating its growth. Spring is the ideal time to divide the clumps. Dig up a portion of the cluster, ensuring a generous amount of roots, and replant the division at the same depth as the original. Space the divisions approximately 2 feet apart. Thoroughly water both the original and transplanted plants.

When grown in optimal conditions and with proper care, Anise Hyssop can spread through rhizomes and self-seeding. Open-pollinated varieties are easily started from seed. Remember to press the seeds into the seed starting mix rather than burying them, as they require light to germinate. Cold, wet stratification can aid germination rates. Typically, the seeds will germinate within 1 to 4 weeks. Collecting seeds from mature blossoms is also a simple process. Allow the flowers to dry on the plant before collecting the ripe seeds in a bag. Additionally, division or semi-ripe stem cuttings taken during the summer can be used to create sterile hybrids.

While Anise Hyssop is generally hardy, it is susceptible to crown/root rot in poorly drained soils. To prevent common issues such as rust, powdery mildew, and leaf spots, ensure proper air circulation and avoid overhead watering. Despite these possible challenges, Anise Hyssop is a resilient perennial that deer tend to avoid. Its ability to attract pollinators and beneficial insects makes it an excellent choice for insectaries and companion planting in orchards. Its fruiting heads also provide a source of food for songbirds. Consider incorporating Anise Hyssop into more informal landscapes, herb borders, edible landscapes, or food forests. It adapts well and can even naturalize in moist, well-drained soils.

Consumption Methods: Anise has numerous applications in both the yard and the kitchen. Bees, butterflies, and hummingbirds are drawn to the nectar of the blooms. Birds, on the other hand, devour any seeds remaining on the stalks as the season progresses. Both the blossoms and the leaves have a strong licorice aroma and flavor. Aromatic leaves can be crumbled in salads, used to make jellies, steeped in herbal tea (like the Cheyenne tribe does to cure depression), or used to potpourris. Seeds can be sprinkled in cookies, muffins, or biscotti batters; dried leaves can be substituted for seeds for a similar licorice flavor.

Warnings: Nausea may be caused at exceptionally high doses.

Beth Root

Birth Root, Wake Robin, Nodding Wakerobin, Indian Shamrock, Lamb's Quarters, Indian Balm, Ground Lily, Cough Root, Jew's Harp Plant, Milk Ipecac, Pariswort, Rattlesnake Root, Snakebite, Three-Leaved Nightshade, Red Trillium, Stinking Benjamin.

Trillium erectum.

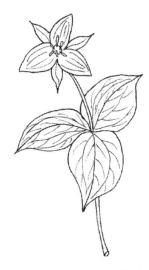

Identification: Beth Root, scientifically known as *Trillium spp.*, is a perennial herb belonging to the genus Trillium in the Liliaceae family. It can be found in temperate regions of North America and eastern Asia, particularly in rich and moist woodland areas with acidic soil.

The root of Beth Root emits a faint turpentine fragrance and has a peculiar aromatic and sweetish astringent taste when chewed, gradually turning bitter and acidic, which may cause salivation.

The stem of Beth Root is simple and can range in height from 3 to 30 inches. It emerges from a blunt tuber-like rhizome. The leaves of Beth Root are net-veined and somewhat mottled, typically measuring between 2 to 15 inches in length.

Beth Root produces flowers during the months of May and June. These flowers consist of three sepals and petals and can exhibit various colors, including white, pink, rose-maroon, red-brown, purple, green, yellow-green, or bright yellow.

Following the flowering stage, Beth Root develops pink or red three- or six-angled berries as its fruit.

Traditional Uses: Among the Iroquois people, beth root was highly regarded for its medicinal properties. The Seneca tribe, in particular, valued this herb for its ability to address gynecological concerns. Women within the tribe would utilize beth root as a natural aid during childbirth, as it was believed to promote healthy contractions and ease labor pains. Additionally, it was employed as a supportive remedy for menstrual irregularities, offering relief from discomfort and aiding in balancing the reproductive system.

Moving further west, the Cherokee Nation held beth root in high esteem for its versatile healing capabilities. This tribe recognized the herb's astringent properties and used it to address various gastrointestinal conditions. Beth root was often prepared as a decoction and consumed to alleviate diarrhea, dysentery, and other digestive disturbances. Moreover, the Cherokee utilized it as a poultice for external applications, finding it effective in treating wounds, cuts, and skin irritations.

The Potawatomi tribe, inhabiting the Great Lakes region, also embraced beth root for its therapeutic qualities. They revered it as a potent remedy for respiratory ailments, particularly bronchitis and coughs. The Potawatomi would prepare a decoction from the root and imbibe it to soothe irritated airways and promote expectoration. This herbal elixir was believed to possess mucolytic and anti-inflammatory properties, offering much-needed relief during times of respiratory distress.

Modern uses: The root includes steroidal saponins, which exert hormonal effects on the body, according to modern studies. These saponins are utilized in obstetric and gynecological treatment.

Solvents: Boiling water, alcohol.

Hardiness Zones: Zone 4-9.

Sourcing: The Eastern United States and Canada are home to Beth Root. It can be found throughout the Midwest and Appalachia, from Missouri to Arkansas. Beth Root grows abundantly in Kentucky, Indiana, Tennessee, and Ohio.

Remember to harvest during the plant's dormant season and carefully extract the underground rhizome while minimizing your impact on the environment. Alternatively, consider cultivating beth root in your own garden from rhizome divisions or purchasing from reputable nurseries.

Gardening Tips: Beth Root (Trillium erectum) thrives in deep, well-drained woods or humus-rich soil, making it ideal for shady and damp locations during the summer. Surprisingly versatile, it can adapt to shade, semi-shade, or even full sun. With an impressive resilience, this plant can withstand extremely low temperatures, enduring frost as severe as -35 degrees Celsius. Luckily, deer and rabbits tend to leave beth root undisturbed, allowing it to flourish without constant protection. The unassuming white blossoms of beth root possess a curious characteristic - a putrefied body-like appearance paired with a nearly scentless nature. If you choose to propagate this herb from seeds, be prepared to exercise patience, as it typically takes around two years for the plants to bloom. Seeds stored for some time should be planted in late winter or early spring for optimal germination. Within a span of 1-3 weeks, you can expect the seeds to sprout and initiate their growth. While the plants develops roots after the first round of cold stratification, shoots may not emerge until the second year and up to three years. To ensure successful overwintering during their early stages, it is recommended to provide young plants with cold frames in the first year. Throughout this period, it is crucial to maintain adequate moisture, avoiding both excessive dryness and saturation.

When it comes to dividing beth root plants after the flowering season, exercise caution to preserve their vitality. Larger divisions can be directly planted in their permanent locations, while smaller pieces thrive in light shade within small pots. Come the following spring, these smaller divisions can be safely transplanted to their designated spots, establishing themselves and preparing for future growth.

Consumption Methods: Creams, salves, and tinctures are the most common uses for Beth Root. Useful in pulmonary conditions, Beth root with the accompanying herbs Slippery elm (*Ulmus fulva*) and a small portion of Lobelia seed (*Lobelia inflata*), in powder form 10-20 grams. One teaspoon of the grounded up root boiled in 1 pint of milk is an expedient help in diarrhea and dysentery.

Warnings: If ingested incorrectly, Beth Root can cause nausea, vomiting, and irritation of the stomach and intestines. Skin irritation has also been reported by some people. It has the potential to cause miscarriage in pregnant women and exacerbate heart conditions.

Blue Cohosh

Squaw Root, Papoose Root.

Caulophyllum thalictroides.

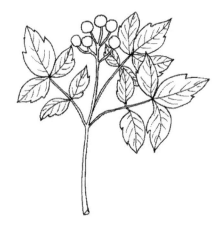

Identification: Blue Cohosh (Caulophyllum thalictroides) is a leafy perennial that reaches a maximum height of around 30 inches. It grows erect from a sturdy, brown-gray rhizome that branches out beneath the soil. The plant's leaves are tri-pinnate, composed of ovate leaflets that are finely divided. Each leaflet features three lobes, tapering to a wedge-shaped base.

During the flowering season, Blue Cohosh reveals its distinct beauty. The flowers emerge from the terminal leaf, displaying colors ranging from yellowish green to purple. Measuring approximately half an inch in width, the flowers consist of six sepals arranged in two rows. The petals are inconspicuous. Within the ovary lie two dark-blue, roundish seeds, each about ⅛ inch in diameter.

Traditional Uses: The Cherokee tribe valued Blue Cohosh for its medicinal properties, particularly for its potential benefits during pregnancy. They believed that the herb could help induce labor and alleviate associated discomfort. Additionally, they utilized Blue Cohosh as a tonic to support women's reproductive health.

Among the Delaware and Iroquois tribes, Blue Cohosh was employed as a women's medicine. It was considered useful for addressing menstrual irregularities and providing relief from cramps and other discomforts associated with the reproductive system.

The Menominee tribe recognized the herb's potential to ease labor pains. They utilized Blue Cohosh as a natural aid during childbirth, believing it could facilitate smooth and efficient contractions.

Modern Uses: Naturopaths and herbalists utilize Blue Cohosh for various purposes. It is commonly employed as an aid during childbirth to support uterine contractions and facilitate labor progression. While anecdotal evidence exists, it is important to note that scientific studies on Blue Cohosh are limited. However, some laboratory studies have explored its potential bioactive compounds and their effects on smooth muscle contractions. Furthermore, a clinical trial conducted at the University of Maryland Medical Center investigated the herb's efficacy in promoting cervical ripening.

Solvents: Boiling water, alcohol.

Hardiness Zones: Zones 3-8.

Sourcing: Shaded places and rich, moist soil are required for blue Cohosh to thrive. It's virtually found only in the Appalachian Mountains' damp woodlands nowadays. Avoid foraging if possible and acquire seeds from a reputable source, otherwise you might opt for propagation from cuttings.

Gardening Tips: Blue Cohosh should be planted outside. Plant the roots 2.5cm deep in damp wood soil with a pH of 4.5 to 7. They are relatively easy to keep once started.

Mulch for the winter. Keep the soil moist at all times by watering. To keep the soil moist, use leaf mulch. Don't bother them once they've settled in.

They should be planted 30 to 40cm apart in shaded regions and spaced 30 to 40cm apart.

Plants can be divided in the early autumn, or cuttings taken from the roots can be used to make more plants (complete with rhizomes).

Plants grown from seed will have to be grown for five years before the root can be harvested.

Consumption Methods: It can be made into a tincture, a lozenge, or a tea. Steep 1 oz. of the root in 1 pint of boiling water; dose, administer 2 tablespoonfuls every three hours. For nervous and sluggish cough it will act as an expectorant, for spasms it may be given more freely.

Warnings: Blue Cohosh used in large quantities can produce nausea, headaches, and high blood pressure.

Cascara Sagrada

California Buckthorn, Bearberry, Yellow Bark, Sacred Bark, Chittem, Chitticum.

Rhamnus purshiana.

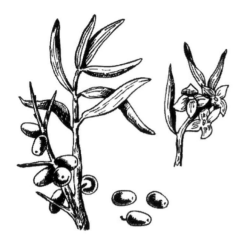

Medical uses: Cascara Sagrada, which means "holy bark" in Spanish, has been utilized as a laxative by Native Americans for millennia. Cascara was first utilized in western medicine in the 19th century, and it is still used in over-the-counter laxatives today, frequently in conjunction with other herbs like Aloe Vera. Other uses include as a treatment for digestive problems, joint and muscle pain, gonorrhea, gallstones, and dysentery. Check out more information in the second volume!

Solvents: Boiling water, alcohol.

Hardiness Zones: Zones 4-9.

Sourcing: Cascara can be found in the wild along the Pacific coast from British Columbia to northern California, as well as in Idaho and Montana. It can be found in moist to dry shade forests and mixed woodlands, as well as floodplains, often along streams or in moist ravines at low to moderate elevations.

Gardening Tips: Cascara Sagrada is a deciduous shrub that thrives in well-drained soil with moderate moisture levels. It prefers partial shade to full sun exposure, although some afternoon shade can be beneficial in hotter climates. When planting, ensure you provide enough space for the shrub to grow and spread, as it can reach heights of 15 to 25 feet. Pruning is best done during late winter or early spring to maintain a manageable size and promote healthy growth. Regular watering is crucial, especially during dry spells, to prevent the soil from drying out. However, be cautious not to overwater, as excessive moisture can lead to root rot. It is important to note that Cascara Sagrada is not a rapid grower and may take a few years to establish itself fully. Patience is key when waiting for its ornamental value to emerge. Although aphids can be an issue for Cascara, and its leaves have been shown to be vulnerable to Phytophthora, it appears that it is typically trouble-free, and its qualities of flexibility, seasons of beauty, and bird appeal much outweigh the hazards.

Consumption Methods: Many options are available, ranging from teas to tinctures, soaps to lotions. As with many of the other herbs in this volume, teas remain a popular option due to ease of access and quick relief. Check the second and third volume for more ideas.

Warnings: Stomach cramps and diarrhea are two common side effects. You should not use it if you have stomach pain, nausea, or vomiting, as you should with any laxative.

Black Chokeberry

Black Chokeberry, Aronia Berry, Aronia, Chokeberry.

Aronia melanocarpa.

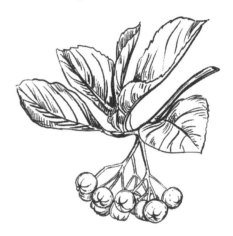

Identification: Black chokeberry grows 3–5 feet tall, is tidy and well behaved, and makes a great ornamental shrub for a traditional garden. The foliage and flower stems are smooth and glossy on most forms. The leaves turn rich saturated shades of red in the fall. Black chokeberry produces clusters of showy white flowers with pink stamens that are presented well as they are set above the leaves. The fruit is inky black when ripe, often beautifully polished in fall, and creates a striking contrast to the red fall leaves. The dried fruit remains on the plant all winter. Black chokeberry can be cultivated in a wide range of soils from sand to clay.

Traditional uses: Fruits were eaten by the Potawatomi, and an infusion of fruits was used to treat colds. The fruits were also eaten by the Abnaki. Hemorrhoids have traditionally been treated with it topically. It's also been used to keep the urinary system healthy, combat bacteria and viruses, improve memory, aid digestion, and treat diabetes and arthritis.

Modern uses: Antioxidants (anthocyanins and flavonoids) are found in greater abundance in Black Chokeberry fruit than in any other temperate fruit.

Solvents: Water, alcohol.

Hardiness Zone: Zones 3-8

Sourcing: Any reputable retailer or online storefront. Easy to find. Chokeberries can be found wild in swamps, drylands, and wet woods.

Gardening Tips: This shrub has a wide range of adaptability and hardiness. It thrives in both wet and dry environments. Furthermore, while the soil pH should preferably be acidic, it can also grow in alkaline soil. While it prefers well-draining soil, it may readily tolerate swampy conditions. When determining how to employ Black Chokeberry in the landscape, take advantage of its versatility. Its tolerance of swampy soil, for example, makes it a great choice for moist locations where many other plants would not thrive.

Because Black Chokeberry is tolerant of a wide range of growth conditions, it spreads quickly throughout the landscape. If you don't want many shrubs to develop a thicket, keep an eye out for suckers around the base of the plant that will sprout additional plants. Aside from that, this shrub requires very little maintenance because it will basically look after itself. It also doesn't have a lot of difficulties with pests and diseases. To keep it in shape, water it during dry spells and prune it once a year.

A Black Chokeberry shrub can be grown in full sun or light shade. However, full daylight, or at least six hours of direct sunshine on most days, will provide the finest flowering and fruiting. In too much shadow, the shrub will likely only flower and fruit sparingly, as well as create feeble growth that could eventually kill it.

This shrub's adaptability to a wide range of soils is one of its strengths. It can grow in either sandy or clay soil but likes to grow in a medium between the two. It can also handle some salt in the soil, making it a good choice for a location along a road where road salt is used.

The water requirements of Black Chokeberry are moderate. It can withstand both drought and flooding on rare occasions. However, giving your shrub some water during long dry spells or very hot weather is preferable.

The cold and hot temperatures of its growing zones are well tolerated by Black Chokeberry. To prevent frost, it blooms late in the spring. However, if there is a late frost, the blossoms may be damaged, and later fruiting for that growing season may be affected. If frost is expected in your location while your shrub is in bloom, consider covering it with a sheet to protect it. Furthermore, as long as there is excellent air circulation around the leaf to prevent fungal diseases, dampness is usually not a concern for the shrub.

Unless your soil is low in nutrients, you won't need to fertilize your Black Chokeberry. You may accelerate the growth of your shrub by mixing compost into the soil when you plant it. After that, put a little coating of compost every spring to ensure ongoing healthy growth.

Pruning the Black Chokeberry shrub will be limited to removing suckers around the base of the plant as needed to prevent undesirable new shrubs from sprouting. Lightly prune the stems after the plant has finished flowering in the spring to shape the shrub to your desire. Remove any dead, damaged, or diseased shrub parts as soon as you notice them.

Consumption Methods: Cascara Sagrada is commonly consumed as a tea, with a recommended dose of one to four cups per day. To prepare Cascara Sagrada tea, steep a tea bag or dried Cascara Sagrada bark in boiling water for 5 to 10 minutes. While the dark fruit of Cascara Sagrada is edible and rich in antioxidants, it is important to note that the primary use of Cascara Sagrada is for its

potential herbal benefits. The fruit itself may have a distinct aftertaste but can be used to make preserves or blended into juices to enhance their flavor profiles

Warnings: The pits of chokeberries can be toxic, especially to certain animals such as livestock. This is due to the fact that Chokeberries contain amygdalin, which the body converts to cyanide, a lethal poison, which is why cherry pits are rarely consumed as they are in the same category.

Echinacea

Echinacea, Black Sampson, Black Susans, Brauneria Angustifolia, Brauneria Pallida, Brauneria spp., Echinacea Anustifolia, Echinacea Pallida, Echinacea Purpurea, Indian Head, Purple Cone Flower, Red Sunflower.

Echinacea.

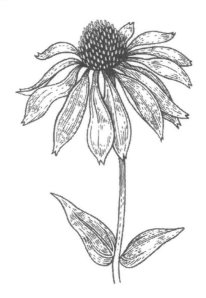

Medical uses: Echinacea, a cherished herb, holds a prominent place in both traditional and modern herbal practices. Among the Plains tribes (such as the Cheyenne, Lakota, and Pawnee), Echinacea was traditionally used for its immune-boosting properties. It was employed to support overall health and well-being, particularly during times of illness or weakened immunity. In modern times, Echinacea has gained popularity as a natural remedy for immune support and is widely used by herbalists and homeopaths, as well as classically trained physicians.

Check out the second volume for more information.

Solvents: Alcohol.

Hardiness zone: Zones 5-8.

Sourcing: Echinacea grows wild from the east to the Midwest of the United States, commonly across prairies and grasslands as a favorite food of foraging animals and birds. Echinacea plants and seeds are commonly available through plant sellers.

Gardening Tips:
There are several varieties of echinacea that you can pick from for your herbal garden. I encourage you to consider planting it if you have the right condition, it's beautiful

and is a panacea, treating from cough, to poultices, to stomach upset.

Echinacea pallida, or pale purple coneflower has sublime early summer flowers drooping straplike ray flower "petals" in a soft, creamy pink, surrounding a spiny orange-brown cone of disc flowers, each dotted with white pollen on top. They attract a wide variety of pollinators. The flowers are set above foliage that is seldom over 12 inches tall; plants may reach 30–36 inches tall. The sharply spiny seed heads turn almost black in winter and hold well all the way until spring. Pale purple coneflower is a denizen of hill, gravel, or otherwise rocky prairies in nature, so give it lean, well-drained garden soils. It is suitable for the perennial border, where it does exceedingly well in droughty locales with poor soil. Plants have failed in traditional landscapes that are fertilized and irrigated.

Echinacea angustifolia or narrow leaf purple coneflower is very similar to pale purple coneflower, perfect for a traditional perennial border in full sun. It demands perfect drainage and tolerates extreme heat and drought.

Echinacea purpurea, or purple coneflower is a popular perennial throughout the Midwest, widely planted in prairie gardens and naturalizing almost everywhere. The showy rosy-pink ray flowers surround an orangish cone of disc flowers, blooming from midsummer and sporadically into fall. The flowers are very rich in nectar, attracting many pollinators, including butterflies. It's a preferred host plant for the silvery checkerspot, whose young caterpillars feast in little armies, prettily skeletonizing some leaves. The fruiting heads are spiny, ripen almost black, and are quite showy in winter, especially when capped with snowfall. American goldfinches seek the seeds as soon as they are formed. Very popular in all styles of landscaping, purple coneflower is often massed in perennial borders. It may self-sow into dense plantings and allowing it to do so is a good idea because it is fairly short-lived. It is stunning mixed with other wildflowers and grasses and is at its best in a semishady natural garden.

Echinacea paradoxa, or purple yellow coneflowers is a paradox in the coneflower clan, as the names aptly describe: its yellow floral pigments are what's behind the outbreak of beyond-purple coneflower hybrids. The leaves may grow about 12 inches high with flowers atop nearly bare stems reaching to 3 feet. The large flower head consists of bright yellow, 3-inch ray flowers that droop like a skirt around a 2-inch cone of rich reddish brown disc flowers. The dark, almost black fruiting head holds well into winter. Yellow-purple coneflower doesn't run; it is well behaved and suitable as a traditional landscape perennial. In nature, this Ozark Highlands endemic grows in thin soil over bedrock. It demands good drainage and does best in full sun and scorching heat. Does not self-sow.

All Echinacea varieties require a minimum of four hours of daily sunlight to thrive. However, considering their native habitat at forest borders, they also appreciate locations with a combination of morning shade and afternoon sun or vice versa, creating a favorable environment for their growth. When it comes to soil preferences, Echinacea can tolerate poor or rocky soil conditions but does not fare well in damp or mucky soil. To provide optimal conditions for the plants, ensure they are planted in well-drained soil. Adding a layer of compost as mulch at the time of planting can promote healthy growth and soil enrichment. Echinacea plants grow in clumps, forming clusters that add a captivating appeal to the garden. While the size of each individual plant may increase, they do not spread aggressively through roots or rhizomes. The final size of the plant clump depends on the specific variety. Therefore, consulting the mature size stated in the plant description is essential for making appropriate spacing decisions. For example, if a variety is expected to reach a width of 18 inches, allowing 18 inches between plants will provide sufficient space for their development.

One important aspect to consider with Echinacea is the presence of deep taproots. Once established, these plants prefer to remain in their chosen location. Transplanting or moving them after they have settled in can be challenging, as they may struggle to re-establish themselves. If transplanting is necessary, it is advisable to do so in the spring, taking care to create as large a root ball as possible to minimize disruption to the plant's root system. Promptly replanting the transplanted Echinacea is crucial for its successful adaptation. Echinacea can be planted in full to part sun, ensuring that they receive adequate light for healthy growth. Spring or fall are suitable seasons for planting. Alternatively, Echinacea can be cultivated from seed, but they require a period of cold, damp stratification to germinate. For successful seed germination, sow them thickly in the fall, after a hard frost in northern regions or before winter rains elsewhere. Lightly cover the seeds to deter birds from eating them. In the spring, the seeds will naturally germinate, and most plants will begin to blossom in their second year, making starting with transplants a recommended approach to enjoy their blooms earlier.

Echinacea is a clump-forming perennial that exhibits an impressive stature. Depending on the specific variety, they can reach a mature height of up to four feet tall and have a width ranging from 12 to 36 inches. The size variations allow for selecting the most suitable Echinacea varieties based on the available space in your garden. The plants bear large, cone-shaped flowers on long, straight stalks, contributing to their captivating visual appeal. Their upright habit adds a structural element to the garden design. When it comes to maintenance, Echinacea plants are hardy and usually do not require frequent staking. However, in partial shade conditions, they may occasionally become tall and floppy. To provide support, individual stalks can be gently tied to a single stake using delicate thread, ensuring the plants remain upright and visually appealing.

Echinacea is considered a low-water plant, though young plants will require regular watering to help establish their new roots. Following a pattern of frequent watering immediately after planting, the frequency can be gradually reduced to a couple of times per week, then once per week, and eventually every other week, depending on the local climate conditions. Once established, Echinacea can withstand drought conditions, making them a resilient addition to the garden. However, in cases of extreme drought, it is advisable to provide supplemental water as needed. Regarding fertilization, most perennials, including Echinacea, have relatively low nutrient requirements and do not require regular seasonal fertilization. Mulching the plants with compost in the spring is generally sufficient, unless the garden has specific nutrient deficiencies. If Echinacea plants are producing abundant leaves but no blossoms or if the leaves exhibit unusual colors like purple or yellow, obtaining a soil test can help identify the specific nutrient deficiencies and guide appropriate treatment.

To encourage soil fertility around Echinacea plants, rather than burying the stem, mulching it with compost in the spring can provide a boost to the surrounding soil.

One unique aspect of Echinacea is that deadheading, or removing spent flowers, is not necessary. Allowing the flowers to remain on the plant and dry naturally at the end of the blooming season offers several benefits. The seeds of Echinacea are a valuable food source for wildlife, attracting birds to your garden. Additionally, the plants may self-sow, providing new seedlings for the following growing season, offering delightful surprises as they emerge.

To control the size and prolong the blooming season, pruning Echinacea plants back to around 30 inches tall in June can be effective. This practice helps manage their height and creates a wonderful, staggered blooming display if selectively applied to some plants while leaving others unpruned.

During the dormant period, typically in winter when the plants are entirely dry and dormant, it is essential to allow them to rest undisturbed. The seed heads serve as a significant food source for birds during this time. However, when tidying up the garden in the middle of winter, it is acceptable to cut back the plants.

Consumption Methods: Roots, leaves, and flowers can be used to make teas, tinctures, decoctions, and much more, check the second and third volume for more information. It's the perfect immune booster, in the colder months one to three cups a day of echinacea tea goes a long way to avoid upper respiratory diseases and flus.

Warnings: While Echinacea (genus Echinacea) is generally considered safe for most individuals when used appropriately, it is important to exercise caution and be aware of potential considerations. Allergic reactions to Echinacea have been reported in some individuals, particularly those with known allergies to plants in the Asteraceae family, such as ragweed. If you have a known allergy or sensitivity to these plants, it is advisable to avoid using Echinacea. Additionally, Echinacea should not be used by individuals with autoimmune disorders or those taking immunosuppressive medications, as it may stimulate the immune system.

Elderberry

Elder, Elderberry, Black Elder, European Elder, European Elderberry, European Black Elderberry.

Sambucus nigra.

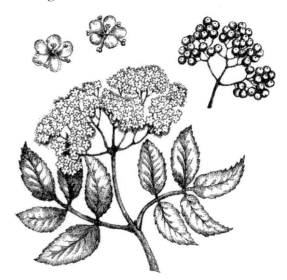

Medical Uses: Elderberry (*Sambucus*) has a rich history of medical uses, with Native Americans valuing various parts of the plant for their therapeutic properties. Elder flower tea was a popular remedy among Native Americans, employed to address a wide range of ailments. It was believed to alleviate fevers, upset stomachs, colds, the flu, headaches, indigestion, twitching eyes, itchy skin, dropsy, rheumatism, and the pain associated with sprains and bruises. The tea was also known for its diaphoretic and diuretic properties, promoting perspiration and urination, and was used to address appendix inflammation as well as kidney and bladder infections. Additionally, elder flowers were utilized in poultices to aid wound healing, improve complexion, soften and tone the skin, and lighten freckles and spots. For those seeking culinary delights, the blooms also impart a delightful clove-like fragrance, which can be used to flavor pancakes, muffins, and cakes. A personal favorite includes dipping the flowers in batter, deep-frying them, and sprinkling them with sugar. Check out the second volume for more!

Solvents: Water, alcohol.

Hardiness Zone: Zones 3-8.

Sourcing: Any reputable retailer or online storefront. Easy to find. Wild elderberries can be found in moist habitats and forested areas, making them easier to find on the East and West coasts of the United States.

Gardening Tips: Elderberry is a fine plant for natural landscapes, bird gardens, edible landscapes, and food forests. The huge, flat clusters of lacy white flowers are gorgeous and often rebloom into summer, finally becoming abundant displays of fruit that ripen to dark purplish black and are attractive in late summer into fall. Mature shrub size is 8–15 feet, usually with multiple stems, although some specimens are almost treelike. The Elderberry is a tree that grows to be a beautiful addition to any food garden.

The Elderberry tree, which is related to the Honeysuckle, can reach a height of 20 feet. Although some types are smaller and single-stemmed, it usually grows in a shrub-like cluster of stems.

Elderberry leaves are serrated and grow in bunches of three to nine along with the twigs. They are staggered and positioned in an opposing configuration, which means they do not line up from one side of the stem to the other. The fragrant blooms bloom in tiny clusters in the spring and are waxy white in color. These help to promote the desirable berries in the autumn, so just harvest a fraction of the blossoms if you want to enjoy the berries as well.

Elderberry trees thrive in wet, well-drained soil with lots of sunlight in the garden. They can also develop runners, so any undesirable branches must be removed, or your garden will be overrun. It's possible that you'll have to wait for 2 to 3 years after planting for your Elderberry to bloom and bear fruit. Cuttings have a lower success rate than seeds when propagating the Elderberry. Fortunately, as numerous berry-eating birds have demonstrated, the seeds take root quickly and build a strong tree.

Elderberry plants are also available at many nurseries. If you have a specific application in mind, make sure to ask if the type you're purchasing is appropriate.

American Elderberry is a low-maintenance shrub that can thrive in various growth situations, from moist soil to rocky terrain, as well as in areas with strong sun exposure or plenty of shade. However, it is crucial to ensure an ample water supply for your plant to flourish and yield a bountiful harvest of berries.

During the initial years of growing American Elderberry, focus on allowing the bush to establish itself. Pruning should be kept to a minimum, with regular inspections to address invasive weeds, which can pose a common challenge for shallow-rooted plants. It's important to note that a significant berry harvest may not be expected until the second or third year of growth.

While the berries of American Elderberry can be fairly sour on their own, they can be used to make delicious jams or pies by adding a generous amount of sugar. Additionally, the plant's small white blooms, arranged in clusters called cymes, can be used to create flavorful wine, cordials, and syrups. For those interested in the plant's medicinal properties, the dried fruits can be used in teas and tinctures.

American Elderberry thrives in a wide range of sun conditions, making it suitable for various positions in your yard or landscaping. While it can adapt to different soil conditions, it is recommended to provide humusy, well-draining soil with a pH range of neutral to acidic. Avoid locations prone to standing water, as the shallow roots of the plant are susceptible to rot. When planting, space each shrub a few feet apart to allow for unrestricted growth.

Watering is crucial, particularly during the peak growing season, and especially in periods of extremely hot or dry weather. Aim to provide about an inch or two of water per week to keep the Elderberry adequately hydrated. As the roots of the plant are close to the surface, monitoring the moisture level of the topsoil is essential.

Overwatering is unlikely as long as the soil has proper drainage.

American Elderberry prefers colder and moister conditions rather than hot and dry environments. While it does not have specific humidity requirements, it appreciates rainfall.

Fertilization is not strictly necessary for American Elderberry, but it can help boost fruit production. Incorporating manure or compost into the soil before planting can enhance nutrient density. Additionally, applying a 10-10-10 fertilizer mixture in the spring can provide supplementary nutrients to support healthy growth.

Keep in mind that American Elderberry has a tendency to produce suckers, which can be beneficial for native gardens but may become invasive in certain situations. If necessary, consult your local garden center for advice on managing and containing the plant.

Pruning is typically done in early spring. Remove any dead, damaged, or diseased canes, as well as those that are over three years old. Trimming encourages new development and helps maintain a tidy appearance for leggy shrubs. Elderberry cuttings can be rooted and used for propagation by storing them in water for at least two months, using rooting hormones to prevent bacterial and fungal issues, and subsequently planting them in a well-draining spot with some shade.

Elderberries have thin roots, making them suitable for container gardening. When potting in the spring, choose a large pot with a diameter of at least 2 feet and a depth of at least 20 inches. Ensure proper drainage holes or create them using a drill. Use nutrient-rich potting soil with a pH of 5.5 to 6.5 and mulch the topsoil with compost. Regular watering is essential to prevent drying.

While growing American Elderberry is relatively trouble-free, common issues may include aphids, mealybugs, elder shoot borers, and scales. Diseases such as canker, leaf spot, and powdery mildew can also affect the plant. Regularly clearing the soil of encroaching weeds is crucial to prevent them from choking out the delicate roots of the Elderberry plants.

Consumption Methods: The fruit (and flowers) are edible, making excellent jellies, syrups, and preserves (but note: stems and foliage are highly toxic). Elderberry tea and decoction are also great option to take advantage of its antioxidants. Taken as a supplement or made as a lotion, soap, or liniment Elderberry can stand on its own as a regenerative remedy great for skin conditions such as eczema and acne. Check out the second and third volume for more information.

Warnings: The raw berries of some elderberry species contain substances that can cause nausea, vomiting, and diarrhea if consumed in large quantities or improperly prepared. Therefore, it is crucial to cook the berries thoroughly before consumption to neutralize these potentially harmful compounds. Additionally, it is important to differentiate between different elderberry species, as some species may have toxic properties. If you are uncertain about the specific type of elderberry you have, it is advisable to consult a knowledgeable source or refrain from consuming the berries altogether. Furthermore, pregnant or breastfeeding individuals, as well as those with underlying health conditions or taking specific medications, should consult with a healthcare professional before using elderberry supplements or products.

Feverfew

Altamisa, Bachelor Button, Camomille Grande, Chrysanthemum Parthenium, Featherfew, Featherfoil, Flirtwort Midsummer Daisy, Midsummer Daisy, Santa Maria, And Tanacetum Parthenium.

Tanacetum parthenium.

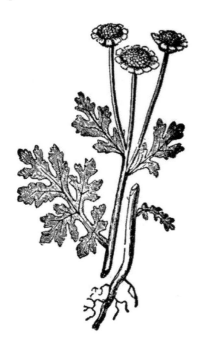

Medical Uses: Feverfew or wild quinine was used as a source of quinine to treat malaria. Some Native American tribes used the leaves to make a salve to cure burns and a decoction to use as a diuretic. Tonic, Aromatic, Astringent, Antiperiodic, Stimulant.

Solvents: Boiling water, alcohol.

Hardiness Zones: Zones 5-9.

Sourcing: Feverfew, as it is a hardy plant, can be found across the continental United States as long as the area is sunny and offers enough water to support it.

Gardening Tips: If you want to spread it from seeds, buy them online if you can't get them locally. Sow them in a seed tray with a well-draining starting mix indoors in early spring. Scatter the seeds on the soil's surface and lightly push them down. Keep the tray in a bright spot by covering it with a plastic sheet or placing it in a plastic bag.

If you want to put seeds directly on the ground, wait until the temperature rises to roughly 60 degrees Fahrenheit (15 degrees Celsius) in the spring, and the last frost date has passed. Until the seeds germinate, keep the soil uniformly moist. Within one or two weeks of seed sowing, germination occurs.

Many gardeners mistakenly perceive this plant as a weed since it settles down by itself in the garden. A full to a somewhat sunny position is ideal for growing Feverfew. Growing Feverfew in pots, railing planters, and window boxes is also doable; you can simply cultivate it on your balcony garden if you keep it away from a windy location.

Feverfew plants prefer moist soil that never totally dries out. Watering on a regular basis is crucial, but overwatering will kill it, so use extra caution while watering in the winter.

Except for thick clay-rich soil, this low-maintenance shrub thrives in all soil types. It thrives in nutrient-dense, well-drained, and loose soil.

If your soil is rich in organic matter, you won't need to use fertilizer to grow Feverfew. You can, however, apply a fertilizer that you use for other flowers on a monthly basis.

Plants of the Feverfew family are grown both as perennials and as annuals. Annual cultivars do not germinate in the winter and die off in the spring. Feverfews are vulnerable to harsh cold and require extra attention during the winter months.

Protect the plant from severe cold in the winter by mulching. Mulching also aids in moisture conservation during the summer.

After the initial blossoming, deadhead the faded blooms and lightly trim the shrub. Pruning encourages the development of fresh blooms. Long, leggy, and unhealthy branches with discolored leaves should be pruned. You can prune the plant down to roughly a third of its original size.

Gardeners who are raising Feverfew plants may encounter issues such as incorrect planting sites and persistent waterlogging in the soil. Slugs, powdery mildew, spider mites, and aphids are among the pests and illnesses that can affect Feverfew plants. Colonize geraniums, garlic, or cress as companion plants to deter pests.

Leaves can be harvested at any time, and flowers can be harvested when the plant is in bloom. The optimal time to harvest Feverfew is when it is just starting to flower. Feverfew should be dried as soon as possible after harvesting. To get the most out of this dried herb, don't keep it for more than 120 days.

Consumption Methods: Feverfew is well recognized for its use in the prevention of migraine headaches and associated nausea and vomiting, which can be achieved by eating the leaves, drinking the tea, or taking a tincture.

Warning: There have been no significant negative effects associated with the usage of feverfew. Nausea, bloating, and digestive issues are possible side effects; chewing the raw leaves can cause mouth ulcers and discomfort. Feverfew can cause allergic reactions in people who are allergic to ragweed and similar plants.

Goldthread

Goldenroot, Yellow Snakeroot, Threeleaf Goldthread.

Coptis trifolia.

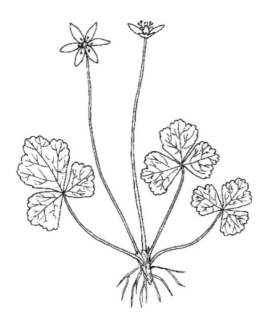

Identification: Goldthread is a native groundcover with glossy evergreen leaves 3-6 inches tall, which produces small, astoundingly beautiful flowers in May. The name refers to the yellow-gold, thread-like undergrounds roots. The beautiful glossy green leaves are compound, divided in three leaflets and fan-shaped. They uncoil every spring like a fern, to replace the previous year's leaves.

Medical uses: The herb was utilized by Native Americans as a digestive aid as well as a treatment for infections and mouth sores. The moniker "canker root" was given to Goldthread as a result of this. Goldthread's usefulness wasn't restricted to therapeutic purposes; because of its beautiful gold color, Native Americans also utilized it to make a yellow dye and flavor beer.

Solvents: Boiling water, alcohol.

Hardiness zone: Zones 4-8.

Sourcing: Native Goldthread is hard to find, as it is teetering on endangered. Do not forage, try to find the seed through a reputable seed saver or seller.

Gardening Tips: Goldthread seeds are easier to come by than ready-to-plant seedlings. They may be treated as general wildflowers that grow in swampy conditions. It prefers shade, moist, and acidic soil. It's an early and quick bloomer, the fragile flowers don't last very long, but make for an extremely attractive groundcover when they do. Seeds should be sown directly outside as soon as they ripe. They will germinate during the first winter and flower after the second.

It may attract ruffed grouse, who enjoy eating it.

Consumption Methods: Dry leaves are good for making tea and tinctures to treat mouth sores. The rhizomes and roots have antibacterial properties and are particularly useful for sore eyes, thrush, and as a tonic.

Warnings: In children, especially babies, Goldthread is extremely dangerous. It contains a substance called berberine, which can raise bilirubin levels in neonates. Bilirubin is a substance produced by the liver. In neonates, too much bilirubin can cause lasting brain damage, especially in premature babies.

Honeysuckle

Honeysuckle, Common Honeysuckle, European Honeysuckle, Woodbine.

Lonicera periclymenum.

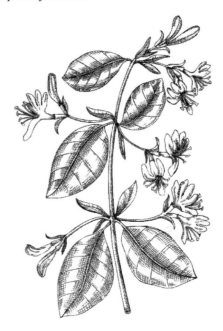

Medical Uses: Honeysuckle has a variety of purposes in Native American culture. Asthma, sore throats, and coughs were treated with leaves that were either dried and smoked or soaked in warm water as tea. When chewed leaves are administered to bee stings, the swelling is reduced. Check the second volume for more information.

Solvents: Boiling water, alcohol.

Hardiness Zone: Zones 5-9.

Sourcing: For live plants, many reputable sellers are available both online and in local nurseries. Difficult to grow from seed.

Gardening Tips: Honeysuckle comes in almost 200 different types. At least 20 of them are native to the northern hemisphere and can be found in North America. Honeysuckle comes in three varieties: vines, shrubs, and bushes.

Honeysuckle Vines are a type of vine that grows in the Honeysuckle family. Honeysuckle vines are a common, easy-to-grow climber with a wide range of variations. Vines can be planted as ground cover, but they're usually trained to cover walls and structures using trellises.

Honeysuckle Shrubs are a type of shrub that grows in the Honeysuckle family. Honeysuckle is an excellent choice for an informal hedge, and numerous types thrive well in pots and containers.

Note that bush Honeysuckle is one of the more invasive varieties of Honeysuckle and should not be planted in your garden or yard. Bush Honeysuckle spreads swiftly, encroaching on other areas of your yard and darkening them out.

Rock honeysuckle is an ideal vine to climb up a small trellis or garden sculpture. Near the branch ends, the paired leaves are fused into what looks like a single 3-inch-round leaf that the stem appears to pierce; these perfoliate leaves can be exquisitely waxy-coated, silvered or bluish, reminiscent of eucalyptus. Each branch end is studded with creamy yellow flowers that age to orange in late spring, followed by orange-red berries in fall. The nectar-rich flowers are visited by many pollinators, from hummingbirds to various bees; birds relish the fruit; and the foliage hosts several unusual caterpillars, most notably the hornworm of the snowberry clearwing, a day-flying sphinx moth that mimics a bumblebee. Planted without support, it can take on a haystack-like growth, making you think it is a shrub. Easy to grow, to 6 feet or more in cultivation, in any well-drained soil. Extremely drought tolerant.

Northern bush-honeysuckle sports nothing spectacular but is a garden-worthy sleeper, more dynamic than many evergreen shrubs. Its flowers reward close inspection, and its foliage is clean and neat, with the new growth of some plants emerging coppery in spring. Fall color is shades of red, from burgundy to scarlet. Plants slowly sucker into a thicket, rarely growing more than 4 feet tall and making a fine low shrub or hedge.

After any fear of frost has passed, plant your Honeysuckle in early April, no matter the type. Essentially, Honeysuckle should be planted in a sunny position where the soil is wet and excess water can drain.

Honeysuckle prefers full sun but may grow in partial shade. Honeysuckle can withstand partial shade, but if it doesn't get enough sun, it won't blossom as much and may lose its leaves.

Make sure your Honeysuckle is planted in organically rich, well-drained soil. It should be moist but not soggy, as overwatered soil can cause issues. They thrive on soil that is acidic to mildly alkaline, with a pH of 5.5 to 8.0 on the pH scale.

Additionally, if you want your Honeysuckle to climb and aren't planting it against a home or other structure, you'll need to put support structures in place. Anything that the plant can grip onto can be installed, such as a trellis, pole, fence, or other robust structure. Before you plant your Honeysuckle, make sure you do this. Plants should be between 6 – 12 inches away from the support once they are set up.

In all reality, after initial setup, they can endure a variety of cool-weather situations, although some varieties may require additional winter care, depending on the kind you plant. The more delicate or tropical types will be the ones to suffer the most from the harsh winter conditions. Pruning carefully, planting close to supports, and mulching thickly around the roots and at the base can all assist in safeguarding your plant.

To train a Honeysuckle vine to climb a pergola, wall, or trellis, carefully attach the plant to the support with plastic tie tape or another stretchy material that allows for development. The material should not cut into the plant as it grows. Make sure the stems don't rub against the supports by constructing a figure 8 with your ties, ensuring sure the crossed section goes between the stem and the support.

As for pruning, other than keeping the shape clean and controlled, you won't need to spend much time pruning your plant.

Whether you have a vine or a shrub to prune will determine how and when you prune. Almost any time of year, vines can be softly trimmed for shaping. If you're trimming an older or aggressive vine, wait until at least fall or winter if you have a dormant variety. Bushes can be clipped as soon as the spring blossoms fade.

Remove any dead, diseased, or damaged stems with bypass pruners. Cut stems just past a leaf node or to the point where they join another stem.

If you've chosen an evergreen kind, keep in mind that it will not fall dormant. To avoid removing fresh buds, prune them after the flowering season has ended.

Lastly, Honeysuckle plants should be watered and mulched regularly (but not excessively). Make sure your soil doesn't get too wet - only water as needed to keep it moist and humid. Each spring, add layers of compost.

Apply organic plant food in the spring to encourage and promote growth. A 2- to 3-inch layer of composted manure can also be added. You may not need to fertilize Honeysuckle if you plant it in fertile soil.

Consumption Methods: Tea is the most prevalent consumption method, steep dried leaves in boiling water for 5 to 10 minutes to make fresh Honeysuckle tea to treat cough as a demulcent. Check the second and third volume for more

Warnings: Drink Honeysuckle tea in moderation, as the leaves are rich in saponins that can cause digestive upset.

Hop Hornbeam

American Hop-hornbeam, Eastern Hop Hornbeam, Hop Hornbeam,
Hop Horn Beam, Ironwood, Leverwood, Wooly Hop hornbeam.

Ostrya.

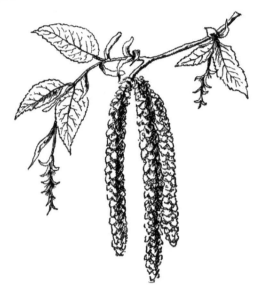

Medical Uses: The wood of this tree is robust, firm, and long-lasting, and it was previously utilized to make sleigh runners. Fence posts, fuel, and tool handles are all made from this material. Native Americans used the interior wood to heal toothaches, weary muscles, and coughs. The wood from the branch's heart was used to make cough syrup and a kidney disease medication by the Chippewa.

Antiperiodic, tonic, alterative.

Solvents: Boiling water, alcohol.

Medicinal parts: inner wood and bark

Hardiness Zones: Zones 3-9.

Sourcing: While larger specimens can be found in deep, well-drained soils within mixed stands of bottom land hardwood, this tree also thrives in dry, rocky woods and sloped areas across upland and mountain regions, including North Carolina and beyond. To acquire Hop Hornbeam for your own landscape, consider purchasing saplings from local nurseries.

Gardening Tips: This stellar tree offers subtle four-season beauty. Pendulous golden male catkins appear in spring before leaves fully emerge; female flowers form pale green fruit that look like hops, mature to brown, and hang on the tree into winter. Cardinals and purple finch eat the seeds of the fruit. Fall foliage is golden brown, the leaves often persisting through winter; I've observed cedar waxwings settle in for the night, snuggled in the rich brown winter leaves. The delicate branching pattern is exquisite in winter, along with the rugged nature of mature trees and their finely longitudinal-striped bark. This species is a superior smaller shade tree for a confined space or under the canopy of other deciduous natives like oaks and hickories. Its winter leaves make it a good windbreak or winter screen in areas where an evergreen cannot be utilized. It's sturdy and long-lived in cultivation; a moist to seasonally dry, well-drained upland site is all that's needed. It's quite easy to grow from purchased saplings as long as they are situated within zones 3-9.

Consumption Methods: The bark should be gathered in August and September, it should be carefully kept in a dark, dry, and cool place and used granulated to make teas or decoctions that are extremely useful in treating intermittent fevers. A tincture has proved effective in treating headaches.

Joe-Pye Weed

Kidney-root, Sweetscented Joe Pye Weed, Sweet Joe-Pye Weed.

Eutrochium purpureum.

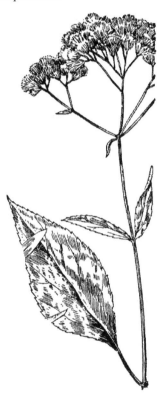

Identification: Perennials to 5' tall in the northern range, and up to 10' in the southern states. It grows from a rhizome on a stout stem, topped with flower heads that are domed to flat topped. Flowers are pink to purple and tubular-shaped disks. Leaves are lance shaped and in whorls, up to seven in a whorl, each leaf toothed, rough and hairy to the touch. Another species is spotted Joe-Pye weed (*E. maculatum*).

Traditional uses: Joe Pye Weed (Eutrochium spp.) has a rich history of traditional use by Native Americans, who recognized its medicinal properties and employed it for various purposes. Native American healers, such as Joe Pye himself (historically spelled Jopi), introduced the plant to colonists for its efficacy in treating typhus fever caused by the Rickettsia bacteria.

Among Native American tribes, Joe Pye Weed was valued as a revitalizing tonic, aiding in relieving constipation and acting as a diuretic for addressing urinary tract problems, including kidney stones. The plant's tea was utilized as a wash for infections, providing cleansing and promoting healing.

In particular, the hollow stems of the Eutrochium maculatum species were ingeniously utilized by Cherokees and other tribes as straws. Meskwakis regarded the root of Eutrochium purpureum as an aphrodisiac, sucking on it during courtship rituals. The roots of Eutrochium purpureum were highly prized for their medicinal properties. A root decoction was employed to treat bed-wetting in children and as a diuretic for congestive heart failure (dropsy). The tea derived from the plant was also used in managing asthma.

Both species of Joe Pye Weed were utilized by Native Americans for treating menstrual disorders, dysmenorrhea, and as a recovery tea for women after pregnancy. Additionally, Cherokees used Eutrochium purpureum to address rheumatism and arthritis, as well as a diuretic. The infusion of the root was known to possess laxative properties.

Other tribes found diverse applications for Joe Pye Weed. Potawatomi utilized fresh leaves as poultices for wound care, while Navajos employed the root as an antidote for poisoning. The Iroquois and Cherokee tribes used the roots and blossoms as a diuretic to address urinary and kidney problems. The roots and leaves could be steeped in hot water to create a tea that was consumed to alleviate fever and inflammation.

Modern uses: While specific studies and research on Joe Pye Weed are ongoing, preliminary findings and anecdotal evidence suggest various potential uses.

One area of interest is Joe Pye Weed's anti-inflammatory properties. It contains phytochemicals such as flavonoids and phenolic compounds that exhibit anti-inflammatory effects, which may have implications for conditions characterized by inflammation, such as arthritis and rheumatism. However, further research is needed to explore these potential benefits and understand the mechanisms involved.

Joe Pye Weed is also believed to possess diuretic properties, potentially aiding in promoting healthy kidney function and assisting in the elimination of toxins from the body. Some herbalists and alternative medicine practitioners recommend its use as a supportive therapy for urinary tract problems, including kidney stones.

Furthermore, Joe Pye Weed has been traditionally used to address menstrual disorders and dysmenorrhea.

Effects: Diuretic, Stimulant, Tonic, Astringent, Relaxant.

Medicinal parts: root and flowers.

Solvents: Boiling water, alcohol.

Hardiness Zones: Zones 4-8.

Sourcing: Do not forage, buy seedlings or seeds from a reputable source.

Gardening Tips: This plant is a striking late-summer bloomer worth adding to your wildflower garden. It can reach heights of 3 to 12 feet (1-4 meters), providing considerable focal attraction. Furthermore, the blossoms have a subtle vanilla scent that intensifies when crushed. The domes of rosy-pink flower clusters atop this plant are its crowning glory, and when the plant is in its late-summer bloom, they form an ideal landing pad for butterflies. The leaves too are notable, whorled in threesomes or foursomes along the purplish or purple-spotted stem, and in fall, the plant is attractively covered in delicate tufted fruits. Spotted Joe-Pye weed can be used in traditional perennial borders, where it grows 4–5 feet tall. It is a solution to a problematic wet site, perfect for a pondside or rain garden, and a must for a butterfly or insectaries garden. Do not fail to include it in the night garden, as it's a magnet for nocturnal moths. Spotted Joe-Pye weed grows well in good garden soil but performs best with adequate moisture and wet conditions. Divide large plants to propagate them. Joe Pye Weeds prefer full sun to partial shade in the garden. They also prefer moist soil that ranges from medium to rich. Joe Pye Weed can withstand damp soil conditions, but not very dry ones. Plant these decorative wonders in somewhat shaded locations in areas with hot, dry summers.

When it comes to planting Joe Pye Weed, the best season is in the spring or fall. Joe Pye Weed is an excellent backdrop plant because of its vast size, but it also requires a lot of space to thrive. In fact, because they will eventually produce enormous clumps, they should be planted on 24 inch (61 cm) centers. In the garden, group Joe Pye Weed with other comparable woodland plants and decorative grasses.

You can usually locate this wildflower in nurseries and garden centers if you don't have it growing on your land already. Many of these Joe Pye Weed plants, on the other hand, are advertised as E. Maculatum. This variety has more foliage and flower heads than the wild version. Because it is a shorter variant, 'Gateway' is a popular cultivar for home gardens.

Joe Pye Weed care requires very little upkeep. When the soil is kept moist, or shade is given, the plant enjoys regular, deep watering and can endure heat and drought fairly well. A covering of mulch will also aid in the retention of moisture. Older plants can be separated and replanted as new growth emerges in the early spring or fall. When the middle of the garden is devoid of Joe Pye Weeds, it's time to divide.

The entire clump must be dug up, with the dead central material cut away and discarded. The separated clumps can then be replanted. Late in the fall, plants die back to the ground. This dead growth can be pruned, or it can be left over the winter and pruned in the spring. Joe Pye Weed plants can be grown from seeds, albeit this is not the most favored method of production. They require ten days of stratification at 40 degrees F. (4 C.).

Do not cover the seeds because they need sunshine to germinate, which takes two to three weeks on average. In the spring, root cuttings can also be taken.

Consumption Methods: Joe-Pye Weed is a common tea, as well as tincture to treat infections, colds, and arthritis. Produces a beautiful scent.

Juniper

Common Juniper.

Juniperus communis.

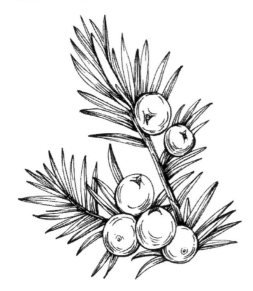

Medical Uses: In many Native American tribes, Juniper plants are associated with protection. Juniper was employed by Interior Salish and Northwest Coast tribes to ward off evil spirits. Junipers were thought to treat 'ghost sickness,' a disease that plagued bereaved relatives or those who handled the bodies of the deceased, among the southern Pueblos. To keep their tepees secure from storms, Plains Indian tribes like the Dakota, Cheyenne, and Pawnee placed Juniper boughs on their tepees or burned them in the campfires. People in various cultures, particularly hunters, would carry a Juniper spring as a protective charm or rub Juniper branches on their bodies before starting on a risky expedition to ward off grizzly bears, monsters, or ill luck. Juniper is one of the most common herbs seen in medicine bundles and amulets. Some tribes in the Southwest and Southern California ate Juniper berries, and Juniper leaves were commonly utilized as medicinal plants. Check out the second and third volume for more information on all the amazing ways you can use it.

Solvents: Boiling water, alcohol.

Hardiness Zones: Zones 3-9.

Sourcing: To source juniper (Juniperus spp.), consider visiting local plant nurseries or specialized garden centers. These establishments often carry a variety of juniper species suitable for different landscapes and gardening needs.

Gardening Tips: Juniper (Juniperus spp.) encompasses a wide range of plants, including low-growing ground cover, edging plants, shrubs, and trees, with over 170 cultivated species. These versatile plants come in various shapes, such as narrow columns, tight pyramids, and rounded forms. They feature fragrant foliage that can take the form of needles or overlapping scales, with some varieties having both types of foliage.

When it comes to juniper shrubs, there are male and female varieties. Male flowers supply pollen for female flowers, which then produce berries or cones after pollination. A single male shrub can pollinate multiple females, resulting in berry production. When planting juniper shrubs, it is important to choose a location that offers full sun or mild shade. Excessive shade can lead to the spreading of branches in an attempt to capture more sunlight, potentially causing irreversible damage to their shape.

For planting shrubs with balled and burlaped roots, fall is the ideal time. Dig a planting hole that is twice as wide and deep as the root ball. Place the shrub in the hole, ensuring that the soil line on the stem matches the surrounding ground. Backfill the hole with the removed soil without any additives, gently pressing down to remove air pockets. After planting, thoroughly water the shrub and top up the soil if it settles. During the first two years, water young plants during dry spells. Once established, juniper is drought-resistant and can rely on natural water sources. Fertilize the shrub with a 10-10-10 fertilizer in the following spring after installation and every other year thereafter.

One notable juniper species is Juniperus virginiana, also known as Eastern red cedar. It is an exceptional evergreen choice for windbreaks and ornamental use, particularly in challenging soils where other evergreens struggle. Eastern red cedar is wildlife-friendly, with female trees producing abundant blue, berry-like cones that attract many birds. It serves as the sole host for the olive juniper hairstreak butterfly. While the fruits are edible to some extent and used as a flavoring in gin, it is worth noting that sweet berries with a gin aftertaste are quite rare. In winter, the foliage takes on reddish-brown or orangish-olive tones, complementing the seasonal hues. The tree trunks display vertical strips that exfoliate, often adorned with white lichens. Juniperus virginiana thrives in well-drained soils and prefers full sun, though it can tolerate heat, drought, and even grow in rocky outcrops with minimal soil.

Consumption Methods: Juniper berries have been used as a seasoning in food and as a flavoring component in alcoholic beverages (e.g., gin); juniper has also been employed in traditional medicine for a variety of purposes. Most commonly, if not made into a tincture, juniper berries can be crushed and ingested directly. Check the third volume for other recipes and the second volume to learn more about it.

Warnings: Irritation, burning, redness, and swelling are some of the negative effects of using juniper on the skin. It should not be used on big skin wounds.

Lemon Balm

Balm, Bee Balm, Cure-All, Dropsy Plant, Honey Plant,
Melissa, Melissa Folium,
Melissa Officinalis, Sweet Balm, Sweet Mary.

Melissa officinalis.

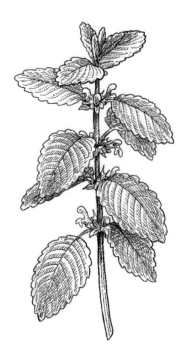

Medical Uses: Balm was dubbed "bee" by a Cherokee elder, or "wa du li si." The leaves are used to produce cold drinks or hot tea, and the herb is used to make salves. It is used to help women with cramps, migraines, and/or anxiety during menstruation. The lemon-like perfume is supposed to be strongest shortly before flowering, making this an excellent time to harvest the plant for usage. It was also used in one of the various recipes for calming the soul of someone who was "behaving strangely." Check out the second volume to learn more about it.

Solvents: Boiling water, alcohol.

Hardiness Zones: Zones 4-9.

Sourcing: This mint-family perennial is native to mountainous parts of southern Europe and northern Africa, but it has naturalized in nearly every warm or temperate climate on the planet. If there's sun and moist soil, you could potentially find some lemon balm growing. Widely available in garden stores and worth having.

Gardening Tips: Lemon balm (Melissa officinalis) is a versatile and fragrant herb that is relatively easy to grow in your garden.

Lemon balm thrives in a location that receives full to partial sun. Choose a well-drained spot in your garden that offers protection from strong winds. The herb can adapt to a variety of soil types but prefers soil that is fertile and slightly acidic to neutral.

You can start lemon balm from seeds or purchase young seedlings from a nursery. If sowing seeds, do so in the spring either indoors or directly in the garden. When transplanting seedlings, space them about 12 to 18 inches apart to allow for healthy growth.

Prepare the planting area by removing any weeds and incorporating organic matter, such as compost, into the soil. This will help improve drainage and provide essential nutrients for the herb.

Once planted, keep the soil consistently moist but avoid overwatering, as lemon balm prefers slightly moist conditions rather than overly wet or dry soil. Regular watering during dry periods is important to ensure healthy growth.

Mulching around the base of the plants can help retain moisture and suppress weed growth. Apply a layer of organic mulch, such as straw or wood chips, around the base of the plants, leaving a small space around the stems to prevent moisture-related issues.

To encourage bushier growth and prevent the plant from becoming leggy, pinch back the stems regularly. This will help promote branching and result in a fuller and more compact lemon balm plant.

Harvest the leaves as needed throughout the growing season. For the best flavor, gather the leaves in the morning after the dew has dried but before the sun is at its strongest. Use the leaves fresh or dry them for later use by hanging small bunches upside down in a cool, well-ventilated area.

Lemon balm is known for its ability to attract bees and beneficial insects to your garden. If you want to deter bees or prevent the herb from spreading too aggressively, consider planting it in containers or using barriers, such as root barriers or underground edging.

Consumption Methods: As with many other herbs, tinctures, supplements, and teas are available. As Lemon Balm is a popular targeted treatment for relaxation and sleep, supplements and tea are the most popular options available.

Warnings: At high dosage, Lemon Balm may cause digestive upset.

Licorice

Black Sugar, Common Licorice, Mulaith, Sweetwood.

Glycyrrhiza glabra.

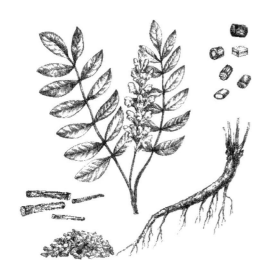

Medical Uses: American Licorice (Glycyrrhiza lepidota) holds a rich history of traditional use among Native Americans throughout the country. The peeled and dried roots of this plant were brewed into a medicinal tea, which was commonly employed to soothe upset stomachs and alleviate diarrhea.

Various tribes had distinct applications for American Licorice. The Cheyenne, Montana Indians, and Northwestern Tribes consumed the delicate spring shoots raw. The Lakotas utilized the plant's root as a remedy for flu, while the Dakotas prepared a topical solution by boiling Licorice leaves in water to alleviate earaches. The Blackfeet brewed a tea from the root to address coughs, chest pain, and sore throats.

The leaves of wild Licorice were skillfully used in poultices to treat sores in both humans and horses. Additionally, the young shoots of the plant were chewed on to maintain a sweet and moist tongue. The Buffalo runners of the Black Foot Indians sucked on the burrs of this shrub as a means to quench their thirst.

Today, our utilization of American Licorice draws inspiration from the practices of Native Americans. This remarkable plant is rich in anti-inflammatory flavonoids, free radical scavenging antioxidants, estrogen balancing isoflavones, and calming saponins. As a result, Licorice extracts are readily available in health food stores and online sites, offering a wide range of potential benefits for treating various ailments. Licorice tea, in particular, remains a popular form of the herb, renowned for its digestive, respiratory, and adrenal gland health-supporting properties.

Check out the second volume for more!

Solvents: Water, boiling water, alcohol.

Hardiness Zones: Zones 9-11.

Sourcing: Licorice root can be found growing wild within its climate zone, preferring full sun and spots with space to be a ground-covering plant.

Gardening Tips: Growing American Licorice (Glycyrrhiza lepidota) in your garden requires patience and dedication, but the rewards are well worth the wait. While commercial harvesting typically occurs when the plants are four to five years old, in a home garden, you can expect a small yield after three years, similar to the first harvest of asparagus.

To grow American Licorice from seed, sow them on the surface of potting compost in mid to late spring or early autumn. Keep the seeds warm, around 20°C (68°F), and expect germination in two to three weeks. Since germination can be unpredictable, it's advisable to sow additional seeds as a backup plan.

Alternatively, you may find one- or two-year-old plants available. From the second year onward, Licorice will produce new shoots from underground stems known as rhizomes, which can be clipped off and used to propagate new plants.

When planting Licorice in your garden, choose a location that mimics its natural habitat—riverbanks with ample water and sunlight. Avoid frost pockets and windy areas. Sandy soil is ideal, but if your soil is heavy, prepare it by excavating a pit at least two spits (the length of a spade blade) wide and deep. Remove stones, incorporate compost, and refill the pit.

Licorice plants are relatively resilient once established and can be planted out after the last spring frost in most regions. In colder climates, planting Licorice in a container and providing winter protection in a greenhouse or sheltered spot is recommended. Ensure the container is deep enough to accommodate the plant's strong roots.

As Licorice matures, it can reach impressive heights of up to two meters (six feet) with a meter-wide spread (three feet). Allow enough space around the plants, especially if you plan to dig up the roots. Licorice's violet or pale blue flowers and ferny foliage make it an attractive addition to the back of a border. Consider surrounding it with shallow-rooted summer annuals like marigolds for added visual appeal.

Licorice, being a legume, benefits from nitrogen fixation in its roots and requires little additional fertilizer. However, mulching can help suppress weeds, retain moisture, and provide some extra nutrients. Keep an eye out for potential pests like slugs, caterpillars, spider mites, and diseases like powdery mildew. Protect your plants from rabbits, as they may find Licorice appealing.

When the time comes to harvest your Licorice plant, dig up the roots. The roots are long, flexible, and have a brownish-yellow exterior with a delicious yellow inside. Harvest the thickest horizontal roots while leaving the deep tap root and thinner horizontal roots to continue growing. In extremely cold climates, consider replanting or bringing the plant indoors for winter.

The Licorice roots can be enjoyed raw, offering a unique sweet and salty flavor. Chewing releases the sap and intensifies the sweetness. The roots can also be dried for later use in teas, baked goods, or flavoring. Keeping a root in a jar of sugar can provide a delightful flavoring for cakes.

Remember to harvest your Licorice plant annually, as the roots can grow to incredible lengths if left unharvested. To avoid overpowering your flowerbed, maintain regular harvests, as Licorice roots can reach up to four meters (13 feet) or even eight meters (26 feet) in length.

Consumption Methods: 1 lb. of Licorice root boiled in 3 pints of water, reduced by boil- ing to 1 quart, is an all-purpose decoction. Check the second and third volume for more!

Warnings: Although Licorice root is typically regarded safe as a food ingredient when ingested in excessive amounts or for long periods of time, it can induce major side effects such as elevated blood pressure and decreased potassium levels. Because the composition of Licorice products vary, it's impossible to establish whether a certain quantity of consumption is safe or not. People with hypertension (high blood pressure), heart disease, or kidney illness should be especially concerned about the effects of Licorice on potassium and blood pressure.

Glycyrrhizic acid, a component of Licorice, is thought to be responsible for some of its adverse effects. Licorice that has had this component removed (known as DGL for deglycyrrhizinated Licorice) may not have as many negative effects.

Premature delivery and health problems in children have been linked to Licorice use during pregnancy. It's unclear whether Licorice root is safe to use while breastfeeding.

Lomatium

Biscuitroot, Indian Parsley, Desert Parsley.

Lomatium.

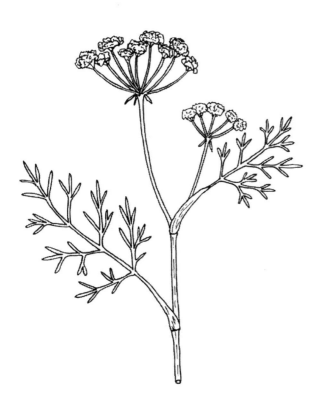

Medical Uses: The importance of Lomatium as a source of food and a therapeutic cure was recognized by many Native American tribes. To make sweet-tasting biscuits, the Lomatium root was peeled, dried, and pounded into flour. Lomatium seeds could be consumed raw, roasted, or processed into flour.

The root was eaten by Native Americans to treat a variety of respiratory diseases. Colds, flu, bronchitis, TB, hay fever, asthma, and pneumonia were all treated with Lomatium. In addition, Lomatium was utilized in a tobacco blend. During rituals, the herb was smoked, and healers used the smoke to treat respiratory infections. When Native Americans were exposed to tuberculosis, and other diseases brought to North America by Europeans, Lomatium was employed.

When the world was faced with the influenza pandemic of 1917–18, Americans used castor oil, tobacco, aspirin, and morphine as treatments. Lomatium was prescribed instead by American herbalists, and the medicine was used with reported success, particularly in the Southwest.

Solvents: Boiling water, alcohol.

Hardiness Zones: Zones 5-12.

Sourcing: Lomatium, also known as biscuitroot, can be sourced from its natural habitat in various regions of the United States. This perennial herbaceous plant is typically found in arid or semi-arid environments, particularly in the western parts of North America. It thrives in well-drained soils, including sandy or rocky areas, grasslands, and open woodlands. Lomatium species can be encountered in states such as California, Oregon, Nevada, Idaho, Utah, and Montana, among others. To source Lomatium, one can explore local nurseries, native plant sales, or specialized seed suppliers that offer region-specific varieties. It is important to respect regulations and guidelines related to the collection and sourcing of native plants, ensuring their sustainability and conservation in their natural habitats.

Gardening Tips: Lomatium thrives on sunny slopes in dryish, rocky soil, with a huge tap root laden with aromatic oleo-gum-resin as its anchor.

Lomatium is a difficult plant to grow. In the fall to early spring, sow the seeds in an outdoor nursery bed, with germination in the spring. Alternatively, sow seed in warm soil after 60 days of cold, wet treatment (in moist peat moss in a plastic bag in the fridge). Plants should be spaced 1 to 2 feet apart. Large umbels of flowers up to 3 feet tall.

Consumption Methods: Make a tincture or tea from the leaves to treat upper respiratory diseases with a sweet taste.

Warnings: Lomatium extracts or tinctures containing the resin (and possibly the coumarins) can induce a full-body rash in certain persons. Some people may experience nausea as a result of using this plant.

Mullein

Great Mullein, Flannel Plant, Candlewick Plant, Hag's Taper, Velvet Dock, Velvet Plant, Clown's Lung-wort, Torches, Our Lady's Flannel, Jacob's Staff, Aaron's Rod.

Verbascum thapsus.

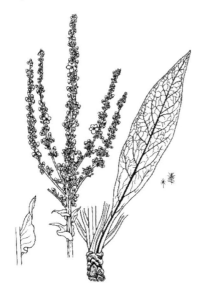

Medical uses: Many of the traditional therapeutic uses of Mullein were comparable in the Old and New Worlds, although it's unclear if European settlers learned about the herb from Native Americans or vice versa. Mullein leaf and flower teas were used by some Native Americans to treat respiratory ailments, but the plant's roots were also employed. For coughs, the Creek Indians drank a decoction of the roots; for asthma, other tribes smoked the roots or dried leaves. To alleviate "prickly rash," the Cherokee massaged Mullein leaves into their armpits. Bruises, tumors, rheumatic aches, and hemorrhoids were all treated using leaf poultices. Mullein flower oil, which is prepared by steeping the blossoms in warm olive oil, is also used to cure hemorrhoids and earaches. Mullein leaves have been used to soften skin, referring to the Quaker habit of putting Mullein leaves on the cheeks to redden them. A yellow dye produced from the blossoms has also been used as a hair rinse and to color fabric since Roman times. Check out the second volume for more information.

Solvents: Water, boiling water, alcohol.

Hardiness Zones: Zones 5-11.

Sourcing: Mullein may grow in a broad range of soil conditions, including dry, gravelly places— the plant is both heat and drought resistant.

Gardening Tips: Mullein seeds sprout best when exposed to cold, damp environments for a period of time (cold stratification). Mullein seed can be sown directly outside in the fall and will germinate the following spring. Seed can also be started indoors six weeks before the last frost in the spring. If you're starting seeds indoors, cold stratify them for 4-6 weeks before planting. Mullein seeds must be exposed to light in order to germinate. Seeds should be sown 8-12" apart on the soil surface and lightly pressed to settle. In 12-15 days, the seeds will sprout. Once the

risk of frost has gone, transplant seedlings outside. Thin seedlings to a spacing of 20-24" between mature plants.

In traditional medicine, all parts of the Mullein plant are employed. With a garden fork, harvest roots in the first fall or the next spring. During the growth season, you can pluck leaves by hand at any moment. When the blooms have fully bloomed, harvest them. Cut the flower stalk's top 3-6" off. Fresh or dried parts can be used.

Select a warm, dry spot for Mullein drying and fully dry pieces before storing them in a paper bag or glass container. Store in a cool, dry place.

Mullein is a biannual flowering plant that blooms, sets seeds, then dies in its second year of life. Allow your plants to overwinter in your garden, and towering flower stalks will bloom the following season. The seeds are ready to harvest in the fall. When the blossoms have dried and become brown, collect the seeds. Seeds should be kept in a cool, dry place. The seeds will last for two years.

Consumption Methods: Use a poultice of mullein leaves on a nettle sting or just rub a leaf on it. The tea of fresh leaves is a useful antispasmodic. Check the second and third volume for more!

Warnings: Contact dermatitis is a skin reaction that causes itching, redness, and irritation in some Mullein species. If you have sensitive skin or are prone to allergic reactions, test Mullein on a patch before applying it to your skin.

Milkweed

Butterfly Flower, Silkweed, Silky Swallow-Wort, Virginia Silkweed.

Asclepias Syriaca

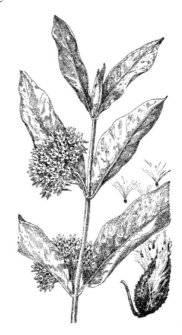

Medical Uses: Milkweed, a plant rich in traditional medicinal uses, has been employed by various Native American tribes such as the Navajo, Iroquois, Cherokee, Blackfoot, Meskwaki, and others across the Americas. In vitro studies have confirmed the antibacterial and antiseptic properties of Milkweed. Externally, crushed

Milkweed leaves were applied to treat skin ulcers, wounds, ringworm, and headaches. The root was often ground into a powder or juice and used topically for treating tumors, wounds, boils, and rashes. The sap was utilized externally to address leprosy, remove warts and freckles, brighten the skin, and treat ear infections. Some tribes employed Milkweed mixtures, while others chewed on the root. Milkweed was also used internally to cure snakebites and employed as a remedy for sore throats, rashes, rabies, hemorrhage, respiratory ailments, toothache, heart disorders, fever, and digestive conditions. Additionally, it was believed to possess contraceptive and abortifacient properties.

Check the second volume for more

Solvents: Boiling water, alcohol.

Hardiness Zones: Zones 4-9.

Sourcing: Milkweed can be sourced from its natural habitat in various regions of the United States. This plant is typically found in open fields, meadows, prairies, and along roadsides. Different species of Milkweed thrive in different regions, such as Common Milkweed (Asclepias syriaca) in the eastern and central parts of the US, and Showy Milkweed (Asclepias speciosa) in the western states. To source Milkweed, one can explore local native plant nurseries, participate in native plant sales, or connect with conservation organizations that focus on preserving native flora. It is important to source Milkweed responsibly and avoid harvesting from the wild to protect its natural populations and provide support for pollinators like monarch butterflies.

Gardening Tips: Milkweed plants play a vital role in supporting a diverse ecosystem. The nectar-rich flowers attract wasps and fritillaries, which collect nectar for sustenance while inadvertently pollinating the flowers. This mutual relationship leads to the formation of fruits containing seeds, ensuring the continuation of milkweed populations. Monarch caterpillars have uniquely adapted to feed exclusively on milkweed, forming a crucial part of the interconnected "milkweed village." Within this village, various creatures like aphids, true bugs, and moth caterpillars with striking coats of hairs coexist, relying solely on milkweed for sustenance. Creating your own milkweed village in your garden is a wonderful way to support these species. Once the risk of frost has passed and the soil has warmed, you can plant milkweed seeds indoors or directly sow them outside. If the plant's appearance is a concern, consider placing milkweed in a secluded yet sunny spot or at the back of a border. By cultivating milkweed, you are providing a vital habitat for a host of fascinating and interconnected organisms.

The Milkweed plant is a tall plant that can grow to be 2 to 6 feet tall (0.5-2 m.). The leaves are huge and green, and they grow from a tall stem, turning a reddish tint as the plant ages. The waxy, pointed, and dark green leaves of young Milkweed detach from the stem, allowing the milky liquid to ooze from the growing plant. As the plant matures, the stems become hollow and hairy. From June to August, the Milkweed flower blooms in a range of colors, from pink to purple to orange.

Butterfly milkweed produces the most vibrant orange (occasionally vermilion red or even golden yellow) flowers of any native plant. They occur in early to midsummer with an occasional flower later in summer. The plant is leafier than most milkweeds. Leaves are narrow, strappy, and fine-textured. Narrow pod-shaped fruits hold well into winter, crowning the stems. Unlike most milkweeds, which are short-lived perennials, butterfly milkweed may live for decades. The activity of all its pollinators adds to its buzz as a masterpiece of art and science. This milkweed is an ideal perennial for a traditional perennial border and grows 24–30 inches tall. It thrives in harsh sites as well, making an excellent plant in a rock garden or other hot, sunny location with good drainage. Butterfly milkweed flourishes in average to well-drained soil that may be rocky, gravelly, or sandy. Some strains even grow in pure clay, but most demand fast-draining soils.

Milkweed does not always start growing in northern gardens in time for butterflies to benefit fully. There, you can start Milkweed seeds indoors so that they are ready to sow once the soil has warmed up.

Before sprouting, Milkweed plants benefit from vernalization, a chilly treatment. They get this when they're planted outside, but you can speed up the process by stratifying the seeds. Place seeds in a damp soil container, cover with plastic wrap and store in the refrigerator for at least three weeks. If desired, plant in containers and place under a grow lamp inside six weeks before soil conditions outside have warmed. Mist the soil to keep it moist, but seeds that sit in soggy soil may rot. Transplant the seedlings to their permanent, sunny home outside when they have two sets of leaves. If planting in a row, space plants about 2 feet (61 cm) apart. The Milkweed plant has a long taproot and dislikes being moved after being planted outside. Mulch can aid in water conservation. Milkweed plants can be used in mixed borders, meadows, and natural settings. To provide more pollen to our flying companions, put Milkweed plants with tubular-shaped, shorter flowers in front of them.

Consumption Methods: As Milkweed can be poisonous, it is more commonly used in creating salves and creams for treating surface wounds and skin ailments.

Warning: Please note that while milkweed has many valuable ecological benefits and supports various species, it is important to handle milkweed with caution. Some species of milkweed contain toxic cardiac glycosides that can be harmful if ingested or if their sap comes into contact with the eyes or sensitive skin. It is advised to exercise caution when handling milkweed plants, especially if you have known allergies or sensitivities. Additionally, milkweed should not be consumed or used for medicinal purposes without proper knowledge and guidance, as certain species may have adverse effects. If in doubt, it is recommended to consult with experts or professionals familiar with milkweed before using it in any form.

Motherwort

Throw-Wort, Lion's Ear, Lion's Tail.

Leonurus Cardiaca.

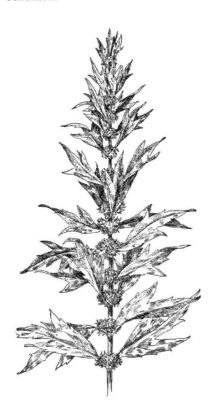

Identification: Motherwort, a member of the mint family, is an erect perennial herb that typically reaches a height of 3.5 feet, although it can be shorter in some instances. Its stem is characterized by its quadrangular shape, grooves, and often hairy and hollow composition. The plant features opposite leaves with long petioles, deeply lobed and coarsely toothed. The upper leaves exhibit three to five lobes, showcasing a dark green color on the top surface and a lighter green shade underneath. Delicate red flowers are arranged in dense false whorls, emerging from the upper leaf axils, adding a splash of color to the plant from April to August, with the timing varying based on latitude and altitude. When the leaves of motherwort are crushed, they release a distinct and peculiar odor, further contributing to its unique characteristics.

Traditional Uses: Motherwort, scientifically known as Leonurus cardiaca, derives its name from its historical use in toning the heart muscle, symbolically represented by the term "lion's heart." This herb has a rich traditional background, utilized by both the Chinese and pioneers for its various medicinal properties. It has been regarded as a tonic for treating conditions such as amenorrhea, dysmenorrhea, urinary cramps, and general weakness. Additionally, motherwort has been credited with its ability to clear toxins from the body. In ancient Greece, it was administered to pregnant women to alleviate stress and anxiety. However, caution is now advised during pregnancy due to its uterus-stimulating effects. Motherwort has also been employed as a remedy for bacterial and fungal infections, both internally and externally. The aerial parts of the plant, including the leaves, flowers, and stems, are gathered during the flowering period and used to prepare infusions for treating conditions like asthma and heart palpitations. With its introduction from Europe, Native American tribes such as the Delaware, Oklahoma, Micmac, Mohegan, and Shinnecock incorporated motherwort infusions into their traditional medicine as a gynecological remedy for "female ills." Additionally, it was used by the Cherokee and Iroquois as a digestive aid, a sedative for nervous and hysterical illnesses, a nerve tonic, and a stimulant to prevent fainting, respectively. Motherwort's multifaceted traditional uses highlight its valued role in various cultures throughout history.

Modern uses: Motherwort has gained recognition in modern herbal medicine for its diverse range of uses. It has received approval from Commission E for addressing nervous heart complaints such as palpitations and thyroid dysfunction. Among herbalists and naturopaths, it is highly regarded as a superior herb for women, known for its uterine and circulatory stimulating properties, making it a potential aid in relieving symptoms of PMS. The plant exhibits various therapeutic effects, including hypotensive, antispasmodic, diuretic, laxative, sedative, and emmenagogue actions. One of the active constituents in motherwort, called leonurine, contributes to toning the uterine membrane and regulating its function. In homeopathy, preparations using motherwort are utilized during menopause. Interestingly, Chinese herbal medicine aligns with the traditional European uses of motherwort as a standalone herb, without the usual combination with other herbs. In China, Leonurus japonicus, a related species, is extensively utilized, and its efficacy is supported by numerous clinical studies. Combining motherwort with passionflower has been suggested for blood pressure reduction. In Chinese medicine, a decoction of dried motherwort herb is employed as a uterine stimulant.

Antispasmodic, Emmenagogue, Nervine, Laxative

Solvents: Boiling water, alcohol.

Medicinal parts: tops and leaves

Hardiness Zones: Zones 4-8.

Sourcing: Motherwort (Leonurus cardiaca) can be sourced in various regions across the United States. This herbaceous perennial plant thrives in a wide range of habitats, including meadows, fields, open woodlands, and neglected areas. It is commonly found in regions with temperate climates, such as the northeastern and central parts of the country. Motherwort prefers well-drained soil and partial shade, although it can tolerate full sun. If you're looking to buy motherwort, you can often find seeds or young plants at local nurseries specializing in herbs or medicinal plants.

Gardening Tips: Motherwort (Leonurus cardiaca) is a versatile and resilient herb that can be grown in the home garden. To cultivate motherwort, stratify the seeds for a few weeks before planting. You can choose to directly sow the seeds in the garden during late fall, allowing them to naturally stratify throughout the winter. Motherwort is a hardy plant that adapts to different light and soil conditions. However, it has a tendency to self-seed abundantly, so be mindful of its spreading nature.

To prevent excessive reseeding, prune the plant back to 3-5 inches after flowering but before the seeds mature. The beautiful purple/blueish blooms of motherwort add a calming and soothing touch to the garden. The unique leaf structure adds visual interest. In the fall, you can divide the roots for propagation. Keep in mind that as a member of the mint family, motherwort can become invasive if not managed properly. After flowering, harvest the entire herb and dry it for storage. The dried herb can be used to make tinctures or brewed into tea. Motherwort attracts bumblebees, which rely on its flowers for pollen and nectar. Additionally, it provides habitat and protection for field sparrows in prairie environments.

Consumption Methods: Motherwort can be made as leaf tea, tincture, and capsule form. To counteract the harshness of motherwort, it is frequently blended with honey, ginger, lemon, sugar, or other strong flavors when drank as tea. Instead of Valerian (Valeriana oflicinalis) the fresh juice of leaves and flowers, 30-40 drops, can be used for calming the nerves and inducing a soothing sleep.

Warnings: Diarrhea, gastrointestinal discomfort, and uterine bleeding are all possible overdose side effects.

Oregon Grape

Oregon Grape-Holly, Holly-leaved Barberry, Holly-leaved Oregon Grape,
Oregon Hollygrape, Mountain Grape.

Mahonia aquifolium.

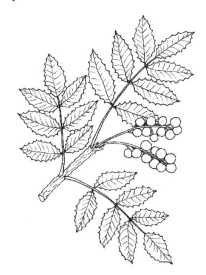

Medical Uses: Oregon Grapes have been utilized by Native Americans for thousands of years as medicine, food, and dye. In 1899, it was designated as the state flower of Oregon. Poor liver function, digestive difficulties, eczema, acne, giardia, herpes, and malaria are all conditions that Oregon Grape has been used to cure. Its anti-inflammatory and antibacterial effects are the most common reasons for its use. Berberine, an alkaloid present in goldenseal and barberry, is the principal active chemical ingredient. This alkaloid is used by plants for the same reason it is used by humans; to protect roots from microbial invasion.

Solvents: Boiling water, alcohol.

Hardiness Zones: Zones 5-9.

Sourcing: Oregon grape (Mahonia aquifolium) is native to western North America, particularly the Pacific Northwest region of the United States. It thrives in a variety of habitats, including forests, woodlands, and scrublands. It prefers well-drained soil and partial shade, although it can tolerate a range of light conditions. It is commonly found in moist, shady areas, such as the understory of forests. When sourcing Oregon grape, be sure to respect local regulations and obtain plants or seeds from reputable nurseries or suppliers who specialize in native plants.

Gardening Tips: Motherwort is a versatile plant that can thrive in various lighting conditions, ranging from full sun to deep shade, although partial shade is preferred. It is adaptable to different soil types but thrives best in humus-rich, slightly acidic soil that is evenly moist yet well-draining. Prior to planting, prepare the soil by incorporating a generous amount of compost into the planting hole. It is advisable to protect the young plants from harsh winter winds for optimal growth.

To propagate Oregon Grape, you can take cuttings from semi-ripe wood in the fall. These cuttings can be used to produce new Oregon Grape plants. Additionally, you can remove sucker growths at the base of the plant and transplant them elsewhere in the spring. If starting from seeds, it is recommended to cold stratify the Oregon Grape seeds for three weeks before sowing them in the garden. This can be done by storing the seeds in a moist medium in the refrigerator. Sow the fully ripened seeds in the fall for germination the following spring. Keep in mind that germination may take up to six months for stored seeds.

If you choose to grow Oregon Grape seeds indoors, cover them with moistened planting mix and refrigerate them for three weeks prior to sowing. Maintain a temperature of around 50°F (10°C) in the growing medium until the seeds germinate, which typically takes about six weeks for fresh seeds. Once the seedlings have emerged, provide them with proper care, including regular watering and appropriate lighting, until they are ready to be transplanted into the garden.

Consumption Methods: While the dark blue to purple berries are a little acidic when eaten fresh, they are delicious when cooked into preserves. The jelly has a gorgeous midnight blue color and a tangy, earthy flavor. Outside of being used as a food, teas, tinctures, and herbal supplements are available.

Warnings: Oregon Grapes are neither poisonous nor allergic. However, eating too many of them at once, as with many other fruits, can create digestive issues. The berries also contain berberine, a natural chemical substance. It's an alkaloid found in plants belonging to the same family as barberry. Excessive berberine use, on the other hand, has been related to brain development problems in fetuses and infants. It's better to avoid berberine because it can pass from the mother's placenta and breastmilk to her child.

Ostrich Fern

Fiddlehead Fern, Shuttlecock Fern.

Matteuccia struthiopteris.

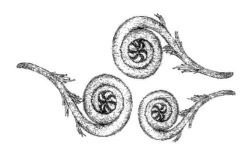

Medical uses: Ostrich Fern fiddleheads are known to be popular in creating a gargling solution for treating sore throat, while other parts of the plant are used for back pain, healing sores, and producing afterbirth effects.

Solvents: Boiling water.

Hardiness Zone: Zones 3-7.

Sourcing: The Ostrich Fern flourishes in wooded areas with plenty of shade, moisture, and nutrient-rich soil. They are frequently observed in the wild along creek banks and thrive in moist soil. In northern latitudes, they may handle partial sun, but in hotter climates, they should be planted in full shade and watered regularly. Basically, they're content as long as they're shaded and wet. As a result, Ostrich Fern can be found all over the United States.

Gardening Tips: There are no particular techniques for growing Ostrich Ferns. While spores can be used to cultivate them, it is preferable to order plants from a trustworthy grower. Your plants will normally come as dormant, bare-root plants packed in moss or wood shavings, ready to be planted. Plant Ostrich Ferns in a shallow hole with lots of room for their roots to expand. Ascertain that the crown is just above the soil level. Fill up the area around the roots with any ordinary soil and water thoroughly—Water Ostrich Ferns on a regular basis for the first year or so. Don't set your expectations too high at first, and don't be alarmed if the plant appears to be slowing down. The initial task for an Ostrich Fern is to build a strong root system. During the first season, the fronds may begin to grow and then die back multiple times. Once planted, the plant expands quickly by underground rhizomes, quickly filling in the available space. Ostrich Ferns require no maintenance other than cleaning up dirt during the dormant season. They'll welcome a little fertilizer now and then, and, of course, keep them properly watered during droughts. Ostrich fern is most beautiful when its fiddleheads emerge in spring; the fresh fronds of vibrant green are widest toward the top and come to an abrupt point. Fully unfurled, plants are vase-shaped and reach 3–4 feet tall. In winter, after the surrounding sterile fronds have died, the stiff, brown plumelike fertile fronds stand around 2 feet tall. This fern requires moist, humus-rich soils and shade; some sun is tolerated in more northern and eastern locations as long as they stay moist. Ostrich fern spreads by ground-hugging rhizomes to create extensive masses; it spreads so quickly and vigorously, it is best used as a tall groundcover in moist, shady sites. Propagate by division. You might want to try harvesting fiddleheads for a springtime dinner treat once you've learned how to cultivate Ostrich Ferns and have a decent bed established. Fiddleheads are the first Ostrich Fern shoots to emerge in the spring, and they get their name from their resemblance to a fiddle's neck. The sterile shoots that will eventually grow into the biggest fronds are these. Take only half of each crown when it is still little and tightly curled. Wash them thoroughly before cooking and discard the brown papery covering.

Consumption Methods: Ostrich, or fiddlehead ferns, as they can be known, as generally prepared as a powder to be directly applied to wounds or cooked to be eaten. Fiddleheads can be boiled or steamed, and they're very delicious when sautéed in bacon drippings with garlic. Make sure to properly fry them and only use Ostrich Fern fiddleheads. Ostrich Ferns can be the right option for filling that damp, shaded location, repairing a problem area with lush and attractive growth, and providing an otherwise pricey delicacy for your springtime table, all while requiring very little care.

Warnings: Ostrich Fern is said to have a sedative effect on some people. It is not suggested for persons who are taking anti-anxiety medications. The tannins in this herb can induce stomach upset in large amounts; therefore, it's not recommended (or required) to use a lot of it.

Partridgeberry

Partridge Berry, Squaw Berry, Two-Eyed Berry, Running Fox.

Mitchella repens.

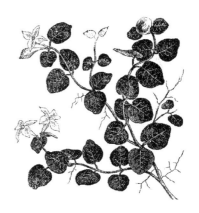

Identification: The shining leaves are roundish or heart-shaped, 3-4 in. long, which sometimes look like clover; they are opposite on the stem and may be marked with white lines, and they remain green throughout the winter. The fragrant white or pink paired flowers, 1 in. long, are joined at the base and usually have four hairy petals; seen in bloom from June to July. The scarlet berry, which remains on the plant all winter, is 3 in. in diameter, containing usually eight bony seeds. The berry is edible but is nearly tasteless.

Medical Uses: The taste of partridge berries is characterized as bland or moderately fragrant at best. Tea produced from the leaves and fruits was used by Native American women, especially the Mohawk tribe, to cure a variety of obstetric and gynecological ailments. Other traditional and historical texts claim that it has additional medical benefits, such as nerve soothing and stomach relief.

Astringent, Diuretic, Tonic, Parturient

Medicinal Part: The whole herb

Solvents: Boiling water, alcohol.

Hardiness Zones: Zones 4-9.

Sourcing: Partridge berry is indigenous to North America and found in dry and swampy woods from south-western Newfoundland to Minnesota, south to Florida and Texas, and in Guatemala. Partridgeberry can be found in open spaces where ground cover is possible, as it is a plant that seeks to spread rather than grow tall. Live plants are available at reputable retailers.

Gardening Tips: If you want to cultivate partridgeberries, you'll need to choose a location with well-draining, humus-rich soil. The vine prefers sandy, neutrally acidic, or alkaline soil. Plant the vines in a location that receives early sun but receives afternoon shade. Plants of Partridgeberry grow slowly but steadily, eventually forming Partridgeberry ground cover. Partridgeberry plants are easy to care for because they are rarely attacked by pests or infected by illnesses. Once established, Partridgeberry plant care essentially consists of clearing garden detritus from the mat. Dig up a segment of existing Partridgeberry plants and transplant it to a new location if you wish to reproduce it. Because the vine usually grows from nodes, this method works nicely.

Consumption Methods: 1 teaspoonful of the herb to 1 cupful of boiling water for menstrual complaints, indigestion, and bladder pains.

Pleurisy Root

Asclépiade, Asclépiade Pleurétique, Asclépiade Tubéreuse, Asclepias tuberosa, Butterfly Weed, Canada Root, Flux Root, Orange Milkweed, Orange Swallow Wort, Pleurisy, Racine du Canada, Racine Colique, Racine de Flux, Racine de Tubercule, Swallow Wort, Tuber Root, Vencetósigo, White Root

Asclepias tuberosa.

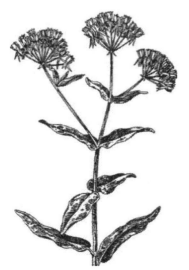

Identification: Pleurisy root (*Asclepias tuberosa*) is an exquisite perennial herb belonging to the Asclepiadaceae family. It can be commonly found thriving in dry, gravelly, and sandy soils across the United States and Canada. This herbaceous plant boasts large, irregular tuberous roots with a distinctive yellowish-brown hue. While fresh roots possess a somewhat nauseous and bitter taste, they develop a more desirable flavor when dried. The stems of pleurisy root are covered in fine hairs and gracefully reach a height of 2-3 feet. They bear lanceolate leaves that are alternately arranged, featuring a hairy texture and showcasing a rich dark green color on their upper surface, while their undersides exhibit a pale hue. The plant graces us with numerous erect flowers, displaying a stunningly vibrant orange-yellow color. These blossoms bloom from June to August and give way to long, narrow, and softly hairy pods that stand upright.

Medical Uses: Native American tribes utilized Pleurisy Root both orally and topically to treat lung infections and wounds. The plant was continuing to be used mostly for lung disorders such as pleurisy and pneumonia by Eclectic physicians in the United States. It was also used to treat infections as a diaphoretic (a drug that produces sweating). From 1820 through 1905, Pleurisy Root was an official medicine in the United States Pharmacopoeia. Native American tribes utilized Pleurisy Root both orally and topically to treat lung infections and wounds. Physicians jumped on these concepts and proceeded to utilize the plant to treat pleurisy and pneumonia, among other ailments. It was also used to treat infections as a diaphoretic, a drug that produces a sweating effect.

Solvents: boiling water

Medicinal parts: root

Hardiness Zones: Zones 4-9.

Sourcing: Pleurisy Root favors sand soil with more shade than sun; hence it can be found along roadsides, fields, and prairies. Butterfly weed grows best in full sun, although it can also thrive in moderate shade. The plant prefers a light, fertile sandy soil that drains well.

Gardening Tips: Pleurisy Root spreads outward and reaches a height of 36 inches. Butterflies, hummingbirds, and other pollinators love it because it produces clusters of distinct orange blooms.

Pleurisy enjoys full sun and thrives in moderately damp to dry, well-drained soil.

Pleurisy is best sown in the fall, just below the soil surface (about 3/8 inch) ") with a light tamping technique. Otherwise, it can be planted in the spring but will need to be cold stratified. Seeds should be blended with wet starting media and stored in the refrigerator for four weeks. Keep an eye on the mixture to make sure it hasn't dried out; keep it moist. If seeds start to germinate, plant them right away.

Seeds can be started in flats in a greenhouse or other warm indoor areas after stratification. Lightly tamp seeds into the soil's surface, or cover with a thin layer of dirt and water. Keep the soil or potting media moist until the seeds sprout. Once the first genuine leaves have appeared, and the fear of a spring freeze has passed, transplant outside.

Consumption Methods: Pleurisy root (Asclepias tuberosa) is valued for its therapeutic properties and can be prepared as a decoction or infusion. It is commonly used to promote perspiration and expectoration, making it beneficial for respiratory ailments such as lung inflammation, catarrhal conditions, and bronchial congestion. This herb is known to alleviate pain and ease breathing difficulties without exerting stimulant effects. Pleurisy root has also been employed in the treatment of acute rheumatism, dysentery, colds, flu, as well as various fevers, including those characterized by biliousness and burning sensations. It is particularly regarded as a suitable remedy for children due to its gentle yet effective action in small doses.

Warnings: If you take more than the prescribed dose of Pleurisy Root, you may get nausea, vomiting, or diarrhea.

Red Root

New Jersey Tea, Jersey Tea Ceanothus, Mountain Sweet, Wild Snowball.

Ceanothus Americanus.

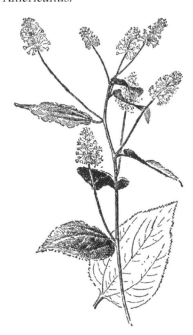

Medical Uses: Red Root has been used in traditional Native American medicine for a long time. Colds, fever, pneumonia, digestive difficulties, toothaches, and urinary tract infections in women were all treated with the root steeped as tea. Check the second volume for more information.

Solvents: Boiling water, alcohol.

Hardiness Zones: Zones 4-8.

Sourcing: Any reputable retailer or online storefront. Easy to find. Red Root can be found wild in swamps, drylands, and wet woods. The plant is native to the northern United States and can commonly be found among other hearty temperate bushes and flowering plants.

Gardening Tips: The Red Root plant prefers a warm, sunny location; however, it may tolerate partial shade. Red Root grows best in limestone or sandy soils, but it can also thrive in bone-dry conditions. However, plants of this variety abhor any sort of disturbance to their underlying foundations, so it's best to simply put them outside in stable regions when they're young. Because this plant despises over-pruning, you should only cut wood that is longer than a pencil off it. If you must prune the plant despite everything, it is advisable to do so in the spring. While the plants are still young, Red Root begins to bloom swiftly—the Red Root plant blooms in its second year, usually at the start of spring. Furthermore, Red Root plants hybridize well with other plants that share a similar diversity of location. Various plants that grow in this type of environment also have a cooperative and beneficial interaction with specific bacteria in the soil, which eventually form lumps on the plant roots and aid in nitrogen fixation. Seeds are commonly used to develop the Red Root plant. After the Red Root seeds have developed and matured, they should be sown in a cool frame as soon as possible. If you're using saved seeds, soak them in warm water for around 12 hours before storing them in cool stratification at 1°C for one to three months. If the seeds are stored at 20°C for one to two months, they should develop normally. An excellent, nutritious seed, easily hand-gathered and added to your bird feeder

Consumption Methods: Tincture or tea made fresh from dried leaves.

Warnings: Some research has indicated that Red Root may cause blood clotting, making it dangerous for those on blood thinners.

Slippery Elm

Grey Elm, Red Elm, Slippery Elm, Soft Elm.

Ulmus rubra.

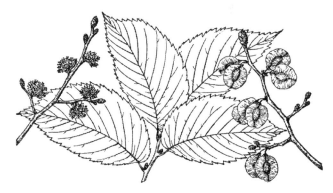

Medical uses: For generations, the weird mucilaginous bark of Slippery Elm has been utilized as a herbal treatment in North America. Native Americans utilized Slippery Elm to treat wounds, boils, ulcers, burns, and skin inflammation with therapeutic salves. Coughs, sore throats, diarrhea, and stomach problems were also relieved by taking it orally. Check out the second volume for all its traditional and modern uses.

Solvents: Boiling water, alcohol.

Hardiness Zones: Zones 3-9.

Sourcing: Slippery elm (Ulmus rubra) is native to the eastern and central regions of North America, particularly in the United States. It can be found growing in a variety of habitats, including moist forests, stream banks, and bottomlands. This deciduous tree thrives in areas with rich, loamy soil and a moderate amount of sunlight. It is commonly found in states such as New York, Pennsylvania, Ohio, and Kentucky. Look for certified organic sources to ensure the highest quality and environmental responsibility. Buy as grown tree or seeds. Harvest only the bark sparingly with small-diameter cutsand the seeds for transplanting.

Gardening Tips: It's not difficult to get started with planting Slippery Elm trees. When the Slippery Elm samaras are mature in the spring, gather them. They can be knocked from branches or swept from the ground. After air-drying the seeds for several days, the next stage in developing Slippery Elm trees is to sow them. Remove the wings if you don't want to risk damaging them. Alternatively, you can stratify them in a wet medium at 41 degrees F (5 degrees C) for 60 to 90 days before planting.

When the seedlings are several inches (8 cm) tall, transplant them into larger containers. You can also immediately plant them in your garden. Choose a location with moist, rich soil, and full sun to partial shade. Prefers alkaline and moist soil, but tolerates dry soil. The woody taproot system will grow deep down in drier soils and develop shallow and wide-spreading in moist soils. Seeds may be produced as early as 15 years of tree age, but 40 years is more normal.

More resistant to Dutch Elm disease than its close cousin American elm tree.

Consumption Methods: A popular tea to treat acid reflux. Check out the dose, other uses, and great recipes in the second and third volume.

Warnings: At high dosage, Slippery Elm may cause digestive upset.

Solomon's Seal

Polygonatum.

Polygonatum biflorum.

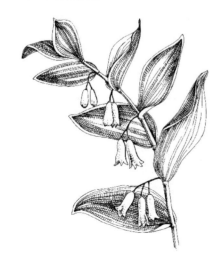

Medical uses: The starch-rich rhizomes of smooth Solomon's Seal were utilized as a "potato-like meal" in soups and bread by Native Americans. The immature shoots can be eaten fresh or cooked to make an asparagus-like dish. In a Chippewa headache cure, a decoction of roots was dusted on hot stones and the smoke inhaled. Find more information in the second volume.

Solvents: Boiling water, alcohol.

Hardiness Zones: Zones 3-9.

Sourcing: Solomon's Seal can be grown or found wild in semi-dappled, dappled, or full shade. It won't grow well in the shade of low-branched trees or in city alleyways. Morning and late afternoon sun are fine for Solomon's Seals, but midday sun scorches and crisps their leaves. In the country wilds across the midwest, you're likely to find some sooner or later.

Gardening Tips: Solomon's Seal is a handsome perennial herb of the Asclepiadaceae family, known for its graceful appearance and versatility in garden settings. It thrives in a variety of soil types, including dry, gravelly, and sandy soils, making it adaptable to different regions across the United States and Canada. The plant features nodding whitish-green elongated bell-shaped flowers that bloom in late spring, attracting bees and hummingbirds with their rich nectar. As fall approaches, the foliage transforms into a stunning golden yellow color, while pendent blue berries emerge at each leaf axil, adding further visual interest.

In addition to its aesthetic appeal, Solomon's Seal has practical uses as well. The short, spreading rhizomes and shoots of the plant are edible, making it a valuable addition to food forests. Its architectural clumps of foliage lend themselves well to traditional shady perennial borders and insectaries, creating a habitat for beneficial insects and birds. Gardeners can incorporate Solomon's Seal into their woodland gardens, taking advantage of its preference for moist and shady environments.

When cultivating Solomon's Seal, it is advisable to provide it with rich soil, preferably with added compost, to support its growth and development. The plant tolerates a wide range of light conditions, from full shade to partial shade, making it versatile for different garden settings. It is a low-maintenance plant, with deadheading unnecessary as the spent blooms naturally fall off. The foliage remains attractive throughout the growing season, reducing the need for constant upkeep.

Solomon's Seal is typically propagated by division, allowing gardeners to expand their plantings. Seeds can also be used, although they may take up to two years to germinate. The plant is hardy in USDA hardiness zones 3 to 9, adapting well to varying climatic conditions. It can withstand cold temperatures and is tolerant of hot, dry climates with proper care, including adequate soil moisture, shade, and protection from scorching winds. Mulching around the plants helps to maintain cool root temperatures and conserve moisture.

While pests and diseases are generally not a major concern for healthy Solomon's Seal plants, occasional fungal issues may arise in wet weather. Ensuring proper air circulation around the plants can help prevent and address these problems. Watch out for slugs and snails, as they can cause damage to the leaves and stems. Natural pest control methods can be employed to mitigate these issues and preserve the health of the plants.

Overall, Solomon's Seal is an attractive and versatile plant that brings beauty, edible value, and ecological benefits to the garden. With its adaptability to different light and soil conditions, it offers gardeners a range of options for incorporating it into their landscape designs while providing habitat and food sources for beneficial insects and birds.

Consumption Methods: Eaten raw, as a decoction, or tincture.

Warnings: There are few warnings other than the fact that intense doses may cause some gastric upset.

Stinging Nettle

Common Nettle, Nettle, Stinger Nettle, Bichu, Feuille d'Ortie,
Graine d'Ortie, Grande Ortie, Ortie, Ortiga, Urtica.

Urtica dioica.

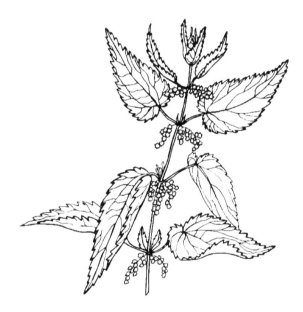

Medical Uses: Throughout history, indigenous cultures have held a deep connection with the Stinging Nettle plant, incorporating it into various aspects of their lives. Tribes such as the Winnebago, Coastal Salish, Omaha, Cupeo, Menominee, and Subarctic peoples utilized nettle fibers to create clothing items like undershirts, robes, cloaks, and ponchos. It was also used in the construction of fishing nets, showcasing the versatility of this plant.

The Native American traditional uses of nettle encompassed not only practical applications but also medicinal and ceremonial purposes. In the spring, several tribes consumed fresh nettle leaves or prepared nettle tonics, which were believed to purify the blood and liver. Pregnant women found benefit in nettle as well, as it was believed to prevent excessive bleeding during childbirth, alleviate labor pains, and strengthen the

uterus and fetus. The styptic properties of nettle, which help control bleeding, made it a popular choice for wound care among different groups. Dried and powdered nettle could be applied to wounds, or fresh leaves lightly pounded and used as a wrap to enhance the healing process.

One of the oldest documented uses of Stinging Nettle is urtication, a practice that involves thrashing one's limbs with nettle stalks. This ancient technique has been employed by indigenous cultures worldwide, including North America, to address arthritic joint pain. While there are differing opinions on its effectiveness, some believe that the sting of the nettle plant may trigger an anti-inflammatory response in the body, helping to alleviate arthritic swelling.

Stinging Nettle also held ceremonial significance for certain Native American groups. In Nevada, nettle leaves were burned in sweat lodges, serving both as an offering and as a treatment for pneumonia and influenza. The Kawaiisu people attributed strong dream-inducing qualities to nettle, and individuals seeking medicinal dreams would walk barefoot through nettle fields as part of their preparation for entering the dream world.

In indigenous folklore, Stinging Nettle is often associated with the coyote, a symbol of trickery and transformation. This connection reflects the plant's ability to both sting and heal, embodying the duality of nature's forces.

Check out the second volume for more

Solvents: Boiling water, alcohol.

Hardiness Zones: Zones 3-10.

Sourcing: Stinging nettle can be sourced in various regions across the United States, as it is a widespread and common plant. It thrives in moist and fertile soils, often found near streams, rivers, meadows, and woodland edges. Whether you choose to wild harvest or cultivate it in your garden, stinging nettle can be obtained by locating patches of the plant in suitable habitats or obtaining seeds or starter plants from reputable sources.

Gardening Tips: Stinging nettle (Urtica dioica) is a fast-growing herbaceous plant that can reach a height of about 4 feet (1 meter). It is known for its small, hollow silica-tipped hairs that can cause a stinging sensation if touched. To grow stinging nettle, you can start seeds indoors four to six weeks before the last frost date or plant them directly in the garden in the spring. Choose a location with rich, moist soil away from other herbs. Sow the seeds in a row about an inch wide and keep the soil consistently moist. Once the nettle seedlings have grown, transplant them into a prepared garden bed, spacing them at least 12 inches (30 cm) apart.

When harvesting stinging nettle, it is important to wear protective gloves and clothing to avoid the stinging hairs. Select the top two or three pairs of leaves from the plant's tops in the early weeks of spring when the leaves are fresh and tender. Harvesting can continue throughout the summer, but be mindful that the stalks and stems can become fibrous. Use sharp scissors or garden shears to cut the nettle leaves outside, or tongs in the kitchen when handling them for cooking.

Stinging nettle can serve various purposes in the garden. It can be used as a natural deer repellent or as a source of nutrient-rich fertilizer. It is a resilient and invasive plant, so it's important to control its growth and prevent it from spreading excessively. Regular monitoring and removal of unwanted plants can help keep stinging nettle in check and prevent it from overpowering other garden plants.

Consumption Methods: Stinging nettle (Urtica dioica) has been used for various medicinal purposes. It is known to possess anti-inflammatory, diuretic, and antioxidant properties. The recommended dose and uses of stinging nettle may vary depending on the specific condition being addressed. It is commonly used to relieve symptoms of allergies, such as hay fever, by reducing histamine production. It is also utilized as a natural remedy for joint pain, arthritis, and urinary tract infections. Stinging nettle can be consumed as a tea, extract, or incorporated into topical preparations for skin conditions like eczema and dermatitis.

Warnings: It's important to distinguish between Stinging Nettle and "White Dead Nettle" (Lamium album).

Sumac (Smooth, Staghorn, And Fragrant)

Red Sumac, Scarlet Sumac, Common Sumac, Western Sumac.

Rhus glabra.

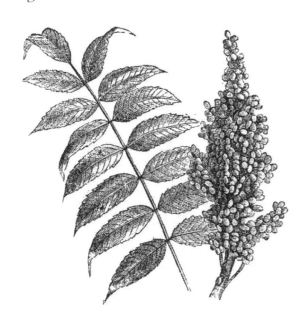

Medical Uses: Smooth Sumac has a long history of medicinal use among various Native American tribes. The medicinal properties of smooth Sumac have been utilized in numerous ways. Tribes such as the Natchez and Ojibwa used different parts of the plant for various therapeutic purposes. Smooth Sumac was employed as an antiemetic, antidiarrheal, antihemorrhagic, and as a treatment for blisters, colds, asthma, tuberculosis, sore throat, ear and eye ailments, ulcers, and rashes. The roots

of fragrant Sumac were specifically used by the Natchez to heal boils, while the Ojibwa drank a decoction of aromatic Sumac root to alleviate diarrhea. Additionally, smooth and staghorn Sumac were valued for their dyeing properties, as their berries, roots, inner bark, and leaves were used to produce a range of vibrant colors. In certain tribes of the plains region, the leaves of fragrant, staghorn, and smooth Sumac were even mixed with tobacco and smoked.

Solvents: Boiling water, alcohol.

Hardiness Zones: Zones 5-8.

Sourcing: Sumac can be sourced in various regions of the United States, where it is commonly found in its natural habitat. It thrives in diverse environments, including woodlands, meadows, and open areas, and is well-adapted to different soil types. Smooth Sumac (Rhus glabra) is native to the eastern and central parts of North America, ranging from the southern United States up to Canada. Staghorn Sumac (Rhus typhina) is also native to North America and can be found in regions spanning from eastern Canada to the central and eastern United States. Both species prefer full sun to partial shade and well-drained soils. When sourcing sumac, it is important to ensure that you are harvesting from areas where it is abundant and legally permitted. Additionally, it is advisable to consult local regulations and conservation guidelines to ensure responsible and sustainable sourcing practices.

Gardening Tips: Fragrant sumac's tiny yellow flowers are relished by the first insects of spring, their bloom coinciding with the emergence of the spring azure butterfly. Female plants produce stunning red, fuzzy fruit that ripens from late spring into midsummer, when they are one of the most ornamental features of any plant, contrasting perfectly with the green foliage. Fruit becomes dark reddish brown by late summer and occasionally persists into winter. Fall color is exceptional on plants originating locally or regionally. Winter twigs, tipped with next spring's flower buds, are a favored browse of deer and rabbits. Larger forms of this popular shrub are occasionally used as focal ornamentals but are mainly seen at the back of the border or as screen plants; smaller cultivars ('Gro-Low', for example) are used as groundcovers. The edible fruits have become trendy for flavorings and teas and are in demand by chefs working with local ingredients. Fragrant sumac grows best in well-drained, limestone-based soils, from pure sand and gravel to clay.

Smooth sumac makes a fine mass planting in well-drained soil on steep embankments or against a woodland or tree planting. The light green flowers, which appear in early to midsummer, are noticeably fragrant. Many insects and woodland butterflies visit the flowers. Female plants produce showy pyramidal clusters of fuzzy reddish fruit which hold through winter. The leaves are dark blue-green above with lighter bluish, luminous undersides that reflect night light; this plant shines in such a situation, near an outdoor seating area or at a front entry, for example. In fall, leaves turn to intense and saturated reds, often with a pinkish overtone. A word to the wise: smooth sumac runs in all directions except toward shade.

Staghorn sumac is the largest and most treelike of the running sumacs, reaching 35 feet or more; it makes an excellent edge-of-the-woods or hedgerow planting in large landscapes. Sumac is best known for its flaming fall color, and staghorn sumac's is yellow, orange, or red, often all on the same plant at the same time. Staghorn sumac has the showiest fruit of the sumacs: it's fuzzy with metallic hairs, ripens red in late summer, and lingers through winter; fruits, on female plants, are exceptionally ornamental when adorned with snow. Its young stems, velvety like a stag's horn, are also quite noticeable and usually red-brown in winter. Plants require moist, well-drained soil. Cut back to the ground to rejuvenate.

Sumac is becoming more popular in the landscape as a result of its spectacular fall color. The leaves of most species become a brilliant red color in the fall, but there are also yellow and orange Sumac variants for gardens. If you want to see a beautiful fall display, choose a deciduous rather than an evergreen type.

Consumption Methods: It's perfect as an winter meals due to its tangy, citrus-like flavor. For medicinal purposes it can be made as a tea or tincture to balance blood sugar and alleviate muscle pain.

Warnings: Sumac has an anti-lipase effect. This, in turn, can lead to rapid weight reduction since it has an impact that partially limits fat absorption in the small intestine while simultaneously speeding up fat breakdown.

Sundew

Catchfly, Dew-Threads, Flypaper.

Drosera.

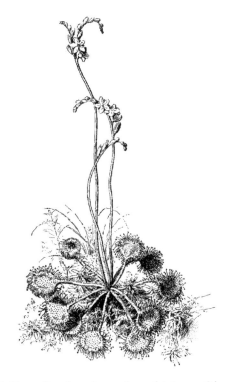

Medical Uses: Sundew has a long history of herbal use, and it's known for its aphrodisiac and strengthening properties. It relaxes the muscles of the respiratory system, making breathing easier and reducing wheezing, and is therefore useful in the treatment of a variety of chest problems. Because the plant has grown scarce, it should not be collected in the wild. Antibacterial, antibiotic, antispasmodic, antitussive, demulcent, expectorant and hypoglycemic are all properties of the flowering plant. The herb is beneficial in the treatment of whooping cough, as it has a unique effect on the respiratory organs. It's also used to treat phthisis in its early stages, chronic bronchitis, and asthma. Corns, warts, and bunions have all been treated with it externally. In the summer, the plant is collected and dried for later use. Use at your own risk. Internal usage of this herb induces a color change in the urine that is completely harmless. Plumbagin, which is antibacterial against a wide spectrum of infections, is found in a plant extract. The leaf juice has been utilized to heal warts and corns because of its protein-digesting enzymes. A homeopathic cure is made from the entire fresh plant, picked just before it begins to flower. It is mostly used to treat coughs and is only effective against whooping cough.

Stimulant, Expectorant, Demulcent, Antispasmodic

Medicinal Part: The whole herb.

Solvents: Boiling water, alcohol.

Hardiness Zones: Zones 9-11.

Sourcing: The plants favor acidic soils and occur in bogs or marshes, where they commonly grow on top of sphagnum moss. Some subspecies are currently threatened with extinction, although others can still be found in Florida's wetlands and the swamps of the southernmost states.

Gardening Tips: Most Sundews grow in typical carnivorous plant soil, which is damp and low in nutrients (often bogs and fens). To compensate for the lack of soil, they catch and eat the juices of insects. Some desert Sundews, on the other hand, can withstand the heat by only developing when it rains.

The finest soil combination for growing Sundews at home is a 1:1 mix of peat moss and sand/perlite. Use a mixture of sand and perlite for other Sundew species that live in hotter climates, such as Australia. Tuberous Sundews are a type of Australian Sundew that thrives in tropical climates.

Most Sundews that dwell in hot climates have adapted to their surroundings; most become dormant during hot weather and resume growth once the rainy season begins.

You may also acquire a soil mix for Sundews that contains perlite and peat moss, such as this.

Choose plastic containers with holes on the bottom for growing Sundews. Sundews that thrive in humid environments can thrive in plastic or glass containers without holes. Keep them in a humid, wet environment. For small Sundews, a pot size of 4 inches is ideal, and for larger ones, a pot size of 7-10 inches is ideal.

Sundew feeding may be a lot of fun. If your environment is conducive to the growth of the Sundew plant, you can leave it outside, and it will feed itself for the most part. Sundews are attractive plants that attract their own prey.

If you keep it indoors (in a terrarium or greenhouse, for example), you can feed it insects or other foods. Houseflies, ants, spiders, gnats, moths, and fruit flies are examples.

If you can't find any live insects, freeze-dried insects such as fly larvae can be purchased. Moisten the food to make it softer, and only feed your Sundews hard-to-digest insects once or twice a week, such as crickets or grasshoppers.

Water your Sundews the same way you would other carnivorous plants. Fill the tray halfway with water and place the pot with the plant in it. When the plants go into dormancy, keep the soil wet to slightly dry.

Only distilled, reverse osmosis, purified, demineralized, or rainwater should be used. Use only distilled or bottled water since tap or mineral water includes minerals that will build up in the soil and damage the plant.

In full light to part sun, most Sundews grow and develop their colors to their greatest potential. A windowsill is the greatest spot to store them if you keep them indoors. Artificial light fixtures can be used to give light in greenhouses and terrariums if necessary.

Consumption Methods: Tinctures made from alcohol are the most common consumption method; however, dried leaves to create teas are available. If not consumed, powdered plant leaves may be made into a salve that is effective against skin conditions.

Warnings: Sundew can be a skin irritant if used prolongedly on healthy skin. If applying topically, watch the area to ensure that Sundew is not applied for longer than needed or accidentally smeared onto healthy skin.

Trillium

Toadshade, Wakerobin, Birthroot.

Trillium cernuum.

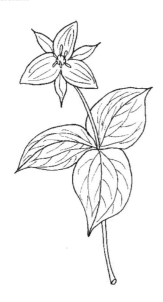

Medical Uses: Trillium, a versatile plant, not only offers edible leaves but also holds medicinal value recognized by Native Americans. The tender young leaves, with a sunflower seed-like taste, make a delightful addition to salads. They can also be cooked as a pot herb, although an abundance of other greens is available during this season. The medicinal properties of Trillium root are notable, as it possesses antibacterial, antispasmodic, diuretic, emmenagogue (to stimulate menstruation), and ophthalmic effects. In alternative medicine, the roots are often utilized. They can be boiled in milk to create a remedy for diarrhea and dysentery, both in fresh or dried form. Grated raw root serves as a poultice to alleviate swelling in the eyes and provide relief to rheumatic joints. For wound treatment and prevention of gangrene, the leaves are boiled in lard and applied as a poultice. Infusions made from the root are effective in relieving cramps, and the plant's common name, birthroot, alludes to its historical use in promoting menstruation. In addition, a decoction of the root bark, when used as ear drops, can help alleviate earaches. Trillium root was highly revered among American Indian women for its ability to facilitate childbirth and address various female ailments, making it a sacred herb known exclusively to their medicine women.

Solvents: Boiling water, alcohol.

Hardiness Zones: Zones 3-9.

Sourcing: Trillium can be found in most damp, shaded areas throughout the temperate regions of North America. Trilliums are difficult to transplant from the wild, and many are endangered; therefore, they should be obtained from a reliable nursery that specializes in their care. They can be grown from seed, though flowering will take some time. In fact, blooming can take up to four or five years.

Gardening Tips: The outward-facing bloom of this beloved woodland wildflower sits on a short pedicel and lasts a long time. It is the showiest flower of our trilliums, with milky white petals and an eye of yellow stamens in midspring; flowers turn rosy pink as they age. Some plants produce flowers with stacked or fully double petals; double-flowering trilliums are highly prized by shade gardeners, but such flowers are sterile, producing no pollen or fruits. Plants reach 12–15 inches tall and are readily cultivated in woodland, shade, or wildflower gardens throughout the Midwest. All trilliums may be propagated by dividing their rhizomes; this is best done as the plant is going dormant in late summer or fall.

When the seedpod has gone from white to russet brown, collect the seeds in late June or early July. Sow the seeds right away, or store them in damp peat moss and keep them in the fridge until you're ready to plant them in a shady outdoor seedbed. Throughout the growing season, the area should be enriched with plenty of humus or compost and maintained evenly moist. It will take two years for seeds to germinate. When the plant is dormant, either in the fall or late winter, rhizome cuttings or division can be used to reproduce it (prior to new growth). Plants should be spaced about ten inches (25 cm) apart and covered with at least two inches (5 cm) of dirt.

Trillium wildflowers require minimal upkeep or attention once established in the garden. You merely need to maintain the soil evenly moist but not soggy, as long as they've been planted in a good spot. In dry weather, they may also demand water. Fertilizer isn't required as long as the soil contains lots of organic matter or compost. However, if desired, you can renew this every year. The outward-facing bloom of the large-flowered Trillium sits on a short pedicel and lasts a long time. It is the showiest flower of our trilliums, with milky white petals and an eye of yellow stamens in midspring; flowers turn rosy pink as they age. Some plants produce flowers with stacked or fully double petals; double-flowering trilliums are highly prized by shade gardeners, but such flowers are sterile, producing no pollen or fruits. Plants reach 12–15 inches tall and are readily cultivated in woodland, shade, or wildflower gardens throughout the Midwest. All trilliums may be propagated by dividing their rhizomes; this is best done as the plant is going dormant in late summer or fall. Prairie trillium grows about 12 inches tall and can be used for naturalizing in woodland gardens. The petals curve upward like a bud; the sepals fall downward. The leaves are beautifully mottled green with burgundy splotches. Despite its common name, prairie trillium does not grow on prairies. It is probably the easiest of our trilliums to grow in a garden and quickly multiplies into a clump of many flowering stems. Propagate by dividing its thick rhizome; this is best done as the plant goes dormant in late summer or fall.

Consumption Methods: Tea and tincture.

Warnings: When consumed in large dosages, trillium can accelerate menstruation or labor, as well as produce nausea and vomiting. External application of this herb may cause inflammation. Trillium is not recommended for use by pregnant women.

Valerian

Garden Heliotrope, Setwall, All-Heal.

Valeriana officinalis.

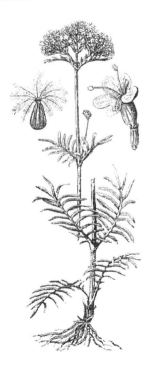

Medical uses: Valerian is an aromatic plant of woodland with sedative effects. Stress-reducing, tension-relieving mild sedative for insomniacs. The roots were decocted in water to treat pain, colds, and diarrhea. A poultice of the root was used to treat cuts, wounds, bruises, and inflammation.

Solvents: Boiling water, alcohol.

Hardiness Zones: Zones 3-9.

Sourcing: Valerian is easy to find across the plains of the United States, as the plant prefers to grow and flower in damp, semi-sunny plains, making them a common plant to find fields, around ditches, and anywhere wildflowers bloom.

Gardening Tips: The plants reach a height of 3 to 5 feet (1-1.5 meters) and produce white, lightly perfumed blooms. Also called garden heliotrope, valerian's a lovely tall flower in the garden, the pinkish white flowers catch your eye, wafting a honeysuckle-like aroma throughout the garden. The robust divided leaves and thick stems resemble lovage. Valerian's mass of small white roots reek of skunk, perfume-y dirt, and stinky feet, which gets worse as they dry, sit out, or are exposed to heat. This plant self-seeds rampantly and tolerates many soil types but really takes over in moist, manure-rich soil. More than once, organic farmers have called me over to dig up ill-behaved plants. When I filled my trunk, they said, "That's all your taking?" In my dry, sandy gardens, it's far better behaved. Be sure your region permits planting valerian.In the fall, harvest the roots by watering the plant and then digging it up. Wash the roots and dry them in the oven at 200 degrees F (93 degrees C) with the door slightly ajar. It may take two growing seasons for the roots to reach harvestable size.

You'll need to water your Valerian herb plant frequently and cover it with mulch to help it retain moisture. A Valerian herb plant will also quickly self-seed. Remove the blossoms before they have a chance to grow and drop seeds if you don't want your plants to spread. It's simple to grow Valerian herbs. The seeds can be planted immediately in the ground when all danger of frost has gone, or they can be started indoors and transplanted outside after several weeks.

In the winter, the roots of a Valerian herb plant will die down to the ground, but the roots should be OK and will sprout new growth in the spring. It thrives in a wide range of situations, including full sun to moderate shade and any well-draining soil, but prefers to be kept moist.

Consumption Methods: Valerian promotes muscle relaxation, which makes it useful for muscle pain including tension headaches and back pain (it will probably make you sleepy). Valerian mildly reduces hypertension by relaxing and dilating the blood vessel lining. Check the second and third volume for more.

Warnings: The use of Valerian comes with the traditional side effect of any herb that helps with the realm of sleep; drowsiness, clouded thinking, daytime fatigue, dry mouth, and headache. Remember, this is a sedative herb. Don't drive or operate heavy machinery after taking it. Many medications (antianxiety, sleep, antidepressant, pain) may synergistically increase sedation alongside herbal sedatives including valerian. Slowly introduce the herb, gradually increasing the dose to make sure it agrees with you and doesn't oversedate. Not everyone feels good with valerian.

Virginia Snakeroot

Birthwort, Dutchmanspipe, Pelican Flower, Sangrel, Sangrel-Root, Serpentaria, Serpentary Root, Snakeroot, Snakeweed, Thick Birthwort.

Aristolochia serpentaria.

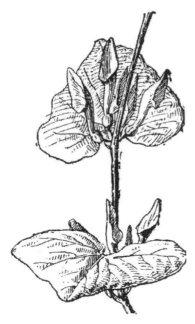

Identification: Virginia snakeroot, a resilient perennial plant, thrives in the wooded hills of Pennsylvania, Virginia, Ohio, Indiana, Kentucky, and southwestern states like Louisiana and Texas. This plant boasts a fibrous root system, exhibiting a rich brown hue, adorned with numerous stem scars. From these roots, a dense tress of branching roots, approximately 3 inches in length, emerges, emanating a distinct gingery aroma that sets it apart. The root possesses a bitter taste. Rising from the base, one or more erect stems with a zigzag pattern reach heights of 1 to 2 feet, displaying a purplish color near the plant's base. The oblong leaves, measuring around 3 inches in length and 1 inch in width, contribute to the plant's elegant appearance. During the months of June and July, the plant adorns itself with a modest number of purple or dull-brown flowers, supported by short stems that sprout from the root, adding a touch of delicate beauty to its surroundings.

Medical uses: Virginia snakeroot has been esteemed by various Native American tribes for its medicinal properties, particularly in treating snake bites, fevers, colds, and as a general painkiller. Different tribes, including the Cherokee, Choctaw, and Shawnee, recognized its efficacy and incorporated it into their traditional healing practices. The root's remarkable ability to swiftly alleviate symptoms garnered its reputation as a potent remedy for snake bites, hence its name. Acting as a potent stimulant, Virginia snakeroot redirects the flow of blood outward, making it valuable in the early stages of eruptive diseases, before the appearance of external manifestations. By inducing perspiration and invigorating the vital forces, it aids in purging the system of any harmful substances. Additionally, as a nerve stimulant, it acts rapidly, finding use in cases of nervous system depression or exhaustion, particularly in the later stages of illnesses such as smallpox, scarlet fever, and pneumonia.

Stimulant, Diaphoretic, Anodyne, Antispasmodic, Tonic, Nervine

Solvents: Boiling water, alcohol.

Hardiness Zones: Zones 8-10.

Sourcing: Virginia snakeroot is typically found in hilly woodland areas across several regions in the United States. Its natural habitat spans from Pennsylvania, Virginia, Ohio, Indiana, and Kentucky, to the southwestern states of Louisiana and Texas. This perennial plant thrives in the rich soils and shaded environments of these regions. When sourcing Virginia snakeroot, it is important to seek out reputable suppliers who specialize in medicinal herbs and botanicals. They may either cultivate the plant in controlled environments or ethically wild-harvest it from its native habitats. It is recommended to consult with local herbalists, native plant nurseries, or medicinal plant organizations for guidance on sourcing Virginia snakeroot responsibly and ethically.

Gardening Tips: Allow 1 quart of peat moss to soak up the extra water and drain. Place the peat moss in a plastic bag for storage. Place the seeds in the peat moss, seal the bag, and store it in the refrigerator's bottom shelf. Mark this date in your calendar 85 days in advance. After three months of cold stratification, the seeds germinate optimally.

Take the Virginia Snakeroot seeds out of the fridge. Examine the seeds for germination. Place the seeds back in the refrigerator for another five days if there are no signs of sprouting. If any seeds germinate, transfer the bag to your potting area and separate the sprouting seeds into separate containers. If germinated seeds are kept in the bag for the full 90 days, they may decay.

Fill a growing container halfway with good potting soil and water thoroughly. Allow for drainage of the soil. Spread the seeds that haven't grown on the soil's surface and press them down. Seeds require sunshine to germinate, so don't cover them.

Place the growing tray in direct sunlight or in a sunny, draft-free spot. Using a fine mist, keep the soil moist until the seeds germinate. Move the seedlings to individual grow pots filled with wet potting soil using a pair of garden tweezers.

Place the seedlings in a bright but not direct-sun area. Keep the soil moist but not soggy; else, your seedlings will perish. Allow the seedlings to grow for the first year in a covered environment.

Consumption Methods: Tincture, teas, and cold infusions to treat pain of various nature.

Wild Ginger

Wild Ginger, American Ginger.

Asarum canadense.

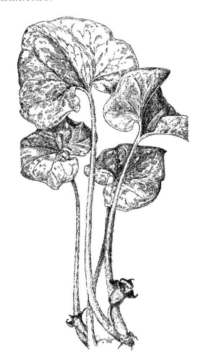

Traditional Uses: Wild ginger has a long history of medicinal use among Native American tribes throughout the United States. The rhizome of wild ginger was highly valued for its various therapeutic properties. It was commonly used to stimulate menstruation and regulate irregular heartbeat. Additionally, the root of wild ginger was employed as a treatment for colds, coughs, and sore throats, thanks to its antiseptic and tonic properties. Native Americans also utilized wild ginger in traditional medicine to address a range of ailments, including scarlet fever, nervousness, vomiting, headaches, and earaches. It was even considered a heal-all, showcasing its versatile nature. For earache relief, the Meskwaki tribe would soak crushed rhizomes in water and administer the liquid into the affected ear. The early European settlers adopted some of these practices, incorporating powdered wild ginger rhizome into tooth powder alongside other botanical ingredients like black alder, bayberry, and black oak bark. Moreover, the use of candied rhizome and syrup to alleviate flatulence and stomach pains likely stemmed from similar uses of gingerroot in their home countries. Another interesting belief tied to wild ginger was the "doctrine of signs," which associated the herb's kidney-shaped leaves with its potential to heal kidney ailments. Additionally, wild ginger was utilized to treat snakebites and induce sweating to alleviate fevers.

Solvents: Water, boiling water, alcohol.

Hardiness Zones: Zones 9-12 (Can grow in others, with conditions met.)

Sourcing: Wild Ginger can be found all over the eastern United States. It thrives in dark deciduous woodlands with rich mesic soils. If you're looking to source ginger, look to your local woodlands.

Gardening Tips: Wild ginger is a unique and attractive groundcover that thrives in shady landscapes and moist woodland gardens. It can be transplanted to a shady area of your garden and serves as a hardy plant that continuously produces roots for culinary use. Growing up to 6-9 inches tall, wild ginger spreads through rhizomes that run along or near the soil surface. In spring, jug-shaped flowers emerge, nestled between two glossy heart-shaped leaves. The outermost whorl of the flower reveals a vibrant madder red color. When selecting wild ginger rhizomes, opt for large and healthy ones measuring 4 to 6 inches long with multiple emerging "fingers."

Choose a planting location in full to partial shade with rich, loamy, and well-draining soil. Wild ginger is a natural understory plant that flourishes in hot, humid environments with dappled sunlight. It can be grown in pots or directly in the ground. If your soil lacks nutrients, amend it with compost or aged manure. Spring is the ideal time for planting, but it can be done at any time in warmer climates.

To plant wild ginger:

1. Separate the fingers from the rhizomes and cut each rhizome portion into 1 to 2-inch pieces, ensuring each piece has at least one bud.

2. Allow the rhizome pieces to dry for 24-48 hours before planting to prevent root rot.

3. Plant the rhizome pieces at least 12 inches apart and no deeper than 1 inch. For commercial cultivation, double rows with a working passage between rows are common.

4. Water the newly planted rhizomes thoroughly.

5. Within approximately a week, you will begin to see the emergence of leaves.

6. Once growth is established, water the wild ginger sparingly but deeply.

As the plant grows, the wild ginger will reach a height of four feet, with many of the roots visible above ground. This is a normal characteristic of the plant. Enjoy your thriving wild ginger groundcover and the delightful culinary and ornamental benefits it brings to your garden.

Consumption Methods: Ginger falls into being an "everything" herb. Products and methods to craft home remedies exist in every form. The most common intake method is through eating ginger as a juice, tea, or part of a prepared meal as a spice. Ginger excels in the kitchen, for sure.

Warnings: Aristolochic acid is a component found in wild ginger. Some health authorities have called out aristolochic acid as a naturally occurring toxin that can cause cancer, human cell mutations, and end-stage kidney failure, according to Health Canada.

Wild Strawberry

Woodland Strawberry, Alpine Strawberry, Carpathian Strawberry, European Strawberry

Fragaria vesca.

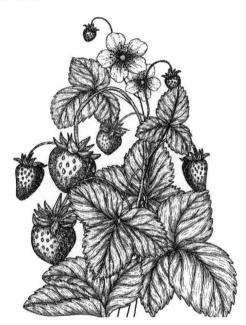

Medical uses: Wild strawberries, cherished by numerous Native American tribes across different regions, have long been valued for their remarkable medicinal properties. The leaves and berries of wild strawberries possess a rich array of beneficial attributes, including astringent, diuretic, laxative, and tonic properties. Native American tribes such as the Cherokee, Iroquois, Ojibwa, and Lakota have utilized these plant parts for various healing purposes.

The leaves of wild strawberries are particularly versatile and widely employed in traditional medicine. They are often brewed into a tea, known for its blood-toning properties and its effectiveness in alleviating diarrhea in both adults and children. The Cherokee and Ojibwa tribes, in particular, have extensively used the leaves to address digestive ailments. Additionally, the leaves are known to possess cooling properties, and a slice of strawberry can be applied externally to soothe sunburned skin, providing relief and promoting healing. Tribes like the Lakota have made use of this natural remedy to alleviate the discomfort of sunburn.

The powdered leaves of wild strawberries, when mixed with oil, form a poultice that has been employed by tribes such as the Iroquois and Cherokee to treat open lesions and wounds effectively. This application helps cleanse the affected area and promote healing. The astringent properties of the leaves contribute to the tightening of tissues, aiding in the healing process. The Iroquois have been known to use the poultice for the treatment of wounds and sores.

The fruits of wild strawberries, containing salicylic acid, offer additional medicinal benefits. This compound is recognized for its anti-inflammatory properties and has been utilized by tribes such as the Ojibwa and Lakota to address liver and kidney problems, as well as to alleviate symptoms of rheumatism and gout. These tribes have incorporated wild strawberries into their traditional remedies for these specific ailments, harnessing the natural healing power of the berries.

Furthermore, the roots of wild strawberries possess diuretic and astringent properties. Tribes like the Iroquois and Ojibwa have used decoctions of the roots as internal remedies to address conditions such as diarrhea and chronic dysentery. Externally, the roots have been employed as a throat gargle to alleviate sore throats. The Iroquois have also recognized the root's efficacy in the treatment of chilblains, a condition characterized by inflammation and itching of the extremities.

Solvents: Boiling water, alcohol.

Hardiness Zones: Zone 3-8.

Sourcing: Rich, loamy soil in temperate areas is where you'll most likely come across a wild strawberry bush. However, select garden centers will sell you wild varieties during the prime growing season. Gardeners who want to raise wild strawberries must propagate the plants themselves because they are rarely seen in commercial nurseries.

Gardening Tips: Wild strawberry occurs in all but the hottest and driest parts of North America, and in cultivation, it thrives in almost any well-drained soil. The spring flowers are shockingly white with a yellow center. Fruits are small and red, as ornamental as they are delicious. The three-parted leaves often turn rich red shades in autumn and persist through winter, hugging the ground. This groundcovering species is as aggressive as vinca or English ivy, quickly filling any space. It makes a tremendous stand-alone groundcover in full sun or even dry shade. It is perfect for a natural landscape, where it may run between existing plants, and it should be plugged into established prairie gardens. Wild strawberries are integral plants for edible landscapes and food forests; they have a more intense flavor than the cultivated strawberries hybridized from them. Note: fruit is produced only on female plants. Wild Strawberry plants will thrive in a gently shaded, fast-draining bed once they have been propagated. To produce a large crop of berries, the bushes must be properly spaced and mulched.

Late spring or early summer is the best time to start fresh wild strawberry plants. Look for a rooted plantlet around the base of an established wild strawberry plant, which is generated when a stem meets the ground and takes root.

Remove the stem that connects the wild strawberry to the rooted plantlet and cut it off. Use a pair of shears that are both sharp and clean. Around the base of the plantlet, draw a 3-inch circle. Using a portable spade, dig down to a 5-inch depth along the 3-inch mark.

Remove the rooted plantlet from the soil and fill in the hole it has created. Fill a 4-inch pot halfway with garden soil and halfway with acidic compost with the plantlet. Place the wild strawberry in a gently shaded spot after fully watering it.

For three to four weeks, grow the wild strawberry in a gently shaded area to encourage it to create a larger, more productive root system. During the summer, move the plants to an area of the garden that gets four to six hours of sun per day. Every week, add 1 inch of water.

In coastal areas, prepare a planting site in the fall, and in inland areas, prepare a planting site in the spring. If possible, use a raised bed or weed a planting area with 12 to 14 square inches of room for each plant. Avoid places with poor drainage or rocky, inorganic soil.

In the top 10 inches of soil, apply a 5-inch layer of gently acidic organic compost. In a raised bed, space the wild strawberries 8 to 14 inches apart, or 12 inches apart in the ground. Make the planting holes 1 inch deeper than the pots, so the plant's base is slightly higher than the soil level.

After planting, water each wild strawberry to a depth of 4 inches. To keep the soil moist, apply a 2-inch layer of mulch around each plant. Between the mulch and the base of the wild strawberry plants, leave a 1-inch gap.

Throughout the growing season, give your plants 1 inch of water per week. Watering should be avoided during wet or cool weather to avoid decay. During extended periods of drought or heat, increase watering to twice weekly.

Consumption Methods: Most will eat the berries raw; however, the raw, dried leaves of strawberries are good for making strawberry tea. It's an incredibly helpful adjuvant in a nutritional therapy for arthritis

Witch Hazel

American Witch Hazel.

Hamamelis virginiana.

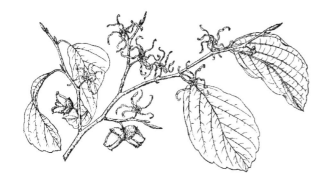

Medical Uses: Witch hazel, a plant revered for its medicinal qualities, has a rich history of traditional use among various Native American tribes and continues to be valued in modern times. Tribes such as the Iroquois, Mohegan, and Cherokee recognized its therapeutic properties and employed it for various purposes. Traditionally, witch hazel was used by the Iroquois to treat swelling and inflammation, while the Mohegan used it to ease sore muscles and joints. The Cherokee utilized witch hazel as an astringent for skin ailments and to alleviate discomfort associated with bruises and sprains.

In recent years, scientific studies have shed light on the numerous health benefits of witch hazel. Research has shown that witch hazel extract possesses anti-inflammatory, antimicrobial, and antioxidant properties.

It has been found to be effective in treating skin conditions such as acne, eczema, and psoriasis, providing relief from itching and inflammation. Furthermore, witch hazel has been studied for its potential to alleviate symptoms of hemorrhoids and varicose veins due to its vasoconstrictive properties.

In addition to its topical applications, witch hazel has also been investigated for its potential use in oral health. Studies have shown that witch hazel mouthwash exhibits antibacterial properties and can help reduce gum inflammation and bleeding. It has also been explored for its potential as a natural remedy for coughs and colds, as well as a treatment for hemorrhoids.

The traditional knowledge of Native American tribes regarding witch hazel has stood the test of time, and current scientific research continues to validate its therapeutic properties. Today, witch hazel is widely available in various forms, including creams, ointments, toners, and extracts, making it a versatile and popular choice in natural medicine.

Check the second volume for more information.

Solvents: Water, alcohol.

Hardiness Zones: Zones 5-7.

Sourcing: Witch Hazel can be found across the United States, generally in well-drained soil near water sources, particularly in craggy areas where shadows can be found during the height of the day.

Gardening Tips: Witch Hazel is a huge deciduous shrub with beautiful, fragrant blossoms in the winter that requires little care and is resistant to most pests and illnesses. Witch Hazels thrive in full sun (or filtered shade in hotter climates), where the blossoms blaze like flaming embers in the low winter sun's backlight. They prefer well-aerated soil and consistent water and are acid or alkaline tolerant.

While most types reach a mature height and width of 10-20 feet, witch hazels can be pruned to keep them smaller once they've stopped blooming. Prune before the summer so that the buds for the following year can grow. Suckering twigs should be trimmed from around the base. Branches can be trimmed and forced to bloom once fresh flower buds form.

Consumption Methods: Witch Hazel falls into the category of a "panacea" herb. For topical use only. A distilled extract of the leafy twigs can be preserved with 14-15% alcohol. The distillate can be used on acne and eczema direct or diluted 1:3 with water. Otherwise 5-10g of dried leaf or bark can be decocted in 250ml water for poultices and wound irrigation. Used also to reduce inflammation in sprains.

Warnings: Because some people may be allergic to witch hazel, it's advised to test it first on a small area of skin and keep an eye on it for 24 hours. It should be okay to apply to a greater region if there is no redness, itching, or irritation.

White Sage

Garden Sage, Meadow Sage, True Sage, Kitchen Sage, Dalmatian Sage.

Salvia apiana.

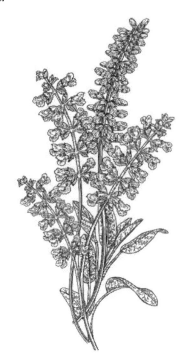

Traditional Uses: White sage holds significant cultural and traditional value among Native American tribes, including the Luiseno, Cahuilla, and Kumeyaay. The Luiseno people used white sage leaves to construct ceremonial hunting fires, believed to bring good luck to their hunts. Additionally, they consumed the young tops of white sage stalks, which were peeled and eaten raw. The Cahuilla tribe harvested white sage seeds and combined them with wheat flour and sugar to make gruel and biscuits, providing a nourishing food staple. For medicinal purposes, white sage was used by the Cahuilla and Kumeyaay tribes to treat fevers. The leaves were either eaten or smoked in sweat-houses, and a cough infusion was prepared from the leaves. The smoke from burning white sage was also utilized to fumigate houses contaminated by measles. The Cahuilla tribe employed crushed sage leaves mixed with water as a wash and conditioner for hygiene purposes. They would also apply the crushed leaf mixture under their armpits to mask odors. Interestingly, the Cahuilla believed that placing white sage on their hunting weapons could reverse any bad luck caused by a woman touching the equipment.

Anti-fungal, antibiotic, anti-inflammatory, calming, cleansing.

Solvents: Boiling water, alcohol.

Hardiness Zones: Zones 8-11.

Sourcing: White Sage plants grow wild in the southwestern United States, close to Mexico.

Gardening Tips: White Sage (Salvia Apiana) is a remarkable plant that can be successfully grown in your garden with proper care and attention. In its native area of California, it is best to sow White Sage seeds outdoors

in the autumn, before the winter rains arrive. If you are within its range and plan to transplant, fall is an ideal time for planting. Fall offers cooler temperatures, creating favorable conditions for establishment. In its endemic zone, the rainy season from January to April provides the best growth environment. However, if you are transplanting White Sage outside of its natural habitat, it is recommended to do so in the spring when temperatures start to warm up.

When cultivating White Sage, it is important to be mindful of its extensive spreading root system. Take caution when filling the landscape with other plants, as digging near the White Sage can disturb its roots.

White Sage is known for its tolerance to dry conditions and can withstand temperatures as low as 10 degrees Fahrenheit (Zone 8). It prefers well-draining, mineral-rich soil with good aeration, such as gritty or loamy soils composed of materials like granite, sandstone, and shale. The plant naturally thrives on dry, clay slopes where the angle aids in drainage.

To ensure the health of your White Sage, provide it with full sun exposure, receiving at least six hours of direct sunlight per day. Regular watering is necessary during the establishment phase, especially if there is limited rainfall. Be mindful of the drying rate of the root ball compared to the surrounding soil, as it may require adjustments in watering frequency.

It is crucial to avoid overwatering White Sage, as excessive moisture can lead to failure, especially outside its native region. During the dormant summer period, White Sage can tolerate minimal precipitation. If you are growing it in an area with frequent summer rains, be prepared for potential challenges.

Fertilization needs for White Sage can vary depending on the soil conditions. If the soil is already rich in minerals and organic matter, the fertilizer applied during mail-order delivery may be sufficient. However, for container plantings, it is recommended to use a balanced fertilizer every two months.

White Sage can be successfully grown in containers, but it is important to choose an appropriately sized pot to prevent overwatering. When repotting, carefully inspect the roots for signs of overcrowding, and transplant into a slightly larger container using a sterilized "soilless" potting mix. This mix should be free from diseases, weed seeds, and toxins, while still containing organic materials. It is important to avoid high sand or vermiculite content, as sand lacks proper aeration and vermiculite can retain excessive moisture.

As a sun-loving plant, White Sage is not suitable for indoor cultivation. It requires full, direct sunlight and adequate air circulation to thrive.

White Sage is characterized by its vertical growth habit and dense basal rosettes of stiff, slightly succulent white-green leaves. Its ability to fold down its leaves during periods of drought helps it withstand prolonged dry conditions. This slow-growing plant can take two to three years to reach its maximum size of 36 inches in both height and breadth. During spring to summer, it can produce flower spikes that can reach a height of 60 inches.

Consumption Methods: Topical applications from poultices, teas, and infusions

Warnings: The chemical thujone is found in some sage plants, including common sage (Salvia officinalis). If you consume too much thujone, it can be fatal. This substance has the potential to cause seizures and harm the liver and neurological system. The amount of thujone in sage varies depending on the species, harvest time, growth circumstances, and other factors.

Wormwood

Green Ginger, Grand Wormwood, American Wormwood,
Western Wormwood, Madder Wort, Wormwood Sage, Sweet Annie.

Artemisia absinthium.

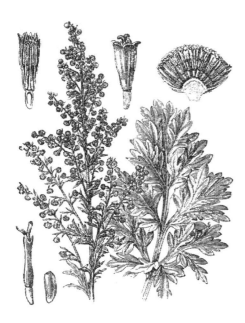

Medical Uses: Wormwood, known for its distinct aromatic properties, has a rich history of traditional and modern uses. Native American tribes such as the Ojibwe, Lakota, and Cheyenne have utilized wormwood for various medicinal purposes. Traditionally, it was employed as a natural remedy for digestive issues, such as indigestion and bloating. The Cheyenne tribe used wormwood to treat fevers and infections, while the Lakota tribe used it as a diuretic and to alleviate menstrual discomfort. In modern times, research has focused on wormwood's potential antimicrobial and anti-inflammatory properties. Studies have shown that wormwood extracts may exhibit antibacterial effects against certain strains of bacteria, including those resistant to conventional antibiotics. Additionally, wormwood has been investigated for its potential use in the treatment of cancer, with some studies suggesting its ability to inhibit the growth of cancer cells. Furthermore, wormwood is a key ingredient in the production of the alcoholic beverage absinthe.

Check out the second volume for other modern and traditional uses.

Solvents: Boiling water, alcohol.

Hardiness Zones: Zones 4-8.

Sourcing: Wormwood plants can be easily bought through online plant wholesalers, or cuttings can be sourced from wildly growing plants that are common in areas east of the cascade mountains in areas that are dry and low-lying, such as pastures.

Gardening Tips: To successfully grow wormwood or sweet Annie, choose a sunny location with well-drained soil as these plants do not tolerate excessive moisture. Spring is the ideal time for planting wormwood, whether you're starting from seeds or transplants. If starting from seeds, sow them in flats and transplant the seedlings into the garden after the last spring frost. Once established, wormwood plants are relatively low-maintenance. They can benefit from annual fertilization and regular watering, but be cautious not to overwater as this can lead to root rot. Light trimming, especially for spreading varieties, can help maintain their growth and prevent them from becoming unruly. Wormwood plants are typically resistant to diseases, except for root rot in excessively damp soil. Their aromatic foliage naturally deters many garden pests.

Sweet Annie, a variety of wormwood, is particularly valued for its feathery and sweet-smelling foliage, as well as its yellow blossoms, which are often used in floral arrangements and wreaths. Although classified as an annual, sweet Annie reseeds easily and can become invasive in some cases. Its fern-like foliage emerges in spring and flowers in late summer. Allow sufficient space in the garden as sweet Annie can reach a height of about 2 feet (61 cm).

To harvest sweet Annie for floral arrangements or wreaths, wait until the blooms develop in late summer. Cut branches and gather them in small bundles, then hang them upside down in a dark, well-ventilated room for two to three weeks until completely dry. To collect seeds, cut the foliage to the ground, leaving some plants for self-seeding. Place the seeds in a paper bag and allow them to dry before gently shaking them loose. Sweet Annie, like other types of wormwood, is easy to grow and can thrive in containers as well as various garden settings. Their fragrant and attractive foliage provides year-round enjoyment while also deterring common garden pests. Once established, sweet Annie plants require minimal maintenance, making them a valuable addition to any garden..

Consumption Methods: The tincture is anthelmintic, antiseptic, antispasmodic, carminative, cholagogue, emmenagogue and stimulant. The bitter taste of the leaves is used to stimulate digestion and to ease wind and bloating.

Warnings: The United States Food and Drug Administration (FDA) considers Wormwood to be dangerous for internal consumption because it contains the poisonous compound thujone. The FDA specifies that all Wormwood products sold in the United States be free of thujone; thus, it's generally safe in food and beVerages (including bitters and vermouth). It is better to use only premade and FDA-approved products if you are unsure of the thujone status before using a product.

Yerba Mansa

Anemia California, Anemopsis californica, Anemopsis de Californie, Lizard's Tail,
Queue de Lézard, Swamp Root, Yerba Manza.

Anemopsis californica.

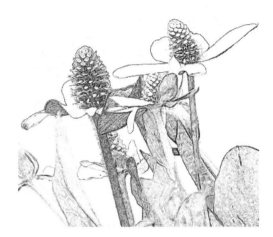

Medical Uses: Yerba Mansa was used by native Americans in southern California for a variety of purposes. The plant was most famously used as a disinfectant. The herb acted as an antibacterial, antifungal, and antimicrobial in general. To keep infected cuts clean, a powder of dried root was sprinkled on them. Yerba Mansa was used by the Cahuilla people of the Mojave Desert to disinfect cuts from knife wounds.

The plant was also used by the Cahuilla to encourage the formation of new skin after a wound. Check out the second volume for more.

Medicinal Part: Leaves

Solvents: Boiling water, alcohol.

Hardiness Zones: Zones 7-10.

Sourcing: This plant grows in marshes and rivers and prefers moist soil and full sun. Yerba Mansa can be found throughout the southern United States and several of its neighboring states. It can be found in Arizona, California, Colorado, Kansas, Nebraska, New Mexico, Oklahoma, Oregon, Texas, and Utah, to name a few. Parts of northeastern Mexico are also home to this species.

Gardening Tips: In containers or in the ground, Yerba Mansa is very easy to grow. It prefers full sun to half shade, making it suitable for a variety of gardens. It doesn't care about the pH of the soil (it prefers a range of 5.0 to 9.0) or the type of soil. It prefers damp soils and will require regular summer watering to stay green. To simulate natural circumstances, we let our wetland plants gradually dry out beginning in September (simply water less regularly).

Yerba Mansa thrives in areas of the garden that are regularly watered. They're commonly used as a ground cover around (and even in) shallow ponds, around fountains, rain gardens, and other naturally damp areas by gardeners. They are well-suited to container gardening and make excellent specimen plants in bog gardens and pots. Some gardeners use them as groundcovers around trees that need to be watered on a regular basis. They're also employed in reclamation operations to improve soils (plants remove salts and decrease soil pH).

In the summer, keep the soil moist; in the fall, reduce the amount of water; in the late fall or early winter, cut back (or even mow) dead plants.

Pruning should be done when the plants have died back; it will not harm the plants. You have the option of using the dead leaves as mulch or not (they decrease the soil pH and add organic material).

Consumption Methods: A decoction goes a long way to treat inflammation of the mucous membranes, swollen gums and sore throat. Acts as a diuretic. It's a welcomed addition to any anti-spasmodic and lung-soothing tea.

Yerba Santa

Yerba Santa, Mountain Balm, Bear's Weed, Gum Bush, Gum Plant, Consumptive Weed.

Eriodictyon Californicum.

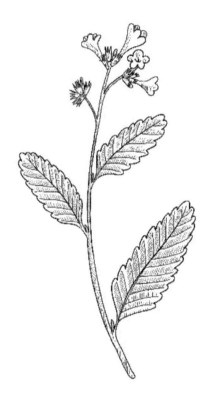

Medical Uses: The Chumash Indians and other California Native Americans have used Yerba Santa to heal lung ailments, boost saliva production, and halt bleeding from minor cuts and scrapes. From the late 1800s through the 1960s, Yerba Santa was formally used in the United States and the United Kingdom for illnesses such as influenza, bacterial pneumonia, asthma, bronchitis, and tuberculosis.

Demulcent, Expectorant, Stimulant

Medicinal Part: Leaves

Solvents: Boiling water, alcohol.

Hardiness Zones: Zones 8-11.

Sourcing: Yerba Santa is a plant that is native to western and southwestern North America, as well as northern Mexico. Obviously, the plant prefers sandy loam and arid climates, faring better in hot, dry locales with plenty of bright sun.

Gardening Tips: Once grown, the Yerba Santa plant is sturdily and consistently productive until the weather cools.

Yerba Santa plant is a perennial herb that dies back in the cold in USDA Zones 8 and 9. When the weather heats up again, it regrows.

It can be grown in pots and brought inside to overwinter. That way, you'll have leaves all year.

Give this plant some afternoon shade and partial sun. Feel free to experiment with the plants, since they may even flourish in full shadow.

Too much heat and not enough moisture might cause the leaves to wilt, but a good watering or shower will bring them back to life.

A soil pH of 5.6 to 6.5 is ideal. The optimum soil is sand or light clay, which drains well but retains moisture. Although the Yerba Santa plant likes water, it does not want its roots to sit in puddles.

The flavor is strongest in the young, sensitive leaves and shoots, but the huge leaves will add enough flavor if used to wrap food when cooking.

Yerba Santa plant seeds are available online or at local specialty stores. Seeds can be planted directly in the garden or in seed-raising pots indoors. Before planting, wait until the spring frost has passed.

Eight weeks before transplanting outside, start seeds indoors.

Lightly sprinkle the seeds on the surface and lightly push them in. Yerba Santa plant seeds require light to germinate, so don't cover them.

Keep the soil moist, and don't let it dry out. Start with a mist sprayer and then gentle watering after you see seedlings emerge.

When the Yerba Santa plant reaches about 12 inches in height, thin it out.

A Yerba Santa plant in a container is a good option, especially if you live in a cooler climate. You'll be able to transfer it when the weather becomes chilly.

Use a 10-gallon container since I don't want to repot my Yerba Santa plant too much. If you wish to keep the plant tiny and repot more frequently, you can grow it in a smaller container.

If the plant has become rootbound, repot every two years. Before replanting in a slightly larger container with fresh potting soil, remove the plant and cut away any dead or damaged roots.

When the weather cools, bring the pot inside, and you'll be well on your way to winter. The Yerba Santa plant survives the winter well indoors.

Another advantage of growing Yerba Santa plants in containers is that they spread quickly in the garden. It will take over an area if you do not keep up with eradicating undesirable spread.

Yerba Santa plants will thrive and have few problems if you follow a few easy guidelines.

Fertilize your plants once every six to eight weeks. Look for an organic fertilizer made exclusively for tropical plants and follow the directions carefully.

Using a tropical fertilizer will keep the foliage green and luscious all year long.

Water is very important to Yerba Santa plants. You don't want the soil or container mix to dry up between waterings, so don't overwater. As much as possible, keep the soil moist.

When my Yerba Santa plant becomes scraggly and leggy, I prune it. It alternates between being perfect and being a shambles.

In zones 8 and 9, hard trim the plant in the winter to encourage spring and summer growth. This helps to control the size and spread of your garden while also keeping it neat.

Prune and tidy up the plant as needed in warm places where it does not die back in the winter. Depending on the weather, it may drop some leaves or remain evergreen all year.

Consumption Methods: Yerba Santa is commonly used as an expectorant to alleviate respiratory issues such as coughs, colds, and bronchitis. Yerba Santa is also known for its anti-inflammatory properties and is used to relieve sore throats, asthma, and allergies

Yerba Santa can be prepared as a tea by steeping 1-2 teaspoons of dried leaves in a cup of hot water for 10-15 minutes. The tea can be consumed up to three times a day. A popular preparation involves making a Yerba Santa syrup. To make the syrup, combine 1 cup of dried Yerba Santa leaves, 1 cup of honey or maple syrup, and 2 cups of water in a saucepan. Simmer the mixture over low heat for about 30 minutes until it thickens. Strain the syrup and store it in a glass jar. This syrup can be taken by the spoonful to soothe coughs and respiratory discomfort.

Warnings: Taking Yerba Santa may increase urination and cause decongestion, meaning nasal drip.

Yucca

Adam's Needle, Common Yucca, Spanish Bayonet, Bear-Grass,
Needle-Palm, Silk-Grass, Spoon-Leaf Yucca.

Yucca filamentosa.

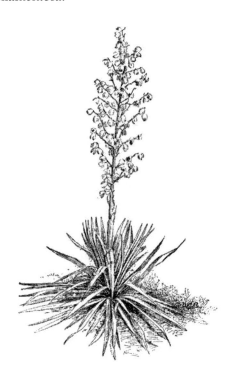

Medical Uses: Yucca, with its versatile properties, has been traditionally used by Native American cultures for various purposes. One significant use among several tribes, including the Western Apaches, is for personal hygiene. The roots of Yucca baccata are pounded to extract beneficial compounds used in shampoo and soap, contributing to their hair and skin care routines. Additionally, the Apaches utilize the fibers from Yucca leaves to create dental floss and ropes, showcasing the plant's practical versatility. Another interesting application of Yucca by the Western Apaches involves the preparation of a gravy by combining pulverized Juniper berries with Yucca fruit. They also ferment crushed Juniper berries with soaked Yucca fruit to produce a unique drink. Yucca soap, known for its cleansing properties, was used by various Native American tribes to address issues like dandruff and hair loss. Furthermore, Yucca plays a vital role in non-medical practices, serving as a material for crafting sandals, belts, textiles, baskets, ropes, and mats, which are still carried out by contemporary tribes like the Hopi, Papago, and Ute Indians. The Zuni people have their own unique tradition of using a mixture of Yucca sap soap and pulverized aster to bathe newborns, believed to promote hair growth. Additionally, the Navajos utilize bundles of Yucca fibers tied together as brushes for cleaning metates, demonstrating the plant's practical applications beyond medicinal uses.

Check out other traditional and modern uses in the second volume.

Solvents: Boiling water, alcohol.

Hardiness Zones: Zones 5-11.

Sourcing: Any reputable retailer or online storefront. Easy to find. Wild Yucca can be found in dry habitats and, making them prevalent in the southwest United States.

Gardening Tips:

Yuccas are stunning plants with a wide range of sizes and characteristics. Smaller varieties can grow to be 2 to 4 feet tall and wide, while larger ones can reach towering heights of 30 feet and span 25 feet wide, forming clumps several times the size of individual plants. Lack of sunlight can lead to spindly leaves and reduced flowering, so it's important to choose a location that receives ample sunshine.

The leaves of Yuccas are typically long, narrow, and sword-shaped, often with sharp spines, arranged in rosettes. Some Yucca species have razor-sharp foliage. Flowers emerge on tall stalks that arise from the plant's core, with some reaching impressive heights of over 10 feet. The flowers are commonly white or cream-colored, sometimes with hints of pink, purple, or green.

It's essential to distinguish Yuccas from yucas (cassava), as they are often confused. Yuccas are unrelated to yucas and do not produce edible tubers/roots like cassava, which are used to make tapioca and cassava flour. The roots of Yucca plants are not suitable for consumption.

Depending on the Yucca type, some varieties bloom in the spring, while others bloom in the mid-to-late summer. Polycarpic perennials, such as Yucca species, bloom every year for the rest of their lives, while monocarpic variants, like Hespero-Yucca whipplei (syn. Yucca whipplei), flower once and then gradually decline and die, similar to their relatives in the Agave family.

Adam's needle yucca can be used in harsh sites and sunny, windswept, rocky landscapes where many evergreens would struggle. Its large flower spike reaches above the spiky basal leaves, forming a spectacular 4- to 6-foot tall candelabrum of white flowers in early summer. It was these glowing flower spikes, along with the fact that Adam's needle yucca was often planted in cemeteries, that inspired the nickname "ghosts in the graveyard." Where its pollinating yucca moths are present, Adam's needle yucca produces seedpods that hold well into winter. It grows in almost any upland soil from clay to sand, has a tenacious root that is nearly impossible to remove, and even survives in light shade, though it doesn't flower in shade.

Soapweed yucca, a Great Plains species, grows in well-drained soils on steep loess, rocky, or gravelly substrates. It is a rugged evergreen for a harsh site where many other evergreens would struggle (but it does make a striking companion to shrubby junipers, if they are already present and thriving); the sunny, windswept, rocky end of my driveway is adorned them. The spiky 2-foot-long narrow foliage grows in a striking tuft and is grayish green all year. In early summer, the plant produces a 2- to 3-foot spike of greenish cream pendent flowers that are followed by up-facing seedpod fruits that ripen blackish and remain into winter. The flowers are pollinated by the yucca moth and nothing else, so plants produce no pods where the moth is absent (unless you hand pollinate the flowers).

For successful cultivation, Yucca seeds can be started indoors at any time of the year or sown outdoors in the spring when temperatures range from 55 to 65°F for hardy varieties and 66 to 75°F for more tender types. Soak the seeds for 24 hours before planting or scarify the surface with sandpaper to aid germination. Plant the seeds at a depth of one to two seed lengths, spacing them one to two seed lengths apart. Germination should occur within 3 to 4 weeks if the seeds are kept moderately moist. After approximately 8 weeks, transplant the seedlings into larger pots or a permanent position. More information about propagation from offsets can be found below. Yucca plants have a slow and inconsistent growth rate, especially when cultivated from seed. It may take a few years for them to reach the flowering stage. Regular maintenance includes clipping dead or damaged leaves, preferably during early spring before the growing season, to manage the plant's size and appearance. Trimming the top section of a trunk can reduce its height, and new offsets will typically develop from the cut site. However, growth patterns may vary at times. Dead or broken leaves near the bottom of stemless rosette varieties can be removed whenever necessary to maintain the plant's tidiness. After flowering, it is recommended to clip the flower stalks back to the base, especially if the appearance of the stem is not desired. Yuccas are not particular about soil type as long as it is well-draining to prevent rot. It is crucial to consider the mature size of Yucca plants when selecting a location, as some varieties can become quite large. Keep them away from pathways and play areas to avoid accidental contact with their sharp, spiky leaves. Over time, Yuccas develop massive root systems that can crack foundations, destroy retaining walls, and invade pools and irrigation pipes. Removing any leftovers can be used to propagate additional Yuccas.

While Yuccas are known for their drought tolerance and ability to thrive on neglect, they benefit from regular watering of about an inch per week during the spring and summer, as well as occasional deep soakings. During the winter, they require less water. Overwatering can lead to yellow foliage and mushy roots, so it's important to strike a balance. Propagation of Yuccas can be done through offsets, root cuttings, or seeds. Remove offsets in the spring, remove any foliage, and plant them. Provide adequate water and protection until the roots establish. Root cuttings can be taken in the winter or spring by cutting a 3-inch portion from the existing root structure, allowing it to dry in a cool, dry place for a few days before planting in potting soil. Place the cutting in a spot that receives indirect light, and roots should start to grow within three to four weeks. While Yuccas are generally hardy plants with few major pest or disease concerns, they can occasionally encounter issues such as cane borers, scale insects, and fungal leaf spots. To prevent brown leaf spots, it's advisable to water at the base of the plant instead of using overhead watering. One common concern with Yuccas is stem rot, which can be avoided by using well-draining soil. Yuccas' spiky and thorny character makes them resistant to deer. Additionally, Yucca blossoms emit a fragrance that attracts Yucca moths, which play a critical role in pollination. The moths rely on Yuccas as their host plants, and in return, they ensure the plant's reproduction. The white-winged Yucca moths blend in with the blossoms they pollinate and lay eggs in, while their caterpillars consume some seeds, leaving behind enough for the plant's regeneration.

Consumption Methods: Yucca plants have been valued for their numerous applications, including medicinal, culinary, and practical uses. In addition to its practical applications, Yucca has been utilized in traditional medicine for various health benefits. The roots of Yucca baccata or Yucca filamentosa, for instance, can be used medicinally.

Yucca root extract has been employed in traditional medicine for its potential anti-inflammatory and analgesic properties. It has been used to alleviate symptoms associated with arthritis, joint pain, and inflammation. Yucca root extract is also believed to support digestive health by aiding in the breakdown of carbohydrates and promoting healthy gut flora.

Moreover, Yucca root has been traditionally used to support respiratory health. It has been utilized as an expectorant to help relieve coughs and congestion. Yucca root extract may also have antioxidant properties, which can help protect against oxidative stress and promote overall well-being.

Aside from its medicinal uses, Yucca can be incorporated into culinary preparations. The flowers, fruits, and young stems of certain Yucca species are edible and have been used by Native American tribes in traditional dishes. Yucca flowers can be consumed raw or cooked, adding a unique flavor to salads or stir-fries. The fruits can be roasted, ground, or used as a thickening agent in soups and stews.

Moreover, the roots of Yucca baccata or Yucca filamentosa can be used to create a potent extract. To prepare the extract, one cubic inch of the roots can be pureed in 2 cups of water. After straining and filtering the mixture, another pint of water can be added to create an organic and water-soluble insecticidal spray.

This natural spray can be beneficial for protecting fruits and vegetables from pests. It serves as an alternative to more toxic insecticides while still effectively deterring unwanted insects. The yucca-based spray is safe for organic gardening and can be an excellent choice for those seeking environmentally-friendly solutions.

Additionally, Yucca plants have been traditionally utilized to make soap. The saponins present in Yucca roots provide natural cleansing properties. To create Yucca soap, the roots can be processed and combined with other ingredients to form a lathering and cleansing bar.

Beyond insecticidal spray and soap-making, Yucca plants have a long history of practical uses. Native American tribes have employed Yucca fibers for creating sandals, belts, textiles, baskets, ropes, and mats. Today, the Hopi, Papago, and Ute Indians continue these traditions, utilizing Yucca fibers in their crafts.

Warnings: Yucca, if consumed in excess, can cause stomach upset.

Conclusion

I hope you have enjoyed reading this book as much as I've enjoyed writing it, and I hope it will accompany you in your ongoing journey to the discovery of Native American herbs and their medicinal uses.

If you found this book useful and are feeling generous, please take the time to leave a short review on Amazon so that other may enjoy this guide as well.

I leave you with good wishes and hopefully a better knowledge of the plants around us and their amazing powers. This volume is part of a seven-books series on Native American Herbalism from foraging and gardening native plants to making herbal remedies for adults and children. Check out the other volumes to gain a deeper understanding of the amazing wisdom and knowledge of our forefathers and to improve not only your health, but the health of our land as well.

The Native American Herbalist's Bible 6

The Gardener's Companion to Native Medicinal Wildflowers

An Illustrated Handbook to Grow a Healing Meadow that will Attract Bees, Butterflies, and Birds

Linda Osceola Naranjo

Introduction

We live in a country where the cure for virtually any disease and ailment is within our grasp. In our forests, meadows, plains, and gardens grow small, seemingly insignificant flowers and herbs, plants that we don't look twice at, and trees of which we don't even bother to learn the name. Yet, they are the key to a better, healthier, and more sustainable way of life.

Our forefathers, more attuned with nature than we could ever imagine to be, understood that, and took carefully and sparingly the gifts that Nature offered to heal themselves and grow stronger.

We have lost that knowledge.

Only starting from the 1970s, a renewed interest in botanic medicine has uncovered the depth of the Native American knowledge of plants and their healing powers. The research has not only helped herbalists, but physicians and scientist as well that re-discovered substances that the Native Americans people knew about for hundreds of years.

This book is the extended edition of the best-selling The Native American Herbalist's Bible: 3-in-1 Companion to Herbal Medicine, offering four more volumes on gardening techniques, growing healing plants and wildflowers, and pediatric healthcare.

This is the unabridged companion to Native American herbs, their traditional and modern use, complete with appropriate doses and usage, gardening tips and techniques for both medicinal plants and wildflowers. The book is completed by a list of simple and effective recipes for the most common ailments for both adults and children.

You don't need to put at risk the delicate natural balance of your body and that of your loved ones by taking drugs and medications, if an easily available natural solution is just outside your door. Harvest carefully or grow your own herbs, learn to know your body and what works best for you, communicate with the nature surrounding you, and you will in a small way bring back a culture that for too long has been treated as inferior.

This book will teach how to find and treat the herbs the way the native American tribes did: from the forest to your herbalist table, but you will have to find your way to listen to your body and the plants around you.

To aid you in your holistic journey, we have decided to divide the book in seven handy volumes.

The first volume will give you a full theoretical approach to Native American medicine and the herbal medicines methods and preparations.

The second volume is a complete encyclopedia of all the most relevant herbs used in traditional Native American medicine, complete with modern examples, doses, and where to find them, making it a very effective field guide.

The third volume is a "recipe book" of sorts: it offers easy herbal solutions to the most common diseases a budding naturopath can encounter. It is meant as a jumping point to find your own way to treat yourself and your fellow man and will come in handy even to the most experienced herbalist.

The fourth volume provides a complete theoretical and practical approach to Native American traditional planting techniques and how they can be implemented in modern gardens.

The fifth volume is the native gardener's almanac for medicinal herbs. Foraging is not always an option and a lot of herbs are handy to have in your garden: this volume will guide you through the herbs that you can and (should) have in your garden.

This sixth volume continues the guide to the plants you can plant in your gardens focusing on healing wildflowers, which are not only good for your health, but for the planet as well, and they are not bad on the eyes either!

The seventh volume focuses on native pediatric healthcare. Treating children is a very delicate undertaking, their physiology is more sensitive to external agents, especially drugs. Natural herbalist treatments are effective and gentle in treating common, less severe, pathologies and they won't needlessly weaken your child's immune system. The herbs listed in this last volume have been carefully researched to specifically treat children and their ailments, avoiding any allergic reaction and boosting their immune system.

I am happy to guide through a life-changing journey in search of lost knowledge, amazing healing plants, and carefully crafted herbal remedies and I hope it will help you nurture a stronger relationship with the nature surrounding us and the many gifts it bestows upon us.

Planting a wildflower garden

This subject has been treated extensively in the fourth volume of this series. Therefore, this is only a brief introduction to planting a wildflower garden, take a look back for more information.

Wildflowers have a remarkable resilience and ability to self-replicate. These plants thrive in the wild, requiring minimal care and effortlessly adapting to their surroundings. One of the greatest advantages of wildflowers is their adaptability to various soil conditions, making them an excellent choice for challenging areas of your land that are hard to maintain. With their captivating beauty and easy maintenance, wildflowers truly offer a match made in gardening heaven.

The benefits of growing wildflowers in your garden extend beyond their effortless nature. By incorporating wildflowers, you can maintain a fresh and natural appearance while reducing your water and fertilizer usage, resulting in cost savings and less effort. The use of perennial wildflowers like agrimony, bird's foot trefoil, or betony ensures long-lasting blooms that will grace your garden year after year.

Wildflowers play a vital role in supporting the environment in multiple ways. These vibrant plants serve as essential pollinator habitats, helping to sustain dwindling bee populations. Unlike many cultivated plants that feature complex petal structures, wildflowers often possess accessible nectar-producing parts that allow pollinators to thrive. By planting wildflowers, you create an environmentally friendly space that attracts a variety of beneficial creatures, including birds, bees, butterflies, and insects, all contributing to the health and visual appeal of your garden.

In addition to their role in pollination, wildflowers offer significant advantages for fruit and vegetable production. Many of our beloved crops, such as strawberries, raspberries, cherries, and apples, rely on insects for robust pollination and bountiful harvests. Incorporating wildflowers into your garden helps maintain a healthy insect population, ensuring optimal pollination for your crops.

Moreover, wildflowers provide invaluable resources for wildlife, offering essential seeds, insects, and other nourishment. They play a crucial role in erosion control and stormwater management, acting as natural filters in croplands and wooded areas. The extensive root systems of wildflowers act as natural filters for groundwater, helping to mitigate the effects of drought. By following the strategies outlined in volume 4, you can create a wildflower patch that attracts a diverse array of wildlife to your garden.

To ensure successful growth, it is recommended to sow wildflowers in the spring, allowing for a long growing season that enables the plants to establish themselves before setting seed. If starting later in the summer, provide a timeframe of at least eight to ten weeks before frost to allow the seeds to self-sow, ensuring a flourishing wildflower display in the following seasons.

Now, the task at hand is finding the perfect location for your wildflower garden. Select an area that receives partial to full sun, as this will provide the optimal amount of sunlight for your wildflowers to thrive. Take into consideration the mature size of the wildflowers, as some species can grow quite large. Position them away from pathways and play areas to avoid accidental contact with their sharp leaves. Over time, the extensive root systems of wildflowers may develop, which can have implications for nearby structures such as foundations, retaining walls, and irrigation systems. However, any leftover roots can be utilized to propagate additional wildflowers, making the most of their self-replicating nature.

Embrace the joy and beauty of wildflowers in your garden. Their resilience, low maintenance requirements, and contribution to the environment make them a delightful addition to any landscape. With their vibrant blooms, they will bring a touch of natural charm and allure to your outdoor space, creating a haven for both you and the many creatures that will be drawn to their abundance.

A little preparation goes a long way

The key to success is proper soil preparation! To make room for your wildflowers to grow and develop, remove weeds, grasses, and other plants (roots and all) from the area. Every planting site has a specific amount of water, nutrients, and sunlight. You risk creating a competitive environment where your wildflowers will be stressed as they compete for resources if you leave other plants in situ before sowing your seeds.

Crowding and competition can result in lanky growth (extra-long, floppy stems) and weak plants, putting your planting's long-term health at risk. We don't recommend dispersing seed without removing other plants in the field or into grass; anyone who has attempted scattering seed without removing other plants has been disappointed when their wildflowers don't bloom.

The better you prepare the place, the easier it will be for two very crucial things to occur:

- Without competing plants shading them out and stealing available food and water, your seeds will germinate faster and stronger.
- Your young wildflowers will be better adapted to compete with weeds and grasses that may try to grow back if they are not stressed by competition early on.
- It's a good idea to plan ahead. You may be able to prepare your soil utilizing labor-saving, cost-effective, and environmentally friendly ways if you have a few weeks, months, or even a whole season to plan ahead of your planting date.

- Ensure that all plant waste and roots of old grass and weeds are removed. Otherwise, they will regrow with vigor!

Preparing the Soil
You have a few potential methods to consider.

Rototilling
A rototiller can be used to break up the ground and soften the soil in greater areas. If you don't possess one, you can usually rent one at a reasonable price.

Rototilling or digging the planting area two or three times, a few weeks apart, is the most thorough method. This allows you to bring weed seeds up, allow them to germinate, and then kill them in the next tilling. The first two passes will focus on removing weeds from the soil, while the last pass will ensure that the soil is properly prepared for your future planting.

If you're tilling a lawn that hasn't been mowed in years, your weed seed count is likely to be low. The initial pass can be done at the deepest depth of 4-6", with subsequent passes at a shallower depth of just 2-3".

Expect plenty of weed seeds in the soil if your location has been an ancient field that has grown and seeded itself for years. Rather than tilling deeply, it is preferable to shallow till 2-3" deep two or three times over the course of many weeks. Allow 2-3 weeks between soil turnings to allow weed seeds to germinate before tilling. Then, before seeding, remove all weeds, plants, roots, and detritus.

Avoid digging deeper than recommended; the deeper you dig, the more dormant weed seeds you'll bring to the surface of the soil, where they can develop faster than your wildflowers.

Rototilling with care is beneficial for three reasons:
1. It loosens the soil and provides a "soft" environment for flowering plants to emerge.
2. It fosters good "seed-to-soil" contact and generates a suitable seedbed for germination.
3. It eliminates nearly all of the grasses and weeds that might otherwise compete with your seedlings.

Smothering and Solarization
Both of these strategies work by placing things over your planting area to kill weeds. It's simple to use in large or small spaces, and it's also a very environmentally friendly solution. Solarization, as the name suggests, utilizes the sun's beams over time. To prevent plant growth, smothering necessitates a thick layer of material that blocks out the sun.

Solarizing Grass and Weeds
Cover your soil with translucent plastic, much to a painting drop cloth. Cover the area for 4 to 8 weeks. The sun will shine down on the plastic, trapping an excessive amount of heat and moisture beneath it, killing any plant life that is already present.

Solarizing has the extra benefit of allowing some weed seeds to grow in the sunlight before being killed by the heat.

Suffocating Weeds and Grass
Smothering can be accomplished by covering the planting area with thick tarps, blankets, cardboard, or several inches of leaves or mulch. Cover the area for 4 to 8 weeks. This deprives plant life of accessible sunshine while also introducing a significant amount of heat. Weed seeds germinate in the dark and sprout under the heavy fabric but die off due to a lack of sunshine.

Smothering has the added benefit of providing the ideal setting for earthworms and other soil organisms to devour the decaying plant growth and loosen the soil.

Classic Hand Tools
The undertaking is similar to preparing a new garden bed for a limited space. Typically, all that is required is a shovel or spade, as well as a rake. Simply pull out all of the plants, stir the dirt, and rake the space smooth and clear of rocks and roots. A wildflower planting won't be bothered by a few rocks or uneven patches.

It's especially crucial to get rid of grass roots so they don't come back alongside your new wildflowers. Use a pickaxe, or a smaller-handed variant known as a mattock, or even a sharp spade if necessary. Then it's time to plant!

Plant-Derived Herbicides
Chemical applications may be used by those who are having difficulty removing stubborn weeds. Most hardware stores and garden centers have organic (non-synthetic) herbicides like acetic acid, vinegar, and various combinations.

Always apply herbicides carefully on windless days to avoid harming the plants you've picked for your landscape.

If you're going to use a natural pesticide to get rid of grasses in your garden, make sure it's one that's designed to control 'monocots,' or single-blade plants. Herbicides designed to destroy 'dicots' (also known as broadleaf plants) are likely to kill a portion of your planned planting.

When using weed killers, keep in mind that they are non-selective, meaning they will harm any broadleaf plant or tree they come into contact with, including wildflowers. It's also critical to provide time for herbicides to be eliminated from the soil prior to planting.

Synthetic herbicides, such as Roundup or glyphosate, are not recommended since they can affect people, pets, wildlife, and plants. Glyphosate, for example, can remain in the soil for up to 60 days or longer after application, depending on environmental circumstances.

Know Your Soil
Your soil is almost certainly ideal for wildflowers! Unless the soil is genuinely sterile, which is uncommon, it's best to utilize it just as you found it. The test is straightforward: If there's anything growing in the area, even if it's simply grasses or weeds, wildflowers should thrive without issue. You can grow wildflowers if you can grow weeds!

There are a few exceptions to this rule. For example, if a chemical spill or pollution occurred in the planting area, if you're planting on a new building site where the topsoil was removed, or if the soil is extremely compacted due to drought, heavy traffic, usage, or neglect. Again, determining what is currently growing in the soil is a straightforward method to analyze it: if nothing grows, you may need to amend the soil or find a new location for the meadow. Wildflowers are versatile, but they won't flourish in a sterile environment. If your soil is compacted clay or sandy, adding organic matter might assist in improving the texture.

As we witness on every roadside, wildflowers are incredibly adaptive and thrive in poor soils.

Compost or other organic fertilizers aren't required for producing wildflowers, and they may actually make the soil too rich, attracting weeds and suffocating the growth of some wildflowers.

Do you want a well-kept, well-designed garden with well-behaved plants, vibrant flowers, and appealing foliage? The difficulty is that the Chelsea gardens and flowers require a lot of upkeep, including fertilizer applications on a regular basis and the liberal application of herbicides and insecticides to keep hungry bugs and weeds at bay.

Recapping, growing a wildflower meadow in your yard is one way to keep things simple and low-maintenance while yet looking lovely. Planting perennial wildflowers will produce results year after year. However, be aware that they prefer to grow in poorer soils only to prevent grass development, which would otherwise out-compete the blooms. You can minimize soil nutrition by first removing the topsoil before planting, but another

alternative is to grow wildflower annuals, which can be planted in richer soil.

It's preferable to stay away from gathering seeds from wild plants because this depletes the natural seed bank. Since the 1930s, the number of wildflower meadows has decreased dramatically, with barely 2% of their former numbers remaining. Instead, you should seek out a reputable wildflower seed seller that can advise you on the optimum seed mix for your local conditions. Native species will self-seed more effectively and help wildflower recovery.

Wildflowers are also the most effective pollinator plants, as they aid in the recovery of diminishing bee populations. Many developed plant species contain faulty pollen and nectar-producing organs, as well as numerous petals that prevent pollinators from entering, which is harmful to the ecology.

Instead of viewing bees as pests in your garden, take a seat and observe these pollinators at work. You'll notice some interesting behavior in the way they agitate the pollen chambers of certain flowers to increase pollen release — a technique known as buzz pollination or sonication.

Young bees and bumblebees must learn how to clasp pollen organs and then swiftly activate their wing muscles to produce a vibration that is substantially greater in frequency and louder than that utilized for flying. The discharge of pollen is stimulated when the correct vibration is established. Certain flowering plants, such as potato and tomato blooms, are especially suited to buzz pollination.

Native Medicinal Wildflowers for your Garden

This is a carefully chosen selection of Native medicinal wildflower that you can grow in your backyard. For each plant are indicated its medical uses, solvents, hardiness zone, pollinators, sourcing and habitat, gardening techniques, and consumption methods. However, for more information on their identification, their traditional and modern uses please refer to the second volume of the series. Whereas in the second volume the plants were chosen for their health benefits, in this volume the plants were also chosen for the benefits they can provide in a garden either because they are endangered species which warrant replication in a native garden, or because they are excellent pollinators. Several wildflowers are only present in this volume: for these plants the traditional and modern uses, as well as the identification have been reported in this volume. Happy reading!

Aconite

Monkshood, Wolf's-Bane, Leopard's Bane, Mousebane, Women's Bane, Devil's Helmet, Queen Of Poisons, Blue Rocket.

Aconitum.

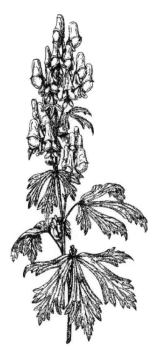

Identification: Mountain wildflower from 2' to 8' tall with dark green leaves, deeply cleft and palmate or deeply palmate with five to seven segments or lobes. Leaves are basal with sharp and coarse teeth. Lower leaves have longer petioles (stems) and leaves are alternate. Numerous flowers, blue to midnight blue, but may vary from purple to white, yellow, or pink. Flowers borne on an erect stalk and lack stipules. Flower appears to be a hood over reproductive parts; this characteristic is distinctive. Also known as monk's hood or wolf's bane.

Traditional uses: The traditional uses of aconite varied among different tribes, each incorporating the plant in their unique cultural practices. For instance, the Shoshone tribe, native to the Great Basin region of the United States, utilized aconite in their traditional medicine. They would prepare aconite roots into a poultice or infusion to treat ailments such as fever, joint pain, and respiratory conditions. Additionally, the Shoshone tribe believed that aconite possessed spiritual properties, and its smoke was used in purification rituals.

In Asian cultures, particularly in China and Japan, aconite, also known as "fuzi" or "monkshood," held a significant place in traditional medicine. In Chinese traditional medicine, aconite roots were processed and used as an analgesic, anti-inflammatory, and to promote circulation. It was often employed topically for conditions like arthritis and rheumatism, as well as internally for cardiovascular and respiratory issues. However, it is important to note that aconite is highly toxic and must be used with extreme caution or under the guidance of a qualified practitioner.

Among the Ainu people of Japan, aconite was used for spiritual and protective purposes. They believed that aconite possessed mystical powers and would use it in ceremonies and rituals to ward off evil spirits and negative energies.

It is essential to highlight that aconite is a potent and toxic plant. Its traditional uses by various tribes were based on their understanding of its properties and their specific cultural contexts. However, due to its high toxicity, the use of aconite in modern medicine and herbal practices requires careful consideration and expert knowledge.

Modern Uses: It is used externally (very toxic internally) to treat sciatica, bruises, shingles, and various forms of neuralgia (Moore, 1993). Plant is cultivated in Europe and used internally by a physician as a sedative and analgesic. In China and Japan aconitum, monk's hood, or Chinese wolf's bane is used to treat shock resulting from heart attack, low blood pressure, coronary heart disease, and chronic heart failure (Zhou, 2014).

Medicinal parts: roots and flowers

Solvents: Alcohol.

Hardiness Zone: Zones 3-8.

Sourcing: These herbaceous perennial plants are primarily found in the Northern Hemisphere's hilly regions, such as North America, Europe, and Asia, where they thrive in the damp but well-draining soils of mountain meadows, shady parts of mountain meadows, drainages, washes, stream edges in moist coniferous forests to 9000'. From the Rockies west to the coast. Often found in the same location as larkspur. It's listed as an endangered species, so please source it from a reputable seed provider or local nursery, do not forage it.

Gardening Tips: A garden flower cultivated for its unusual beauty. In the autumn, sow Aconitum on the soil surface with a 20 to 25 cm spacing for smaller species and up to 100 cm spacing for larger species. Wolfsbane grows best in partial shade, although it may also be planted in full sun if maintained moist.

With a pH of 5 to 6, the soil should be cool and moist. Aconitum plants take anywhere from 5 to 250 days to germinate, so start your seeds in a flat against a north-facing wall before transplanting.

In the summer, Aconitum and similar species demand regular watering. It's also a good idea to stake the plant to protect it from the impacts of bad weather. To sustain development, the plants should be trimmed down each autumn and split every four years.

Consumption Methods: Do not use internally, very toxic. Use only topically under the supervision of a healthcare professional

Warnings: Extremely toxic! Neurotoxin found throughout aerial parts and root. Poisoning similar to rabies; no effective antidote. Employ gastric lavage and/or emesis followed by 2 mg atropine; maintain blood pressure and apply artificial respiration.

Baneberry

Bugbane, Cohosh.

Baneberry rubra.

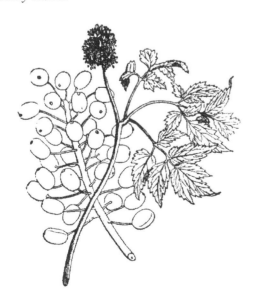

Identification: Red baneberry, scientifically known as Actaea rubra, is a captivating and potentially dangerous herbaceous perennial shrub that adds a touch of beauty to shady landscapes. This flowering shrub typically reaches a modest height of about 1 foot and spreads to approximately 1 foot in width. It can be found flourishing in various habitats, including moist soils, deciduous forests, mixed coniferous forests, open woodlands, swales, stream banks, and swamps. Red baneberry thrives in humus-rich and damp environments, often favoring stony woods.

This remarkable plant features a unique growth structure, boasting glossy, erect stems that reach heights of 1 to 2 feet. These stems, characterized by their triangular shape, provide an elegant framework for the vibrant foliage and enchanting flowers. The leaves of red baneberry are a deep shade of green and possess a smooth texture, enhancing their overall allure.

One of the distinguishing features of red baneberry is its striking fruit. The plant produces egg-shaped berries that can range in color from bright red to a deep shade of purple. These berries, although visually appealing, contain cardiogenic toxins that can have a sedative effect on myocardial tissues in humans. It is important to exercise caution and avoid ingesting or handling the berries or any other parts of the plant.

Red baneberry's toxic properties serve as a defense mechanism in the natural world, deterring potential predators from consuming its fruit or coming into contact with its potent compounds.

Medical Uses: Despite its deadly characteristics, the plant was once utilized to heal a number of diseases by numerous native American tribes.

For colds and coughs, the Blackfoot, for example, utilized a decoction of roots. For sores, the Cheyenne use a decoction of roots. An infusion of the roots was used as a rheumatism wash by the Iroquois. The plant was reputedly used to cure rattlesnake bites by Canadian tribes.

Pollinators/Wildlife: As the flowers are sweet and attractive, it will attract pollinators, such as bees, flies, beetles, and small insects. The berries are food for many birds, especially the American Robin.

Solvents: Boiling water, alcohol.

Hardiness Zones: Zones 3-8.

How to source it: In the Midwest's understory woodland habitats, there are two types of baneberry. White baneberry (*A. pachypoda*) is found largely in the eastern and Midwest in zones 3-8, while red baneberry (*A. rubra*) is found throughout much of North America in zones 3-7 except in the southeastern U.S.

Gardening Tips: Fruits ripen in upstate New York from late August to September. When the seed matures, the color of the baneberry fruit changes. Dolls Eye grows a few weeks before Red Baneberry. White baneberry turns porcelain white, while Red baneberry turns crimson red. After the fruit begins to change color, you can collect it at any moment. The fruit will stay on the plant for several weeks before rotting.

When the fruits have turned a different hue, it's time to harvest them. Each fruit has a number of seeds. Collecting immediately after the color change, rather than waiting a few weeks, may assist in speeding up germination. By macerating the fruits and floating off the pulp and skins, the seeds can be removed. Sound seed sinks to the bottom of the pond. Small batches of fruit can be macerated by hand, while larger amounts can be processed in a food processor. Sow the seeds right away or start stratifying them for storage. After cleaning the seed, don't allow it to dry out.

After harvest, most Baneberry seeds will germinate in the first or second season. Because germination rates are high, some seeds may take an extra year or two to germinate. A cooling period of one to two months is required for seed; the seed sown outside in the fall will meet this need. Before planting, stratified seed should be exposed to outside temperatures or kept in the refrigerator for one to two months. Early spring through mid-summer is when seedlings germinate. By the fall, they will have grown into little plants. During the second growing season, the plant should blossom. Sow seed 12" deep on the surface of the soil. Any soil from medium to rich will suffice. Remove the leaf litter, sprinkle seeds on the soil, and then replenish the leaf litter in natural conditions.

Baneberry is simple to grow and propagate from seed woodland species. The fruits are plentiful, easy to pick, and the seed germinates quickly. Baneberry thrives on moist to moderately wooded soils and grows in part sun to full shade. It may grow in a variety of soil and horticultural situations. Baneberry thrives in soils that are rich, deep, and well-drained. Doll's eye grows in both moist and dry mixed woodlands. pH that is in the middle of the range. Baneberry is only a small part of the herb layer in which it thrives. Sugar maple and basswood are good trees to look for if you want to know where the baneberry will thrive. False Solomon Seal, Zig-zag Goldenrod, Bloodroot, and Wild Geranium are all common herb companions. The two Baneberries are frequently found growing side by side, and they occasionally hybridize, yielding fruits that are a mix of the two parents' colors.

Consumption Methods: One common application is the preparation of a tea using the root. This herbal tea has been traditionally used to alleviate stomach pains, coughs, and colds. It is also believed to be beneficial in regulating menstrual irregularities and relieving post-partum pains. Additionally, it has been used to stimulate milk flow in nursing mothers. However, it is crucial to note that the root of red baneberry is a potent purgative and should be used with great caution, particularly when consumed internally.

Externally, a poultice made from the root of red baneberry can be applied topically to address itchy skin. This natural remedy is believed to provide relief and promote healing. However, it is advisable to use caution when applying the poultice to avoid any potential irritation.

Due to its purgative, irritant, and emetic properties, it is essential to approach the internal use of red baneberry with extreme care. The potent nature of the rootstock requires proper knowledge and guidance from experienced herbalists or healthcare professionals.

Warnings: Red baneberry (Actaea rubra) is a highly toxic plant, and caution should be exercised when dealing with it. All parts of the plant, including the berries, contain cardiogenic toxins that can have severe effects on human health. Ingesting any part of the plant, especially the rootstock, can lead to serious poisoning symptoms, including gastrointestinal distress, vomiting, diarrhea, and potentially life-threatening cardiac effects.

It is essential to remember that red baneberry should never be consumed or used internally without proper knowledge and guidance from trained professionals. The plant's purgative, irritant, and emetic properties make it unsuitable for self-medication or home remedies by laymen.

Furthermore, the berries of red baneberry are attractive but extremely toxic. They should not be mistaken for edible berries and should be avoided by children and pets. Accidental ingestion of the berries can result in severe poisoning and should be treated as a medical emergency.

When handling red baneberry, it is recommended to wear protective gloves to prevent any contact with the skin. In case of accidental contact or ingestion, immediate medical attention should be sought. It is advisable to keep this plant out of reach and to educate yourself and others about its toxicity to prevent any potential harm.

Bellwort

Merrybells, Strawbells.

Uvularia grandiflora.

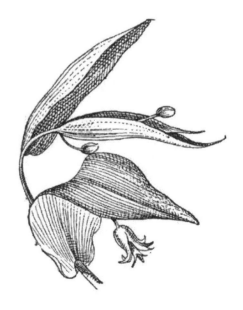

Identification: Bellwort develops a perennial, creeping root-stalk, and a stem 8 to 14 inches tall, dividing into 2 branches topside. The leaves are elliptical, clasping-perfoliate, acute at the apex, rounded at the base, 2-3 inches long, broad, smooth, and glaucous underneath. The flowers are single, pale yellow, approx. 1 inch long, pendulous from the end of one of the branches.

Medical Uses: Native Americans and early pioneers both employed bellworts for medicinal purposes. The herb has traditionally been used to cure snakebites, reduce swellings, and as a poultice for other skin wounds and inflammations.

The usage of the Uvularia genus plants for medical purposes by early colonists had its origins, at least in part, in their use by Native Americans for a number of medical illnesses other than sore throat tea. The roots were used as a poultice to cure boils, wounds, ulcers, and broken bones by the Haudenosaunee Indians (also known as the Iroquois). The roots were also administered internally to promote the repairing of bone fractures. Treatment for diarrhea, blood purification, as a backache infusion, as a wash for sore eyes, and as an emollient for tight muscles were among the other uses. It was also utilized by the Menomini to treat edema.

Native Americans and early colonists both ate bellwort plants as part of their diet.

Tonic, demulcent, and nervine.

Pollinators/Wildlife: You'll see a variety of pollinators, from many types of bees to smaller insects. Offers a larger nectar reward than the Bloodroot or Rue Anemone which flower around the same time and is therefore a prized attraction for the large Mining bee (*Andrena Melandrena*). Also interesting for tiny sweat bees (*Lassioglossum*)

Solvents: Boiling water, alcohol.

Medicinal part: root

Hardiness Zones: Zones 4-9.

Sourcing: Bellwort with large flowers grows in damp deciduous forests in the Eastern United States and Canada. Deer browsing is a threat to this forest floor species. It's also vulnerable to habitat loss due to construction and non-native species like buckthorn and garlic mustard displacing it. Bellwort, a sign of a healthy forest floor ecology, can be restored by removing invasive plants.

Gardening Tips: This quintessential native for the woodland garden blooms in spring and becomes a 2-foot-tall foliage plant that holds through the growing season (with adequate rainfall). The plants emerge upward but bend over as they grow, a botanical ballet producing nodding, light to golden yellow flowers, themselves shaped like a drooping pinwheel. The emerging foliage is bluish or purplish but matures true green, holds clean through the summer, and turns golden in fall or if stressed by summer drought (in the wild, plants go dormant during summer droughts). Ants collect the ripe seeds for food (as with many spring-flowering woodland ephemerals, they are coated in a fatty elaiosome), inadvertently transporting and planting the seed. Ideally, give large-flowered bellwort (aka merrybells) limestone-based, well-drained, humus-rich, loamy soils. Large clumps are easily divided as the plants go dormant in late summer or fall.

Bellworts thrive in areas that have been permitted to keep a good tree canopy or in temperate damp environments, such as the Pacific Northwest. USDA plant hardiness zones 4 through 9 are suitable for bellwort wildflowers. Provide them with protection from the sun's rays as well as enough water, and you'll have bright blossoms for years to come.

Bellwort plants are best started from division. Don't go out into the woods to gather flora. They are widely accessible from nurseries once again. The seeds' beginning is finicky, to say the least. The germination rate is not optimal, and the plant must rely on environmental cues to sprout. Growing bellwort from divided roots or stolens is a tried and true method of propagation. In late winter or early spring, just dig up the plant and divide it into two halves. The stolens or sprouting stems that the plant sends out from the base plant organically multiply the plant. It's similar to strawberries in that you can easily detach rooted stolens and start a new clump of the wildflower.

Bellwort prefers damp, rich soil that isn't too wet. Make sure the area you're planting in is well-drained. To a depth of at least 6 inches, work in substantial amounts of organic compost or leaf litter (15 cm.). Choose regions under trees or densely populated shrubby areas where you can find shade from the sun. In the fall, mulch around the plants in cooler zones. Because the foliage dies back and grows back in the spring, no pruning or trimming is required. Keep an eye out for slug and snail damage, as well as excessive dampness. Aside from that, these small wild herbs are an excellent complement for a natural forest garden.

Consumption Methods: To prepare bellwort tea, steep 1 to 2 teaspoons of dried bellwort leaves or flowers in a cup of hot water for about 10 minutes. This herbal infusion can be consumed for its potential benefits, such as promoting relaxation and soothing respiratory discomforts like coughs and congestion.

Another traditional use of bellwort is as an eye wash. Infusions or decoctions made from bellwort can be used externally as a gentle eye wash to alleviate eye irritation, redness, or discomfort. It is important to prepare the eye wash solution properly by steeping the bellwort plant parts in warm water and straining before use.

Warnings: Few side effects are recorded; however, dizziness has been noted in some when taking larger doses.

Boneset

Throughwort, Common Boneset, Ague-weed, Indian Sage.

Eupatorium perfoliatum

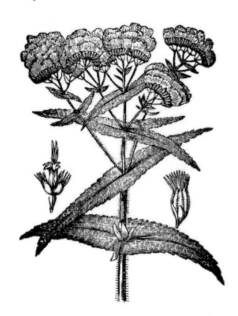

Medical Uses: The Chippewa tribe commonly used boneset as a medicinal herb for treating fevers and colds. They would prepare a hot infusion or decoction from the leaves and stems of the plant and administer it to reduce fever and alleviate symptoms associated with respiratory illnesses. On the other hand, the Iroquois tribe utilized boneset as a remedy for aches, pains, and muscle injuries. They would prepare poultices from the leaves and apply them externally to soothe sore muscles and promote healing.

Check out the second volume for more information!

Pollinators/Wildlife: Bees of all types, larger flying insects, mostly wasps. The most common visitors will be digger bees, small carpenter bees, and sweat bees. It also attracts scollid wasps and late-flowering boneset offers refuge to monarch butterflies that migrate southbound.

Solvents: Boiling water, alcohol.

Hardiness Zones: Zones 4-8.

Sourcing: It's relatively simple to grow Boneset plants. The plants naturally grow in wetlands and along stream banks, and they thrive even in extremely moist soil. They prefer partial to full sun and make excellent forest garden plants.

Gardening Tips: It's relatively simple to grow Boneset plants. The plants naturally grow in wetlands and along stream banks, and they thrive even in extremely moist soil. They prefer partial to full sun and make excellent forest garden plants. In fact, it shares many of the same rowing conditions as Joe-Pye Weed. The plants can be grown from seed, but it will take two to three years for them to bloom.

I personally think it looks beautiful against a backdrop of phlox and black-eyed Susan.

Consumption Methods: Boneset has been used as a medication for ages, and it is thought to have anti-inflammatory qualities. The plant's aboveground parts can be collected, dried, and steeped to make tea. It should be noted, however, that it has been demonstrated to be toxic to the liver in several studies.

Warnings Boneset can cause gastric upset and liver damage.

Black Cohosh

Black Snakeroot, Macrotys, Bugbane, Bugwort, Rattleroot, Fairy Candles.

Actaea racemose.

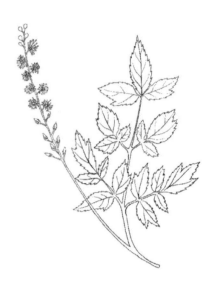

Medical Uses: Native Americans grew Black Cohosh plants for a variety of medical ailments, including snake bites and gynecological difficulties. The Chippewa tribe traditionally used black cohosh root as a remedy for various women's health issues. It was commonly used to alleviate symptoms associated with menstrual discomfort, including cramps and irregularities. Additionally, it was utilized during menopause to ease hot flashes, mood swings, and other related symptoms. The Iroquois tribe also valued black cohosh for its medicinal properties. They used it as a tonic to support women's reproductive health and to address menstrual problems. The root was often prepared as a decoction or tea and consumed to promote balance and overall well-being. In addition to the Chippewa and Iroquois, many other tribes valued black cohosh for its medicinal properties. For example, the Cherokee tribe used black cohosh root as a remedy for women's health issues, including menstrual cramps and menopause symptoms. The Algonquin tribe utilized it for treating rheumatism and as a general pain reliever. The Delaware tribe used black cohosh as a diuretic and to promote sweating during fevers. The Mohegan tribe regarded it as a powerful emmenagogue and employed it to regulate menstrual cycles. The traditional knowledge and uses of black cohosh by these tribes reflect its versatility and effectiveness in addressing various health concerns.

Check out the second volume for more.

Pollinators/Wildlife: Black Cohosh is a mesic to dry woodland plant that thrives in high-base-element soils. The flowers have a sweet/fetid odor that attracts pollinators such as flies, gnats, beetles, and bumblebees. Bumble Bees, Sweat Bees, and Leaf-cutter Bees are the most likely visitors. It's rabbit-resistant.

Solvents: Boiling water, alcohol.

Hardiness Zones: Zones 4-8.

Sourcing: It's a native medicinal plant that can be found from Maine to Ontario, south to Georgia, and west to Missouri and Indiana in lush hardwood forests. It can be found in North Carolina at heights of up to 4,000 feet and is most abundant in the state's western region. You can either buy seeds from a reputable nursery or collect your own Black Cohosh seeds to grow in your home garden. It is over-harvested, therefore avoid foraging it.

Gardening Tips: To grow Black Cohosh (Actaea racemosa) in your garden, start by collecting the seeds in the fall when they have dried out in their capsules and are beginning to break open, producing a rattling sound. Sow the seeds right away.

For successful germination, stratify the Black Cohosh seeds by exposing them to a warm/cold/warm cycle. Keep the seeds at 70°F (21°C) for two weeks, then at 40°F (4°C) for three months. This stratification process helps break seed dormancy. Once the seeds have been stratified, plant them 1 to 2 inches (4-5 cm) apart and 1/4 inch (6 mm) deep in moist, high-organic-matter soil. Cover them with a 1-inch (2.5 cm) layer of mulch.

Black Cohosh thrives in shade but can also tolerate full sun, although the plants may appear lighter in color and the leaves may be more prone to scorching. In harsh climates, you can choose to sow the seeds in a cold frame for germination in the following spring. Alternatively, you can propagate Black Cohosh through division or separation in the spring or fall, but wait at least three years after planting before doing so.

Keep the soil consistently moist as Black Cohosh plants dislike drying out. Consider staking tall flower stalks to provide support. These perennials may take some time to establish, but they will add visual appeal to your landscape. Even the spent seed casings can be left in the garden over winter to create texture and interest.

Consumption Methods: Tea and tincture, check the second and third volume for more recipes.

Warnings: Black Cohosh overdoses can cause gastric upset. Use in moderation.

Bloodroot

Boloroot, Coonroot, Large-Leaved Bloodwort, Large-leaved Sandwort, Panson, Pauson, Puccoon, Puccoon-Root, Red-Indian Paint, Red-Puccoon, Redroot, Snakebite, Sweet Slumber, Tetterwort, White Puccoon.

Sanguinaria canadensis.

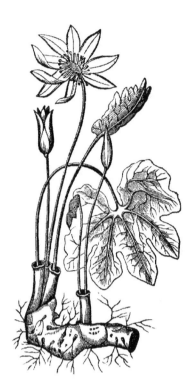

Medical Uses: Bloodroot has long been used by Native Americans to induce vomiting in order to cleanse the body of toxic poisons and to help with menstrual problems. Alternative medicine practitioners claim that it can treat a wide range of medical ailments. The plant is most commonly employed as an expectorant and antibacterial in respiratory infections, as well as a debriding agent in dental health in western herbal therapy. Check out the second volume for more information

Pollinators/Wildlife: As the weather warms, the flowers open, announcing their presence to early flying pollinators – the earliest bees of the season, plus flying insects that make their way out early in the spring. The petals attract pollinators but do not offer any nectar, relying partly to pollinate on the hopeless search of the bees that transfer the pollen without getting the reward. Once the bees are done, the ants take over (this symbiotic relationship is called myrmecochory), and harvest the seeds that cointain oil and sugar, as they carry the seeds they help propagation.

Solvents: Boiling water, alcohol.

Hardiness Zones: Zones 3-8.

Sourcing: Bloodroot is a spring wildflower endemic to North America, growing in rich woodlands from Nova Scotia to Florida, and west to Alabama, Arkansas, Nebraska, and Manitoba. Bloodroot loves moist forests with plenty of warm sun during the day.

Gardening Tips: Bloodroot (Sanguinaria canadensis) is a captivating wildflower that brings beauty to woodland or shade gardens. Its early spring blooms are a sight to behold, with pure white petals delicately encircling a cluster of vibrant yellow stamens, all centered around a green pistil. In cooler temperatures, the flower buds often display a charming pink tinge, further enhancing their allure. The foliage of Bloodroot is equally stunning, characterized by exquisitely shaped leaves adorned with deep undulating lobes, creating a distinct shield-like form around the flowers and developing fruit. Beyond its aesthetic appeal, Bloodroot also serves as a valuable source of pollen for bees during the spring season.

To successfully grow Bloodroot in your garden, it is essential to replicate its preferred natural habitat. This includes providing a well-draining soil that is rich in organic matter, particularly humus. Bloodroot flourishes in loamy soils, which mimic the conditions found in woodland areas. Additionally, planting the flowers in shaded areas, preferably beneath the canopy of deciduous trees, mimics the dappled sunlight they receive in their native habitats.

When it comes to propagation, Bloodroot offers two viable options. The first method involves collecting seeds from mature Bloodroot plants. As the flowers fade and the seedpods develop, gently shake them over a paper bag to collect the seeds. These seeds should be sown as soon as possible, preferably in mid to late spring when they have reached maturity. Plant the seeds at a shallow depth, allowing them to germinate in the following spring.

The second method of propagation involves root division. This can be done at any time, but it is generally recommended to undertake this process when the plant is dormant. Carefully divide the root sections and plant them approximately 1 to 2 inches (2.5 to 5 cm) deep in soil that is acidic and rich in organic matter. Choose an area that receives dappled sunlight, ensuring that the plants are not exposed to direct, intense sunlight.

To ensure the optimal growth and health of your Bloodroot plants, it is crucial to provide consistent moisture to the soil. Water the plants regularly, aiming for twice a week to maintain a moist environment throughout the summer. This practice will help the leaves stay vibrant and prevent the plant from entering dormancy prematurely. As fall approaches and winter sets in, gradually reduce watering to allow the plant to naturally go dormant.

Once your Bloodroot plants have established themselves and reached their second year of growth, you can consider feeding them with a balanced fertilizer. This will provide the necessary nutrients to support their ongoing development and ensure continuous blooming in the years to come.

With proper care and attention to its specific needs, Bloodroot will not only thrive in your garden but also create a stunning display of delicate blooms and captivating foliage.

Consumption Method: Bloodroot exudate thinned with water is an excellent natural mosquito repellent, the moniker "red skin" given to the Native American tribes by the colonizers is most likely due to the skin coloration of the application of bloodroot. Bloodroot is a component in black salve; a corrosive skin salve used to help in the ridding of warts and problematic sores. Check out the second and third volume for more uses and applications.

Warnings: As with other ingestible herbs, overdosing can cause gastric upset.

Blue Vervain

Simpler's Joy, Holy Herb.

Verbena hastata.

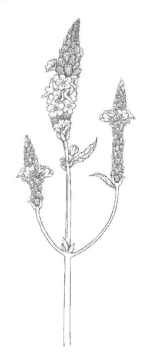

Identification: Blue vervain (Verbena hastata) is a captivating and resilient native wildflower that thrives in the enchanting landscape of riverbanks. With a preference for partial shade and moist, rich soil, this perennial herbaceous plant adds a touch of elegance to its surroundings. Rising tall and erect, blue vervain reaches heights of 2 to 5 feet, commanding attention with its striking presence. Its square stems, covered in fine hairs, can display shades of green or red, adding to its visual appeal.

The lance-shaped leaves of blue vervain progress in pairs along the stem, their toothed edges lending an interesting texture to the plant. These leaves, measuring approximately 6 inches in length and 1 inch in width, enhance the overall beauty of the plant. But it is the magnificent flowering spikes that truly captivate observers. Displaying a mesmerizing shade of purplish-blue, the elongated panicles of blooms create a spectacle, reaching up to 5 inches in length. Each individual bloom, around 1/4 inch across, proudly showcases conspicuous lobes, adding intricate details to the overall floral arrangement.

Blue vervain graces the landscape with its vibrant blooms in the mid to late summer, bringing a burst of color to the natural surroundings. As the blooming period concludes, each flower gives way to four oblong nutlets, tinged in reddish-brown. These triangular-convex nutlets contribute to the plant's reproduction and further its spread.

The growth and expansion of blue vervain are facilitated by rhizomes, horizontal roots that produce new plants. Through this means of propagation, blue vervain gradually colonizes its preferred habitats, enriching riverbanks with its graceful presence.

Medical Uses: Early American herb doctors relied on this New World native regularly for a wide range of conditions. Eventually it was forgotten and is now experiencing a resurgence of appreciation, particularly for its ability to quickly release both emotional and physical tension. Blue vervain helps create balance. The herb was traditionally used to ease gastrointestinal irritation, act as an expectorant, and produce sweating. Early European settlers adopted indigenous peoples' practices. Despite its extensive and long-time use in herbal medicine in North America, little research has been done on this common native plant. It contains the iridoid hastatoside, which has anti-inflammatory and analgesic properties. An ethanolic extract has been found to have antidiarrheal and gastrointestinal motility-inducing properties.

Pollinators/Wildlife: The seeds of this wildflower provide sustenance to an array of avian friends, including the cardinal, swamp sparrow, field sparrow, song sparrow, and slate-colored junco. Delicate caterpillars of the verbena moth gracefully traverse its leaves, finding sustenance in its green foliage. Notably, the blue vervain serves as a vital host plant for the development of the enchanting common buckeye butterfly, as its leaves become a nurturing shelter for the butterfly's larvae.

The significance of blue vervain extends beyond its role as a food source. It also beckons a variety of pollinators to partake in its nectar-rich blossoms. Among the buzzing visitors are a diverse range of bees, including both long and short tongued bee species, the intriguing epoline cuckoo bee, the specialized verbena bee, and the diligent halictid bee. In addition to bees, the vibrant blooms of blue vervain attract the elegant three-waisted wasps, the enchanting thick-headed flies, and the golden soldier beetles, all of which contribute to the intricate web of life surrounding this remarkable wildflower.

Solvents: Boiling water, alcohol.

Hardiness Zones: Zone 8.

Sourcing: It is native to most of the 48 contiguous United States and neighboring Canada, where it can be found in fields, thickets, and damp soils. Blue vervain thrives in damp environments with full to partial sun. It grows in a variety of habitats, including damp meadows, thickets, and pastures, as well as riversides, marshes, ditches, and river-bottom prairies.

Gardening Tips: This tall, majestic plant adds architectural beauty to your garden as well as attracting a variety of pollinators. Staking is rarely required for this plant. It can withstand minor floods and standing water, making it an excellent choice for a rain garden. When cut, the small tubular flowers bloom from bottom to top and last a long time. It is a self-seeding perennial with a short life span.

The optimal conditions for blue vervain are full sun and moist, well-drained, moderately rich soil. In late October, sow blue vervain seeds immediately outside. The seeds' hibernation is broken by cold temperatures, allowing them to germinate in the spring. Remove weeds and lightly cultivate the soil.

Sprinkle the seeds over the soil's surface, then cover them with a rake to a depth of no more than 1/8 inch (3 ml.)—lightly mist with water.

This pest- and disease-resistant plant requires little maintenance once established. Maintain a moist environment for the seeds until they germinate. After that, one thorough watering each week during the summer is generally plenty. If the top 1 to 2 inches (2.5 to 5 cm) of soil feels dry to the touch, water deeply. The soil should not be permitted to become too wet, but neither should it be allowed to become too dry. During the summer, a balanced, water-soluble fertilizer is administered monthly to blue vervain. A mulch layer of 1 to 3 inches (2.5 to 7.6 cm) thick, such as bark chips or compost, keeps the soil moist and inhibits weed development. In chilly winter climes, mulch also protects the roots.

Consumption Methods: Blue vervain is safe for most people, including children; however, it's incredibly bitter, which makes it unpalatable in tea and nauseating in large doses. Often, just a few drops of the tincture will work its magic. Use internally for depression, fever, cough, cramp, jaundice, and headache. It can be used externally as a poultice to treat acne and ulcers.

Warnings: Blue vervain has been traditionally used for its potential sedative and relaxing properties. It may cause drowsiness and impair cognitive function, so it is important to avoid activities that require alertness, such as driving or operating machinery, after using blue vervain. Additionally, it may interact with certain medications, including sedatives, antidepressants, and blood thinners, leading to adverse effects or reduced efficacy.

Individuals with underlying health conditions, including liver or kidney disorders, should exercise caution when using blue vervain, as it may affect these organs. It is advisable to consult with a healthcare professional before using blue vervain, especially if you are pregnant, breastfeeding, or have any pre-existing medical conditions.

As with any herbal remedy, allergic reactions are possible. If you experience any adverse effects or allergic symptoms, such as rash, itching, or difficulty breathing, discontinue use immediately and seek medical attention.

Comfrey

Lack Root, Blackwort, Bruisewort, Common Comfrey, Gum Plant, Healing Herb, Knitbone, Prickley Comfrey, Salsify, Slippery Root, Wallwort.

Symphytum officinale.

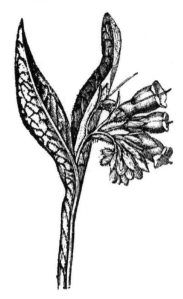

Identification: Blue vervain (Verbena cerulea) is a perennial plant that displays a remarkable growth habit. Its foliage emerges in spring, forming a basal rosette of leaves from which a sturdy, upright stem emerges, capable of reaching heights of 4 feet or more. The leaves of blue vervain are characterized by their wrinkled and rough texture, with the basal leaves exhibiting a more ovate shape, while the upper leaves are long and broadly lance-shaped, measuring between 8 to 12 inches in length. Atop the stem, clusters of pale purple to violet flowers grace the plant, arranged in dense, hanging cymes. These exquisite flowers feature a fused calyx with five distinct tips and a fused five-tipped corolla, adorned with a pentangular tube.

Medical Uses: Comfrey has a rich history of traditional uses among indigenous cultures worldwide. The leaves of this remarkable plant are often brewed into a soothing tea and incorporated into the diet of various indigenous communities. In Japan, comfrey is widely cultivated and pickled, although its consumption as a food is not recommended due to the presence of liver-toxic pyrrolizidine alkaloids, which are most concentrated in the roots of the plant. Externally, comfrey poultices have been applied to bruises, swellings, sprains, burns, and even to promote the healing of broken bones. The infusion of comfrey leaves, known as leaf tea, has been utilized to address ailments such as ulcers, hemorrhoids, bronchitis, and congestion. Notably, comfrey extract is approved by the Commission E for its effectiveness in treating blunt injuries. Scientific research has also revealed its anti-inflammatory properties, particularly in the context of rheumatism. Comfrey is classified as a mucilaginous and cooling herb, containing a compound called allantoin, which is believed to stimulate cell growth and is often found in wound-healing skin creams. Under medical supervision, the leaf tea is still employed to address chronic bronchial problems, ulcers, colitis, arthritis, and rheumatism. It is worth noting that allantoin extracted from comfrey is available as a separate product at pharmacies, providing a safer alternative to using the whole comfrey plant and avoiding potential exposure to toxins. Furthermore, clinically proven comfrey salve has demonstrated efficacy in alleviating pain and reducing swelling in muscles and joints.

Pollinators/Wildlife: Comfrey (Symphytum officinale) is not only a valuable plant for its medicinal uses but also a fantastic pollinator attractor. Its long tubular flowers, which only allow access to long-tongued insects, make it a favorite among pollinators. You can expect to see an array of buzzing visitors, including Garden Bumblebees (Bombus hortorum), Common Carder (Bombus pascuorum), Early Bumblebee (Bombus pratorum), and Buff-tailed Bumblebee (Bombus terrestris). These diligent bees play a vital role in the pollination of comfrey, aiding in its reproduction and supporting biodiversity in your garden or food forest.

However, it is important to note that recent research has discovered a potential concern for beekeepers. Bees that pollinate comfrey flowers have been found to carry trace amounts of toxic pyrrolizidine alkaloids back to their hives. These alkaloids can also be detected in honey derived from comfrey nectar. As a precaution, beekeepers may want to consider avoiding comfrey as a forage source for their bees to prevent the presence of these alkaloids in honey.

Nonetheless, for gardeners and permaculturists, comfrey remains a valuable addition due to its fertilizer capabilities. The plant's deep taproot absorbs nutrients from the soil and stores them in its leaves, which can be harvested and used as a nutrient-rich mulch or compost. This natural fertilizer enhances soil fertility and provides nourishment to surrounding plants, contributing to the overall health and productivity of your vegetable garden or food forest.

Medicinal parts: leaves, roots

Solvents: Boiling water, alcohol.

Hardiness Zones: Zones 3-9.

Sourcing: Comfrey (Symphytum officinale) is primarily a garden plant but can occasionally be found in the wild, where it has escaped to waste grounds and roadsides across the country. While it may not be commonly encountered in natural habitats, its adaptability allows it to thrive in various conditions, be it in shady areas or under full sun. One notable characteristic of comfrey is its aggressive and spreading nature, which can make it a resilient and fast-growing plant in the garden landscape.

For those interested in cultivating comfrey, it can be conveniently obtained from nurseries or herb cottages, where it is readily available for purchase.

Despite its reputation for being a garden plant, it is important to exercise caution when introducing comfrey to natural habitats or areas where it can potentially become invasive. Due to its vigorous growth and ability to self-seed, it has the potential to outcompete native plants and disrupt local ecosystems.

Gardening Tips: Comfrey is a low-maintenance plant that adapts well to a wide range of growth environments. Mature plants have a complex root system that includes a deep taproot. Those roots travel deep, break off easily, and new plants can sprout from remaining root bits — don't even think about rototilling it! This permits them to extract nutrients and moisture from the soil more efficiently. However, if you ever want to get rid of Comfrey plants, this makes it tough. So, plan carefully where you want to plant it, because once it's established, it's almost impossible to remove. As its leaves decay, it's a fantastic natural fertilizer and garden amendment. Plant it around fruit trees or cultivate a stand to chop and add to leaf mulch, compost piles, and make compost tea fertilizer. After you dig up a plant, any small bit of the root left in the soil will most certainly sprout a new plant. If you want to keep the plant from spreading too far, grow it in a container or raised garden bed rather than in the ground.

If you remove the wasted blooms as soon as possible, you can prevent the plant from distributing its seeds. Reblooming can also be induced by cutting down the stems after the plant has finished flowering. Comfrey, like all rapid plants, needs a lot of nitrogen to look good and flower well. As a result, it's critical to ensure that the soil contains enough organic matter. Apart from requiring water during long dry spells, Comfrey is usually self-sufficient.

Plants of the Comfrey family are generally free of pests and diseases. Comfrey rust, for example, can overwinter in the roots of the plant, weakening its growth and flowering. It is, however, uncommon in most locations. Slugs and snails can also wreak havoc on the plants, although deer tend to ignore them.

Comfrey may thrive in full sun to moderate shade, although on most days, it needs at least three hours of direct sunshine. Plant it where it will obtain protection from the hot afternoon sun in the hottest areas of its growing zones.

The plant may grow in a variety of soil types, including clay and somewhat sandy soil. It does, however, prefer organically rich, loamy soil with good drainage. It prefers a little acidic to neutral soil pH, but it may also survive slightly alkaline soil.

Comfrey plants prefer a consistent level of moisture in the soil. Once established, they can withstand some drought, although they like at least a modest amount of precipitation. Keep the soil of young plants moist but not waterlogged at all times when the top inch or two of soil begins to dry up, water mature plants.

Within its growing zones, Comfrey is resilient to both severely cold and extremely hot conditions. Once frost and freezing temperatures hit in the late fall, it will die back. The roots, however, will stay, and the plant will reappear in the spring. Comfrey doesn't mind being humidified as long as there's enough moisture in the soil.

The ideal way to feed Comfrey is to add organic amendments to the soil on a regular basis, such as a layer of compost in the spring. Comfrey's extensive roots are good at accessing deep nutrients in the soil, so it doesn't require any further feeding.

Comfrey can be grown from seed, but it needs to be chilled over the winter to germinate. It's also very uncommon for seeds to be sown and not germinate for two years. As a result, root cuttings are more commonly used to propagate the plant. Roots should be cut into 2- to 6-inch lengths and planted horizontally above 3 inches deep. Plant them deeper in sandy soil than in clay soil. Keep the soil moist (but not waterlogged) until you see signs of development.

Avoid cultivars, especially prickly comfrey, which has proven to be weedy and invasive.

Consumption Methods: Comfrey soothes with mucilaginous compounds as well as allantoin, which improves skin integrity. Comfrey rapidly heals wounds, sometimes too fast and not as well as calendula, St. John's wort, and gotu kola. I prefer to use comfrey on old scars, for aches, pains, bumps, bruises, and general skin health. Add it to rash and fungal formulas to promote skin healing and integrity. Use the fresh poultice on small burns and nettle stings for fast, soothing, cooling relief.

Even though we often make comfrey leaves into comfrey oil, its wound-healing constituent allantoin is more soluble in hot water. Make a decoction tincture using fresh or dried comfrey roots with a final 20 to 25 percent alcohol (comfrey's mucilage repels high-proof alcohol) — just an hour or two of simmering will do, no need to concentrate it down unless you want to. We call topical tinctures "liniments," and this should only be used topically because of comfrey root's potential liver toxicity when taken internally. Comfrey promotes rapid wound healing, helps with old scars, and eases aches and pains. I don't use it in deep wounds because it can trap in infection (it's not antimicrobial) and increase the scarring in new wounds (it's fast, not sophisticated). The liniment makes a great ingredient in calendula-comfrey cream (to heal rashes from eczema and other conditions) and in antifungal blends (to promote healing alongside herbs with direct antifungal activity like thuja and chaparral).

Comfrey also makes an extremely effective liquid fertilizer.

Warnings: Consumption or internal use of comfrey is not recommended due to the presence of liver-toxic pyrrolizidine alkaloids, which can cause serious harm.

Elecampane

Elfwort, Elfdock, Horseheal, Yellow Starwort.

Inula helenium.

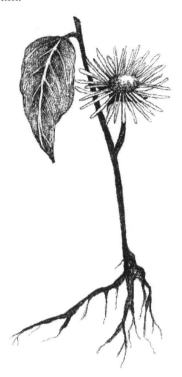

Identification: Elecampane is among the many wild sunflower relatives, but it has the distinction of producing unique aromatic medicinal roots. In the first year, the scrappy rosette with its large, flat leaves could easily be mistaken for a docklike weed. It looks completely different in its blooming years, reaching 4 to 7 feet tall with robust leaves and branching stalks of yellow blossoms. It prefers damp, rich loamy soil yet tolerates garden beds without irrigation.

Medical Uses: Elecampane, a powerful herb used in herbal medicine worldwide, has a rich history dating back to ancient Greece. Legend has it that Helen of Troy herself, as she embarked for Troy, held the vibrant yellow flowers of this shrub in her hands. Native to Southeastern Europe, elecampane made its way to North America with European colonists, where it was embraced by Native Americans, particularly the Iroquois Indians, who continue to use it as a cough remedy. Combined with comfrey root and spikenard root, elecampane has been employed by Native American herbalists to address lung and bronchial infections. In Contemporary Chinese Medicine, elecampane remains a popular treatment for respiratory problems. With its expectorant properties, elecampane facilitates the expulsion of deep-seated mucus from the lungs and boasts potent antiseptic and antibacterial effects. It has been effectively used to address chronic bronchitis, chronic asthma, and whooping cough, especially in cases characterized by yellow or green mucus. Elecampane is traditionally relied upon to promote productive coughing and the clearance of obstructed mucus, expediting the recovery process and restoring clear respiratory passages.

Carminative, warming bitter, antimicrobial.

Pollinators/Wildlife: Attracts bees, moths, and butterflies. It's pollinated mostly by *Inula royleana.*

Solvents: Boiling water, alcohol.

Hardiness Zones: Zones 4-9.

Sourcing: Elecampane may thrive in a variety of climates and temperatures, but it prefers warm summers and frigid winters. It thrives from the midwest to the eastern seaboard since it does not grow well in particularly hot and humid climates.

Gardening Tips: Elecampane needs a lot of space to grow, so space them out 12 to 30 inches apart. It's simple to cultivate from seed and can be divided once it's fully grown. Elecampane spreads by underground "runners" that carry both roots and upward-climbing shoots. Unlike many other rhizomatous plants, elecampane is a more muted spreader that rarely becomes invasive. It may self-seed and generate new plants from falling seeds in optimal conditions. Large plants can be divided every few years if desired.

Elecampane has minimal major insect and disease concerns, as one would expect from a plant that rapidly naturalizes.

Elecampane thrives in partial shade, although it can also thrive in full sun.

Elecampane does not require specific soil conditions as long as the land is well-drained. The plants may grow in a variety of soil types, including sand and clay. It's best to use a moist, semi-fertile loam.

Keep the soil moist but not wet by watering as needed. Elecampane does not require a specific watering schedule because it is a wildflower, but proper, thorough watering will assist in establishing healthy roots for harvesting.

Elecampane may thrive in a variety of climates and temperatures, but it prefers warm summers and frigid winters. It does not thrive in extremely hot and humid climates.

There's no need to use commercial fertilizers or flower food on elecampane blooms, and organic feeding is preferable if you wish to harvest the roots for medicinal purposes. In the spring, simply top-dress the soil with compost.

When using gathered herbs for medical purposes, exercise caution. Elecampane is commonly mixed with other herbs in commercial herbal formulations to make supplements that assist respiratory health. The roots are cleansed, diced, and utilized in teas or tinctures when used alone. However, there is evidence that consuming huge amounts of this plant might make you sick; therefore, it is not a plant to use lightly.

Harvest the roots of elecampane in the spring or fall, starting in the second year of the plant's life or later. It has a huge and sturdy taproot that must be dug up to be harvested. Because the roots and rhizomes form an octopus shape, dig a wide area to keep as much of the root as possible. A pitchfork can help loosen the soil without causing too much damage to the roots, but a shovel will suffice.

If desired, you can harvest the entire plant. Alternatively, if the plant is huge, you can divide it and harvest only a piece of the root and foliage growth. In any case, the foliage will have died back and isn't worth saving.

Cut off the foliage and thoroughly clean the roots after harvesting the plant. Hand-squeeze the root's stiff outer layer to break it apart, then peel it away to reveal the clean, white interior. As desired, prepare the inside of the root.

After harvesting the root, propagate elecampane with cuttings in the fall. Choose a healthy root that is about 2 inches long and has a bud or eye on it. Each cutting should be planted about 12 inches deep and at least 12 inches apart. Ensure that the area is well-watered until the earth freezes. Water sparingly in the spring to keep the soil moist. In two years, the resulting plant should be ready to harvest.

Elecampane seeds are simple to grow. If sowing in the garden, wait until all risk of frost has passed before planting. Alternatively, a few weeks before the final frost, you can plant them indoors, in a greenhouse, or in a cold frame. Because the seeds require sunshine to germinate, sow them on the surface or under a thin layer of soil that allows sunlight to pass through. Keep the soil moist at all times. In around two weeks, the seeds should germinate. Once the seedlings have sprouted two sets of leaves, transplant them to the garden.

Consumption Methods: Elecampane has a potent, complex flavor with bitter, aromatic/perfumey, balsam, and pungent notes. In the respiratory system, it moves mucus, warms and opens the lungs, and fights infections, particularly in cold, stagnant, congested states. Perfect for cough syrup.

Although best known as a lung herb, elecampane also makes a superb digestive bitter, stimulating digestion while fighting chronic dysbiosis and intestinal infections. It has a unique reputation as a warming bitter (most bitters, like artichoke leaf, are considered energetically cold). It also contains inulin, a starch that feeds beneficial bacteria. Elecampane can be added to animal feed as an antimicrobial and deworming agent.

Warnings: Few side effects are recorded; however, dizziness has been noted in some when taking larger doses. This is not a plant for high doses, which may cause nausea, yet it is quite safe in low to moderate amounts. People with gastric irritation or who are already hot and dry may not be a good fit for elecampane unless it is formulated with cool, moist herbs like mullein or marshmallow.

Evening Primrose

Evening Star, Sundrop, Weedy Evening Primrose, German Rampion, Hog Weed, King's Cure-All And Fever-Plant.

Oenothera.

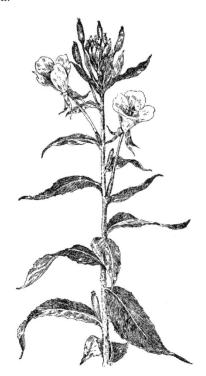

Medical Uses: Evening Primrose, a versatile plant, offers edible components throughout its various parts. Native Americans in Utah and Nevada consumed the seeds as a food source, while the young leaves were enjoyed either raw or cooked as a potherb. To mitigate bitterness, boiling the leaves in multiple changes of water was a common practice. The nut-flavored roots of Evening Primrose were highly valued in English and German gardens as early as 1614, where they were boiled akin to parsnips. English settlers in America later introduced Evening Primrose seeds to the British Isles. Notably, the plant's resemblance to rampion, a bellflower with edible roots and basal leaves, prompted its reintroduction to North America in the mid-nineteenth century, where it was known as German rampion and utilized as a vegetable. Additionally, Evening Primrose held medicinal significance among Native Americans. The Ojibwa poulticed the entire plant to alleviate bruising, while the Cherokee brewed a tea from the root to aid in weight loss. The Forest Potawatomi considered the seeds a valuable remedy, although detailed records of their specific uses have been lost. European settlers in the eighteenth century also recognized the medicinal properties of Evening Primrose. The leaves or roots were applied externally to promote wound healing, and a tea derived from the leaves and roots was employed to soothe upset stomachs.

Check out the second volume for more information.

Pollinators/Wildlife: Evening Primroses, known for their enchanting fragrance, have developed a fascinating relationship with various pollinators. Hawkmoths and bees, including Sweat bees and others, diligently assist in the pollination of the plant's flowers. However, Evening Primroses also have an intriguing connection with parasitic moths, whose caterpillars feed on the blossoms and seeds. This unique symbiotic relationship has likely played a significant role in the evolutionary process of the primrose, which boasts over 400 species in the United States alone. Alongside these interactions, the plant attracts moths such as the Little Glassywing, contributing to its diverse ecological impact. Furthermore, the seeds of Evening Primroses serve as a delightful addition to bird feeders, attracting an array of feathered friends, including finches, sparrows, and various other avian species. Eastern Goldfinches, in particular, hold a special fondness for this plant, benefiting from the abundance of seeds it generously provides.

Solvents: Boiling water, alcohol.

Hardiness Zones: Zones 4-9.

Sourcing: This plant, which is native to Missouri, Nebraska, Kansas, Oklahoma, Texas, and Mexico, thrives in barren soil with little water and full light.

Evening Primrose grows well in hot weather and tolerates drought. It blooms in pink, pale lavender, or white and pink and grows 18 to 24 inches tall. You can find Primrose anywhere amongst wildflowers, but particularly so in the southwest.

Gardening Tips: If the invasive nature of Evening Primrose doesn't dissuade you (not to mention the fact that you'll be sleeping while its lovely blossoms are out), you're in luck because this herbaceous perennial can be grown by even the most inexperienced gardeners. Your Evening Primrose plants will thrive as long as you provide them with lots of sunshine and well-draining soil.

Evening Primrose plants, in addition to being a lovely, vivid addition to your garden or landscape, have a long history in the medical world; several of the plant's common names, such as cure-all or fever plant, allude to these holistic benefits. It was first found by Native Americans, who used it to cure wounds and skin disorders (such as sunburn or eczema), and then by Europeans, who used it to treat asthma, whooping cough, and other ailments. It's most typically found as a herbal supplement or oil these days, and it's used to treat skin problems as well as pain from conditions like multiple sclerosis and rheumatoid arthritis. The blossoms are edible, both fresh and cooked, and are frequently used in salads.

Evening Primrose, contrary to popular belief, is a sun-loving plant that only blooms at night (which makes it ideal for moon gardens). It should be planted in full sunlight (or partial shade) and in a location where the plant may get at least six to eight hours of warm sunlight per day.

Another important prerequisite for successful Evening Primrose cultivation is well-drained soil. It should, however, retain moisture rather than becoming waterlogged. Consider covering the soil with a heavy layer of mulch to help keep the roots cool during the summer.

Evening Primrose thrives with regular watering and may require a little more if cultivated in a particularly hot region during the summer. If you observe any yellowing or browning on your Evening Primrose's numerous leaves, it's a sure sign that it's getting too much water and is likely suffering from root rot or a fungal disease.

Even though it blooms and grows best in the summer, Evening Primrose loves cooler temperatures. In order to flower successfully in the summer, the plant must become established (i.e., produce roots and foliage) during the chilly early spring months. Early in its life, too much heat might cause the plant to become leggy or look like a weed.

Fertilizer is not required as part of your Evening Primrose care regimen; it will thrive without it. If you're working with exceptionally terrible soil, however, you can add some organic material to your mix.

Evening Primrose is normally produced from seed, and while seeds may be purchased online, seeds can also be collected from wild plants growing along the roadside or in public gardens. Once you have your Evening Primrose seeds, plant them in the fall or early spring in an area with full sun and previously cultivated soil. Sow the seeds on top of the soil and give them plenty of water. After the seedlings have germinated, thin them down to about one foot apart.

Evening Primrose does not flower in its first year of life, instead of producing a green rosette at ground level. In the second year, a long, stiff blossom stem emerges from the base. Secondary branching occurs around halfway up this flower stem, and the leaves get smaller as you travel higher up the flower stalk. The four-petaled blooms, which appear at the beginning of summer, are about an inch wide. They'll eventually die and generate seeds, which will be dispersed across the area by weather conditions or eaten by wild birds.

Varieties Evening Primrose leaves are eaten by beetles, but they don't inflict enough harm to kill the plant. Aside from mealybugs, spider mites, and aphids, you may expect to see a variety of other common garden pests on a regular basis. If your plants show signs of infection, use insecticidal soap or oil like neem oil to treat them.

Consumption Methods: Evening primrose oil is great for treating PMS

Warnings: Primrose overdoses can cause gastric upset. Use in moderation.

Goldenrod

Common Goldenrod, Canada Goldenrod.

Solidago Rugosa.

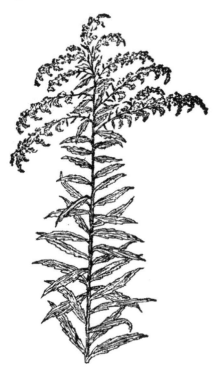

Medical Uses: Goldenrod is a widely distributed plant. It can be found throughout Europe, Asia, North Africa, and North America, among other continents. Goldenrod is a flower that grows in a number of states. It is Kentucky's state flower. There are over a hundred species of the flower, with about thirty of them found in Kentucky Goldenrod has traditionally been used to treat a variety of ailments: a carminative for digestion, gas, and bloating; a mild antimicrobial for respiratory and urinary infections; an anti-inflammatory; a diuretic for hypertension formulas; a rich source of bioflavonoids for blood vessel health; and more. The genus name Soledago means "to make whole." It's been used to treat wounds, diabetes, and tuberculosis, among other things. It is now mostly utilized to aid with the body's water loss. The leaves are used to treat a variety of ailments. They may be dried and used to make a tea that has been shown to have relaxing properties. It's been used to alleviate depression and stress. Check out the second volume for more information.

Pollinators/Wildlife: Goldenrod is a one-stop shop for all kinds of pollinators. It is a major resource for honeybees, but also long-horned bees, sweat bees, bumble bees, and several types of digger bees which are more active in the fall. A research conducted in New England showed that there are 11 species of solitary bees that specialize in goldenrod. They also attract monarch butterflies.

Quite astoundingly tall goldenrods have a defensive behavior that no other plant has showed which has prove quite effective against insect pests: instead of developing chemical toxins like many other plants, the emerging buds nod downward when the flies approach to lay gall-inducing eggs, they literally duck to avoid them! They most likely sense the mate-attracting pheromones of the flies, but it is not yet quite clear how they do it.

Solvents: Boiling water, alcohol.

Hardiness Zones: Zones 3-9.

Sourcing: This vibrant and resilient plant is commonly found in meadows, fields, prairies, and along roadsides throughout North America, including the United States, Canada, and Mexico. It flourishes in a range of habitats, from sunny open areas to woodland edges and even disturbed sites. Goldenrod's adaptability allows it to grow in different soil types, including dry, sandy, or loamy soils.

To source goldenrod, one can explore the countryside, parks, nature reserves, or even their own backyard, depending on the region. In the eastern and central parts of North America, such as the Appalachian Mountains, Great Lakes region, and the Midwest, goldenrod is abundant. In the western regions, it can be found in the Rocky Mountains, Great Plains, and along the Pacific Coast.

During the late summer and early fall, goldenrod displays its vibrant yellow flowers, making it easier to spot. Look for clusters of tall, erect stems adorned with densely packed blossoms. Be cautious when harvesting goldenrod, as it may grow alongside other plant species, including those with similar-looking flowers. It is essential to correctly identify goldenrod to ensure proper sourcing.

While goldenrod can be sourced from the wild, it's important to practice sustainable foraging and respect local regulations. When gathering goldenrod, only take what you need and be mindful of the plant's role in supporting pollinators and wildlife. If unsure about the legality or sustainability of harvesting goldenrod in a specific area, it is advisable to seek guidance from local conservation authorities or consult with experienced herbalists or foragers.

Gardening Tips: If you're looking to enhance your garden with a plant that offers numerous benefits and easy care, consider incorporating goldenrod. Opt for tall goldenrod or zigzag goldenrod and mix it with rough blazingstar for a stunning color display. These plants attract migrating butterflies and bees with their nectar, encouraging pollination in your garden and keeping pests away from your prized produce. Not only do I adore goldenrod for its many advantages, but also for its vibrant blooms and delightful fragrance.

Goldenrod is a magnet for beneficial insects, which in turn can help deter harmful pests as they seek out the plant's food source. These self-seeding wonders require minimal water and can thrive without the need for fertilizer. With over a hundred different types available, including many indigenous to the United States, there's a goldenrod variety for every environment. These clump-forming perennials add a golden glow to your landscape, blooming with magnificent yellow flowers in late summer and fall.

Growing goldenrod is a breeze as it adapts to various conditions, although it thrives best in full sun. It can tolerate different soil types as long as the soil is well-draining. Once established, goldenrod requires little maintenance and returns year after year. It's drought-tolerant, reducing the need for regular watering. Every four to five years, it's advisable to divide the clumps to maintain their vitality. In spring, you can easily obtain cuttings and plant them in your garden to expand the goldenrod's presence.

Not only does goldenrod bring beauty to your landscape, but it also acts as a beacon for butterflies and beneficial insects. By incorporating this remarkable plant into your garden, you're creating a harmonious ecosystem while enjoying its stunning display of colors.

Consumption Methods: Goldenrod offers fantastic antihistamine and mucus-thinning and -moving properties for allergies, sinus congestion, and sinus infections. Harvest the tops just as they're beginning to bloom. Use the flowers in combination with tulsi to make a mild tea to protect from allergic reactions. A liniment made from leaves and flowers can be applied to wounds. Check the second and third volume for more.

Warnings: Goldenrod is a herb that must be taken in moderation. It may produce major adverse effects such as excessive perspiration, nausea, vomiting, diarrhea, tremors, rapid heartbeat, and confusion if overdosed. You may think it is the reason for your hay fever due to its thick pollen, but the real culprit is ragweed which blooms at the same time.

Goldenseal

Berberine, Eye Balm, Eye Root, Goldenroot, Ground Raspberry, Hydrastis Canadensis, Indian Plant, Jaundice Root, Orange Root, Yellow Root.

Hydrastis canadensis.

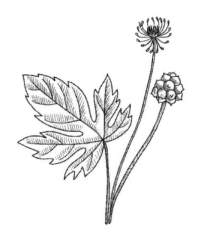

Medical Uses: Goldenseal was a multi-purpose medicinal plant utilized by Native Americans. It was used by the Cherokees to heal skin disorders and painful eyes, and a powder prepared from the root was mixed with bear fat to make an insect repellant. It was also used as a diuretic, stimulant, and cancer treatment.

Goldenseal was traditionally utilized by Native Americans in general to treat skin diseases, ulcers, fevers, and other ailments. It was embraced as a medicinal herb by European settlers, who used it to treat a range of ailments. Check out the second volume for its traditional and modern uses.

Pollinators/Wildlife: Small polylactic bees and small flies tend to favor the blooms of this plant, especially *Dialictus* and *Evylaeus,* but also Syrphid flies and some larger bees. The fruits are inedible for humans but tasty food for all sort of birds, especially Red-winged Blackbirds who also act as seed disperser.

Solvents: Boiling water, alcohol.

Hardiness Zones: Zones 3-8.

Sourcing: Goldenseal grows from southern Quebec to northern Georgia and west to Missouri. It's native in rich, heavily shaded deciduous forests. Reproduces clonally via rhizomes that can be find in the wild, but should preferably be sourced from reputable seed savers or local nurseries. They are overharvested for its medical uses and at risk due to development and logging. Avoid foraging, it's a great option for cultivation.

Gardening Tips: Goldenseal, a valuable medicinal plant, thrives in rich, wet, loamy soil with a pH ranging from 5.5 to 6.5. Excellent water drainage is essential, as Goldenseal does not tolerate soggy conditions. Growers often choose slightly sloped areas to ensure proper water flow. For cultivation in open areas, shade structures such as wood lath frameworks or polypropylene shade structures are recommended to provide the necessary 70 to 75 percent shade. Forest culture can benefit from tall hardwood trees like basswood, hickory, tulip poplar, or white oak, which provide natural shade along with companion plants like Black Cohosh, Bloodroot, ginseng, mayapple, and trillium. Raised beds are particularly useful for clay-rich soils, and adding compost or organic material improves soil fertility. If the soil pH is below 5.5, lime application can help stimulate growth, while rock phosphate is suitable for soils deficient in phosphorus. Nitrogen requirements can generally be met with organic products like compost.

It's important to avoid areas where soilborne diseases have previously caused issues to ensure the health of Goldenseal plants. Propagation can be done through rhizome fragments, root cuttings, or seeds. To grow from seeds, ripe fruits should be harvested and mashed, allowing the seeds and pulp to ferment in water until they can be separated. Ensuring the seeds remain moist is crucial throughout this process. After cleaning and rinsing, sow the seeds one-quarter to one-half inch deep in a shady nursery bed, spacing them 1 to 2 inches apart and covering with leaf mulch to prevent soil drying. Germination of Goldenseal seeds can be slow and irregular, sometimes taking up to two seasons.

Rhizome pieces are the most common and reliable method of propagation. Cut the rhizomes into half-inch or larger pieces, ensuring each piece has at least one large bud and intact fibrous roots. Plant the rhizome pieces just below the soil surface, with the bud pointing upright in a well-prepared bed. Rows should be spaced 6 to 12 inches apart, with 6-inch spacing between rhizome pieces. Mulching the area with hardwood leaves or crushed bark helps retain moisture and control weeds. Before plants sprout in spring, the mulch should be scraped back to a depth of 1 to 2 inches.

Regardless of the chosen propagation method, it is crucial to keep the beds weed-free, especially during the initial years of establishment. Effective weed management is essential for the successful growth of Goldenseal plants.

Consumption Methods: As a bitter, goldenseal and other berberines stimulate digestive juices and improve gastric function, but they have the additional benefit as antimicrobials that are particularly well suited to fight intestinal infections, chronic diarrhea, dysbiosis, and small intestinal bacterial overgrowth. Check out the second and third volume for more uses and recipes.

Warnings: Goldenseal is known to be totally safe at moderate dosage.

Hepatica

Common Hepatica, Liverwort, Kidneywort, Pennywort.

Hepatica nobilis var. *obtusa.*

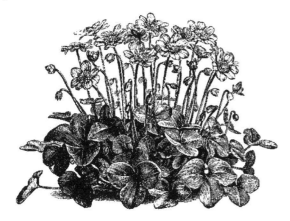

Identification: Hepatica, a small perennial plant that can reach a height of up to 5 feet, exhibits distinctive characteristics. It features basal leaves that remain evergreen, providing year-round interest. The differentiation between the two species, H. nobilis var. acuta and H. nobilis var. obtusa, is determined by the shape of their leaves. The former displays sharp lobes, while the latter showcases round lobes. When stems and leaves emerge, they are covered in fine hairs. The flowers of H. var. acuta bloom in shades of violet to blue, while H. var. obtusa produces whitish blossoms, each adorned with six to ten sepals. Commonly known as American liverwort, this charming plant is among the first to bloom in the spring, typically gracing gardens with its vibrant display in March or April.

Traditional Uses: The plant was named for its previous use as a liver cure, and its ingredients include pharmacologically active flavonoids and saponins. Abdominal pains, poor digestion, constipation, and gynecological concerns were all treated using native species by Native Americans.

Hepatica was used in a variety of ways by Native Americans. Cherokees, Chippewas (Ojibwa), Iroquois, Menominis, Potawatomis, and Sac and Fox were among the tribes who employed this herb. The plant was used to purify the blood. Tea made from the roots and leaves was used to alleviate vertigo, coughs, and sore throats. Root tea was used to cure children's convulsions as well as diarrhea. Coughs were relieved by chewing the roots.

Poor digestion and constipation were treated with leaf tea. Tea was also used to heal abnormalities like twisted jaws and crossed eyes as a wash. Hemorrhoids were treated with a poultice made from the plant.

H. nobilis var. obtusa, in particular, was infused and utilized as an emetic, laxative, and even as an abortifacient. The infusion of H. var. obtusa was believed to have contraceptive effects. The Menominee tribe employed leaf infusions and root decoctions to address issues such as diarrhea and vertigo. Additionally, the liver-like appearance of the leaves led to the belief, following the Doctrine of Signatures, that hepatica could be used to treat liver problems. Folk practitioners would administer small amounts of the roots and leaves to alleviate indigestion, as well as disorders of the kidney, gallbladder, and liver. Another variety, sharp-lobed hepatica (H. nobilis var. acuta), was used in decoctions to aid digestion and alleviate labor pain in pregnant women. It was also regarded as a tonic and blood purifier. The decoction was employed as a uterine stimulant to induce childbirth, while the infusion was utilized to alleviate abdominal pain and as an emetic and laxative. In fact, in 1884, hepatica was considered one of the most widely used "medicinal" herbs. Hepatica was employed as a love potion by some tribes. The female would dust her love interest's garments with powder made from dried leaves. To "bewitch" their desired love interests, some females chewed on the herb.

Hepatitis was utilized as a good luck charm by other tribes. The roots were planted near or on fur-bearing animal traps. The roots were also thought to have the ability to predict fortunes.

Modern uses: Still used by herbalists to cure liver disorders, especially gallstones.

Tonic, Demulcent, De-obstruent, Mild Mucilaginous, Astringent.

Pollinators/Wildlife: The bright flowers white to deep-blue violet attract pollinators early in the blooming season. They are the spring harbingers in the North American woodlands. They attract mostly dipteras and solitary bees. However, because Hepatica can self-pollinate, these visitors aren't required to generate seeds, which is important when pollinators are hampered by cold weather.

Solvents: Boiling water, alcohol.

Medicinal Part: The whole plant

Hardiness Zones: Zones 4-9.

Sourcing: Hepatica is a tiny evergreen herb that grows in rich woodlands from Minnesota to Maine and north to Alabama. The flowers are most typically blue or lavender, though white versions, especially in southern locations, and various colors of pink may be seen. They thrive in a variety of climatic zones.

Gardening Tips: Round-lobed hepaticas, one of the first wildflowers to bloom each spring, are botanical gems native across the Northern Hemisphere. The variation in flower colors and leaf patterns these diminutive plants offer makes them beloved and increasingly popular perennials—hepaticas are on the verge of becoming mainstream in U.S. gardens and landscapes, seen everywhere from containers to woodland and rock gardens to perennial border edges. In the wild, round-lobed hepatica is usually found in more sandy, acidic soils; however, it is tolerant of a range of soil types and pH levels in cultivation. Its flowers are virtually identical to those of sharp-lobed hepatica. The leaves are similarly three-parted but with rounded lobes, and they retain a fuzzier look through the season, sometimes showing an imaginative array of burgundy and silver patterning that is unmatched by any evergreen woodland perennial.

The early spring flowers of the sharp-lobed hepatica are something to look forward to; young plants will produce only a few flowers, but a mature clump can be crowned with them. The three-parted leaves with pointed tips are liver-shaped (hence liverleaf, another common name). The leaves are evergreen but usually turn burgundy in winter. This is a premier plant for an open shady woodland garden or edge of a woodland perennial border. As it grows just 6 inches tall, it's best displayed on rock walls or outcrops and planted with diminutive companions like moss, sedges, and smaller ferns. It makes a prime container plant for shade. Cultivate sharp-lobed hepatica in moist, shaded sites in calcareous soils. Larger plants can be divided. Hepatica thrives in moderate to full shade and makes a great specimen plant for under and around trees or in forest settings. This plant prefers well-drained soil, although, in low-lying locations, it may withstand wet soil. Only a few plants can withstand heavy soils as well as liverleaf Hepatica. They're one of the easiest plants to grow in this book.

In the summer, sow seeds for blooming the following spring. Summer planting helps the plant to establish itself before winter sets in and store nutrients for next year's flowers. Hepatica plant care is rarely required once it has been planted, especially if proper Hepatica growing conditions have been given. After the flowers have faded, separate the clumps of plants that have multiplied to propagate them and add them to another area of your garden.

Consumption Methods: Tea or tincture. Use in moderation. It may cause dermatitis externally.

Warnings: When used by mouth, it can produce a variety of adverse effects, including diarrhea, stomach discomfort, and renal and urinary system inflammation. Fresh liverwort can cause discomfort, itching, and pus-filled blisters when applied directly to the skin. If applying topically, perform a patch test first.

Lady's Slipper Orchid

Moccasin Flower, Camel's Foot, Squirrel Foot, Steeple Cap,
Venus' Shoes, Whippoorwill Shoe.

Cypripedium.

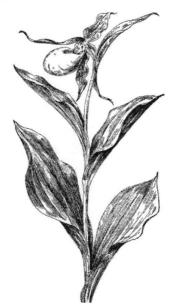

Medical Uses: Fevers, headaches, menstrual cramps, and labor pains were all treated using Lady Slippers by Native Americans. The Yellow Lady Slipper, Cypripedium parviflorum, was the most popular species, with Cherokees in Georgia and Ojibwe in Canada all favoring it. The Pink Lady Slipper was also utilized by the Wisconsin Menominee and the Northeast Penobscots. The orchid's greatest characteristic, though, was its ability to soothe, which European-descended settlers learned to value.

Insomnia, anxiety, and overall emotional tension were treated with tinctures of Lady Slipper roots. In the fall or early spring, Native Americans would gather the roots, dry them, and grind them into a powder. They generally used some sort of alcohol instead of water because many of the active compounds didn't dissolve in it. Check out the second volume for more information

Pollinators/Wildlife: Lady Slippers can be a bit devious. Pollination is required for Lady Slippers. Bees are drawn inside the flower pouch through the front slit by the beautiful color and delicious aroma of the flower. Once inside, the bees discover that there is no reward and that they are confined with only one way out, no reward for the bee, but plenty of pollination for the flower. They are pollinated by megachilid bees, but also other bees, wasps, and ants, as well as moths, flies, and butterflies who are all susceptible to its deception. They also attract a non-native butterfly, the European skipper, who get trapped in the flower and prevents pollination, which might be one of the reason for this beautiful flower quick demise.

Solvents: Alcohol.

Hardiness Zones: Zones 2-5.

Sourcing: This orchid thrives in forested or open marshes and moist forests, forming enormous clumps in limy environments at low to moderate elevation, making them easier to find in the bogs of the Midwest and eastern states. They are an endangered species, do not, under any circumstance harvest it. Buy only from reputable sources.

Gardening Tips: While Lady Slipper is rare in the wild and difficult to grow, with the right care and conditions, it is feasible to grow this cool-climate orchid in the garden.

Dig a hole twice as big (or more) as the Showy Lady Slipper's root ball, whether planting in a shadier yard or a rock garden. Work the mixture into the earth you dug out of the hole. Place the plant over the hole and hold it there. Allow the orchid's base to be level with or just below the ground level. Fill with the potting soil. Firmly pack. Only use enough of the potting mix to support the orchid's base.

Plant Lady Slipper orchids in partial shade or dappled sunlight. Replicate natural habitat conditions such as circumneutral peatlands or sunny openings in mossy woodlands found from Newfoundland to North Dakota and Manitoba and south to Georgia in the Appalachians.

This orchid flourishes in moist deciduous forests and rocky outcroppings with rich organic soil that is likely alkaline or limestone-based. Plants can thrive in a pH range from acidic to neutral.

Give this orchid well-drained soil, as with all Cypripedium species. Allow it to thrive in a consistently damp, humus-rich habitat, and it will blossom into a jewel in any forest garden.

Each time you water, make sure the soil is well saturated. Then, before watering again, let the top two inches of the plant dry off.

Feed it an orchid fertilizer or one with organic elements like fish emulsion. Throughout the growing season, apply every two weeks.

Working a time-release fertilizer into the soil at the start of the growing season is another approach to feed the Lady Slipper. It's important not to over-fertilize the plant because this can harm it.

Don't try to pull a wild Lady Slipper out of the ground. The wild populations of this orchid have drastically reduced as a result of people collecting it in its native habitat. Because plants take 15 years to flower, they take a long time to reappear after being uprooted.

Plants dug up in the wild are also noted for not surviving as well as store-bought specimens, and they've been difficult to cultivate until the late 1990s when researchers improved their understanding of the small seeds borne on the plant's upcoming fruits.

It's better if the seeds are planted at least two inches deep. If you're dividing by rhizome, do it cautiously in the early to mid-spring and then transplant with part of the soil from the root ball right away. Plants that are properly cared for can survive for up to 50 years.

If you're going to plant in a container, choose one that's just big enough to accommodate the growing roots for two years. Make sure the bottom and sides of the pot have drainage holes. Allow extra water to drain when watering.

One part perlite, one part charcoal, three parts coarse sand, and three parts peat can be used. Add a small amount of water until the soil is damp but not wet.

Keep an eye out for slugs and snails. To avoid infection, remove any additional mulch or leaves. To keep snails and slugs away from the orchid, fill a shallow pan halfway with beer and place it in the ground nearby.

Rust, gray mold (Botrytis), and Cercospora leaf spots can all be seen on the Lady Slipper. When the orchid is dry, remove the affected leaves, clean up any dirt around the base, and, if necessary, use a professional leaf spot cure.

Consumption Methods: You may make a tincture with the plant, but it is better if you leave it alone and take comfort in its beauty.

Warnings: Most warn that Lady Slipper may cause mild skin irritant effects such as redness, itching, and breakouts if bare skin is exposed to it for a prolonged amount of time.

Lily of the Valley

May Bells, Our Lady's Tears, Mary's Tears.

Convallaria Majalis.

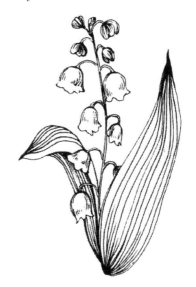

Identification: Lily of the valley is an extraordinary perennial herbaceous plant that showcases a captivating display of foliage and flowers. Its basal leaves are gracefully shaped, oval, and smooth, with a vibrant medium to dark green hue. These leaves, which measure 5-10" in length and 3-5" in width, exhibit a slight glaucous sheen and lack any hair. Emerging amidst the foliage is a charming raceme of flowers, typically ranging from 4-9" in length. The raceme, though shorter than the leaves, elegantly curves and showcases 6-16 exquisite blossoms. Each flower boasts a bell-shaped corolla, approximately 1/3" in both length and width, adorned with 6 dainty lobes that gracefully arch outward. The blooming period, a delight for the senses, spans about 3 weeks from late spring to early summer, during which the flowers emit a captivating fragrance. To ensure the development of its distinctive red berries, measuring 6-8 mm in diameter and containing a few minuscule seeds, successful cross-pollination is required from genetically distinct plants. Beneath the surface, the plant's rootstalk manifests as a fibrous and rhizomatous structure. This robust rootstalk gives rise to dense colonies of clonal plants, forming an interconnected network of rhizomes that often dominate the surrounding landscape, outcompeting other plant species in their vicinity.

Medical Uses: Heart disorders, such as heart failure and irregular heartbeat, are treated with lily-of-the-valley. It's also used to treat UTIs, kidney stones, labor contractions that aren't strong enough, epilepsy, fluid retention (edema), strokes with paralysis, eye infections (conjunctivitis), and leprosy.

Convallotoxin, convallatoxol, convalloside, convalloside, convalloside, convalloside, convalloside, convalloside, convallarin, glucoconvalloside, and convallamarin have comparable effects to digitalis, but the effect is less cumulative, making it safer for senior patients.

Pollinators/Wildlife: The Lily of the Valley blooms in May, and the blossoms have a strong, sweet perfume that attracts honeybees and bumblebees, which pollinate the plant, but not always get nectar in return.

Solvents: Boiling water, alcohol.

Hardiness Zones: Zones 3-9.

Sourcing: Lily of the Valley is recognized for its beautiful white, bell-shaped blossoms and incomparable scent. This shade-loving plant is also hardy and dependable ground cover that may be found practically anywhere in the United States due to the fact it only truly requires some water and decent shade.

Gardening Tips: Once planted, this plant requires minimal effort to thrive. During dry spells, make sure to water. Also, if elder plants' flowering has slowed, it's generally a good idea to dig them up and divide them to stimulate new development. Replant them in an area where they will have more room. They make for an excellent groundcover since the rhizomes reproduce clonally.

Plant Lily of the Valley in a sunny or shady location. The plant can tolerate direct morning sunlight, but it need cover from the intense afternoon sun. Full shade is best if you dwell in a warmer portion of its growing zones.

Lily of the Valley prefers organically rich, well-drained soil. It may, however, grow in a variety of soil conditions, including clay. It prefers soil that is acidic to neutral in pH, but it may even survive slightly alkaline soil.

This plant prefers damp soil that isn't too wet. When the soil begins to dry out due to a lack of rain or hot weather, water it. The plant's growth and blossoming will be hampered if the soil is too dry.

Lily of the Valley prefers mild weather with a moderate amount of humidity. The optimum temperatures are between 60 and 70 degrees Fahrenheit. In dry, hot regions, the plant does not thrive. It may also die back during the hottest summer months, even in temperate areas. However, this usually does not kill the plant, and it will usually come back the next spring.

Unless you have poor soil, the Lily of the Valley doesn't require fertilizer. In the spring, if your soil is lacking in nutrients, you can use an organic slow-release granular fertilizer.

Consumption Methods: You can make it into teas, tinctures, salves, oils, and liniments, which are also quite fragrant. They are perfect cut-flowers for tiny bouquets to scent the house in May and June.

Warnings: Lily of the valley contains potent cardiac glycosides, including convallatoxin and convallarin, which can be highly toxic if ingested. These compounds have a strong effect on the heart and can lead to severe cardiac arrhythmias, decreased heart rate, and even heart failure. It is crucial to avoid consuming any parts of the Lily of the valley plant, as it can pose a significant risk to human health. In case of accidental ingestion or contact, seek immediate medical attention.

Lobelia

Blue Cardinal Flower, Cardinal Flower, Indian Tobacco, Lobelia.

Lobelia erinus.

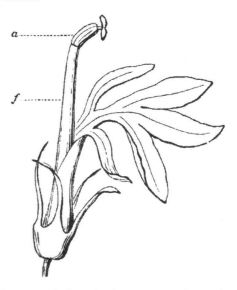

Medical Uses: Lobelia, also known as Indian tobacco, has a rich medicinal history specifically in the treatment of respiratory conditions such as asthma, bronchitis, pneumonia, and cough. Native Americans traditionally smoked Lobelia to alleviate symptoms of asthma. During the 19th century, American physicians frequently used Lobelia to induce vomiting, earning it the nickname "puke weed" due to its emetic properties. Today, Lobelia is recognized for its ability to help clear mucus from the respiratory tract, including the throat, lungs, and bronchial tubes. Although limited scientific research exists on Lobelia, some herbalists incorporate it into comprehensive asthma treatment plans. The active compound in Lobelia, lobeline, was once considered to have a similar effect on the body as nicotine. Consequently, lobeline was utilized as a substitute for nicotine in various anti-smoking treatments and aids designed to assist individuals in quitting smoking.

Lobelia was used extensively by Native American peoples in their ceremonies, much like tobacco, as a Ceremonial (Emetic) in religious rites by several Native American tribes. The plant was thought to be able to ward against storms when smoked. It was also used in rain dances and placed on gravestones. The herb was also utilized by Native Americans to make love potions and as an antidote to such love charms. The Lobelia has practical purposes as well; it was frequently burned to keep gnats away from a location. An infusion of the plant was used to induce vomiting and to treat tobacco or whiskey addictions, as well as as a love or anti-love medicine. To counteract sickness caused by witchcraft, an infusion of the herb was taken. Some native North American Indian tribes thought that if the finely crushed roots were hidden in the food of an arguing couple, they would fall in love again. Long before Samuel Thomson, who is credited with its discovery, the plant was known to the Penobscot Indians and was commonly used in New England. Check out the second volume for more uses.

Pollinators/Wildlife: Hummingbirds, bumblebees, and other long-tongued bees are drawn to the nectar and pollen of the blooms. Due to the depth of the nectar storage, it takes a long-nose pollinator to enjoy the Lobelia flower. Blue lobelia attracts sweat bees, small carpenter bees, yellow-faced bees, and bumble bees.

Solvents: Boiling water, alcohol.

Hardiness Zones: Zones 10-11.

Sourcing: Lobelia, both the annual and perennial varieties, is a versatile plant that can be found in a wide range of locations. Annual Lobelia seeds can be sown directly in the garden or started indoors for later transplantation. These plants thrive in full sun but can tolerate partial shade in certain circumstances. They prefer moist and nutrient-rich soil for optimal growth. Lobelia is a common sight in the prairies and roadside ditches across the United States, showcasing its adaptability. This diverse plant species can be found from coast to coast, with variations in size and abundance depending on the region. In the western mountains, high-altitude Lobelia species are smaller in size and commonly found near or above the tree line in the Sierras and Coastal Ranges. If you wish to introduce Lobelia to your garden, L. siphilitica can be easily transplanted to a moist, semi-shaded area, providing a beautiful addition to your landscape.

Gardening Tips: Annual Lobelia can be found in almost any place. Lobelia seeds can be planted directly in the garden or brought inside to be transplanted later. These plants like full sun but will take partial shade in some cases. They also prefer soil that is moist and nutritious. Start inside around 10 to 12 weeks before your region's latest frost date.

Water thoroughly after scattering the tiny seeds on top of the soil. Place them in a well-lit, warm environment. Within a week or two, the seedlings should emerge, and you may begin thinning them out. Transplant the plants to the garden once the threat of frost has passed and they are at least 2 to 3 inches (5-7.5 cm) tall, spacing them approximately 4 to 6 inches (10-15 cm) apart.

The Lobelia plant is low-maintenance once it is established. During hot, dry months, however, Lobelia care necessitates frequent watering, especially for those grown in containers. If desired, a general-purpose liquid fertilizer can be used once a month or once every four to six weeks.

Lobelia should begin blooming in your garden around mid-summer and continue until the first frost. You can deadhead Lobelia plants to keep them looking tidy; however, it isn't necessary.

Make sure you get the native species and not a cultivar which won't produce enough nectar for hummingbirds. Here are a two great options:

Lobelia cardinalis: I'm not sure any flower is redder than this. The long flower spikes bloom from the bottom up for six weeks in late summer and early fall, during migration of hummingbirds. A profile of this exquisite flower perfectly fits the head of ruby-throated hummingbirds, its primary pollinator, and a few butterflies with long proboscises, such as the spicebush swallowtail and cloudless sulphur, visit to nectar on the flowers. Cardinal flower grows 3–5 feet tall, and its fruiting heads add interest to the landscape in late fall. It's best in natural gardens along a stream or river; plants self-sow in bare, moist soils. It's often planted in rain gardens and perennial borders, and it's a quintessential plant for a hummingbird garden. Separate the basal offshoots of this short-lived perennial each May, and plant them singly to keep a planting thriving indefinitely. Do not mulch except as a protective covering in winter.

Lobelia siphilitica: This lobelia produces tall showy spires of light to rich blue flowers in late summer, a bloom season that coincides with that of cardinal flower, but great blue lobelia is pollinated by bees, mainly bumblebees. Plants grow about 3 feet tall and are tolerant of a wide range of soils, as long as they are not dry. Like cardinal flower, this rather short-lived perennial needs to be divided or allowed to self-sow to persist. This adaptation makes great blue lobelia best suited to a natural garden—or a close-to-home perennial bed where you can easily keep an eye on it and give it extra attention.

Consumption Methods: Teas and decoctions have proven effective in treating psychostimulant abuse and eating disorders. A tea made from the fresh leaves is analgesic and febrifuge and the poultice can be applied to the temples to treat headaches.

Warnings: While Lobelia has been historically used in herbal medicine for respiratory ailments, it is important to note that its safety and effectiveness have not been extensively studied. It may cause adverse effects and interact with certain medications. Overuse or misuse of Lobelia can lead to nausea, vomiting, sweating, and other uncomfortable symptoms. Individuals with certain medical conditions, such as heart disease, high blood pressure, or seizure disorders, should avoid using Lobelia. Pregnant and breastfeeding women should also refrain from its use due to potential risks.

Marigold

Pot Marigold, Marygold, Poet's Marigold, Scotch Marigold, Scottish Marigold.

Calendula officinalis.

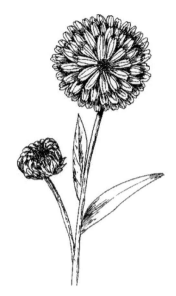

Medical Uses: The Marigold grows in marshy places, hardwood swamps, and alongside ponds. Native Americans utilized its roots to treat colds and wounds, induce vomiting, defend against love charms, and help with delivery.

Marigold has been used to cure a number of health ailments for generations, in addition to its aesthetic value. Marigold has been used for similar therapeutic purposes in Chinese, Mexican, European, and Native American medical traditions, including the treatment of general pain.

Antiseptic, astringent, cholagogue, diaphoretic , stimulant and vulnerary. Used in external preparations for bites, stings, sprains, fungal infections, wounds etc. Check out the second volume to discover more traditional and modern uses.

Marigolds were first used by the Aztecs, who believed they had magical, religious, and therapeutic virtues. Marigolds were originally mentioned in 1552 in the De La Crus-Badiano Aztec Herbal. Marigolds were used to heal hiccups, lightning strikes, and "for one who wishes to safely cross a river or water." The final application validates Marigolds' magical properties.

The Marigold was developed by the Aztecs to have larger blooms. Early Spanish explorers are said to have collected native Marigold seeds from the Aztecs and brought them to Spain in the 1500s. Marigolds were produced on the grounds of monasteries throughout Spain.

Pollinators/Wildlife: Up until and through the early frosts, Marigolds are proving to be excellent in attracting and feeding pollinating insects. They continue to bloom profusely thus late in the season, providing pollen and nectar as well as or better than just about any other garden flower. Consider them to be open 24 hours a day, seven days a week. They'll keep pollinators coming to your garden even as the season starts to close. You'll most

likely want to grow *Calendula officinalis* for a medicinal herb garden and the good news is that they also attract bees and offer quite a lot of nectar at that. Marsh marigold is also medicinal and attracts bees and hoverflies.

Mountain and French Marigold attract butterflies, especially American Painted Ladies.

Marigold is also a well-known insect repellant and therefore a welcomed addition to any vegetable patch. It deters whiteflies, aphids, and soil nematodes when interplanted among vegetables, potatoes, and roses.

Solvents: Boiling water, alcohol.

Hardiness Zones: Zones 2-11.

Sourcing: Marigolds are members of the Tagetes genus, which includes 40 species that are all annuals. All are endemic to the Western Hemisphere and can be found in the wild from the Southwestern United States to Argentina's Central and South America. Mexico has more species than any other country. Marigolds thrive on moderately fertile, well-drained soil; however, they will grow in practically any soil. Remember that they're used to warmer climes, so they'll be simpler to find in the drier southern states. If these conditions are met, look for patches of wildflowers, and you just may find some growing amongst the masses of other beautiful flowering flora. Of course, seedlings are available in almost every nursery, so you don't have to start them from seed if you really want to get your flower garden off to a fast start, be careful to get native species and avoid seeds mix which are most likely cultivars.

Gardening Tips: Marigolds, with their vibrant blooms and pest-resistant nature, are a gardener's delight. These hardy annuals require minimal maintenance once established and provide continuous blossoms throughout the summer until the arrival of frost. To ensure a profusion of flowers, regular deadheading is recommended.

When choosing a location for your Marigolds, opt for a spot with full sunlight as it promotes optimal growth and abundant blooms. While Marigolds are not too particular about soil conditions, they thrive best in well-drained garden soil with a pH of at least 6.0. They can tolerate a leaner environment with moderate organic matter, making them suitable for various soil types.

Proper watering is essential for young Marigold seeds or seedlings. Ensure they receive frequent watering, especially during the initial stages of planting. If the weather is hot and sunny, daily watering may be required. As the plants establish a robust root system over a few weeks, they become more drought-tolerant but benefit from weekly watering to maintain vibrant blooms.

Unlike some perennial flowers, Marigolds are true annuals, requiring replanting each year. However, their adaptability to different temperature ranges allows them to thrive across various planting zones. Be cautious of powdery mildew, which can develop in damp or humid summers. To prevent this issue, select a location with ample airflow and adequate sunlight.

Feeding your Marigolds may not be necessary unless your soil is exceptionally poor. Regular deadheading is the key to keeping the plants in continuous bloom. Removing spent flowers redirects the plant's energy towards producing new blooms.

Growing Marigolds from seeds is a breeze, and their large, easy-to-handle seeds make them an excellent choice for school projects involving children. While starting seeds indoors 6 to 8 weeks before the last frost date is an option, Marigolds germinate quickly when sown directly in the garden. The direct-sown plants catch up with the indoor-started seedlings as they begin to grow once the weather warms.

Marigolds make attractive border plants, adding vibrant colors to the garden. To create visually appealing combinations, consider pairing them with complementary hues such as yellow and orange daylilies or purples like salvia and verbena. Their compact size makes them ideal for front-of-border plantings or container gardens.

In addition to the popular annual Marigolds, there is also a fascinating perennial variety called marsh-marigold. This spring ephemeral emerges quickly as soon as the ground thaws, gracing wetland habitats with its stunning molten yellow flowers. It creates enchanting rivers or masses of gold in springs, seeps, and fens. Marsh-marigold can reach a height of 2 feet and thrives in constant moisture, even during dormancy. To propagate marsh-marigold, division is the recommended method.

Whether you choose the classic annual Marigolds or the captivating marsh-marigold, these plants bring beauty and versatility to your garden. Their cheerful blooms and ability to ward off pests make them a valuable addition to any landscape. Enjoy their vibrant colors and the ease with which they can be cultivated, providing you with a season filled with floral delight..

Consumption Methods: Antiseptic marigold flowers and leaves poultices can be used for bruises, burns, cuts, sore and inflamed skin. Infused oil or ointment for burns, wounds, athlete's foot. Marigold has resinous flowers and leaves which can be used to treat successfully skin conditions, such as dermatitis and acne.

Warnings: Marigolds carry very few warnings other than the typical advice to take any remedy in moderation and stop use if the skin under the application area becomes irritated or shows signs of a reaction.

Mayapple

American Mandrake, Wild Mandrake, Ground Lemon.

Podophyllum Peltatum.

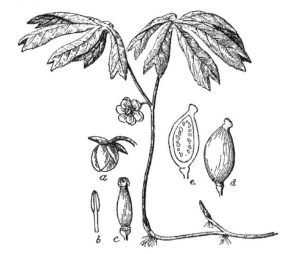

Medical Uses: Mayapple roots were employed as a purgative, emetic, "liver cleanser," and worm expeller by Native Americans and early settlers. Jaundice, constipation, hepatitis, fevers, and syphilis were all treated with roots.

Mayapple was used by the Penobscot Indians as a treatment to treat wart tumors on the skin. The Hurons and Iroquois used it to commit suicide as well. The herb was utilized as an antirheumatic, cathartic, dermatological assistance, ear medication, pesticide, and laxative by Cherokee Indians. Other Cherokee utilized the root as a purgative, vermifuge, anthelmintic, and for the treatment of warts. For other traditional and modern uses check out the second volume.

Pollinators/Wildlife: The blooms don't have any nectar, but the native bees and bumblebees that visit them get a lot of pollen. The flower has a strong or musky aroma to it. Even though there is delayed anthesis (pollen shedding) and receptiveness of the stigma if pollination has not been performed, the frequency of successful pollination in Mayapple flowers is generally low. Queen bumblebees are drawn to Mayapple blooms, in particular, to collect pollen for their raising workers and thus may be major pollinators. This plant isn't going to be popular all the time, but it's still useful.

Solvents: Boiling water, alcohol.

Hardiness Zones: Zones 3-8.

Sourcing: In deciduous woodlands, mayapple is a common native plant. Mayapple is a native forest plant that grows in zones 3 to 8 across most of eastern North America, from Maine to Texas. Talk a walk in the woods within these zones, and you'll likely come upon a patch of these plants. When it blooms, it's time to pick morels.

Gardening Tips: Mayapple plants are native to both damp and dry wooded areas of eastern North America (zones 3 to 8) and thrive in comparable environments. Choose a location with well-draining soil and enough space for the plants to create a small colony. Established colonies may withstand some drought, but young plants should be planted in damp loam that has been supplemented with compost.

Remember that this is a spring ephemeral that will become dormant at some time over the summer when using it in your landscaping. As a result, it'll be most useful throughout the spring and early summer. It also implies that it will leave a hole in its place, which you may want to cover with something different for the rest of the summer. Mayapple should not be planted in an area where continuous color is required.

A place with complete shade is excellent near the southern end of the mayapple's range. They can, however, take some sun in the north, especially if they get enough moisture.

Mayapple plants prefer moist, well-drained soil with a pH that is somewhat acidic. It can grow in moist or dry soil as long as it is humusy and well-drained.

Mayapple needs damp soil, although, like many other woodland wildflowers, it can tolerate dry circumstances if it is in a sheltered spot. In general, a healthy amount of organic matter in the soil aids in moisture retention.

Mayapple tolerates a wide range of temperatures and humidity levels throughout its hardiness range; however, it will die back by mid-summer.

Mayapple does not require any fertilization because it obtains all of its nutrients from organic matter in the soil. Compost amendments will benefit plants in poor soils.

Mayapple can be grown by root division or by sowing the fruit's seeds. However, because seeds take four to five years to mature, root division is the more popular and recommended approach. When the plant is dormant in the fall or early spring, simply dig it up, divide it, and replant it where you want a wide ground cover that even wildlife will avoid owing to its tart leaves.

In the spring, mayapple can acquire a disease called mayapple rust. Yellow or light green dots appear on the top side of the leaves, and rust-colored spores or pustules appear on the underside. The plant tolerates the puckering and dropping of leaves nicely. The disease does not usually kill the plant and does not necessitate treatment.

Consumption Methods: See the second volume!

Warnings: Mayapple contains toxic compounds, including podophyllotoxin and other related substances. These compounds can be harmful if ingested or applied improperly. Mayapple should never be consumed or used without proper guidance and supervision from a qualified healthcare professional.

Ingesting any part of the mayapple plant, including its fruits, roots, or leaves, can lead to severe gastrointestinal distress, such as nausea, vomiting, and diarrhea. In some cases, it can cause more serious symptoms, including liver and kidney damage.

Furthermore, the sap of the mayapple plant can cause skin irritation, blistering, and dermatitis upon contact. Direct exposure to the sap should be avoided, and protective measures, such as wearing gloves, should be taken when handling the plant.

It is important to note that although certain compounds found in mayapple have pharmaceutical uses, such as in the treatment of certain cancers, these applications should only be pursued under the guidance of a healthcare professional.

Prairie Wild Roses

Pasture Rose, Prairie Rose, Wild Rose, Dog Rose, Eglantine, Sweetbriar, Scotch Briar.

Rosa arkansana.

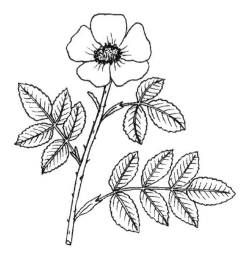

Medical Uses: Native Americans have always used various components of a Prairie Rose for a variety of purposes. They figured out how to make the most of a plentiful supply of diverse treatments and foods

Rose hips form near the base of the bloom and turn a vivid red later in the summer, containing the seeds. The hips of the flower contain several times more vitamin C than a lemon, so the Native Americans would keep them and consume them fresh or make jelly with them when food was limited. Younger stems and leaves were frequently selected and steeped in tea.

They crushed the leaf galls and used them as an ointment for burns, and the roots and hips, steeped, were an efficient remedy for eye irritations.

Pollinators/Wildlife: Prairie Roses are wild flowering plants that provide pollinators with a wide range of pollen, bird nesting sites, and seclusion for small mammals. Their fruits, or hips, are both delectable treats for wildlife and a potent source of antioxidants for humans. Food forests and land restoration efforts rely heavily on native Roses. Bees pollinate the Roses, which have fragrant blossoms that also attract birds and butterflies.

Solvents: Boiling water, alcohol.

Hardiness Zones: Zones 5-10.

Sourcing: Prairie Rose is an open-land plant that can be found in and around grasslands, forests, and savannas, as well as fencerows and thickets. It can be found on the outskirts of woodlands. Look to the fields of the midwest!

Gardening Tips: Prairie wild rose can replace any climbing rose in a traditional landscape. Around the summer solstice clusters of flowers open rich pink but fade to light pink, creating a two-toned effect. The abundant round hips, the most beautiful of any wild rose, are showy in the winter landscape. It makes a large 5-foot-high haystack of arching stems and can climb to 8 feet or more when rambling over other plants or when trained on a trellis. It does not sucker, and its stems do not root where they touch soil. Prairie wild rose thrives in moist, well-drained soil and is more resistant to blackspot than most landscape roses. Prune out dead canes, as you would any climbing rose, to keep the shrub vigorous; if not pruned annually it is best reserved for a natural landscape, where it makes prime wildlife habitat and is a favorite shrub for nesting songbirds—a great replacement for nonnative and invasive multiflora rose.

Growing Prairie Roses are all own-root Roses, which means they develop on their own root systems without the use of grafting, which is used by man to enable some modern Roses to grow well in a variety of climates. In reality, Prairie Roses are the Roses from which all other Roses we have today were bred; thus, they have a special place in any Rosarian's mind and heart.

Prairie Roses flourish in conditions of neglect and are extremely hardy. These hardy Roses thrive in a variety of soil conditions, with at least one of them thriving in moist soil. If left on the bushes, these exquisite Roses will yield lovely Rose hips that will last into the winter and offer food for the birds. They can die well down in the winter because they are their own root bushes, and what comes up from the root will still be the same lovely Rose.

Prairie Roses plants are not difficult to grow. Prairie Roses bushes can be planted in the same way as conventional Rose bushes and perform best in regions with plenty of light and well-drained soil (as a general rule). Rosa palustris, popularly known as the swamp Rose, is one variation that does well in moist terrain. Do not overcrowd Prairie Roses in your Rose beds, gardens, or general landscaping. Prairie Roses of all kinds require space to flourish and reach their full potential. Crowding them, like with other Rose bushes, reduces airflow in and around the bushes, making them more susceptible to disease.

These robust Rose bushes will survive with minimal care once their root systems are established in their new homes. It's not required to deadhead them (remove old flowers), and doing so will reduce or eliminate the lovely Rose hips they produce. They can be pruned to preserve a desired form, but be careful not to overdo it if you want those lovely Rose hips later!

Swamp wild rose usually grows in a clump, forming a 5- to 6-foot-tall upright vase-shaped shrub with pendent branches. The thorny, arching stems create habitat for nesting songbirds. This native shrub produces typical pink wild rose flowers in midsummer (later than most wild roses) and rose hips in fall that hang on the plant through winter, adding a touch of bright interest to the winter garden. It's a fine suckering shrub for a rain, pondside, or wetland garden. It will grow in good garden soil but prefers a moist to wet soil with a lower pH and may even tolerate standing water.

Consumption Methods: When it comes to vitamin C and bioflavonoids, nothing compares to prairie roses hip. Best fresh, rose hip lose much of their vitamin C during drying, cooking, and storing, though bioflavonoids remain. Jam is more effective than tea to keep vitamin C intact.

Warnings: Rose overdoses can cause gastric upset. Use in moderation.

Prunella

Common Self-Heal, Heal-All, Woundwort, Heart-Of-The-Earth, Carpenter's Herb, Brownwort, Blue Curls.

Prunella vulgaris.

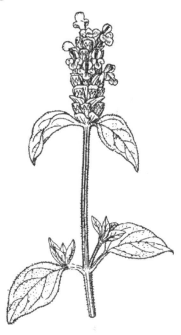

Medical Uses: Prunella is utilized by Native Americans, Europeans, and Asians for a variety of ailments, including thyroid disorders, conjunctivitis, TB, arthritis, and cancer. Isn't that ludicrous, or at the very least exaggerated? Except that Prunella is one of the more widely studied herbs, and even scientific studies show that it can help with a wide range of conditions, including anti-inflammatory pain, gingivitis, osteoarthritis, HIV, herpes, diabetes, high blood pressure, and even tuberculosis, liver cancer, and endometriosis. Check the second volume under Heal-All.

Pollinators/Wildlife: Bees, small butterflies, moths, and skippers are attracted to the blossoms of this perennial, which have no noticeable floral aroma. However it produces a lot of nectar and is very attractive to honeybees, short-tongued bumblebees, and even solitary bees. The leaves are eaten by some moth larvae, but mammalian herbivores dislike the bitter flavor; therefore, the feast is short-lived.

Solvents: Boiling water, alcohol.

Hardiness Zones: Zones 4-9.

Sourcing: Avoid foraging and harvesting, buy seeds or seedlings from local nurseries. Otherwise propagate from cuttings.

Gardening Tips: Prunella, also known as self-heal, is a distinctive low perennial with tall spikes of many flowers and hairy bracts that overlap. The thick, cylindrical, purple flower spikes continue to extend even after blossoming, adding to its unique appearance. Often regarded as a weed in lawns and shady areas, a specific variety that flowers at just 2 inches (5 cm) tall has gained popularity. Its common name, self-heal, reflects its widespread use as an herbal remedy for throat problems.

In its preferred habitat of damp fields, gardens, pastures, and forest borders, especially in the eastern and southern parts of Texas, prunella thrives. While it can be cultivated in various locations, it does require some additional water in extremely dry conditions. If you live in a hot climate, it is advisable to provide prunella with a shaded position to protect it from the scorching afternoon sun.

Prunella is adaptable and can grow in a variety of environments, but it truly thrives in situations resembling its natural habitat, such as woodland margins and meadows. It prefers cool to mild temperatures and can tolerate both sun and partial shade.

To propagate prunella in the spring, you can divide existing plants or plant new ones. Prepare the soil by adding organic matter and plant prunella at a depth of 4 to 6 inches (10-15 cm), with spacing between plants of 6 to 9 inches (15-23 cm). If starting from seed, lightly cover them with soil and trim the seedlings as necessary after they emerge. Indoor seed starting can be done approximately ten weeks before the spring planting season. Since prunella is related to mint and has a tendency to spread, consider using containment measures, such as bottomless pots, in flower beds or borders.

Mature prunella plants, reaching a height of 1 to 2 feet (31-61 cm), may fall over and form new roots in the soil. Therefore, it is advisable to avoid placing the pot flush with the ground to prevent this from happening.

After the blooming period, it is recommended to trim back prunella plants to prevent reseeding and maintain their overall appearance. Regular deadheading promotes more flowering. At the end of the growing season, prune the plant back to ground level.

If you intend to gather prunella for medicinal purposes, cut the blooming tops and dry them upside down in small bunches. Store them in a cool, dry, and dark place until ready for use.

Consumption Methods: Alterative, antibacterial, astringent, carminative, diuretic, styptic and vulnerary. Used as a poultice for wounds, ulcers, sores. Also internal use for disorders such as diarrhoea and sore mouth. Leaves are a welcomed addition to salads and along with the stems they can be added to soups and stir-fries, but make sure to wash-off the tannins.

Warnings: Overdoses can cause gastric upset.

Purple Coneflower

Hedgehog Coneflower.

Echinacea purpurea.

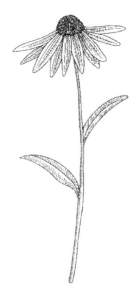

Medical Uses: The purple coneflower, often known by its Latin name Echinacea, is a North American native wildflower that is revered by many American Indian tribes. Coneflowers are connected with elk and given the name "elk root" by Western cultures like the Utes, who believe that wounded elk seek them out as medicine. Many tribes, particularly in the Great Plains and Midwest, employed coneflower roots as traditional therapeutic herbs to cure a variety of swelling, burns, and pain. During sweatlodge ceremonies and the Sundance, coneflower has also been chewed ritually. The Navajo tribe considers the coneflower to be one of their holy Life Medicines. Check the second volume under Echinacea

Pollinators/Wildlife: Purple coneflowers are pollinated mostly by long-tongued bees and butterflies. The sticky pollen gathers on their legs and bodies when they approach the bloom to drink nectar. The first step in cross-pollination is taken here. Some of the bees you might see are Green Metallic bees, Honeybees, and Bumble Bees. It also attracts monarchs, eastern tiger swallowtails, silver-spotted skippers, and black swallowtails.

Solvents: Boiling water, alcohol.

Hardiness Zones: Zones 5-8.

Sourcing: The plant is endemic to the eastern United States, including Iowa and Ohio, as well as Louisiana and Georgia. They reach a height of 2 to 4 feet and have dark green foliage. They are quick growers who self-sow a lot of seeds. These midsummer bloomers will bloom from midsummer till frost in the fall!

Gardening Tips: Purple coneflower thrives in poor or weak soil conditions. Rich or heavily amended soil can result in lush foliage but poor flowering. Ensure that purple coneflowers receive ample sunlight, with at least six hours of full sun each day. In southern regions, morning sun exposure may yield optimal results, while providing late afternoon shade can protect the plants from scorching.

To start purple coneflower plants, you can use either seeds or root division. If you wish to save seeds for future harvests, collect them before birds consume them. Place a brown paper bag over the seed head, turning it upside down to allow the seeds to fall into the bag. Some experienced growers recommend stratifying (freezing) the seeds in moist soil for a few weeks after planting to encourage more abundant blooming. In regions with warm year-round weather, this method can be attempted. Alternatively, planting purple coneflower seeds in autumn in areas with cold winters allows for natural chilling of the seeds.

Root division can be performed in the fall to start new purple coneflower plants. However, it is advisable to divide plants only after they have been in the ground for three years or more. Younger coneflower plants may not have developed a sufficiently large root system for successful division. Repeat the root division process every three to four years.

Growing purple coneflower from seeds is straightforward, making it suitable for novice gardeners, while experienced gardeners appreciate its easy care requirements.

Once planted and established, purple coneflowers require minimal care. Additional watering is generally unnecessary during seasons with normal rainfall, as they are drought-tolerant and thrive in hot, dry summers. Limited fertilization may be required, but it is not always necessary. If flowers appear small or underdeveloped, adding a small amount of well-composted material to the soil around the plants can help.

When late summer blooms start to look weary or ragged, cut back purple coneflower plants by a third. This revitalizes the plant and often leads to a new display of beautiful blossoms that continue until the onset of colder weather. With such simple maintenance, purple coneflowers will reward you with a bountiful crop of flowers year after year..

Consumption Methods: Always a welcomed addition to any self-respecting herbalist's garden. Check out the second and third volume for all its uses.

Warnings: It may cause congestion in the chest and disorders of the liver and gallbladder. When applied directly to the eyes, it may cause irritation. Use in moderation.

Roseroot

Golden Root, Rose Root, Roseroot, Aaron's Rod, Arctic Root,
King's Crown, Lignum Rhodium, Orpin Rose.

Rhodiola Rosea.

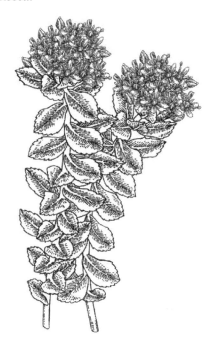

Identification: Tall perennial species with huge flower clusters that can be used in borders or pollinator gardens. Low-growing plants are commonly planted for their foliage and spread by rooting stems, and they perform well on a slope, ground cover, hanging baskets, and even green roofs.

Medical Uses: Roseroot is widely used as a herbal supplement, with effects ranging from relieving anxiety to curing altitude sickness. This plant was used by Alaskan Natives for both medicinal and culinary purposes. It's been used for a long time to lift one's spirits and relieve despair. It's also been shown to boost physical and mental performance, as well as reduce fatigue, stress, and worry.

Modern research has revealed fascinating insights into the effects of Roseroot (Rhodiola rosea) on the body's response to stress. This remarkable herb has been found to enhance the body's resilience and ability to cope with various forms of stress by regulating hormonal responses. One of the key mechanisms through which Roseroot exerts its beneficial effects is its impact on serotonin and dopamine in the brain.

Studies suggest that Roseroot may have a protective effect on these neurotransmitters by inhibiting the enzymes that degrade them and preventing their depletion caused by excessive release of stress hormones. Serotonin and dopamine play crucial roles in regulating mood, emotions, and overall well-being. Maintaining optimal levels of these neurotransmitters is vital for mental and emotional health.

By modulating the activity of stress hormones and supporting the integrity of serotonin and dopamine, Roseroot offers potential benefits in managing stress-related conditions such as anxiety, depression, and fatigue. It is believed to help restore a sense of balance and promote emotional stability.

Moreover, Roseroot has also been investigated for its adaptogenic properties, meaning it helps the body adapt to various stressors, both physical and mental. This adaptogenic action can enhance overall resilience, boost energy levels, and promote cognitive function.

Pollinators/Wildlife: it requires pollination by bees or flies.

Solvents: Boiling water, alcohol.

Hardiness Zones: Zones 2-9.

Sourcing: Roseroot grows in fissures on mountain cliffs and along sea cliffs. It's also an ornamental that grows along stream banks, snow-bed locations, and rock shelves. It thrives in the Arctic and coastal regions of North America, Asia, and Europe, including the United Kingdom. You might be in luck if it's cold and rainy.

Gardening Tips: Roseroot grows best in sandy or sandy-loam soils that are deep, fairly rich, and well-drained. Cleaning the rhizomes is tough in peat soil, while harvesting is difficult in stony soil. Because Roseroot is a high-altitude plant, it requires extra care and attention when grown at lower elevations. Its growth necessitates a high level of dampness. When grown professionally, it requires 500-600 mm of rain. It won't be able to withstand the scorching heat of summer. It can, however, withstand exposure to the sea. When planted 30 cm (12 in) apart, it can be used as a ground cover.

Root division, cuttings, and seeds can all be used to propagate Roseroot. If you want seeds, you'll need a female and a male plant because it's a dioecious plant.

Root division, cuttings, and seeds can all be used to propagate Roseroot. If you want seeds, you'll need a female and a male plant because it's a dioecious plant.

Start in the spring by surface planting it in a sunny position in a greenhouse or cold frame for the greatest results. Keep the soil moist at all times. Germination should take 2-4 weeks at 10 degrees Celsius (50 degrees Fahrenheit). Continue to grow them in a greenhouse until they're big enough to plant in the garden. Some people recommend keeping it in a greenhouse until the following year's early summer.

From August through October, divide your plants. Plant the larger divisions in their permanent placements, and pot up smaller divisions and cultivate them in a cold frame in light shade until they are well established. Late spring or early summer is the best time to plant them.

When the basal shoots are about 8-10 cm (3-4 in) above ground and have plenty of underground stems, harvest them. Plant them in individual pots in a cold frame or greenhouse and keep them in light shade until they are fully rooted. Summer is the best time to plant them.

Consumption Methods: A decoction of the flowers and leaves is helpful in treating indigestion, as well as having a calming effect, and aiding sexual potency. It can also be used to flavor vodka.

Warnings Few side effects are recorded; however, dizziness has been noted in some when taking larger doses.

Rue Anemone

Windflower, Crowfoot.

Thalictrum thalictroides.

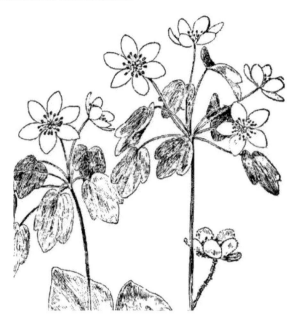

Medicinal Uses: Rue Anemones were employed by Native Americans for a number of medical uses, despite the fact that they were moderately toxic. Anemone-infused tea was used by the North American Indians of Quebec to treat a variety of diseases, including boils, lung congestion, and eye trouble. Meskwaki Indians used seeds to create smoke in order to resuscitate people who were unconscious. Rue Anemone roots were used to treat vomiting and diarrhea as an antiemetic.

Herbalists still utilize Rue Anemone in the treatment of headaches, gout, leprosy, eye inflammations, and ulcers.

Pollinators/Wildlife: Cross-pollination is aided by Rue Anemone's collaboration with early flying bees and flies, especially dark sweat bees, but also large *Andrena* bee. Rue Anemone, like certain other early spring wildflowers such as Hepaticas (Hepatica nobilis) and Bloodroot (Sanguinaria canadensis), has evolved to tempt pollinators with solely pollen. It produces seeds that contain elaisomes which are extremely helpful in the diet of ants that eat the elaisomes and discard the seed, aiding propagation. Deer-resistant due to its toxicity.

Solvents: Boiling water.

Hardiness Zones: Zones 4-8.

Sourcing: Rue Anemone (Thalictrum thalictroides) is a delicate and charming perennial herb that can be found in various regions across North America.

When sourcing Rue Anemone, it is important to consider the specific region and climate. It can be found in different parts of North America, including the eastern United States and parts of Canada. Look for areas with a suitable habitat for Rue Anemone, such as deciduous forests or shady, moist areas with well-drained soil.

In terms of collection, it is recommended to obtain Rue Anemone from reputable nurseries or specialized plant suppliers. They often cultivate and propagate this species, ensuring healthy and well-established plants for transplanting. This approach helps preserve the natural populations of Rue Anemone in their native habitats.

Gardening Tips: Despite their delicate appearance, Rue Anemones (Thalictrum thalictroides) can bloom abundantly in spring if they are not exposed to excessive sunlight or moisture. These resilient plants prefer loamy, well-drained, and somewhat damp soils, avoiding direct sunlight. Urban environments with high pollution levels may hinder their ability to flower.

Native to eastern North American woodlands, Rue Anemones thrive in shady locations. They flourish in partial shade during spring but can tolerate full shade when dormant. Planting them beneath deciduous tree canopies provides the dappled light they prefer during their active growth phase. Even when the tree canopy is dense and blocks much light during summer dormancy, they can still survive. Loamy or sandy soils that are loose and rich in humus are ideal for Rue Anemones, although they can adapt to various soil conditions. They do not tolerate standing water or overly wet conditions and require good drainage. Planting them under trees benefits from the organic debris that helps retain moisture, while a light mulch layer on dry soils aids in moisture retention and protects against spring frosts.

While drought-tolerant, Rue Anemones thrive in mesic conditions with reasonable moisture levels to ensure prolonged blooming in spring. They can withstand dry periods without much additional watering, especially if the area is mulched. Excessive moisture can cause their tuberous roots to rot, while overly dry conditions may lead to early dormancy. When planted beneath well-established trees, Rue Anemones benefit from the drought tolerance of the trees' extensive root systems, which absorb much of the available moisture. Despite their fragile appearance, these resilient plants can withstand strong spring frosts while continuing to bloom.

Rue Anemones are not suitable for hot, sunny, or humid locations. They prefer cooler and shadier environments. The tiny tuberous roots of Rue Anemone can be dug up and divided, or root cuttings can be used to propagate new plants. Early spring, when the plants emerge from dormancy, is the best time to divide them.

While Rue Anemones can be grown from seeds, it is easier to propagate them through division or root cuttings. Collecting seeds from mature plants in early summer and allowing them to dry completely before sowing is recommended. A cold stratification period, by keeping the seeds moist in the refrigerator for a few months, enhances germination success. However, flowering may not occur in the first season after germination.

Consumption Methods: To be used in moderation, due to its toxicity. However, a mild tea is helpful in treating diarrhea and vomiting.

Warnings: Anemone includes protoanemonin, an acrid component that irritates the mouth, gastrointestinal mucosa, and skin. Toxic doses can cause nausea, vomiting, diarrhea, low blood pressure, and respiratory distress if eaten in high enough concentrations.

St. John's Wort

Amber, Barbe de Saint-Jean, Chasse-diable, Demon Chaser, Fuga Daemonum, Goatweed, Hardhay, Herbe à la Brûlure, Herbe à Mille Trous, Herbe Aux Fées, Herbe Aux Mille Vertus, Herbe Aux Piqûres, Herbe de Saint Éloi, Herbe de la Saint-Jean, Herbe du Charpentier.

Hypericum perforatum.

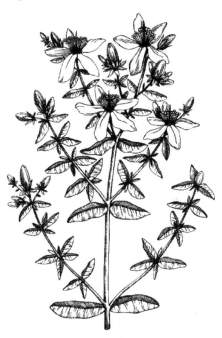

Medical Uses: St. John's Wort was utilized by several Native American tribes to cure wounds, fevers, gastrointestinal problems, nosebleeds, and snakebite. It was also said to be effective in the treatment of ulcers, cancer, and sleeplessness. A must-have plant in self-respecting herbalist's apothecary cabinet and garden! Check out the second volume for all its uses and the third volume for recipes.

Pollinators/Wildlife: Bumblebees are the major pollinators of shrubby St. John's Wort, but honeybees also visit the blooms to collect pollen on a regular basis. Bumblebees and honeybees are frequently seen gathering large baskets of bright yellow pollen, which they transport back to their colonies and use as brood food. Leafcutter bees will also use its leaves for nesting material. It deters herbivores, such as the larvae of rattlebox moth, by producing hypercalin which is fatal to the predators, but incidentally is the same substance that attracts pollinators.

Solvents: Boiling water, water, alcohol.

Hardiness Zones: Zones 5-10.

Sourcing: Rangelands, farms, roadsides, and forest clearings are all teeming with St. John's wort. It prefers well-drained, coarse-textured soils that are slightly acidic to neutral in pH. It probably already grows somewhere nearby your house. Grow it from semi-hardwood cuttings or seeds, add it to your garden, and allow it to spread it for its many medicinal uses, biological activity, and beautiful appearance

Gardening Tips: St. John's wort is a simple to grow plant that can withstand a variety of situations. As a result, many gardeners consider it to be a weed, they should know better! Its Achilles heel, if there is one, is too damp soil. St. John's wort may need to be babied for a while, but once established, it will thrive on its own. In fact, keeping established plants in check will be your primary maintenance task.

For the best flower output, grow St. John's wort in full light in the north. In the South, though, a little shade is beneficial to the plant.

Although it requires well-drained soil, the plant may endure compacted soil

When you're first trying to establish this perennial, keep it well-irrigated. It can withstand drought after it has reached maturity.

Although it tolerates low soils, St. John's wort thrives in fertile soils. For optimal results, amend the soil with compost once a year.

Consumption Methods: As St. John's Wort is so easy to source and safe to use, every consumption method imaginable is readily available, from soaps and creams to teas and supplements, usually from the neighborhood drug store or supermarket.

Warnings: As St. John's Wort can be gastrically powerful, it is important to keep this in mind when dosing, as taking too much can induce upset.

Sunflower

Common Sunflower.

Helianthus annuus.

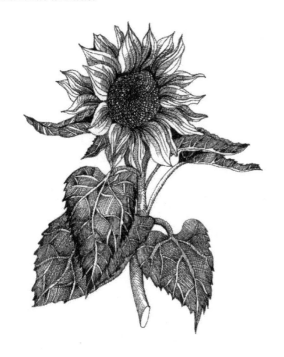

Identification: Belonging to the vast composite genus Helianthus, this plant is commonly known as the Sunflower. Its name derives from the golden-rayed flowers that resemble the sun. One fascinating characteristic of Sunflowers is their ability to track and face the sun from morning to night, a phenomenon known as heliotropism. This unique trait may contribute to the nutritional richness of Sunflower seeds.

Sunflowers (Helianthus annuus) have a long history of cultivation in pre-Columbian America as robust annuals. These plants possess an extensive root system that reaches deep into the soil, allowing them to extract essential trace minerals that may not be readily available in the topsoil. The leaves of Sunflowers are numerous, rough, and quite large, displaying a somewhat heart-shaped form. The broad and brownish disc at the center of the flower consists of tubular florets that develop four-sided, oil-rich achenes. Unlike many other seeds, Sunflower achenes do not burst open when ripe.

The vibrant yellow petals of Sunflowers exhibit a daisy-like pattern, adding to the plant's overall visual appeal. With a towering height of up to 15 feet, Sunflowers are often planted as a concealing border, providing both beauty and privacy to gardens and landscapes.

Traditional Uses: The captivating story of Sunflowers begins with their cultivation by Native Americans in what is now New Mexico and Arizona, dating back to around 3,000 B.C. Archaeological evidence suggests that Sunflowers were farmed even before corn plants were domesticated. However, the wild Sunflower of that time looked quite different from the familiar single-headed, single-stemmed variety we know today. Native American "plant breeders" are credited with the remarkable achievement of increasing seed size by a staggering 1,000 percent through selective breeding.

For Native Americans, Sunflowers held immense significance beyond their agricultural value. The seeds were a vital source of nourishment, and the plants and flower heads were used for medicinal and ceremonial purposes. In fact, the Aztecs of Peru worshipped the Sunflower, adorning their temples with gold-plated Sunflower statues and crowning their princesses with vibrant yellow blossoms.

Native Americans creatively incorporated Sunflowers into their cuisine, making bread and cakes from crushed and ground seeds. They mixed the seed meal with vegetables like corn, beans, and squash, and enjoyed cracked Sunflower seeds as a snack—a tradition that continues to this day. Sunflower seeds provided valuable fats in their predominantly lean meat-based diets. The seeds were even transformed into a type of butter called "seed-balls," similar to peanut butter, which served as a convenient and portable food source.

Roasted Sunflower husks were used to make a coffee-like beverage when steeped in hot water, while the seed's oils found their way into the breadmaking process. The vibrant yellow and purple pigments derived from Sunflowers were used for non-food applications such as dyeing fabrics, coloring pottery, and body painting. Moreover, the Sunflower plant possessed various medicinal properties, offering remedies for wart removal, sunstroke, snakebites, ointments, cauterization, wound healing, and chest ailments. In some cultures, dried Sunflower stalks were even used as a building material.

Native Americans employed Sunflowers as a medicinal resource. The Dakota tribe used it to alleviate chest pains and respiratory problems, while the Cherokee people consumed Sunflower infusions to aid with kidney issues. The Paiute tribe utilized Sunflower roots to treat rheumatism. Sunflower oil was believed to be beneficial for skin problems, and different tribes employed Sunflowers for various medicinal purposes. Some Native American groups viewed Sunflowers as symbols of bravery, carrying Sunflower cakes into battle or sprinkling Sunflower powder on their garments to boost their spirits.

The intriguing journey of Sunflowers continued with their introduction to Europe. Spanish explorers are believed to have brought Sunflower seeds from North America around 1500, which then made their way to Madrid, Spain, where they were cultivated in decorative gardens circa 1510. Later, Sunflowers were imported into Europe by the English and French, marking their presence in the New World.

It is worth mentioning that Native Americans also recognized the mineral-grasping properties of Sunflower roots, using them in combination with other roots for snakebite treatment. Additionally, a warm decoction of Sunflowers was employed as a wash for rheumatism and inflammations, showcasing the diverse applications of this remarkable plant.

Diuretic, Expectorant, Nourishing.

Pollinators/Wildlife: The bee is the Sunflower's primary pollinator, but other insects, animals, people, and even the wind aid in the production of seeds for agricultural and residential purposes. Sunflowers really are a catch-all pollinator.

Solvents: Boiling water, alcohol.

Hardiness Zones: Zones 4-9.

Sourcing: Sunflowers can be found in all 50 states of the United States, with the majority of them flowering in the summer. They have a native range that includes Canada, Northern Mexico, and Central America. Dry, open regions such as prairie lands, plains, and meadows are the Sunflower's natural habitat.

Gardening Tips: Cultivating Sunflowers requires attention to specific factors for optimal growth and flowering. These remarkable plants have a rich history and provide a delightful addition to any garden. Here's a comprehensive guide on how to source Sunflowers, with additional information and tips:

Sunflowers have relatively simple needs, primarily sunlight and well-drained soil. When choosing a location for planting, it is advisable to select a spot that is sheltered from strong gusts of wind to prevent these towering plants from toppling over. Planting Sunflowers in groups is beneficial as they can support each other against wind and rain. Taller varieties may require staking to keep them growing upright, as their flower heads can become quite heavy. One common method of staking is planting

them along a fence, while sturdy bamboo stakes can also be utilized. Care should be taken not to damage the plant's delicate root system when placing the stakes.

Weeding is essential as Sunflowers do not appreciate competing with unwanted vegetation. Mulching around Sunflowers serves multiple purposes: it helps retain moisture in the soil, suppresses weed growth, and maintains a favorable growing environment. Additionally, young Sunflower seedlings are often attractive to wildlife. To protect them, row covers or screens can be used until the plants reach a height of 1 to 2 feet.

For the best flowering and strong stems, it is crucial to plant Sunflowers in full sun, ensuring they receive at least six hours of direct sunlight each day. Sunflowers are heliotropic, meaning their flower heads follow the sun's path throughout the day. Ample sun exposure helps prevent them from bending excessively towards the strongest light source.

Sunflowers exhibit excellent adaptability to various soil types, including poor and dry soils. However, they thrive best in well-drained soil with sufficient organic matter. While they are drought-resistant, regular watering is necessary to encourage blossoming. During dry spells, it is advisable to allow the top 1 to 2 inches of soil to dry out between waterings. If Sunflowers appear droopy and the soil is dry, it indicates the need for more water.

Sunflowers generally prefer temperatures between 70 and 78 degrees Fahrenheit. However, they exhibit heat tolerance as long as their moisture requirements are met. They can withstand cold conditions, provided they receive adequate sunlight. Extreme humidity is also tolerable, provided there is proper air circulation and well-draining soil to prevent root rot and other diseases.

To support the growth and blooming of Sunflowers, they benefit from a fertilizer rich in phosphates and potassium. If the soil is rich and loamy, additional fertilization may not be necessary. However, if the soil is poor, a slow-release fertilizer can be applied in the spring according to the label instructions. It is crucial to avoid overfeeding, as excessive fertilization can lead to spindly stalks.

Sunflowers can be sourced by collecting and saving their seeds. Harvesting is typically done in early fall when the blossoms start to mature. The heads will shift downward, and the central disk florets will begin to wither. To determine if the seeds are ready for harvest, a few can be pulled out and opened. If the seed kernels inside the shell are plump, they are ready to be collected. To preserve the seeds, the entire flower head can be cut off the stalk and hung in a warm, dry, well-ventilated area away from insects and rodents. Covering the seed heads with cheesecloth or a paper bag with small holes for air circulation helps collect any stray seeds. Once completely dry, the seeds can be easily removed from the flower head. It is recommended to select the largest and plumpest seeds for planting, storing them in a cool and dry place until spring.

If Sunflower seed heads are left on the stalks during winter, they can provide food for birds and result in volunteer seedlings the following spring. These seedlings can be thinned out as needed to establish a new Sunflower patch.

While most Sunflowers are cultivated from seeds, they can also be propagated through cuttings. However, the simpler and more common method is to directly sow the seeds. Seeds can be planted in the garden once the threat of frost has passed in the spring, or they can be started indoors three to four weeks before transplanting. Starting seedlings indoors in peat or paper pots allows for seamless planting without disturbing the sensitive root systems.

When planting Sunflower seeds, they should be sown 1 to 2 inches deep in a shallow trench, with a spacing of 6 inches between them. It is crucial to keep the soil moist (but not wet) until germination, which usually takes seven to ten days. Taller varieties should be thinned to a distance of 1 to 1.5 feet, while dwarf varieties can be spaced approximately a foot apart.

Sunflowers are susceptible to various pests and diseases. Birds and rats are particularly attracted to Sunflower seeds, so covering the flower heads with netting can protect them when saving seeds for sowing. The Sunflower moth lays its eggs on the plant, and the resulting larvae tunnel into the flower heads, causing damage. Appropriate pesticide application can help control moth infestations. Additionally, insects and caterpillars may feed on the leaves, and fungal diseases such as powdery mildew and rust can affect the plants. Ensuring adequate air circulation and using garden fungicides at the first signs of infection can help prevent these issues.

Maximilian sunflower is a conspicuously showy perennial, with early fall flowers of a rich, true yellow produced along much of the length of its tall flowering stem, not just at the top. The leaves too are very handsome: narrow and folded, arched downward, and an unusual gray-green. This less-aggressive sunflower does form a clump and is suitable for gardens, where it will grow well in any well-drained soil. It grows 5–6 feet tall in dry soil but will be taller in good garden soil. It is a perfect sunflower for a natural landscape or prairie garden, with the larger grasses as competition; however, it is a bit too seedy for traditional perennial borders.

Western sunflower is one of those less-aggressive sunflowers you can wholeheartedly welcome to your garden. Its wide basal leaves are a beautiful rich green from spring through fall. Its 2-inch flowers, borne on thin stems that are nearly leafless, open earlier than most wild sunflowers, in late summer. Western sunflower is of short stature, for a sunflower, and even in a garden setting, its smaller size makes it easier to control and prevents it from smothering most plants. Its flowering stems rise no more than 3 feet above low foliage. This perennial is suitable for planting in a poor, dry site in scorching sun, from "hell strips" to rock gardens. In rich soils, it will be overwhelmed by other plants.

Consumption Methods: Too many to count, it really warrants a book of its own! It suffices to say that the seed are a great nutritional sources for both essential amminoacids, vitamin D, magnesium, potassium, fluorine, iodine, and iron.

It makes a great carrier oil, but gets rancid fast.

To administer medicinally 2 oz. of Sunflower seeds to 1 quart of water; boil down to 12 oz. and strain; add 6 oz. of Holland gin and 6 oz. of honey. It's a good tonic and immune booster for the colder months, to be administered at 1~2 teaspoons 3~4 times a day.

Trout Lily

Yellow Trout Lily, Yellow Dogtooth Violet, Adder's Tongue.

Erythronium americanum.

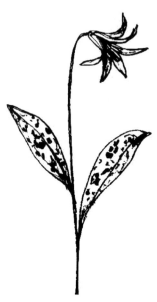

Identification: This enchanting plant, belonging to the Lily family, is a delightful sight as one of the earliest spring flowers, blooming from April to May. It can be found in various locations across the United States, including moist meadows and lightly wooded areas.

It has bulb-like root system, the plant's root extends below the surface, with a white interior and a fawn-colored exterior. From the bulb, delicate feather-like roots emerge, contributing to its overall structure and nutrient absorption.

The stem of this plant gracefully supports two lanceolate leaves, which are pale green in color and adorned with purplish or brownish spots. One of the leaves is nearly double the width of the other, creating an intriguing asymmetrical display. Interestingly, the leaves are more dynamic and active compared to the bulb, showcasing their importance in the plant's growth and survival.

The captivating flower of this plant boasts a vibrant yellow color, with its petals elegantly swept away from the downward-facing center. This unique positioning enhances the flower's allure and creates an eye-catching display. It is worth noting that the petals have the remarkable ability to partially close during nighttime and cloudy days, further adding to the plant's mystique. As the summer heat intensifies, this plant gradually diminishes, resting until its next spring bloom.

Completing its life cycle, the plant produces a capsule-like fruit. This fruit serves as a vessel for housing and dispersing the plant's seeds, contributing to its reproductive success and propagation.

Traditional Uses: The Cherokee and Haudenosaunee peoples employed trout lily for a variety of therapeutic purposes, including reducing fever, healing wounds, and even preventing conception. Trout Lily was used medicinally by Native Americans, who drank root tea for fevers, made poultices for wounds and splinters, and even ate the uncooked leaves for contraception.

Modern uses: According to current studies, the plant's water extracts are antibacterial.

Emetic, Emollient, and Antiscorbutic when fresh. Nutritive when dry.

Pollinators/Wildlife: Spring bumblebees and large mining bees are the primary pollinators of the Trout Lily. Early in the spring, a queen bee emerges in quest of nectar to feed her workers. The nectar of the Trout Lily feeds the hive and acts as an adhesive to adhere pollen to the foraging queen.

A bee visiting a Trout Lily flower normally extracts half of the pollen available in one visit. It frequently pauses in the middle of pollen collection to groom itself and pack the pollen into pollen baskets on its hind legs, as if it is not in a rush. It immediately returns to its hive to unload the pollen. Cross-pollination is hampered for the Trout Lily as a result of this, as the amount of pollen reaching other Trout Lily blooms is severely limited. Trout Lily compensates by having two sets of anthers, one of which opens one day and the other the next, preventing a bee from collecting all of the pollen from a specific flower in one day and allowing other insects to cross-pollinate.

Solvents: Water, alcohol.

Medicinal Parts: The bulb and leaves.

Hardiness Zones: Zones 3-9.

Sourcing: Trout Lily thrives in the Adirondack Mountains of upstate New York's northern hardwood woodlands. It flowers, develops fruit, and dies back before the canopy trees leaf out in the spring. Southern Ontario to Georgia, west to Kentucky, Missouri, and Oklahoma, and north to Minnesota are all places where it can be found. They can be difficult to discover in the wild since they bloom selectively. Source from a reputable local nursery. Trout Lily, like most native wildflowers, should not be transplanted from their natural habitat. If you want to add trout lily to your garden, make sure you get it from a nursery that uses wildflower propagation methods.

Gardening Tips: The tubers of the trout lily, like those of other garden lilies, lack a hard outer skin, making them susceptible to drying. As a result, it's critical to plant the tubers as soon as possible after purchasing them.

Because the trout lily is self-pollinating, two plants are not required. Trout Lily, on the other hand, is best placed in an area where it can naturally grow. Make sure not to destroy the corms that develop from the plant when weeding around it. They will bury themselves in the earth, which will sprout more lilies.

Many ants in or around the plants is a good indicator because trout lily has a symbiotic relationship with ants, who assist the plant naturalize by spreading the seeds. Leave the leaves in place as a natural mulch throughout the winter once it has died back in the summer.

Trout Lily is a member of the lily family; therefore, the popular name dogtooth violet is inaccurate (Liliaceae). The plant's name comes from the toothlike form of the underground rhizomes.

An east-facing area with morning sun is ideal for growing trout lily. Trout Lily thrives beneath deciduous trees like oaks and maples in its natural habitat. This site provides adequate sunlight in the early spring before the trees have leafed out, which the plants require to thrive and bloom.

Later in the summer, dappled shadow should provide protection from the scorching midday and afternoon sun.

Trout Lily may grow in any bright, moist, humus-rich soil that is comparable to that of its native habitat.

During the spring growing season, the plant requires around one inch of water each week from rain or irrigation. After the trout lily has gone dormant in the summer, it requires drier conditions and does not require irrigation.

The trout lily is a cold-hardy plant that thrives in a temperate area.

The plant does not require any additional fertilizer. Instead, plant trout lily in rich soil and top it with organic matter every spring before new growth begins.

Because the trout lily is difficult to grow from seed, it is best propagated via division. It's time to divide the plants after a few years when they've grown into leafy clumps. In the spring, mark their location, so you know where to dig the bulbs in the late summer. Replant the bulbs three inches deep and thoroughly mulch them.

Consumption Methods: When brewed as a tea, Trout Lily and Horsetail grass create a potent remedy for various conditions, including bleeding or ulcers of the breast, bowels, and tumors. This herbal tea can effectively address inflammation and promote healing in these areas.

For immediate relief from nosebleeds, a poultice or liniment made from Trout Lily and Horsetail grass can be applied. This application not only helps stop the bleeding but also aids in soothing sore eyes when used as an eye compress.

Simmering the fresh roots and leaves of Trout Lily and Horsetail grass in milk offers multiple benefits. This preparation is particularly effective in relieving dropsy, hiccups, vomiting, and bleeding from the lower bowels. Its soothing properties can alleviate discomfort and promote overall digestive well-being.

Another method involves infusing the juice of the Trout Lily plant in apple cider. This infusion has been found to be helpful in addressing the aforementioned conditions, providing additional support for healing and symptom relief.

Furthermore, boiling the Trout Lily plant in oil yields a powerful solution that is believed to be a panacea for wounds and inflammation reduction. This infusion can be applied topically to promote healing and soothe inflamed areas.

Warnings: Trout Lily is safe to use in moderation.

Turtlehead

Balmony, Bitter Herb, Codhead, Fish Mouth, Shellflower, Snakehead, Snake Mouth, Turtle Bloom.

Chelone glabra.

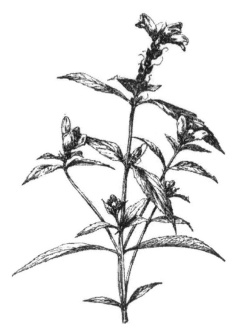

Identification: Wetland dweller from 3' to 5' with a white, showy flower (with pink tinge) that blooms in late summer. Flower, 1.5" to 2" long, is two-lipped, snapdragon-like, and looks like the shell of a turtle. Leaves are opposite, coarsely toothed, lance shaped and dark green on a smooth stem. Seeds are round and bitter.

Medical Uses: Native Americans employed Turtleheads as a mild laxative, similar to senna, rather than the harsh purgative, jamalgota, in their traditional medicinal systems. It's a bitter plant, similar to white horehound, with a mild tea flavor. A decoction of the entire herb was and is still used as a drink for ingestion, gall bladder disorders such as gallstones, liver complaints such as jaundice, nausea, and vomiting, and colic. It was thought to be an anti-depressant and to promote appetite; therefore, it could be useful in the treatment of anorexia nervosa.

The herb was applied externally to piles, irritated breasts, tumors, ulcers, and other skin inflammations in the form of an ointment.

Cherokee used the plant to treat worms. Smashed roots infused to yield anti-witchcraft potion. Also used as a dietary aid to increase appetite due to its bitter taste. Various eastern Native American nations used the herb to reduce fevers and as a laxative (Moerman, p. 154). The ointment of the aerial parts of the plant was used to treat ulcers, painful breasts, and inflamed tumors.

Modern uses: Homeopathic preparation of above-ground parts of plant are used by homeopaths to treat liver and digestive orders to include worm infestation.

Anthelmintic, Cathartic, and Tonic.

Pollinators/Wildlife: This plant is used by the Baltimore Checker Spot butterfly to lay its eggs, making it an important conservation plant. They rely almost exclusively on bumblebees for pollination. A favorite of butterflies and even hummingbirds might visit.

Protect it from deers and small mammals

Solvents: Boiling water, alcohol.

Hardiness Zones: Zones 4-8.

Sourcing: Turtlehead is a perennial that may be found across much of the eastern United States. It grows to a height of 2 to 3 feet and is commonly found near stream banks and moist terrain; obviously, this makes finding wild Turtlehead an easier task along wet streams and riverbanks.

Gardening Tips: The Turtlehead plant is a captivating addition to any garden, boasting pale pink blooms and a mature height ranging from 2 to 3 feet (61-91 cm). Its adaptability makes it a practical choice for gardeners. This plant thrives in moist environments but can also tolerate dry soil conditions. It prefers well-drained soil with a neutral pH and can be grown in full sun or partial shade. Turtlehead flowers can be established from seeds indoors, by direct sowing in wetlands, or by dividing immature plants. When harvesting the beautiful blooms, it is important to do so sparingly and refrain from foraging from the wild. In a vase, Turtlehead flowers can last approximately a week. These plants are deer-resistant, making them a great choice for planting around the edges of vegetable gardens. Additionally, the late summer blossoms attract butterflies and hummingbirds, providing a delightful touch of wildlife to the garden. Turtlehead is easy to divide, allowing for effortless propagation. Applying a thick layer of organic mulch around the plants helps retain moisture and suppress weeds. Suitable for USDA planting zones 4 through 8, Turtlehead thrives in various regions but is not well-suited to desert-like environments.

White turtlehead: the showy spikes of milky white flowers bloom in late summer and early fall, and the seedpod fruits ripen brown and stand tall for winter interest. Turtleheads do best on the edge of a pond or stream, or in a wetland garden. They spread slowly by rhizomes, forming clumps, so are suitable for traditional perennial borders that remain moist. Plants usually grow around 3 feet tall in a garden setting. White turtlehead is the sole host plant for the dazzling Baltimore checkerspot butterfly across most of the Upper Midwest, where it overwinters in leaf litter as a caterpillar. You may see the butterfly at the Minnesota Landscape Arboretum's gardens and wild wetlands in midsummer. White turtlehead thrives in continually moist garden soil—it languishes in dry conditions. Propagate by division.

Rose turtlehead is the perfect native for a traditional perennial border in wet conditions, or at least one that stays moist. Like white turtlehead, it prefers wet soils but will grow in continually moist garden soil—it languishes in dry conditions. Plants usually grow around 3 feet tall in a garden setting. The showy flowering spikes bear rosy pink flowers that are shaped like the heads of turtles and protrude from the stem. Hummingbirds and large bumblebees that are able to open and enter the flowers are responsible for pollination. The seedpod fruits ripen brown and stand tall for winter interest. Propagate turtleheads by division.

Consumption Methods: Turtlehead is a bitter tonic and among the best medicine there is for improving appetite. When the stomach action is weak, Turtlehead has a stimulating influence. A tea of the leaves is given to correct the inactivity due to the sluggish flow of liver fluids. Is used for jaundice, chronic malarial complaints, dyspepsia, constipation and during convalescence from febrile and inflammatory diseases. Balmony is a vermifuge and is regarded by some herbalists as having no superior in expelling worms. An infusion of 1 oz. of the leaves to 1 pint of boiling water may be taken frequently in wine glass amounts.

Warnings: As Turtlehead can be gastrically powerful, it is important to keep this in mind when dosing, as taking too much can induce upset.

Virginia Bluebells

Virginia Cowslip, Lungwort Oysterleaf, Roanoke Bells.

Mertensia virginica.

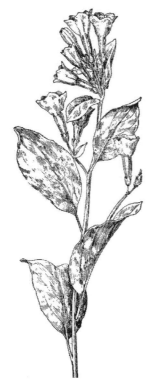

Medical Uses: It was used by Native Americans to cure whooping cough and T.B., and its roots were used as a therapy for venereal disease and as an antidote to poisons, either alone or in combination. This herb was utilized by the Cherokee Tribe to treat whooping cough, tuberculosis, and other respiratory illnesses. This plant's roots were utilized by the Iroquois to treat venereal disease.

Pollinators/Wildlife: Because of the trumpet form of the blooms, butterflies are the most common pollinators of Virginia Bluebells, which may land on the flower's edge and reach the nectar. Pollination is more challenging for bumblebees since they must hover in front of the flower. As you can tell, due to their abundance of nectar and unique shape, they're a favorite of pollinating insects.

Solvents: Boiling water, alcohol.

Hardiness Zones: Zones 3-8.

Sourcing: As you venture through the spring woods, prepare to be enchanted by the captivating display of Virginia Bluebells. These exquisite flowers bloom in a true blue hue, creating a stunning carpet of color that brings joy to any observer. Virginia Bluebells are native woodland wildflowers, thriving in damp woodlands and river flood plains across a wide range. From New York to Minnesota and even extending into Canada (Ontario and Quebec), as well as from Kansas to Alabama, these flowers grace the landscapes with their beauty. Their preference for moist and warm environments makes them particularly fond of southern climates, where they can be found in woodlands and marshes. The native range of Virginia Bluebells encompasses a vast area in eastern North America, spanning from Quebec and Ontario in the north to Mississippi, Georgia, and Alabama in the south. They even reach as far west as the Mississippi River, with Kansas being the westernmost state where these captivating blooms can be found. If you wish to cultivate Virginia Bluebells, it is advisable to obtain seeds from reputable nurseries or consider foraging them responsibly in the wild, avoiding the transplantation of established plants.

Gardening Tips:

The flowers of Virginia bluebells mature from pink buds yet are mainly shades of blue, from soft smoky blue to medium porcelain blue—no photograph can do them justice. Plants grow 1–2 feet tall and may be used in traditional landscapes like any bulb that has spectacular spring flowers and then goes dormant by early summer. They are an essential component of natural woodland and shade gardens and perfect naturalized in a lawn or included for seasonal color in a traditional perennial border. Virginia bluebells thrives in deep loamy soils; it languishes in poorly drained clays or poor dry soils. Propagate by dividing the fleshy rhizome after the plant goes dormant. Self-sows readily. Virginia Bluebells may be deemed invasive in some locations. It's crucial to be aware of how easily this wildflower self-seeds even in its natural range. It will quickly spread, forming dense clumps and colonies.

The first step in effectively producing Virginia Bluebells is to know where to place them. A woody portion of your yard is ideal because they require dappled sun or some shade. With a lot of rich, organic stuff, the soil should drain efficiently while being consistently moist. You shouldn't have to do anything to keep Bluebells alive if you live in the correct climate. Plants can be propagated via seed or division, but if possible, avoid transferring them. They form a large taproot and dislike being transplanted. Dig up your existing plants only when they are dormant, in the fall or very early spring, to propagate them.

Warnings: As they contain glycosides, they can cause gastric upset and diarrhea.

Yarrow

Milfoil, Thousandleaf, Soldier's Woundwort, Bloodwort, Nose Bleed, Devil's Nettle, Sanguinary, Old-Man's-Pepper, Stenchgrass.

Achillea millefolium.

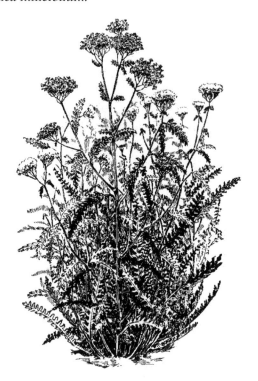

Medical Uses: Yarrow plants are not native to North America, according to certain texts, especially older botanical literature, and were introduced by early Europeans. Although we are not botanists, we find that allegation difficult to believe because we are familiar with indigenous Yarrow words in a variety of Native American languages; yet, we are unaware of any Native American Yarrow words taken from English, French, or Spanish. (Most European-introduced plants and animals are in the exact opposite position.) Yarrow also has a more important and long-standing role in traditional Native American herbalism than dandelions and chicory, which are more recent herbal arrivals. Recent botany literature appears to acknowledge various Yarrow subvarieties more frequently, implying that there were minor genetic variations between Old World and New World Yarrow types and that most Yarrow growing wild in North America today is a hybrid variety of the two. Check out the second volume to discover more uses and recipes.

Pollinators/Wildlife: Pollinators attracted to Yarrow include bees and beetles, but it also draws in butterflies. Yarrow attracts miner, digger, bumble, leafcutter, mason, and sweat bees.

Solvents: Boiling water, alcohol.

Hardiness Zones: Zones 3-7.

Sourcing: Yarrow, also known as Achillea millefolium, is a resilient perennial herb that can be found in various habitats across the globe. It has a wide distribution, growing in meadows, pastures, open woodlands, and disturbed areas. Yarrow is native to Europe, Asia, and North America but has naturalized in many other regions.

In terms of habitat preference, yarrow thrives in well-drained soils with full sun exposure. It can tolerate a range of soil types, including sandy, loamy, and clay soils. Yarrow is drought-tolerant and can withstand dry conditions, making it suitable for arid environments. It is also adaptable to different climates, from cool temperate regions to hot and dry areas.

When it comes to sourcing yarrow, there are several methods to consider. One option is to grow yarrow from seeds. Yarrow seeds can be obtained from reputable seed suppliers or collected from mature plants. Sow the seeds in early spring or fall, ensuring good soil contact but not burying them too deep. Keep the soil moist until the seeds germinate, which typically takes around 14 to 21 days.

Another way to source yarrow is through division. Established yarrow plants can be divided in early spring or fall when they are dormant. Carefully dig up the plant and separate the root clumps into smaller sections, ensuring each division has sufficient roots and foliage. Replant the divisions in well-prepared soil, water them thoroughly, and provide appropriate care to support their growth.

In addition to growing yarrow, it can also be foraged in the wild. Harvest the aerial parts of the plant, including the leaves, stems, and flowers, during the blooming season. Cut the stems above the basal leaves, leaving the

Because Yarrow is commonly grown by division, the easiest option is to purchase your Yarrow as a plant.

Gardening Tips: To ensure proper spacing, it's recommended to plant multiple yarrow plants about 12 to 24 inches (30-60 cm) apart. Alternatively, you can grow yarrow from seeds, which can be started indoors about six to eight weeks before the last frost date. Use moist potting soil and lightly cover the seeds with a thin layer of soil.

Create an ideal environment for germination by placing the yarrow seeds in a sunny and warm location. It typically takes around 14 to 21 days for the seeds to germinate, but this can vary depending on the conditions. To retain moisture and accelerate germination, cover the pot with plastic wrap. Once the seeds sprout, remove the plastic wrap to prevent excessive humidity.

Yarrow plants thrive in full sun, regardless of whether they were grown from seeds or purchased as mature plants. While yarrow is adaptable to various soil types, it prefers well-drained soil. It's impressive how yarrow can thrive even in poor, dry, and low-fertility soils.

However, it's important to exercise caution when growing yarrow, as it has the potential to become invasive under certain conditions. Keep an eye on its growth and take necessary control measures if needed to prevent it from spreading uncontrollably.

Once established, yarrow requires minimal attention. It doesn't require regular fertilization and only needs to be watered during prolonged drought periods. Yarrow is generally low-maintenance; however, it can be susceptible to a few diseases and pests. Common issues include Botrytis mold or powdery mildew, which leave a white powdery coating on the leaves. Treating them with fungicides can help. Additionally, occasional attacks by spittlebugs have been observed on yarrow plants.

Consumption Methods: See the second volume!

It also makes for an easily grown long-lasting cut flower.

Warnings: Yarrow doesn't carry too many harsh side effects but can cause drowsiness.

Conclusion

I hope you have enjoyed reading this book as much as I've enjoyed writing it, and I hope it will accompany you in your ongoing journey to the discovery of Native American herbs and their medicinal uses.

If you found this book useful and are feeling generous, please take the time to leave a short review on Amazon so that other may enjoy this guide as well.

I leave you with good wishes and hopefully a better knowledge of the plants around us and their amazing powers. This volume is part of a seven-books series on Native American Herbalism from foraging and gardening native plants to making herbal remedies for adults and children. Check out the other volumes to gain a deeper understanding of the amazing wisdom and knowledge of our forefathers and to improve not only your health, but the health of our land as well.

The Native American Herbalist's Bible 7

A Companion to Holistic Pediatric Healthcare

How to make and use gentle native herbs and herbal remedies to soothe common children's ailments

Linda Osceola Naranjo

Introduction

We live in a country where the cure for virtually any disease and ailment is within our grasp. In our forests, meadows, plains, and gardens grow small, seemingly insignificant flowers and herbs, plants that we don't look twice at, and trees of which we don't even bother to learn the name. Yet, they are the key to a better, healthier, and more sustainable way of life.

Our forefathers, more attuned with nature than we could ever imagine to be, understood that, and took carefully and sparingly the gifts that Nature offered to heal themselves and grow stronger.

We have lost that knowledge.

Only starting from the 1970s, a renewed interest in botanic medicine has uncovered the depth of the Native American knowledge of plants and their healing powers. The research has not only helped herbalists, but physicians and scientist as well that re-discovered substances that the Native Americans people knew about for hundreds of years. This book is the extended edition of the best-selling The Native American Herbalist's Bible: 3-in-1 Companion to Herbal Medicine, offering four more volumes on gardening techniques, growing healing plants and wildflowers, and pediatric healthcare.

This is the unabridged companion to Native American herbs, their traditional and modern use, complete with appropriate doses and usage, gardening tips and techniques for both medicinal plants and wildflowers. The book is completed by a list of simple and effective recipes for the most common ailments for both adults and children.

You don't need to put at risk the delicate natural balance of your body and that of your loved ones by taking drugs and medications, if an easily available natural solution is just outside your door. Harvest carefully or grow your own herbs, learn to know your body and what works best for you, communicate with the nature surrounding you, and you will in a small way bring back a culture that for too long has been treated as inferior.

This book will teach how to find and treat the herbs the way the native American tribes did: from the forest to your herbalist table, but you will have to find your way to listen to your body and the plants around you.

To aid you in your holistic journey, we have decided to divide the book in seven handy volumes.

The first volume will give you a full theoretical approach to Native American medicine and the herbal medicines methods and preparations.

The second volume is a complete encyclopedia of all the most relevant herbs used in traditional Native American medicine, complete with modern examples, doses, and where to find them, making it a very effective field guide.

The third volume is a "recipe book" of sorts: it offers easy herbal solutions to the most common diseases a budding naturopath can encounter. It is meant as a jumping point to find your own way to treat yourself and your fellow man and will come in handy even to the most experienced herbalist.

The fourth volume provides a complete theoretical and practical approach to Native American traditional planting techniques and how they can be implemented in modern gardens.

The fifth volume is the native gardener's almanac for medicinal herbs. Foraging is not always an option and a lot of herbs are handy to have in your garden: this volume will guide you through the herbs that you can and (should) have in your garden.

The sixth volume continues the guide to the plants you can plant in your gardens focusing on healing wildflowers, which are not only good for your health, but for the planet as well, and they are not bad on the eyes either!

This last volume focuses on native pediatric healthcare. Treating children is a very delicate undertaking, their physiology is more sensitive to external agents, especially drugs. Natural herbalist treatments are effective and gentle in treating common, less severe, pathologies and they won't needlessly weaken your child's immune system. The herbs listed in this last volume have been carefully researched to specifically treat children and their ailments, avoiding any allergic reaction and boosting their immune system.

I am happy to guide through a life-changing journey in search of lost knowledge, amazing healing plants, and carefully crafted herbal remedies and I hope it will help you nurture a stronger relationship with the nature surrounding us and the many gifts it bestows upon us.

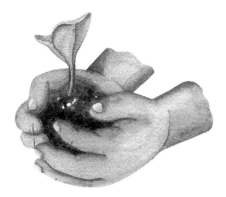

Children are unique creatures with sensitive, highly reactive bodies that are still evolving. They have a big heart, are forgiving, and have a lot of energy. The source of our lives' illumination. They are human, and they, like us, become sick from time to time. When this happens, keep in mind that their delicate bodies require a cautious approach to mending. It's understandable that the first thing we want to do is call the doctor. We want to make our children feel better as quickly as possible. It's heartbreaking to witness your child suffering from a cough that keeps them awake at night or having trouble breathing due to congestion. A doctor will usually prescribe a pharmaceutical treatment, an over-the-counter medication, or tell you to relax and drink plenty of water. A more holistic doctor may suggest medicinal plants as an alternative to other pharmaceuticals that have adverse effects and often contain questionable chemicals.

Medicinal herbs are plants that contain substances and elements that help the body heal in a variety of ways. For at least 60,000 years, people have been using plants in this way. Plants have long been used as medicine in every culture on the planet. Much of that information has been lost or forgotten over time. Fortunately, we now have access to a wealth of information at our fingertips. This makes it simple to determine which plants we may use and why. Scientific research has proven, and continues to prove, what people have known for a long time: medicinal herbs work. As I previously stated, children are delicate and require a gentler approach; thus, not all herbs are suitable for children. However, there are many that work well with children; some are referred to as "children's herbs," and they are all safe and without adverse effects. As a result, there are herbal medicines for children that are both safe and effective!

Hopefully, this information will assist you and your family in achieving holistic health. Please keep in mind that the information provided is not meant to replace or substitute for the advice of a medical professional or physician. Always check with your doctor first since some herbs may be harmful to you depending on your circumstances. It is always recommended to take on additional study so that you can feel secure about using medicinal herbs with your family because you have the greatest information.

The Benefits of Herbal Treatments for Children

You might be a bit skeptical about treating your children with herbal remedies, after all we are more willing to put on the line adults' health to try unknown herbal treatments rather than children's, for whom we might prefer "tried-and-tested", scientifically-proven, Western medicine treatments. However, we mustn't forget that herbal treatments have been around for much longer than supposedly safe chemical agents and drugs. The benefits to using herbal medicine on children are the same as in adult:

- Using natural herbal remedies and treatments are a boost to overall holistic health.
- There is no requirement for a prescription.
- Side effects are reduced and not as pronounced as in the case of using pharmaceutical medicine.
- Herbal treatments can be foraged, home-grown, and are extremely cost effective.

With the added benefit that treating your children with herbal medicine will boost their immunity system and make them less reliant on chemical antibiotics and antivirals for all their life.

Children's bodies are more sensitive than adults. Herbs are a very safe and effective way to boost your children's immune system and treat minor ailments without having to rely on chemical antibiotics and drugs. They are usually gentler than pharmaceutical alternatives, and they provide therapeutic properties without disrupting children's delicate equilibrium. Colds, flu, chickenpox, measles, and even teething problems can all be treated with herbs. They assist children with inflammation, digestion, and other issues. There largely isn't a condition that herbal remedies can't help to solve.
Just to get some perspective, let's consider some interesting statistics.

Did you know that every year in the United States, there are over 1,500 accidental deaths caused by legally prescribed prescription drugs? It's shocking to think that these drugs, which are intended to heal, can sometimes have devastating consequences. In fact, prescription drugs are now the fourth leading cause of death in the nation. And when we add over 1,000 deaths caused by the side effects of drugs, we're looking at a staggering 2,500 medication-related deaths per year.

Now, let's shift our focus to herbs. How many calls do you think the American Association of Poison Control Centers (AAPCC) receives about poisoning from herbs and herbal remedies? You might be surprised to learn that the AAPCC receives so few calls in this regard that they don't even have a special category for herbs.

Consider this: in 2019, the AAPCC reported a total of 2,100 exposures to herbal products among children under the age of six. However, the majority of these exposures resulted in minimal or no effects. In fact, the AAPCC's annual report stated that there were no deaths reported due to herbal exposures in that year. This stark contrast to the thousands of deaths caused by prescription drugs highlights the safety and low risk associated with herbs. It's important to recognize that both traditional herbal medicine and modern allopathic medicine offer tremendous gifts of healing, and they can complement one another. While herbs excel in addressing common ailments, nourishing the body, and promoting overall wellness, allopathic medicine is often the superior choice for life-threatening illnesses and acute symptoms that require rapid intervention.

While allopathic medicine may work quickly and efficiently, it's important to acknowledge its limitations. Pharmaceuticals are potent substances, especially in the small bodies of children, and they can have unintended side effects. On the other hand, herbal remedies, when used appropriately, are gentle, time-tested, and offer a holistic approach to healing. They not only effectively address various health concerns but also have ecological benefits, as they do not pollute waterways and soil like some modern drugs do. It's worth noting that using herbs and allopathic medicine together can be a harmonious and effective approach to healthcare. However, it's crucial to ensure that your doctor or healthcare provider is familiar with both systems and can provide guidance when determining the appropriate use of herbs and pharmaceuticals in specific situations.

The herbs mentioned in this book have been carefully selected for their safety and compatibility with pharmaceuticals. However, as you explore other herbs and natural remedies, it's advisable to seek the guidance of a knowledgeable holistic healthcare provider who can help you navigate potential interactions and ensure the best outcomes for your child's health. In addition to the health advantages, introducing children to the world of herbs can foster a deeper appreciation for the natural world. By opting for herbal treatments whenever possible and teaching them about the value of plants, we can help children develop a stronger connection to nature. Opting for native herbal remedies can also serve as an opportunity to educate them about the complex workings of soil, water, and pollinators that contribute to the growth and healing properties of plants. By incorporating herbal medicine into your family's healthcare routine and collaborating with a holistic pediatric healthcare provider, you not only promote better health but also instill in your child a sense of compassion and mindfulness towards their own bodies and the natural world around them. It's a journey that empowers them to take an active role in their own well-being while respecting and cherishing the bountiful offerings of nature.

A word of caution

Herbs can be your go-to solution for a wide range of simple ailments that children commonly experience, such as colic, rashes, teething discomfort, and everyday bumps and bruises. They can also effectively address common childhood illnesses including ear infections, colds and flu, stomach bugs, and even chicken pox. For these everyday health concerns, herbs can be used with confidence as safe and effective remedies.

However, if you find that herbal remedies aren't providing the desired results or if a more complex health issue arises, it may be time to consider allopathic treatment as the next step. Allopathic medicine, with its focus on emergency and crisis situations, excels in serious and life-threatening conditions. It's crucial to establish a relationship with a pediatrician, preferably one who takes a holistic approach to healthcare. Build this rapport in time, checking in regularly while your child is well, so that the physician is familiar with your children's conditions and preferences and you'll be prepared should a situation arise that requires medical attention.

There are certain signs and symptoms that indicate it's time to seek medical help for your child. It's important to be vigilant and responsive to these indications:

- If your child isn't responding to the herbal treatments you're using, it may be a sign that a more serious intervention is necessary.
- Signs of serious illness, such as a high fever greater than 102°F/39°C, persistent low-grade fever, hemorrhaging, delirium, severe dizziness, unconsciousness, or severe abdominal pain, should not be ignored.
- If your child appears lethargic, weak, unresponsive, or difficult to awaken, seek medical attention promptly.
- Complaints of a stiff neck and headache, coupled with an inability to touch the chin to the chest, or a bulging fontanel (soft spot on top of the head) in babies, could be early signs of meningitis, a condition that requires immediate medical attention.
- Recurring ear infections in your child should be evaluated by a medical professional.
- Difficulty breathing or a bluish color around the lips are signs of respiratory distress and should be addressed urgently.
- Dehydration is a serious concern. Look out for dry lips, a dry mouth, and the absence of urination for over six hours as warning signs.
- If your child exhibits signs of a severe allergic reaction, especially after a bee sting or ingestion of a new food, such as difficulty breathing or swallowing, flushing or redness of the face, swelling of the face or tongue, nausea or vomiting, severe abdominal pain, palpitations, anxiety, or any other unusual responses, seek immediate medical attention.

- Red streaks on the skin extending from a point of infection could indicate blood poisoning and require medical intervention.
- A severe burn, a burn that covers an area twice the size of your child's hand, or any burn that appears to be infected should be assessed by a healthcare professional.

Remember, while herbs are valuable allies for many health concerns, knowing when to seek medical help is essential. By remaining attentive to your child's symptoms and seeking appropriate care when needed, you're ensuring their well-being and giving them the best of both worlds: the benefits of herbal remedies and the expertise of allopathic medicine when necessary.

Patch test

Patch testing or skin allergy testing can be a valuable tool to determine the suitability of a new remedy for your specific needs. This simple yet effective test helps identify any potential skin allergies, ensuring a safe and favorable experience with the product. The best part is, you can easily perform a patch test in the comfort of your own home.

Whether you're considering tinctures, raw herbs, creams, lotions, facial products, oils and serums, shampoos and conditioners, moisturizers, toners, or eye care, conducting a patch test is a wise approach to safeguard your skin's well-being. Even if you've had sensitivities to certain compounds in the past, a patch test can provide you with vital information.

Let's go through the step-by-step process of conducting a patch test at home:

1. Begin by placing a small amount of the substance you wish to test in your mouth. Monitor for any adverse reactions for a few minutes. If no reaction occurs, you can proceed to the next step.
2. Prior to applying the product, ensure that the designated area on your skin is clean and completely dry. If you've recently taken a hot shower, it's advisable to wait approximately 15 minutes before initiating the patch test. This precaution allows any residual heat and humidity to dissipate, ensuring accurate test results.
3. Apply a small amount of the product to the inside of your upper arm, selecting a spot where any potential reaction will be readily visible. To prevent any external factors from interfering, cover the area with a bandage after applying the product.
4. Allow a minimum of 24 hours for the patch test to run its course. During this time, it's crucial to ensure that the patch remains dry. Avoid activities such as swimming, showering, intense exercise, or exposure to excessive heat, as they may compromise the integrity of the test.

5. After the 24-hour period, carefully inspect the patch test site for any reactions. Take note of any itching, redness, swelling, burning sensations, rashes, or stinging. If no adverse reactions occur, it indicates that the product is safe for further use.

Allergic Reaction vs. Irritant Reaction

Allergic reactions occur immediately after using a new product, and some individuals may experience symptoms such as itching, redness, or a mild stinging sensation. It's important to note that allergic reactions involve the immune system and can vary in severity. While mild symptoms are common, more severe reactions can manifest as swelling, hives, difficulty breathing, or even anaphylaxis.

Anaphylaxis is a severe and potentially life-threatening allergic reaction that requires immediate medical attention.

On the other hand, irritant reactions are relatively minor and short-lived. They typically last for about ten minutes and do not recur upon subsequent use of the product. Unlike allergic reactions, irritant reactions do not involve the immune system. However, they can exacerbate pre-existing skin conditions such as eczema, leading to discomfort and potential flare-ups.

In the rare instance that a patch test triggers respiratory symptoms or anaphylactic shock, it's essential to seek immediate medical attention. Individuals who have previously experienced anaphylactic shock are at a higher risk of it occurring again. Therefore, if you have a history of anaphylactic shock, it's advisable to consult with your doctor before conducting a patch test, ensuring your safety and well-being.

When it comes to children's health, it's always important to consult with a pediatrician before using herbal remedies. Finding a healthcare provider who understands and supports your holistic approach to your child's well-being is key. Maintaining a cooperative and respectful relationship with your child's doctor enables them to build trust and establish a strong rapport with medical professionals, ensuring comprehensive and effective care for your little ones. By working together, you can navigate the best treatment options for your child and promote their overall health and wellness.

Everything in moderation

It's understandable that if you've come across reports regarding the potential toxicity of herbs, it may seem alarming when even seemingly harmless herbs like chamomile and peppermint end up on sensationalized "black lists." However, it's important to understand that problems don't arise by the simple act of incorporating herbal remedies in your child's care, but rather from the way herbs are sometimes used in excessively concentrated dosages that go beyond common-sense guidelines.

In the past, herbal remedies were primarily consumed as teas, syrups, and tinctures. These traditional preparations contained modest dosages of the whole herb, which inherently balanced their effects. However, with the advent of herb capsules, large amounts of herb material can now be packed into small pills, allowing for much higher dosages. Additionally, standardized preparations have emerged, offering highly concentrated extracts of specific plant constituents rather than the whole plant. These concentrated forms can surpass the natural concentrations found in nature. While these concentrated dosages have become more readily available in recent times, it's essential to approach them with caution.

Rest assured, with millennia of experience behind the use of medicinal herbs, their safety for your child and your entire family is well-established. However, it's crucial to be a discerning and informed user of herbal remedies. Here are some key principles to keep in mind:

1. **Use herbs with a proven track record of safety**. Stick to well-known and widely used herbs that have been traditionally relied upon for their medicinal properties.

2. **Follow appropriate dosage guidelines**. If you are unsure about the correct dosage for your child, it's always best to consult with a medical professional or a qualified herbalist who specializes in pediatric care.

3. **Pay attention to any idiosyncratic responses**. If you suspect that an herb may be causing an adverse reaction in your child, it's wise to discontinue its use and consult with a healthcare professional to explore alternative options.

4. Whenever you have doubts or your child doesn't seem to be responding as expected to herbal remedies, **seeking guidance from a holistic healthcare professional** is highly recommended. They can provide expert advice tailored to your child's specific needs and guide you in making informed decisions about herbal treatments.

By adhering to these guidelines and consulting with knowledgeable practitioners, you can navigate the world of herbal remedies safely and effectively, harnessing their potential for your child's well-being. Remember, herbs have a rich history of use, and when used judiciously and with respect, they can provide valuable support for your child's health journey.

Gentle Medicinal Native Herbs for Children

When it comes to using herbs for children, it's important to consider their unique physiology and adjust the dosage accordingly. In general, almost any herb that is safe for adults can be used for children as long as the dosage is appropriately tailored to their smaller size and weight. However, for children, it is recommended to focus on herbs that have a "gentler" action to accommodate their constitution.

The herbs listed in this chapter have been carefully selected as they are commonly recommended for children. These herbs are widely recognized as safe and gentle, without causing residual buildup or side effects in the body. While they may be gentle in action, these herbs possess remarkable power and effectiveness. They work in harmony with the body, supporting the immune system, strengthening the nervous system, and nurturing the body's innate ability to heal itself. These gentle herbs should serve as the foundation of herbal healthcare for children. There is often concern about using stronger-acting medicinal herbs such as goldenseal, valerian, or St. John's wort for children. However, in my experience, they can be exceptionally useful and effective when used judiciously. It is important, though, to exercise sensible caution. When employing stronger-acting herbs, it is advisable to use them in much smaller amounts for shorter durations. It is also beneficial to combine them with milder herbs to create a balanced and well-rounded approach to herbal treatment.

For example, goldenseal, a potent immune-supportive herb, can be administered to children in smaller doses for a limited period of time when needed. Valerian, a herb with calming effects, can be used in moderation to support restful sleep or manage occasional anxiety in children. Similarly, St. John's wort, with its proven record of mood-balancing qualities, can be employed cautiously and briefly under the guidance of a healthcare professional for children facing emotional challenges. It is certainly less dangerous, with lesser side effects, and more effective than the psychopharmaceuticals, that are all too often prescribed to children, without much care of the consequences.

By employing a thoughtful and balanced approach, integrating gentle herbs as the mainstay of children's herbal health care while judiciously incorporating stronger-acting herbs for specific needs, we can harness the power of herbs to support our children's well-being in a safe and effective manner. As always, it is advisable to consult with a knowledgeable healthcare practitioner or herbalist who specializes in pediatric care to ensure optimal outcomes for your child's health.

Most of the plants were already discussed extensively in the previous volumes and are discussed hitherto for their benefits on children's health and their safe administration in younger patients.

Aloe

Aloe Vera is an excellent natural remedy for children due to its mild and fast-acting properties. From scrapes and scratches to insect bites, sunburns, and stomach issues, Aloe Vera is a must-have in every natural medicine cabinet. Families across the globe have relied on this ancient herb for thousands of years, and it is both safe and soothing for children of all ages, from toddlers to teenagers.

One minor drawback of Aloe Vera is its softening and detoxifying effect on the stool. If this occurs, simply reduce the daily amount consumed. Rest assured, this adjustment will not cause any other health issues, such as electrolyte imbalances.

Aloe Vera contains no harmful chemicals and is particularly gentle for children. High-quality Aloe Vera products, particularly those derived from whole leaves or concentrated extracts, contain phytonutrients. These active ingredients, numbering over 100, quickly alleviate stomach upsets and may support regular bowel movements without acting as a harsh laxative like prune juice. For a more in-depth understanding of how herbs work for overall wellness, there are excellent books available that delve into the traditional uses accumulated over thousands of years. Aloe Vera plants come in various types and sizes, with over 300 known varieties across different continents. While there may be slight variations, many of these Aloe Vera plants share common active components.

For centuries, Aloe Vera has been used on the skin of both children and adults. This mineral-rich herb, abundant in sulfur, boasts natural growth factors, antimicrobial agents, and anti-inflammatory compounds. Together, these substances work wonders in soothing irritation and maintaining healthy skin. Aloe Vera's remarkable properties make it an effective remedy for sunburns and other skin problems, offering quick relief. Aloe Vera's ability to balance the skin's pH is believed to contribute to its efficacy in soothing skin rashes. When combined with a moisturizing lotion, Aloe Vera helps restore the skin's optimal pH, which can be disrupted by a poor diet or impaired digestive function. Incorporating Aloe Vera into your child's skincare routine and utilizing it for common ailments can provide simple and effective relief.

Safe administration

Use the gel as much as necessary to treat sunburns, itchy skin, dermatitis, and other skin conditions.

Anise

The fruit of an evergreen plant with the fancy name Illicium verum, Anise is a mesmerizing, mahogany-colored, 8-pointed star. It is native to southern China and northern Vietnam. The seeds nestled within each arm of this magical fruit possess a distinctive flavor reminiscent of Licorice and Anise, although they are unrelated to the Fennel Anise commonly known in the West. The deep and nuanced taste of Anise complements meat dishes, broths, poached fruits, mulled wine, and, of course, masala chai, which I personally indulge in every morning. Anise is typically used in its whole, dried form, and occasionally ground. In fact, it plays a vital role in Chinese Five Spice powder, a staple in dishes featuring Chinese pork or poultry.

While there is currently limited scientific evidence supporting the use of Anise as a digestive aid, ancient wisdom has long recommended its benefits in this regard. However, it's essential to note that the FDA has issued warnings against the use of Anise tea in babies and children due to serious and potentially harmful side effects. These adverse effects are likely the result of cross-pollination between Chinese Anise and the dangerous Japanese variety, which is not intended for consumption but rather as incense. To ensure the safe use of Anise, it is advisable to purchase whole Anise from reputable brands and incorporate it into food and beverages in appropriate proportions to enjoy its flavor and potential benefits.

Anethole, a compound found in Anise, has shown promising anti-cancer properties in laboratory studies, particularly against breast and prostate cancer cells. Additionally, linalool, another bioactive chemical present in Anise, may enhance the body's natural defense against cancer by boosting cancer-specific immune function. However, further research is needed to explore these effects in animals and humans. Anethole in Anise exhibits estrogen-like effects, which explains its historical use in promoting lactation, regulating menstruation, and addressing infertility. Nevertheless, excessive estrogenic activity can have negative impacts on the body. To ensure safe usage, incroporate Anise into food in appropriate proportions rather than in concentrated forms.

Furthermore, anethole has antibacterial and antifungal properties, particularly against gram-positive bacteria like Staphylococcus aureus.

Interestingly, Anise contains shikimic acid, a chemical that serves as the starting point for the production of Tamiflu, a widely recognized antiviral medication. However, it's important to note that shikimic acid alone has limited antiviral activity. When combined with quercetin, a compound found in the outer layers of red onions and various plants, it exhibits potent antiviral properties. It's worth mentioning that Fennel and ginger also contain shikimic acid.

Safe administration
The tea is sweet and you can add a bit of anise to other herbal teas to make it more palatable for your children. A ginger and anise tea is an easy, delightful, and effective remedy for an upset stomach. Remember to use whole anise from a reputable source and try testing it as a syrup, yummy and healthy!

Astragalus

Astragalus, a remarkable plant known for its immune-enhancing properties and long-standing medicinal value, has captivated the attention of herbal enthusiasts and health practitioners alike. This perennial herb, scientifically known as *Astragalus membranaceus,* belongs to the legume family and is native to the grasslands of China, Mongolia, and other parts of Asia. With its delicate yet vibrant yellow flowers and slender leaves, astragalus thrives in diverse climatic conditions, displaying its resilience and adaptability. Renowned as a tonic herb, astragalus has earned the reputation of being the "young person's ginseng" due to its adaptogenic nature and rejuvenating effects. It has been an integral component of traditional Chinese medicine for centuries, celebrated for its ability to enhance vitality and promote overall well-being. While there are over 2,000 species of astragalus, *Astragalus membranaceus* is the most commonly used variety in herbal preparations.

One of the key attributes of astragalus lies in its remarkable influence on the immune system. Unlike other immune-supporting herbs that primarily target the body's initial defense mechanisms, astragalus delves deeper into strengthening the immune system's core. It achieves this by replenishing the bone marrow reserve, which plays a vital role in producing immune cells and maintaining the body's protective barrier against pathogens. By nurturing this essential aspect of immunity, astragalus helps fortify the body's natural defenses, making it more resilient to various illnesses and stressors. Moreover, astragalus exhibits potent antioxidant and anti-inflammatory properties, offering additional protective benefits for overall health. It contains an array of beneficial compounds, including polysaccharides, flavonoids, and saponins, which contribute to its therapeutic effects. These bioactive constituents not only support immune function but also contribute to the herb's potential in promoting cardiovascular health, maintaining healthy aging, and supporting liver function.

Incorporating astragalus into your health regimen can be a wise choice, particularly during times when immune support is of utmost importance. Its time-honored use, backed by scientific research, makes it a valuable ally in maintaining optimal wellness.

Safe administration
When it comes to astragalus root, its dried and sliced form resembles a wooden tongue depressor. One of the quickest ways to utilize this potent herb is by preparing a nourishing tea, a method you'll come across frequently in this book for various herbs. Children may even enjoy chewing on a slice of astragalus, much like a licorice stick. Additionally, you can incorporate astragalus into soups and broths by adding a whole or chopped root to the pot and allowing it to simmer for several hours. Before serving, remember to remove the astragalus. Despite its presence, it won't affect the taste of the dish, yet your family can reap the immune-boosting benefits infused into the cuisine. In the event that you're unable to find astragalus in local stores, it is readily available for online purchase, often in shredded dry form. For oral consumption, a recommended dosage of 2 to 6 grams per day is typically suggested.

Calendula

Calendula, also known as marigold, is a remarkable herbal ally for children's health, offering a multitude of positive effects and therapeutic properties. This vibrant and cheerful flower belongs to the Asteraceae family and is native to the Mediterranean region. With its vibrant orange and yellow petals, calendula blooms bring a burst of color to gardens and landscapes, making it a delight for both the eyes and the body.

Calendula possesses powerful anti-inflammatory, antimicrobial, and soothing properties, making it an excellent choice for a variety of childhood ailments. It is commonly used to alleviate skin irritations, such as rashes, eczema, and minor wounds. The flower's gentle yet effective nature makes it suitable for even the most sensitive skin, providing relief and promoting healing without causing further irritation. Calendula can be prepared as a gentle herbal infusion or incorporated into salves, creams, or oils for topical application.

Internally, calendula is beneficial for digestive health. It supports the digestive system, soothing inflammation and promoting healthy gut function. Calendula tea can be prepared by infusing the dried petals in hot water, allowing its therapeutic compounds to be extracted. This mild and soothing tea can aid in relieving digestive discomfort, including colic and stomach cramps. It can be sweetened with a touch of honey for added palatability.

Growing your own calendula is a rewarding experience and allows for a readily available supply of this beneficial herb. Calendula is an easy-to-grow plant, thriving in both garden beds and containers. Its bright flowers attract pollinators and add beauty to any garden. By growing calendula at home, you have control over the cultivation methods, ensuring the purity and quality of the plant. The flowers can be harvested at their peak and dried for future use in teas, infusions, or herbal preparations. Encouraging children to participate in the gardening process instills a deeper connection with nature and fosters an appreciation for the healing gifts provided by plants, check out the final chapter of this volume for more ideas on how to involve children in gardening activities!

Whether applied topically or consumed internally, calendula is a gentle yet effective herbal remedy for children's health. Its versatility, safety, and natural healing properties make it a valuable addition to any natural medicine cabinet. From soothing skin irritations to supporting digestive well-being, calendula offers a holistic approach to promoting children's overall health and wellness.

Safe administration
Make a simple Calendula flower infusion with coconut oil, which is also anti-inflammatory, antibacterial, and antifungal. Even a small amount goes a long way!

Catnip

Catnip, also known as Nepeta cataria, is a fascinating herb that holds numerous benefits for children's health. This herb, a member of the mint family, is renowned for its unique effects on feline friends, but its uses extend beyond playful encounters with our beloved pets. Catnip has a long history of traditional use and is native to Europe and parts of Asia.

Catnip offers a range of positive effects when used for children. It is well-known for its calming properties and is often used to soothe restlessness, nervousness, and anxiety. The herb's gentle sedative action can help promote relaxation and peaceful sleep, making it particularly helpful for children who struggle with bedtime routines or occasional sleep disruptions. Catnip can be prepared as a mild tea or incorporated into herbal preparations such as tinctures or infused oils for topical use.

Additionally, catnip has been found to have digestive benefits. It can aid in relieving stomach discomfort, colic, and indigestion in children. The herb's antispasmodic properties can help soothe the digestive system, reducing cramping and easing gastrointestinal distress. Catnip tea can be administered in small amounts to support healthy digestion, and it is often well-tolerated by children due to its mild flavor. Growing catnip in your own garden can be a delightful and practical endeavor. This perennial herb is easy to cultivate, with its lush green leaves and small white or lavender flowers adding beauty to any garden space. Catnip plants are known to attract butterflies and bees, making it a wonderful addition for encouraging pollinator activity. By growing catnip at home, you have direct access to its fresh leaves and flowers, which can be harvested and used in teas, infused oils, or as an ingredient in homemade remedies. It's important to note that while catnip is generally safe for children, individual sensitivities may vary. It's advisable to start with small amounts and observe your child's reaction before increasing the dosage. If your child exhibits any unusual or adverse reactions, discontinue use and consult with a healthcare professional.

Safe administration
Catnip holds a secret ingredient called nepetalactone, which contributes to its soothing effects. This herb acts as a herbal sedative, similar to valerian, and can offer remarkable relaxation benefits for children. The calming properties of catnip tea may help improve sleep quality, reduce anxiety and worry, and enhance overall mood. When tensions rise, catnip can be your go-to herbal ally. It can be served as a tea throughout the day to alleviate teething discomfort in little ones. Keep in mind that catnip has a bitter taste, so it can be blended with pleasant-tasting herbs like oats and lemon balm or mixed with fruit juice to enhance its palatability.

Catnip also serves as a valuable digestive aid. Offering a few drops of catnip tincture before meals can help support healthy digestion in children. Moreover, when bedtime approaches and your child is feeling fussy, a few drops of catnip tincture can help calm their restlessness and promote a more peaceful sleep. The sedative properties of catnip can work wonders in soothing an agitated child, providing a sense of tranquility and comfort.

One of the notable uses of catnip is its ability to help reduce childhood fevers. It can be employed in two forms for this purpose: as a tincture and as an enema. The catnip tincture can be administered orally, while the enema can be used externally. Both methods aim to harness the fever-reducing properties of catnip, providing relief and comfort during periods of illness.

You'll find the preparation method for tea in the recipe section of this volume.

Chamomile

Chamomile, including the well-known European variety (*Matricaria chamomilla*) and the native North American variety, Wild American chamomile (*Matricaria discoidea*), which has been discussed at lengths in the second volume of this series, is a remarkable herb that offers numerous benefits for children's health. With its delicate flowers and feathery foliage, even the aspect of chamomile exudes a sense of calm and tranquility.

Chamomile is celebrated for its soothing properties and its ability to promote relaxation and support healthy sleep patterns in children. A warm cup of chamomile tea, prepared by infusing dried chamomile flowers, can be a comforting and calming beverage that aids in restful sleep.

Both varieties of chamomile also provide digestive benefits. They possess gentle anti-inflammatory and antispasmodic properties, which can help ease gastrointestinal discomfort such as colic, indigestion, and stomach cramps in children. Chamomile tea or herbal preparations can be administered orally to support healthy digestion and provide relief.

Furthermore, chamomile is known for its beneficial effects on the skin. It can be used topically to soothe minor skin irritations, including rashes, eczema, and insect bites. Chamomile-infused oils or creams offer a gentle and natural solution for promoting skin healing and providing comfort.

Safe administration
To harness the calming properties of chamomile for children, serving chamomile tea sweetened with a touch of honey can be a wonderful choice. This soothing beverage can be offered throughout the day to help calm a stressed or nervous child, promoting a sense of relaxation and tranquility.

In addition to tea, chamomile can be used in the form of an essential oil for its calming effects. Creating a massage oil by blending chamomile essential oil with a carrier oil, such as sweet almond oil, allows for gentle application on the skin. Massaging this oil onto your child's body can provide soothing and calming sensations, helping to alleviate any muscle soreness or tension.

Additionally, chamomile can be used in bathwater to create a calming and therapeutic experience, particularly for soothing skin irritations or promoting relaxation.

Furthermore, chamomile tincture can be used to support healthy digestion in children. By administering a few drops of chamomile tincture before feeding time, you can aid digestion and promote optimal digestive function. This can be particularly helpful for little ones who experience digestive discomfort or have a sensitive stomach.

Remember to start with small amounts when introducing chamomile to your child, especially in essential oil or tincture form, to observe their individual response. If any adverse reactions occur, discontinue use and consult with a healthcare professional.

Warning: Caution should be exercised when using chamomile for children. While it is generally safe, there is a small risk of allergic reactions, especially for those with known plant allergies. Chamomile may also interact with certain medications, and its sedative properties may cause drowsiness. Some children may experience digestive sensitivity. Ensure chamomile is sourced from reputable suppliers, and consult with a healthcare professional before use, especially if your child has underlying medical conditions. By being aware of these considerations, you can safely incorporate chamomile into your child's routine for its calming and digestive benefits.

Comfrey

It's not only a vulnerary, but it's also a demulcent, which is useful when applying a poultice to a wound or burn. It also has the ability to reduce external bleeding. One of the oldest documented usages was by the Greeks, who used it to stop bleeding. It's also an astringent herb, which tightens and tones tissues to minimize fluid loss, as well as an anti-inflammatory and antiseptic.

Comfrey is cooling and moistening, but because it is an astringent, it also has a secondary drying effect. So, it's also a demulcent (slippery and moistening) at first, but it gradually becomes an astringent (drying) to maintain fluids where they belong; hence the energetic term "drying."

Safe administration
External usage of Comfrey is completely safe. When applying Comfrey to wounds externally, keep in mind that it encourages tissue regeneration so well that it can close a wound at the surface before the wound has healed from the inside out.

Warning: Because Comfrey can trap infection inside a wound, make sure there are no signs of infection before applying it.

Dill

Dill, from the old Norse word "dilla" meaning "to lull," has a long-standing reputation for its calming and comforting effects on infants and children. This herb not only aids digestion but also has a remarkable ability to alleviate gastric stress, colic, and nervous digestion in young ones. Rich in essential nutrients such as manganese, magnesium, iron, and calcium, dill offers additional health benefits beyond its soothing properties.

One of the prominent uses of dill is its efficacy in treating various digestive issues. It can help stimulate appetite, relieve gas in the intestines (flatulence), and address liver disorders and gallbladder problems. Dill has also been traditionally employed to address urinary tract problems, including renal disease and conditions associated with painful or difficult urination. Furthermore, dill exhibits a range of therapeutic applications. It can be utilized to manage fever and colds, alleviate coughs and bronchitis, and even provide relief from hemorrhoids. Its antibacterial properties make it effective in combating infections, while its antispasmodic qualities help alleviate spasms and nerve discomfort. Dill is also known for its potential to address genital ulcers and soothe mouth and throat inflammation.

While dill offers numerous health benefits, it is important to use it in moderation and consult with a healthcare professional if your child has any underlying health conditions or if you have any concerns. By harnessing the therapeutic properties of dill, you can provide natural support for your child's digestive health, respiratory well-being, and overall comfort.

Safe administration
If you are not growing it in your garden, Dill is easily found in your local grocery store away, dried, or fresh.

When incorporating dill into your child's health routine, consider various methods of administration. Dill can be used as a flavorful addition to meals, incorporated into soups, stews, or salads, or prepared as a herbal infusion. Additionally, dill essential oil can be diluted and applied topically for localized relief. Dill carries an excellent flavor, so it is particularly easy to sneak into foods all through the year. Meats, soups, anything under the sun can benefit from the tangy, herbal flavor of Dill. There is no recommended dosage for Dill other than to take Dill in moderation.

Echinacea

Echinacea, also known as Purple Coneflower, is a powerful herb native to the United States with a rich history of use by American Indian healers for centuries. Belonging to the daisy family, which includes other plants like ragweed, marigolds, chrysanthemums, and sunflowers, Echinacea is highly regarded for its medicinal properties. Both the root and the flower of the plant are commonly used to create Echinacea supplements, harnessing their beneficial compounds. One of the key benefits of Echinacea is its ability to support the immune system in combating infectious diseases. By enhancing the activity of immune cells that target and eliminate bacteria, fungi, and viruses, Echinacea helps minimize the severity and duration of various illnesses. It has gained significant popularity in recent times for its role in preventing and treating colds, flu, and other respiratory ailments. Echinacea achieves this by increasing the activity of macrophage T-cells, fortifying the body's first line of defense against infection. As a result, it stands as one of the most vital herbs for stimulating the immune system and fighting infections. The remarkable aspect of Echinacea is its potency and effectiveness, while also being safe for children. It is a natural and well-tolerated herb with no known side effects or residual buildup. This makes it a suitable choice for supporting children's immune health without compromising their overall well-being.

In one study, children aged 1 to 5 years old were administered an Echinacea and Vitamin C supplement. For 12 weeks, the children were given the product twice a day. A different set of parents administered a placebo to their child. When compared to the placebo group, the children who took the Echinacea product caught 54% less colds. This implies that combining Echinacea and Vitamin C may help to prevent colds and flu in children and teens.

With its immune-stimulating and infection-fighting properties, Echinacea serves as a valuable herbal ally for both prevention and treatment of respiratory illnesses. By incorporating this herb into your child's wellness routine, you can harness its natural benefits and provide them with additional support for a healthy immune system.

Safe administration
When administering Echinacea, it is advisable to ensure it is taken on a full stomach or with a large glass of water to prevent any potential strain on the stomach. The recommended dosage for ingestion is typically 2 to 6 grams per day. However, it's important to note that Echinacea works best when taken at the onset of an infection or when precautions are warranted, such as when there is a high risk of illness exposure, such as in daycare settings. In such cases, it is recommended to keep your child home and administer Echinacea.

At the first signs of a cold or flu, Echinacea can be taken in the form of tea or tincture to boost the immune system and help fend off the infection. For optimal results, it is beneficial to take frequent but small doses. For adults, this may involve consuming 1/2 teaspoon of tincture or 1/4 cup of tea every 30 to 40 minutes. The dosage should be adjusted accordingly for children based on appropriate dosage charts.

Echinacea can also be utilized as a tea or tincture to address respiratory and bronchial infections in children. Additionally, it can be used as a soothing spray to alleviate sore throats. For conditions like sore gums and mouth inflammation, the tea or diluted tincture can be used as a mouthwash, flavored with peppermint or spearmint essential oil for added comfort.

While the primary use of Echinacea is internal consumption, it can also be beneficial externally. In the form of a wash or poultice, Echinacea can be applied externally to treat skin infections.

Warning: Caution should be exercised when using Echinacea. While it is generally safe and well-tolerated, some individuals may experience allergic reactions, particularly those with known allergies to plants in the daisy family. It is advisable to start with a small dosage and monitor for any adverse reactions. Additionally, Echinacea may interact with certain medications, such as immunosuppressants. If your child has any underlying health conditions or is taking other medications, it is recommended to consult with a healthcare professional before incorporating Echinacea into their regimen. As with any herbal supplement, it is important to use Echinacea responsibly and follow recommended dosages for optimal safety and effectiveness.

Elder

Elder blossoms possess valuable properties as a diaphoretic and relaxant, making them particularly beneficial in managing fevers. These properties help promote tissue relaxation and enhance blood circulation to peripheral areas of the body, such as the skin and limbs. As a result, the pores in the skin open up, facilitating sweating. Sweating not only aids in releasing tension from the body but also assists in cooling it down. Elderflower tea can be a helpful remedy in this regard. Elderflower is a nervine, contributing to relaxation and calmness without causing sedation. In addition to its calming effects, elderberries are rich in vitamin A and C, playing a crucial role in supporting immune system health. They also contain significant amounts of flavonoids and anthocyanins, which offer protective benefits for the heart and contribute to immune enhancement. Both the berries and the flowers of the elder plant possess important antiviral properties. While commonly associated with colds and flu, elder can also be useful in addressing upper respiratory infections. It is frequently combined with echinacea in remedies designed to bolster the immune system.

Safe administration

To prepare Elderflower tea, start by bringing water to a boil. Once boiled, pour the hot water over a spoonful of Elderflowers in a cup or teapot, then cover and set it aside for approximately 5 minutes to steep. For added sweetness and flavor, you can incorporate some raw or local honey. Allow the tea to cool to a suitable temperature for your child to drink comfortably. Elderflower tea has a delightful taste, and the addition of honey will make it even more appealing to your child. Don't be surprised if you find yourself enjoying a cup or two as well! When children experience fever, they can feel quite miserable. Elderflower tea, as described above, can provide relief in such situations. The cooling properties of Elderflower not only help children relax but also promote sweating, which aids in the body's natural cooling process. Elderberries are not only delicious but also have impressive medicinal benefits. They can be transformed into a delightful syrup that not only tastes great but also serves as an effective remedy. Additionally, Elderberries can be used to create a vibrant and immune-stimulating tea. To make the tea more appealing to children, you may need to sweeten it or mix it with fruit juice.

2 to 6 grams per day is the recommended dosage if being ingested.

Warning: Caution should be exercised when using elderberries, as not all varieties are safe for consumption. It is crucial to distinguish between different types of elderberries, particularly the edible Sambucus nigra species and the potentially toxic Sambucus ebulus or Sambucus racemosa species. Only the Sambucus nigra species should be used for culinary and medicinal purposes.

When sourcing elderberries, it is recommended to purchase them from reputable sources or harvest them under the guidance of an experienced forager. Consuming unripe or uncooked elderberries may cause digestive upset and discomfort.

Elecampane

Elecampane is a powerful herb useful for both children and adults alike.

Many respiratory illnesses, such as bronchitis, cause the bronchial tubes to grow red and bloated, making breathing difficult. The phytochemicals helenalin, helenin, and, most crucially, inulin are abundant in Elecampane root. Inulin coats and soothes the bronchial tubes while also working as an expectorant, reducing bronchial secretions and clearing congestion from the lungs.

Elecampane, in addition to its expectorant properties, reduces the irritation and inflammation caused by coughing, as well as functioning as a cough suppressant. Another active chemical identified in the root of this herb, alatolactone, is likely to be responsible for the antitussive effect.

It is especially effective for coughs when mixed with echinacea, licorice, and/or marsh mallow root. If the cough is particularly spastic or repetitive, add to the mix a little valerian, a muscle relaxant. If a respiratory or bronchial infection isn't responding readily, try treating it with a mixture of elecampane and pleurisy root; this combination is generally effective for even the most tenacious lung infections.

Elecampane also contains sesquiterpene lactones, which have a natural antibacterial action and may be effective in the treatment of bacterial respiratory infections.

Elecampane roots contain the phytochemicals alantolactone and isoalantolactone, which have anthElmintic and anti-parasitic effects. Roundworms, pinworms, hookworms, whipworms, and threadworms are among the parasites that these chemicals can kill and remove from the intestine

Elecampane root has a remarkable 44 percent inulin content, which is a prebiotic molecule. Prebiotics are one of the favorite foods of probiotics like Bifidobacteria and Lactobacillus because they promote and nourish healthy gut flora. In the stomach, colonies of these good bacteria assist in fighting infections, reducing inflammation, and promoting regular bowel movements.

Elecampane increases nutrient absorption and encourages healthy digestive system function in the case of loss of appetite and sensations of tiredness caused by poor nutrient absorption

Safe administration

The medicinal use of Elecampane primarily focuses on its root. You can find Elecampane root available in various forms such as dry powder, liquid extract, or loose tea at stores. Alternatively, you may purchase dried slices of the root and crush them into a powder or boil them to create a homemade hot tea. It's important to note that Elecampane root has a rather strong and not particularly pleasant taste, so it may require some creativity when preparing it for children.

To make Elecampane tea more enjoyable for children, consider mixing it with other flavorful herbs like licorice and/or marshmallow root. Adding a touch of cinnamon and sweetening it with honey or maple syrup can also help improve the taste. If using an Elecampane-pleurisy blend, simply combine the tinctures in equal amounts and serve them in water, tea, or fruit juice.

When it comes to Elecampane root supplements, there are different dosages available. The recommended daily intake typically ranges from about 1/4 to 1/2 teaspoon (0.5 to 1 gram) of Elecampane. However, it's always wise to follow the instructions provided on the specific product you're using or consult with a healthcare professional for appropriate dosage guidance.

Fennel

Fennel is a fragrant herb that originated in the Mediterranean and is now available all over the world. Potassium, antioxidants, calcium, iron, magnesium, manganese, and dietary fiber are all abundant in this fruit. Fennel seeds can help with a variety of health problems, including clearing nasal passages during a cold, constipation, asthma, and more. Adults frequently take it after a meal to alleviate dyspepsia.

A well-known carminative and digestive aid, this licorice-flavored plant is renowned for its ability to increase and enrich the flow of milk in nursing mothers. Fennel is also an effective antacid; it neutralizes excess acid in the stomach and intestines and also clears uric acid from the joints, helping to reduce inflammation and the pain of arthritis. It is an excellent digestive aid, stimulating digestion, regulating appetite, and relieving flatulence.

Fennel seeds have been shown to help with a variety of digestive issues, including constipation in youngsters. Fennel seeds are a laxative that promotes regular bowel movements. It softens the feces, making it easier to pass and less painful for the baby. This spice helps a growing baby's digestive tract stay healthy.

Colic is a cramping ache in the abdomen that causes newborns to wail for hours at a time. The digestive tract of babies continues to develop every day, resulting in intestinal cramping. One of the most typical signs of colic is a bloated abdomen. Fennel seeds have digestive qualities that can aid in the relief of cramps. To relieve colic, feed the baby Fennel water, which is created by soaking Fennel seeds in water overnight. The amount, on the other hand, is determined by the child's age.

Fennel seeds are high in magnesium and phosphorus, two important nutrients for children's bone formation. All bone-destroying cells are slowed down by them. Feeding your youngster one teaspoon of Fennel water every other day will aid in their bone development.

Antioxidants, also known as free-radical scavengers, help to protect the body's cells against pollution, U.V. ray exposure, and inflammation. The aging process is also slowed by these nutrients. Fennel seeds are high in antioxidants, which aid in the development of a child's immune and overall health.

Fennel seeds can help with a wide range of respiratory issues. Cineole, an essential oil that helps to keep nasal passages clear, is abundant in them. Use Fennel seeds to treat your child's symptoms if he suffers from bronchitis, asthma, cough, or lung abscesses on a regular basis.

Potassium is abundant in Fennel seeds. They boost the brain's electrical activity, resulting in a well-functioning brain. Regularly consuming a modest amount of Fennel seeds helps to improve the supply of oxygenated, nutrient-rich blood to the brain.

Safe administration

Fennel makes a wonderfully tasty tea for treating colic, improving digestion, and expelling gas from the system. Nursing mothers can drink two to four cups of tea daily to increase and enrich their milk flow. It is also effective in treating eye inflammation and conjunctivitis; use a wash of warm fennel tea that has been strained well through a fine-mesh strainer. Because of its sweet licorice-like flavor, fennel is often blended with other less flavorful herbs to make them more palatable.

Babies aren't likely to be able to chew the seeds, so Fennel extract can be given as a liquid. Soak a tablespoon of Fennel seeds overnight in a cup of water. Filter the water and give your child a spoonful or two of it whenever you need to.

Warning: If administered in the proper amount, Fennel tea is generally safe for newborns. Fennel tea, on the other hand, may cause allergic responses in certain newborns. Do a patch test to see if the spice causes an allergic reaction in your youngster. Give her a small amount of Fennel water and wait two to three days to see if she reacts. Continue to feed your baby Fennel water as needed if the baby shows no signs of allergies, such as rashes.

Hawthorne

Hawthorn is a herb that can be used in a variety of ways. The dried berries, leaves, and flowers, in addition to being used as a food source, have a place in the prepared herbalist's toolbox as extracts, teas, and capsules. Rich in antioxidants, hawthorn helps build a healthy immune system. It is considered a superior heart tonic, strengthening and nourishing the heart. Hawthorn is outstanding both as a preventive to keep the heart healthy and as a remedy to treat heart disease, edema, angina, and arrhythmia

Hawthorn has also earned a reputation as a nervine, or a herb that helps the nervous system and maintains a healthy emotional range. As a result, it has earned a spot in my herbal emergency pack as a helpful herb for the emotional aftermath of a sudden emergency or unexpected occurrences, such as an accident or the death of a loved one. Hawthorn, with its affinity for circulation, might be helpful when we're feeling down and need to "take heart" after an upsetting experience. It is useful during times of grief and can help us weather the sad times of life. Hawthorn is excellent when we are in restless, angry emotions, sometimes with difficulty focusing, in addition to when we feel the need to "take heart." It's safe for kids, and it can be taken alone or in conjunction with other nervine herbs and proper support to help relax and calm hyperactive children. It can be a reassuring herb for those dealing with long-term illness and the feelings of pessimism that sometimes accompany a lengthy recovery period.

Safe administration

Hawthorn, when prepared as a sweetened syrup or jam, offers a delightful treat for children. Another option is to create a flavorful tea by combining Hawthorn with herbs like hibiscus, oats, and lemon balm. It's important to note that Hawthorn has a distinctive astringent taste, which may require some adjustment for young palates.

In terms of dosage, the recommended intake of Hawthorn for children ranges from 2 to 6 grams per day if being ingested.

Hibiscus

Hibiscus, known for its vibrant and beautiful flowers, thrives in hot climates and offers a range of health benefits, especially for children. This immune-boosting flower is particularly beneficial for kids who are dealing with a cold or excessive phlegm.

Rich in vitamin C, bioflavonoids, and antioxidants, hibiscus flower plays a vital role in restoring and maintaining overall health. Its immune-supporting properties help strengthen the body's defense against colds, flus, and other illnesses. Additionally, hibiscus flower is beneficial for treating mild cases of anemia and improving poor circulation due to its high content of bioflavonoids and vitamin C.

The bright red coloring of hibiscus flower is not just visually appealing but also indicates its rich anthocyanin content, which promotes vascular health. In North African traditional medicine, hibiscus flower has long been used to support respiratory health. It is employed in various forms to treat respiratory infections and soothe sore throats.

Apart from its health benefits, hibiscus tea is a delightful natural beverage that children often adore. Its pleasant taste and vibrant color make it an appealing choice. However, it's important to exercise caution when using hibiscus, as it can have mild laxative effects. It's recommended to use hibiscus in moderation and adjust the dosage based on individual needs.

Safe administration

The striking, large hibiscus flowers yield a vibrant ruby red tea with a delightful tart flavor and a sweet aftertaste. While children may prefer it sweetened, the natural taste is already quite enjoyable. For a fun twist, try making a thick hibiscus syrup and adding it to sparkling water for a delicious and refreshing beverage that not only tastes great but also provides numerous health benefits.

Hibiscus tea and extract can be found as nutritional supplements in health food stores, offering convenient options for incorporating this beneficial flower into your child's routine. The dosage may vary depending on the specific product and desired use. A typical serving of hibiscus tea contains approximately 1.5 grams of calyx, the part of the flower used for making the tea. However, research studies have utilized higher doses, with up to 10 grams of dried calyx and extracts containing up to 250 milligrams of anthocyanins.

When consumed as tea, hibiscus is generally considered safe. However, further research is needed to determine appropriate dosages for specific populations, such as pregnant or breastfeeding women, children, and individuals with liver or kidney conditions. It's always advisable to consult with a healthcare professional before incorporating hibiscus or any new herbal supplement into your child's routine.

Lemon Balm

Lemon Balm, a delightful member of the mint family, holds a special place in the herbal world. Its scientific name, Melissa, translates to "honey bee," a fitting name for a herb that can bring a sense of calm and relaxation, especially for active little bees. Lemon Balm is a wonderful choice for children who are constantly on the go but occasionally become irritable and overworked.

Research has shown that Lemon Balm has the potential to reduce anxiety and improve focus, making it beneficial for irritable social butterflies who may not get enough downtime or overstimulated extroverts struggling with concentration. A warm cup of sweet-tasting Lemon Balm tea in the afternoon can have a soothing and centering effect on children experiencing mild anxiety or attention deficit hyperactivity disorder (ADHD). Additionally, a slightly higher dosage of Lemon Balm at night can aid children in falling asleep peacefully. In fact, when combined with valerian root, Lemon Balm has been found to promote better sleep in children under the age of 12.

Lemon Balm offers a gentle and safe herbal option for children's emotional well-being and sleep support. It can be enjoyed as a comforting tea, and its pleasant lemony aroma and flavor make it appealing to young palates. By incorporating Lemon Balm into their daily routine, children can experience the soothing benefits of this remarkable herb and find moments of tranquility amidst their active lives.

Remember, it's always best to consult with a healthcare professional or a qualified herbalist to determine the appropriate dosage and usage for your child's specific needs. With Lemon Balm by their side, children can find balance, relaxation, and renewed energy to navigate the joys and challenges of growing up.

Safe administration

Though lemon balm dries well, its flavor is best fresh. It can be tinctured or encapsulated, but because of its refreshing pleasant flavor, lemon balm is most often served as a tea. The tea can be served with lemon and honey throughout the day to alleviate stress and anxiety, and also as a preventive for herpes, shingles, and thrush (all related viral infections). It is an important remedy for any viral infection, including measles and mumps. For a delicious nervine tonic tea, blend equal amounts of lemon balm, oats, and chamomile. To support a person during a time of grief, add hawthorn to this blend. Add St. John's wort to the blend to treat mild to moderate depression. Fresh lemon balm makes an excellent syrup, which can be added to sparkling water for a refreshing spritzer or all-natural soda. Lemon balm, a supremely delicate herb, poses no safety issues when used as a tea or a tincture.

Licorice

True Licorice, not the red and black imitations seen in the candy aisle, is rich in antiviral properties, making it an excellent remedy for any viral infection, including herpes, shingles, thrush, measles, and mumps. It is often combined with lemon balm for this purpose. Its high mucilaginous content and antiviral and anti-inflammatory properties make it a soothing and healing remedy for sore throats, respiratory infections, viral infections, and gastrointestinal inflammations such as ulcers. It also has mild laxative properties that can help with mild cases of constipation.

Safe administration

Licorice is very sweet and is often combined with other herbs to make them more palatable. On the other hand, licorice root by itself is often too sweet and so is blended with other herbs to tone the sweetness down. Licorice makes an excellent syrup, which can be added to sparkling water for a tasty soda. Children enjoy chewing on licorice sticks, and you can even give a "stick" of licorice root to a teething baby to chew on — though you may have to give the root a few "chews" yourself to soften it enough that the young one can begin to chew on it. It can usually keep the teething baby busy for a little while, at least.

Big amounts of the root can cause headaches, weariness, salt and water retention, potassium loss, high blood pressure, and even cardiac arrest if consumed in large quantities. At most, 4-5 grams per day. The easiest way to dose Licorice is through Licorice teas, many of which are readily available over the counter; however, they are also easy to create at home using Licorice root if you want a pure tea with no other herbs or flowers added. 2 to 6 grams per day is the recommended dosage if being ingested.

Warning: Though children don't usually suffer from these ailments, licorice should not be used by those with hypertension or kidney/bladder problems, by anyone undergoing steroid therapy, or by anyone who is taking medication for a heart or kidney ailment.

Marsh Mallow

Marsh Mallow root is a brown, fibrous husk that comes from the Marsh Mallow plant. The Marsh Mallow plant's flowers, roots, and leaves are all edible.

The therapeutic effects of Marsh Mallow root are derived from the plant's mucilage, or sap-like material. Marsh mallow can be used like slippery elm as a soothing, cooling demulcent in herbal remedies, and it is much more readily available and easy to grow. Marsh mallow root has both antibacterial and anti-inflammatory properties. It is especially soothing to inflamed, irritated membranes and is often used in tea blends and tinctures for sore throat, respiratory infections, and digestive irritation.

The plant's mucilage includes antioxidants, and studies show that it forms a layer over the skin and digestive tract. It may aid with skin irritation and digestive difficulties like ulcers by doing so.

Because Marsh Mallow root's mucilage was initially used to make this dessert, it was given the name Marsh Mallow candy. Candy Marsh Mallows today, on the other hand, are usually devoid of the herb. Rather, they're made of sugar and gelatin.

Children who received a herbal mixture containing Marsh Mallow and other herbs such as chamomile and common mallow had a less acute cough and fewer nightly awakenings than those who got a placebo. However, because this study did not look at the effects of Marsh Mallow root alone, other plants in the blend could have been to blame for the therapeutic effects. (This emphasizes how important it is to know your herbs!)

Children who received a herbal concoction containing Marsh Mallow root and other therapeutic herbs had fewer and shorter-lasting respiratory infections, according to the findings of a small-scale trial.

Safe administration

Serve as a tea for sore throat, digestive irritation, bronchial inflammation, or diarrhea or constipation. Marsh mallow is very soothing to the urinary tract and is often recommended for urinary tract and bladder infections. It also has external applications: Mix it with water into a thick paste to soothe burns and irritated skin, or combine it with oatmeal as a soothing wash or bath for irritated, itchy dry skin.

Marsh Mellow is another easy-to-get-your-hands-on herb, as there are many applications from popular throat teas to ground root available at most health stores. Most aim for 1,200 milligrams daily.

Nettle

Stinging Nettle, a remarkable medicinal herb, has long been valued in children's health treatments for colds and asthma. This herb is truly a treasure trove of vitamins and minerals, offering a wide range of health benefits. It is particularly renowned for its high content of iron and calcium, making it an excellent choice for replenishing these essential minerals in pregnant and nursing mothers. Combining Stinging Nettle with raspberry leaf, another nutritive herb and female reproductive tonic, can provide added support during this special phase of life.

Nettle is an exceptional source of easily assimilated calcium, which plays a vital role in stress relief and nerve repair. Its combination with green milky oats is especially effective in soothing and healing nerves. Additionally, Nettle is valuable for its ability to support tissue and bone repair. When combined with oats and horsetail, it becomes a potent remedy for promoting healthy bone growth and alleviating growing pains in young children.

One of the notable benefits of Stinging Nettle is its effectiveness in addressing allergies and hay fever. Many individuals have reported significant relief from these conditions through the use of Nettle. Its historical use also extends to the prevention and treatment of eczema, gout, anemia, urinary tract infections, and joint discomfort. Stinging Nettle can be used on its own as a tincture or tea, or it may be incorporated into various blends and combinations to enhance its therapeutic effects.

When it comes to children's ailments such as sprains, strains, insect bites, joint problems, and tendonitis, Nettle creams and compresses have proven to be valuable herbal remedies. Their application provides targeted relief and supports the body's natural healing process.

As with any herbal remedy, it is advisable to consult with a healthcare professional or experienced herbalist to determine the appropriate dosage and method of administration for children. By harnessing the healing power of Stinging Nettle, we can support children's overall health, address specific health concerns, and promote their well-being in a gentle and natural way.

Safe administration
Stinging nettle offers various options for consumption, including teas, tinctures, fluid extracts, freeze-dried leaf capsules, and lotions. While nettle has a taste reminiscent of spinach, it requires thorough steaming to eliminate the stinging sensation caused by the small hairs filled with formic acid on the underside of the leaves and stems. These hairs can cause a painful and itchy rash if not handled properly. It is important to exercise caution when handling nettle, wearing gloves and avoiding direct contact. In case of a sting, applying a plantain leaf poultice can help draw out toxins and alleviate discomfort.

For allergies, freeze-dried nettle capsules are often found to be most effective, although combining them with nettle tea and/or tincture can enhance the overall impact. However, it is essential to be mindful of the diuretic properties of both the nettle root and leaf, as excessive consumption may lead to dehydration. Watch out for symptoms such as dry mouth, sunken eyes, and lethargy in children. Moreover, in some individuals, Stinging Nettle may interfere with blood clotting, potentially hindering wound healing.

2 to 6 grams per day is the recommended dosage if being ingested.

Oats

Avena sativa, commonly known as oats, holds a fascinating history and therapeutic potential often overlooked. While we primarily recognize oats as a nutritious grain, the medicinal properties of other parts of the plant should not be disregarded.

Milky Oats refer to the oat tops harvested when they have reached the milky stage. During this period, a white, milky sap is released when the tops are pressed. Capturing the bioactive constituents of Milky Oats is best achieved by tincturing them while still fresh. Alternatively, they can be dried and utilized as a nutritional tonic or added to tea blends, providing both nourishment and a delightful flavor.

Oat straw, on the other hand, refers to the stem of the oat plant harvested during the milky oat stage, when it is still green. To create an infusion that extracts the nutritive and therapeutic benefits of oat straw, combine one ounce of dried oat straw (along with dried milky oat tops, if desired) with four cups of boiling water and steep for 4-12 hours. The resulting beverage is a light, refreshing infusion with a grassy and slightly sweet taste, packed with minerals, trace nutrients, alkaloids, protein, and vitamins.

Oat straw infusion, along with dried milky oats, provides an excellent source of bioavailable vitamins and minerals for regular consumption. It is particularly rich in calcium and magnesium, which contribute to bone strength. Herbalists often prefer green milky oats, harvested before full ripening, as they contain desirable properties. The term "milky" stems from the tiny droplets of milk that emerge when the oats are pressed. However, fully ripe oats also have their uses, as oatmeal made from them offers both nutrition and soothing qualities, making it an ideal choice for individuals recovering from illness.

Calcium, magnesium, and vitamin B found in oats are known for their calming and nerve-strengthening effects. Oats are highly regarded as a nourishing food for the nervous system, especially during periods of stress or when dealing with nervous system weakness or exhaustion caused by factors like depression, overwork, or emotional trauma. Symptoms such as irritability, persistent fatigue, difficulty concentrating, loss of libido, and heart palpitations can potentially be alleviated with oatstraw infusion, which improves mood, reduces anxiety, combats the effects of daily stress, and aids in obtaining a restful sleep.

Safe administration
Oats are perfectly safe in moderation; if sensitive to gluten, options such as an oatmeal bath may be a better choice. Both the milky green oats and oat stalks make a tasty tea, either alone or blended with other herbs such as lemon balm, hawthorn, and hibiscus. It is delicious when brewed double to triple strength and then mixed with fruit juice. Oat tea is recommended for children who are nervous, hyperactive, and stressed and/or are constantly agitated or irritated. Because of its rich mucilaginous content, oatmeal baths are wonderfully soothing for dry itchy skin and for skin irritations.

Peppermint

Peppermint is widely used as a flavor, disinfectant, and food. Peppermint is well known as a medication for its effects on the stomach and intestines. Perhaps you've experimented with the different "tummy teas" offered to alleviate stomach discomfort. Irritable bowel syndrome, intestinal cramps, or indigestion can cause gas, nausea, and stomach pain. Peppermint can help.

Peppermint is a carminative, which means it relieves gas and bloating in the digestive tract, as well as an antispasmodic, which means it relieves stomach and intestinal cramps. Peppermint is safe for infants with colic and can be used to treat hyperacidity (excess stomach acid) and gastroenteritis (nausea and stomach distress, also known as stomach flu).

If the baby accepts it, a teaspoon of Peppermint tea or a cloth soaked in warm Peppermint tea can be applied to the infant's belly to relieve tummy cramps.

Peppermint is often applied topically to the skin for its cooling and calming properties. Peppermint oil is used in a variety of muscle massages and "ices" to relieve pain, burning, and inflammation. Peppermint oil, like other volatile oils, is reasonably well-absorbed and can have a short pain-relieving impact on cramped and spasming muscles and organs. Before using this oil on your skin, dilute it like you would any other essential oil.

Peppermint can also temporarily relieve itching. Apply a drop of diluted Peppermint oil to insect bites, eczema, and other itchy skin conditions, such as poison ivy rash. Peppermint can help relieve headaches, and you can apply Peppermint oil to your temples or scalp for a soothing treatment.

Peppermint's analgesic, antibacterial, antispasmodic, decongestant, and cooling properties are attributed to menthol, the essential oil in the herb. Menthol also aids in the suppression of many disease-causing bacteria, fungi, and viruses, but because stronger herbal antimicrobials are available, herbalists rarely employ Peppermint to treat serious illnesses.

Peppermint tea can be used as a mouthwash for babies with thrush (mouth yeast) or pregnant mothers who choose to avoid stronger herbs and drugs.

Safe administration
The world is your oyster when it comes to Peppermint. In this case, the method can truly be based on your preference. Use for children when they have tummy aches or sluggish digestion, or when they just need a little radiant energy. Peppermint can be made into a tea, tincture (diluted), and mouthwash. It also makes a delicious syrup, which can be added to sparkling water for a cooling drink. I like to introduce children to this plant in the garden and often have them nibble its refreshing, tasty leaves. The essential oil of peppermint is also very healing and useful; however, because of its concentration, be careful with it, especially when using it with children. A drop of the essential oil added to a little water makes a refreshing and stomach-settling mouthwash for a child who's experiencing a bout of vomiting and helps clear the mouth of foul taste.

When it comes to itching, peppermint oil can provide temporary relief. By diluting peppermint oil and applying a drop to insect bites, eczema, or other itchy skin conditions like poison ivy rash, you can experience a soothing effect that helps alleviate discomfort.

Peppermint is also renowned for its potential to relieve headaches. For a calming treatment, you can apply peppermint oil to your temples or scalp. The cooling sensation of peppermint can help ease tension and provide a soothing sensation, assisting in headache relief.

It's important to note that when using peppermint oil, it should always be properly diluted to avoid skin irritation or adverse reactions. You can dilute it with a carrier oil, such as jojoba or coconut oil, before applying it topically.

2 to 6 grams per day is the recommended dosage if being ingested.

Red Clover
Red Clover, a wild plant belonging to the Legume family, holds a variety of therapeutic properties. Cattle and other animals graze upon its vibrant foliage. This remarkable herb has been utilized for centuries to address numerous health concerns, ranging from cancer and whooping

cough to respiratory disorders and skin inflammations like psoriasis and eczema. Traditional remedies often involve the use of Red Clover ointments, which have been applied topically to alleviate skin problems such as psoriasis and eczema. Moreover, Red Clover has been employed as an effective remedy for children's coughs. Recent research has also indicated potential psychological benefits for women associated with Red Clover consumption. This remarkable herb is believed to possess blood-purifying qualities, acting as a diuretic to eliminate excess fluids, an expectorant to clear phlegm from the lungs, and a circulatory stimulant to enhance blood flow and promote liver cleansing. Renowned as an exceptional respiratory tonic, Red Clover is frequently administered to children experiencing chronic chest complaints, including persistent coughs, recurrent colds, and other respiratory issues. Notably, Red Clover boasts an impressive mineral profile, notably rich in calcium, nitrogen, and iron, which further contributes to its therapeutic potential.

Safe administration
Use red clover to make a delicious sweet-flavored tea. Blend it with other respiratory tonic herbs such as mullein and elecampane to treat persistent respiratory problems. Red clover combines well with oats and lemon balm for treating skin disorders and with hawthorn and hibiscus for treating blood and heart issues. As a blood purifier, red clover tea or tincture is recommended in cases of congestion or growths on or in the body, such as cysts, tumors, and fibroids. It is also helpful in alleviating hay fever and allergies and is often combined with nettle for this purpose.

2 to 6 grams per day is the recommended dosage if being ingested.

Red Raspberry
Red Raspberry, scientifically known as Rubus idaeus, is a beautiful plant belonging to the rose family. It is native to Europe and Asia and is widely cultivated for its delicious berries. However, the benefits of Red Raspberry extend beyond its sweet fruit. This versatile herb is not only cherished by women but also holds great value for children's health. Red Raspberry is a renowned blood-nourishing tonic that is gentle and safe for young ones. It is known for its ability to strengthen the uterine wall during pregnancy, providing support and reducing discomfort during childbirth. Moreover, it aids in the prevention of false labor pains and assists in reducing postpartum bleeding and uterine edema. Its potent astringent properties make it a valuable remedy for alleviating menstrual cramps and regulating menstrual flow. In addition to its female-specific benefits, Red Raspberry has been found to be helpful in addressing vomiting in young children and treating conditions such as dysentery and diarrhea in infants. With its rich nutritional profile and therapeutic properties, Red Raspberry stands as a remarkable herb for promoting the well-being of both women and children.

Safe administration
Because of its astringent properties, raspberry leaf as a tea or tincture is helpful for relieving diarrhea and dysentery. Raspberry leaf mixed with white oak bark

and/or spilanthes is an effective mouthwash for sore or infected gums.

The recommended dosage is 5 to 10 mg of the crushed leaf for 240 mL of water. Take up to 6 times a day, or up to 12 g of dry leaf per day.

Rose

The exquisite Rose is more than just pretty on the outside. Roses, especially wild prairie roses, have long been treasured as a herbal treatment and have been utilized to help calm and mend humanity's ills. Gentle Rose is a relaxing nervine, as well as a beneficial respiratory and immunological ally and a topical treatment. Bring the healing properties of Rose into your house and share them with your family.

Rose is a soothing nervine that can be used by the whole family. Rose's moderate antidepressant and sedative characteristics can assist boost emotions while creating a sense of relaxation, and it has long been used to comfort and quiet the heart. Rose can help you get through difficult periods in your life when your emotions are tumultuous. It is used by herbalists to treat sadness, anxiety, anger, grief, and broken hearts. Rose may also aid in the relief of tiredness and sleeplessness. All of this makes it an excellent herb to turn to at the end of a long day for grumpy, overtired children and their parents!

Roses are nourishing and can be used in dishes to aid in overall health. Rosehips, the fruits of the Rose, are incredibly high in immune-boosting vitamin C, far more so than citrus fruits when compared; they also include beta carotene, as well as vitamins K and E, which are beneficial to the body.

Rose can provide soothing treatment to those suffering from colds and flu. Rose-petal rinses, gargles, and tea soothe irritated eyes, a swelling sore throat, seasonal allergies, and infections with excessive nasal discharge thanks to the astringent and anti-inflammatory characteristics of Rose petals. The petals and hips combine to make a great cough syrup. When there is heat contained within the body, such as with fevers, inflammation, or headaches, Rose can aid to promote coolness. The tea and syrup are effective cures for upset stomachs caused by diarrhea. Furthermore, the gorgeous Rose is a superb plant for ladies, especially when it comes to P.M.S., which is characterized by mental stress and unpleasant cramps during menstruation.

When crafting remedies to replenish your natural medicine cabinet, don't forget to include Rose. To have Rose petals and hips on hand when you need them, add them to tea blends, syrups, and honey.

Safe administration
2 to 6 grams per day is the recommended dosage if being ingested. Rose hip jam is a sweet and vitamin C packed options for delicious breakfasts in the colder months. Rose hips also make a much loved, mild and sweet tea.

Slippery Elm

Slippery Elm, derived from the inner bark of the Ulmus rubra tree, is a remarkable herb revered for its exceptional ability to provide relief for a sore throat. This ancient Native American remedy has been utilized for centuries due to its soothing properties. The secret lies in the mucilage, a natural substance found in Slippery Elm. When combined with water, the mucilage transforms into a slippery gel-like consistency. This gel acts as a protective coating, gently enveloping and soothing inflamed mucous membranes in the throat. By doing so, it helps alleviate discomfort and irritation caused by a sore throat. Additionally, Slippery Elm has the remarkable ability to suppress cough receptors in the throat and larynx, providing further relief. The gel's coating action extends along the digestive tract, offering a soothing effect to the entire pathway.

Safe administration
Throat lozenges containing Slippery Elm are available for older children to take. It's also available as a powder that you may mix with orange juice to cover the taste. The sweet flavor of slippery elm combines well with licorice, fennel, and cinnamon and makes a tasty, soothing throat and digestive tea. To make the tea, soak the bark in cold or cool water overnight, or simmer for 10 to 15 minutes. Powdered slippery elm can be added to oatmeal to make a very soothing, easily digested, and healing gruel for those who are debilitated or ill. Add boiling water to two tablespoons of powdered bark and steep for 3 to 5 minutes. Buy only from reputable sources and use sparingly preferring other herbs, it is in the United Planet Savers at-risk list.

Spearmint

Not to continue to drum on Peppermint, but Peppermint and Spearmint are both gentle plants that might aid digestion. Cooling, refreshing, and uplifting, spearmint is one of the most popular mints. Children often appreciate spearmint more than peppermint, as spearmint is a bit milder. It makes a delicious and refreshing tea, useful for lifting a person's mood and brightening the spirits. If you need to sweeten something, pure honey is a fantastic option.

Safe administration Use spearmint to "sweeten" the stomach and breath after sickness, especially vomiting. Just add a drop of the essential oil to water or brew a cup of fresh tea and use it to rinse the mouth several times. Spearmint makes a lovely syrup, which can be added to sparkling water for a light, uplifting drink; it's also wonderful in iced tea, as are the fresh leaves. The fresh leaves can be added to honey to make spearmint honey: Layer a few inches of fresh spearmint leaves on the bottom of a pint jar. Pour warmed honey over the leaves. Put on a lid and let sit in a warm, sunny window for several days, or until the honey has the scent and taste of spearmint. You can scoop the leaves out or leave them in the honey. Use this honey as an "instant tea" by adding a spoonful or two to hot water. Or use the honey to sweeten and flavor other teas. As with Peppermint, there are countless options on the market, from tinctures and teas to cough drops and herbal seasonings on the shelves at your local health food store.

Easy herbal Remedies for Common Children Ailments

Allergies

Allergies can be quite common among children, and they occur when the immune system reacts strongly to certain substances that are typically harmless. Picture your immune system as a superhero with a super-sensitive radar. Sometimes, this radar gets a bit confused and starts flagging things like pollen, pet dander, or even certain foods as dangerous villains. When your child comes into contact with these allergens, their immune system goes into overdrive, trying to protect them from what it mistakenly perceives as a threat.

Depending on the child and the specific allergy, the reaction can happen in different parts of the body. For some kids, it might cause itchy and watery eyes, sneezing, or a runny nose. Others might experience coughing, wheezing, or difficulty breathing. Sometimes, allergies can even lead to tummy troubles like nausea, vomiting, or diarrhea.

It's important to remember that allergies can vary in severity. Some children may have mild symptoms that are more of an annoyance, while others may experience more severe reactions. In rare cases, certain allergies can even trigger a potentially life-threatening emergency called anaphylaxis. This is why it's crucial for parents and caregivers to be aware of their child's allergies and have an action plan in place in case of an emergency.

While there is no cure for allergies, there are ways to manage and alleviate the symptoms. The first step is identifying the specific allergens that trigger your child's reactions. This can be done through allergy testing with the help of a healthcare professional. Once you know the culprits, you can take steps to avoid them as much as possible. This might mean keeping furry friends out of certain areas, using allergen-proof bedding, or reading food labels carefully to avoid allergenic ingredients.

Remember, allergies don't have to dampen your child's spirits or keep them from enjoying life. With the right knowledge, preparation, and support from healthcare professionals, you can help your child navigate allergies and find ways to thrive. Encourage open communication, teach them how to recognize their triggers, and empower them to take charge of their own well-being. Together, you can conquer allergies and ensure that your child's adventures are full of joy and excitement, without the worries of allergy symptoms holding them back.

Supportive Herbs:
- Agrimony
- All-Heal Leaf and Flower
- Barberry Root
- Calendula Flower
- Goldenrod Leaf and Flower
- Goldenseal
- Ground Ivy
- Marigold
- Milk Thistle Seed
- Mullein Leaf
- Nettle Leaf
- Oregon Grape Root
- Oxeye Daisy
- Pearly Everlasting Flowers
- Plantain Leaf
- Yerba Sante

Allergy Nettle Tea
- 1 cup dried Nettle Leaf
- 1 cup dried Goldenrod Leaf and Flower
- ½ cup dried Mullein Leaf
- ½ cup dried Calendula Flower
- ½ to 1 cup Marsh Mallow Leaf
- 2 to 4 tablespoons dried Licorice Root

Combine these herbs (or as many as you have on hand!) and steep. Once the tea has steeped for ten minutes, it's time to drink up. If this is for your child, it's advisable to add honey in order to sweeten the tea's herbal flavor.

Keeping your pot covered while the herbs steep will result in more effective treatment. You can make your tea in the evening and let the herbs simmer overnight if you use a quart jar. In the morning, strain your tea and drink it all day.

You can use any of the herbs in the allergy tea blend on their own.

Drink about 32 ounces of tea each day for the best results. The best time to begin is before allergy season, as the herbs function best as a preventive. It's not too late to start if you've already experienced your first sniffles.

Tip: If you're on blood-thinning medication, skip the Nettle Leaf and up the Goldenrod.

Capsules
The combination of freeze-dried Nettle Leaf capsules and Milk Thistle Seed capsules provides immediate allergy relief. Choose a high-quality brand and take two of each every four hours with lots of water, four pills every four hours.

Allergy Herbal Tea
- 1 teaspoon dried leaves of Oxeye Daisy
- 1 teaspoon dried everlasting Pearly Flowers
- 1 teaspoon dried leaves of Yerba Santa
- 3 cups boiling water

1. In a glass jar, combine the herbs and cover with water; soak for 30 minutes; drain.
2. Take one-half to one cup every six hours to get the most out of it.

Bruises

Bruises are like colorful badges that show your child's adventures and explorations, but they can sometimes be a bit painful and worrisome. When your child bumps into something or takes a tumble, the blood vessels underneath their skin can get damaged. This damage causes a small amount of blood to leak out and collect under the skin, creating that familiar blue, purple, or yellowish mark we call a bruise. Bruises can be quite common in children, especially those who are constantly on the move. And the good news is that most bruises are harmless and will heal on their own over time. First, let's talk about comfort. Applying a cold compress, like an ice pack wrapped in a soft cloth, to the bruised area can help reduce swelling and provide some relief. Encourage your child to take it easy and rest the affected area, especially if it's causing discomfort.

Another helpful tip is to elevate the bruised body part if possible. For example, if it's a bruised knee, propping it up on a pillow while your child relaxes can help minimize swelling and promote faster healing.

Arnica, a plant-based remedy, has been used for centuries to help with bruises. You can find arnica creams or gels at your local pharmacy or natural health store. Gently apply the arnica to the bruised area, following the instructions on the packaging, and let its soothing properties work their magic. It's important to note that if your child has a particularly large or painful bruise, or if they experience other concerning symptoms like difficulty moving the affected area or persistent pain, it's a good idea to consult with a healthcare professional to rule out any underlying issues. While it's impossible to shield your child from every bump and fall, there are steps you can take to minimize the risk of bruises. Encourage them to wear appropriate protective gear during activities like biking or skating, and create a safe environment for play with cushioned surfaces and clear pathways. Teach your child about being aware of their surroundings and taking their time when engaging in physical activities. Building their coordination and balance through activities like yoga or martial arts can also help them develop better body awareness, reducing the likelihood of accidents.

Remember, bruises are a natural part of childhood, and they often signify the adventures and experiences that shape your child's growth.

Supportive Herbs:
- Arnica
- Aloe Vera
- Comfrey
- Yarrow
- Chamomile
- Frankincense
- Witch Hazel

Aloe Vera Paste

You can't go wrong with this homemade Aloe Vera bruise cream, which can genuinely address that problem; you get to choose your favorite ingredients based on your preferences, and it's completely chemical-free, cheap, and simple!

- 2 tablespoons Aloe Gel (can be extracted from a live plant)
- 5-6 drops vegetable oil
- 5 milliliters of chosen essential oil from herbs and flowers above.
- 2-3 drops Vitamin E oil
- 1-2 vegetable glycerin

Follow these steps to create the paste:
1. Add the Aloe Vera Gel to a small glass basin or container.
2. Add the oils and stir, whisking until creamy.
3. Transfer to a useful container and store in a cold location.

Arnica Salve

Any natural first aid kit should include Arnica salve. Arnica is useful for bruises, pains, sprains, strains, and even arthritis flare-ups since it lowers pain and inflammation. Arnica is also useful for reducing the inflammation caused by bug bites. Arnica preparations are widely available at health food stores, so why not make your own? I'm delighted to share my recipe for arnica salve, which is simple to make and effective.

- 1 cup dried Arnica
- 2 tablespoons of dried St. John's Wort
- 2 tablespoons of carrier oil
- 1/2 cup unbleached beeswax
- 20-40 drops essential oil of Wintergreen, Spearmint, or Peppermint

Just follow these steps:
1. Infuse the herbs into the oil using a double boiler – place the herbs and oil into a heat-safe boil placed over a pot of boiling water.
2. Remove the herbs and drain them; remove the oil from the heat.
3. Fill a jar halfway with the infused oil.
4. Beeswax should be added at this point to be melted in the next step.
5. In a small pot of water, melt the beeswax in the oil over low heat.
6. Remove the pan from the heat.
7. If used, add the essential oil. Add the drops before the solution begins to solidify.
8. Seal and allow to come to room temperature to firm up.

Vinegar Fix

In a 2:1 mix with water, add the mix to a cloth and apply to the bruise site, leaving the cloth in place for 10-20 minutes.

Colic

Colic can be an overwhelming experience for both parents and infants, as it is often accompanied by painful spasmodic contractions in the immature digestive tract or trapped air and gas in the intestines. The digestive system of an infant takes time to mature, usually around three months, and while most cases of colic resolve within this period, some may persist longer. It's important to understand that colicky children can be extremely sensitive to their environment, and as parents, we play a crucial role in creating a calm and soothing atmosphere.

Parents' emotional and physical well-being can greatly contribute to easing colic. During mealtimes, playing quiet and peaceful music can be helpful. Nursing mothers can benefit from drinking warm nervine teas like chamomile, lemon balm, and passionflower before nursing, promoting a sense of relaxation. Feeding time should ideally be a quiet and restful moment shared between parent and child. If parents are feeling stressed or tense, the infant may respond with similar energy. While not all colicky babies have stressed-out parents, creating a peaceful environment can positively impact the child's well-being.

Nursing mothers should also be mindful of their diet and avoid foods that could potentially irritate the infant's digestive tract. While each child's system is unique, there are some common irritants to be aware of. Foods from the brassica family, such as cabbage, broccoli, cauliflower, kale, and collards, are high in sulfur, which can cause gas and discomfort in both infants and adults. Hot and spicy foods should be avoided, as infants' systems may not be ready to handle them. Additionally, chocolate, peanuts, and foods high in sugar can slow down digestive action, congest the digestive tract, and contribute to colic symptoms. It can be beneficial to observe the correlation between the mother's diet and the baby's colicky symptoms to identify potential food triggers.

Reducing or eliminating coffee consumption is another consideration. While the amount of caffeine in a daily cup of coffee may seem minimal to adults, it can have a strong stimulating effect on a child's young and sensitive system. Coffee is also acidic and may adversely affect the immature digestive system of an infant, exacerbating colic symptoms.

Probiotics, such as Acidophilus, are highly recommended for infant colic. These beneficial bacteria naturally occur in the human digestive system and can be supplemented to support the growth of healthy intestinal flora and digestive enzymes. Acidophilus preparations specifically designed for children can be found in most natural foods stores. Doubling the recommended amount on the product label is recommended for treating colic. If the child is eating solid foods and not lactose-intolerant, including daily servings of yogurt, kefir, and buttermilk can provide additional probiotics. Fermented foods like sauerkraut and miso are also beneficial for restoring beneficial gut flora. Nursing mothers can consume several servings of these cultured foods daily to support their colicky infant.

Certain herbs have proven helpful in relieving colic symptoms. Slippery elm, fennel, anise, dill, and catnip are among the most beneficial. Infants can be given teas made from these herbs to alleviate acute colic symptoms, or the herbs can be ground into a powder and added to the infant's food. Nursing mothers can also include these herbs in their own diet if they are breastfeeding, providing potential relief for the colicky infant.

Remember, colic can be a challenging time, but with patience, understanding, and these natural remedies, parents can help ease their child's discomfort and create a soothing environment. If colic persists or is accompanied by concerning symptoms, it is always advisable to consult a healthcare professional for further evaluation and guidance.

Supportive Herbs:
- Angelica
- Catnip
- Elderberry
- Peppermint
- Sassafras

Chamomile Tea

Chamomile has antispasmodic and sedative effects, so it can help reduce intestinal cramping while also relaxing you. Chamomile, in fact, includes 19 antispasmodic and five sedative components.

To prepare a cup of tea, follow these steps:
1. Fill a cup halfway with hot water and 1 teaspoon of Chamomile Flowers.
2. Allow for 10 minutes of resting time after covering. Strain and give to the baby in a bottle while it's still warm or at room temperature.

Use around a teaspoon of dried Chamomile Flowers per cup of tea to prepare tea. Place the Chamomile Blossoms in a tea infuser, then pour boiling water over them and steep for 5 minutes. If you're using freshly harvested Chamomile, double the amount.

Tip: Unless she is allergic to pollens, a nursing mother can drink the tea. Instead of flowers, you can use prepackaged Chamomile tea bags.

Pain Tincture

There are a few herbs that can be used here, mainly the list above; however, the steps to create the tincture itself remain the same.
1. Mix one teaspoon of your selected essential oil well with a teaspoon of carrier oil, usually olive or coconut.
2. Once combined, rub the tincture directly onto the pain point.

Simply Add Spices

Studies have shown that babies taking in herbs through food can be efficient as well. Thyme, Paprika, and Turmeric are popular additions, as their flavors lend well to being into food.

Common Cold

The common cold is an all too familiar illness, especially in children. It is caused by a viral infection that affects the nose, throat, and upper respiratory tract. Children are particularly susceptible to colds due to their developing immune systems and increased exposure to germs in school or daycare settings. While colds are usually mild and self-limiting, they can still cause discomfort and disrupt daily routines. Rest and hydration are crucial during a cold. Encourage your child to get plenty of sleep to aid in the healing process. Make sure they drink enough fluids, such as water, herbal teas, and warm broths, to stay hydrated and help thin mucus secretions. Adequate hydration can also help soothe a sore throat and relieve congestion.

Symptoms of a common cold in children may include a runny or stuffy nose, sneezing, coughing, sore throat, mild headache, low-grade fever, and general malaise. Nasal congestion is a common symptom of the cold, and it can make breathing difficult for young children. Saline nasal drops or sprays can help loosen mucus and alleviate congestion. These can be used several times a day to provide relief. Steam inhalation is another effective method to ease nasal congestion. Simply sit with your child in a steamy bathroom or use a humidifier to add moisture to the air.

Fortunately, there are several natural remedies and strategies that can help alleviate symptoms and support your child's recovery. Honey has been used for centuries as a natural remedy for cough and sore throat. For children over one year old, a spoonful of honey can be given as needed to soothe coughs and provide temporary relief. However, it is important to note that honey should not be given to infants under one year of age due to the risk of infant botulism. Herbal teas can also provide comfort and relief during a cold. Chamomile, ginger, and peppermint teas can help soothe sore throats, ease congestion, and provide a comforting warmth.

Echinacea, a popular immune-supporting herb, can be used to strengthen your child's defenses against the common cold. It is available in various forms, including teas, tinctures, and supplements. Good hygiene practices play a crucial role in preventing the spread of the common cold. Teach your child to wash their hands frequently with soap and water, especially before meals and after using the restroom. Encourage them to cover their mouth and nose when coughing or sneezing, preferably using a tissue or their elbow, to minimize the spread of germs. While natural remedies can help relieve symptoms, it's important to monitor your child's condition closely. If their symptoms worsen, they have difficulty breathing, experience high fever, or show signs of dehydration, it is recommended to seek medical attention promptly.

Supportive Herbs:
- Balsam Fir
- Bayberry
- Black Elder
- Blue Vervain
- Canadian Fleabane
- Cayenne
- Cinnamon Bark
- Coltsfoot
- Comfrey
- Echinacea
- Ginger
- Goldenrod Leaf and Flower
- Indian Root
- Licorice Root
- Marsh Mallow
- Osha Root
- Sage Leaf
- Prunella Vulgaris and Flower
- Seneca Snakeroot
- Slippery Elm
- Sumac
- Wild Cherry
- Witch Hazel
- Yerba Sante

Rosemary Nasal Wash

If you've ever purchased the salt solution that comes with your neti pot, you're aware of how expensive it can be. Especially if you suffer from sinus problems and use the neti pot frequently, the treatment, on the other hand, can easily be amplified and replicated at home for a fraction of the cost.
- 1/2 cup non-iodized salt.
- 10 drops of Rosemary essential oil.
- 8 drops of Tea Tree essential oil.

The steps are simple:
1. Combine the salts and essential oils in a glass container. Mix thoroughly, then cover with a lid to keep it safe.
2. To use in your neti pot, mix a pinch with warm distilled water.
3.

Herbal Gargle

Sage is an aromatic astringent that kills rhinovirus, which is the virus that causes many colds. Its benefits are enhanced when combined with vinegar and salt. If you have a dry sore throat, you may wish to have a cup of Marsh Mallow tea afterward to help calm the sore throat.
- 8 fluid ounces of water
- 2 tablespoons dried Sage Leaf
- 8 fluid ounces apple cider vinegar
- 3 teaspoons kosher salt

Follow these steps:
1. Bring the water to a boil in a small pot over high heat. Remove it from the heat and stir in the Sage. Cover securely and set aside for 20 minutes to infuse.
2. Straining, pour the liquid into a container.
3. Shake the container well after adding the vinegar and salt.
4. Gargle a few times a day using this solution.

Sweetened Cough Drops

- 1 teaspoon leaves of dried Goldenrod
- 1 teaspoon Wild Cherry Bark
- 1 teaspoon dried Licorice Root
- 1 teaspoon dried Yerba Santa Leaves
- 1 teaspoon dried Slippery Elm Bark
- 2 cups water
- 2 cups sugar
- 3 tablespoons corn syrup

Just follow the steps:

1. In a pan, combine the herbs listed above and cover them with water. Bring the mixture to a boil, then reduce to low heat and cook for 20 minutes.
2. Remove the pan from the heat and set it aside to cool. Strain the mixture and stir in the sugar and corn syrup.
3. Return to high heat, bring to a boil, then lower to low heat. Cook until the mixture reaches a temperature of 300°F (hard-crack stage).
4. Pour the syrup onto a large, oiled baking sheet and set aside to cool before breaking into one-inch pieces.
5. Use as though it were a store-bought cough drop.

Constipation

Constipation can be a frustrating issue for both children and parents. It refers to irregular or infrequent bowel movements, and the frequency can vary based on individual factors such as diet, body composition, and lifestyle habits. While the average child has a daily bowel movement, some may experience constipation and go without one for two days or more. When waste products stay in the colon for longer periods, they become drier and more compact as more water is absorbed.

There are various factors that can contribute to constipation, including a poor diet, inadequate water intake, stress, lack of physical activity, medication use, irregular bathroom habits, and excessive reliance on laxatives. It can also be associated with certain medical conditions such as thyroid problems, circulatory issues, and disturbances in the colon, such as inflammation, polyps, blockages, or tumors. If constipation persists, it is advisable to seek guidance from a holistic healthcare provider. In children, constipation can also be influenced by psychological factors. Some children may be hesitant or unwilling to use the toilet due to distraction, inattentiveness to their body's signals, previous negative experiences, or a lack of privacy in public settings. It is important to monitor your child's bathroom habits regularly and address any concerns early on to prevent long-term difficulties with elimination. Certain dietary factors can contribute to constipation as well. Foods high in fat, wheat, eggs, and refined processed foods are common culprits. If your child develops constipation, it is advisable to avoid foods that contribute to the issue, such as refined wheat products (e.g., pasta, bread, and crackers) and hard cheeses. Nursing mothers whose babies experience constipation should also consider avoiding these foods. Instead, incorporate foods that promote healthy elimination, such as fruits, vegetables, whole grains, liquids, molasses, dried fruits (particularly apricots and prunes), and moist, cooling foods like oatmeal and Marsh Mallow Gruel. If your child is bottle-fed cow's milk, switching to goat, rice, or soy milk may be worth trying. Certain herbs can offer support for constipation. Carob powder, marshmallow root or slippery elm bark, flaxseed, psyllium seed, licorice root, and Irish moss are among the herbs that can be powdered and added to your child's meals. The recommended dosage is 1 to 4 teaspoons three or four times daily, adjusted for younger children under the age of 10. These herbs provide necessary bulk in the diet and can help regulate bowel movements without acting as direct laxatives.

It's important to note that each child is unique, and what works for one may not work for another. If constipation persists or worsens despite dietary and herbal interventions, it is advisable to consult with a healthcare professional for further evaluation and guidance.

Supportive Herbs:

- Angelica
- Barberry
- Boneset
- Cascara Sagrada
- Cayenne
- Chicory
- Dandelion Root
- Ginger
- Marsh Mallow
- Milk Thistle Seed
- Oregon Grape
- St. John's Wort leaf and flower
- Sunflower

Constipation Tinctures

This combination of tinctures will help to get things moving.

- 12 fluid ounces of Dandelion Root Tincture
- 12 fluid ounces of St. John's Wort Tincture
- 12 fluid ounces of Angelica Root Tincture
- 12 fluid ounces of Ginger Tincture

1. Combine the tinctures in a small container. Cap and label the bottle.
2. Apply 2–4 drops every 20 minutes till you feel better.

Softening Tea

If your child is having digestive upset with your constipation, this tea should help to provide a one-two punch to help soothe any lasting digestive worries.

- 2 tablespoons of Sagrada Cascara
- 3–4 Ginger Root slices (in some ways, to taste)
- 1 tablespoon Cayenne Pepper (a little more, if tolerable)
- 1 teaspoon dried Oregon Grape Root

1. In a saucepan, combine the aforementioned herbs and two cups of boiling water.
2. Steep for 30 to 45 minutes, cool, and drain. Take up to two cups each day, one tablespoon at a time.

Let it flow Tea

This is an excellent treatment for the type of constipation that typically afflicts those with dry constitutions, and it's a little nicer than a single Marsh Mallow. This is for children have hard-to-pass, dry, tiny "rabbit pellet" bowel motions. Every day, drink a quart or more of water.

- 1 cup dried Linden Leaf And Flowers
- 1 cup dried Marsh Mallow Root
- 1/4 cup Cinnamon Bark
- 1/4 cup dried Licorice Root

If fresh, double the amount.
1. Combine all of the herbs in a medium mixing dish. Keep the container sealed.
2. Make a cold infusion by combining 2 to 4 tablespoons of herbs with 1 quart of water in a mason jar or a French press. Before filtering, pour in cold or room-temperature water and soak for 4 to 8 hours.

Cuts

A cut, or laceration, is when the skin gets broken or has a hole in it. It can happen when children accidentally bump into something sharp or get a scrape from falling. Cuts can vary in severity, from shallow ones that only affect the top layers of skin to deeper cuts that may involve tissues like muscles or tendons. Puncture wounds, on the other hand, happen when something sharp, like a nail, knife, or tooth, pierces through the skin. These wounds may not always look serious on the surface, but they can go deep into the tissues underneath. If your child gets a cut or puncture, it's important to clean the area gently as soon as possible. Use warm water and mild soap to wash around the wound and remove any dirt or debris. Remember to wash your hands before taking care of the cut. If there is bleeding, you can help stop it by applying gentle pressure with a clean cloth or bandage. Most cuts and punctures will heal on their own with proper care, but if the cut is deep, has jagged edges, or shows signs of infection like redness or swelling, it's a good idea to get it checked by a doctor or nurse.

Sometimes, the healthcare provider may need to use stitches or other techniques to close the wound and help it heal properly. They can also give you advice on how to take care of the cut at home, like using bandages or applying antibiotic ointment. Remember, keeping the cut clean and protected is important for healing. Encourage your child to avoid picking at the scab and remind them to wash their hands regularly. If you have any concerns or questions about the cut, don't hesitate to reach out to a healthcare professional who can provide the best care for your child's specific needs.

Supportive Herbs:
- Calendula Flower
- Chamomile Flower
- Goldenrod Leaf and Flower

- Kelp
- Marsh Mallow
- Pine
- Plantain Leaf
- Rose
- Prunella Vulgaris and Flower
- St. John's Wort Leaf and Flower
- Yarrow Leaf and Flower

Pine Wound Wash

- 1 teaspoon inner bark of White Pine
- 1 teaspoon bark from Wild Cherries
- 1 teaspoon dried root of Wild Plum
- 2 cups water

Follow these easy steps:
1. In a pan, combine the herbs listed above and cover them with water.
2. Bring to a boil, then reduce to low heat and cook until the bark and roots are tender.
3. Allow to cool, then strain. Allow to cool and thicken on its own.
4. Apply the solution to the afflicted region with a clean cloth.

Liquid Wound Wash

- 1 teaspoon dried Pleurisy Root
- 1 teaspoon Grated Ginger
- 2 cups water

Then follow these steps:
1. In a saucepan, combine the above herbs and cover with water; bring to a boil and cook for 20 to 30 minutes, then strain. The liquid will not thicken – it will be a liquid consistency.
2. As needed, apply topically, using a cloth to wash the area.

Pine Salve

For wounds that have healed or were never extremely deep, pine resin salve is the best option. You can also use the resin from other conifers. Resin can be collected straight from the trees; whitish globs of it can be found along the stem where branches have fallen off. Leave enough on the tree to keep the wound sealed—the tree creates a scab with this resin! It will almost certainly contain fragments of bark, dirt, bug parts, and other debris; don't worry, you'll filter that out during processing.

After collecting resin, wash your hands with a little oil instead of soap and water. Simply pour a small amount of any liquid oil into your hands and scrub as if it were soap. As the resin softens, it will separate from your skin. Then you can wash it away with soap and hot water.

You can infuse your resin with basic oil, but starting with a herb-infused oil ensures that you get the benefits of all of these plants, not just the ones that the resin provides.

- 6-8 ounces Pine Resin or similar Conifer Resin
- 8 fluid ounces Plantain-infused oil, Calendula-infused oil, or Goldenrod-infused oil
- 1 ounce chopped or grated beeswax

Just follow these steps:
1. Combine the resin and infused oil in a small saucepan over low heat and heat gradually, stirring often. The resin will soften and disintegrate, releasing its benefits into the oil.
2. Pour over a cheesecloth. Wrap the remaining mass in a towel and squeeze it as hard as you can to extract as much oil as possible.
3. Use this resin-infused oil to make a salve (see here for complete instructions).
4. Apply to the wound multiple times a day, each time using new, tidy bandages.

Diaper Rash

Wet or infrequently changed diapers, diarrhea, new diets, and antibiotics have all been associated with diaper rash.

A red rash on the buttocks is the most common sign. Fever and a broad rash are common symptoms in severe instances.

After a few days of at-home treatment with over-the-counter ointment and more regular diaper changes, most rashes start to improve. A doctor visit is required if the condition does not improve or if fever and rash develop.

Supportive Herbs:
- Burdock
- Calendula Flower
- Comfrey
- Echinacea
- Evening PrimRose
- Goldenseal
- Kelp
- Licorice Root
- Marsh Mallow
- Oregon Grape
- Plantain Leaf
- Rose
- Prunella Vulgaris and Flower
- Slippery Elm
- St. John's Wort Leaf and Flower
- Strawberry
- Uva-Ursi Leaf
- White Oak
- Yarrow Leaf and Flower
- Yellow Dock

Rash Wash
- 1 teaspoon dried Comfrey Root
- 1 teaspoon white Oak Bark or dried Leaves
- 1 teaspoon Slippery Elm Bark
- 2 cups water

Follow these steps:
1. Fill a container halfway with water and add the herbs; bring to a boil and cook for 20 to 30 minutes; cool and drain.
2. As needed, use as a topical wash.

Skin Soothing Tea
- 1 teaspoon dried Burdock Root
- 1 teaspoon dried Echinacea Root
- 1 teaspoon dried Oregon Grape Root
- 1 teaspoon dried Yellow Dock Root
- 2 cups water

Follow these steps:
1. In a pan, combine the herbs listed above and cover them with water. Bring to a boil, then reduce to low heat and cook for 10 to 15 minutes, until cool enough to drain.
2. Start with a tablespoon and work your way up to half a cup every day.

Homemade Diaper Rash Cream
- 1/4 cup beeswax
- 1/4 cup coconut oil
- 1/4 cup zinc oxide powder

Whip up the cream easily using these steps:
1. In a pot, gently melt the beeswax and coconut oil. Allow to cool after thoroughly mixing.
2. Stir in the zinc powder until it is completely dissolved.
3. Apply liberally to rash several times each day, storing in a glass jar to keep it fresh.

Diarrhea

Oh no, it's the dreaded D-word: diarrhea! Dealing with your little one's upset tummy can be challenging, but don't worry, we've got you covered. Diarrhea can be caused by various things, like viruses or eating something that doesn't agree with your child's stomach. In some cases, it might even be a symptom of an underlying condition.

When your child has diarrhea, you'll notice frequent, loose, watery poop and they might complain of stomach aches. It's important to remember that diarrhea can quickly lead to dehydration, especially if your child isn't drinking enough fluids. So, keeping their fluid intake up is crucial. Keep an eye on how much they're drinking and consider giving them warm baths, as it can help their body absorb liquid more effectively. And in case your little one is at risk of dehydration, a warm enema can provide quick hydration.

During this time, it's best to focus on liquids for your child's diet. Herbal teas, vegetable broth, and chicken or miso soup can be great options to keep them nourished. Solid foods can be hard on their sensitive tummy and may contribute to more runny diapers. However, if your child expresses interest in eating, you can offer gentle foods like yogurt, kefir, buttermilk, cottage cheese, potato soup, mashed potatoes (without gravy or butter), and Marsh

Mallow Gruel. These options are easier to digest and can contribute to the healing process. While dairy products can sometimes worsen diarrhea, cultured options like yogurt, kefir, and buttermilk can introduce beneficial bacteria that support the digestive system. You can also try giving them acidophilus, a probiotic that helps restore healthy gut flora and boosts their immune system. Just follow the recommended dosage on the supplement specifically formulated for children.

Remember, staying hydrated is crucial, so consider using commercial pediatric electrolyte solutions like Pedialyte to prevent dehydration. These solutions are specially designed to replenish fluids and electrolytes lost during diarrhea. In certain cases, if an infection is causing the diarrhea, antibiotics may be necessary. Severe cases of dehydration may require intravenous fluids administered by healthcare professionals. Although dealing with diarrhea can be challenging, it's usually a temporary condition that resolves on its own with proper care and plenty of fluids. However, if you're concerned about your child's well-being or if their symptoms persist, it's always wise to consult with a healthcare professional for guidance and support.

Supportive Herbs:
- Agrimony
- Alumroot
- Angelica
- Barberry
- Blackberry
- Black Currant
- Canadian Fleabane
- Catnip
- Cayenne
- Cinnamon Bark
- Ginger Root
- Marsh Mallow
- Meadowsweet Flower
- Mint
- Pine Bark
- Plantain Leaf
- Raspberry
- Rose
- Prunella Vulgaris and Flower
- Strawberry Leaf
- Witch Hazel
- Yarrow
- Yellow Dock

Cinnamon Capsules

Cinnamon's demulcent property is highlighted when it is extracted into water as an infusion or decoction. If you take a capsule containing the powder and ingest it, the capsule dissolves in your G.I. system, releasing the dry powder, which absorbs excess water and acts as an astringent on the intestinal lining. This is a great way to stop diarrhea. This recipe benefits greatly from the use of the Capsule Machine, a handy manual capsule-filling equipment.

- 20 to 24 empty size "00" gelatin capsules
- 2 teaspoons Cinnamon Powder

Follow these steps:
1. Place the Cinnamon Powder in the capsules.
2. If you have diarrhea, take 1 to 3 capsules. If you don't feel better within an hour, take another dose.

Stomach Tea

- 2 tablespoons dried Alumroot Powder
- 2 tablespoons dried Blackberry Leaves
- 2 tablespoons Angelica Powder
- 1 teaspoon dried Oregon Grape Root
- 2 cups heated water

Next, follow these steps:
1. In a nonmetallic container, combine the plants listed above.
2. Cover the herbs with boiling water and steep for 30 minutes; strain; drink as needed, up to one cup per day.

Stomach Relief Tincture

- 1/2 cup dried Prunella Vulgaris Flowers and Leaves
- 1/2 cup dried Meadowsweet Flowers
- 1/4 cup Rose Petals
- 1/2 cup high-proof alcohol (vodka, gin, rum, brandy, and grain will work well)

Follow these steps:
1. Add your preferred herbs and flowers to a mason jar with your preferred alcohol and allow to steep. The solution is usable after a few days; however, it is best after a few weeks.

Earaches

I know how uncomfortable and painful an earache can be for your little one and all you want to do is just make the pain go away, but you should proceed with caution! Earaches are often caused by excess fluid and infection that affect the inner or outer ear, making it difficult for your child to hear properly. Did you know that the ear canals in young children are not fully developed until they're around three or four years old? This means that the canals don't drain as efficiently, especially when your child has a cold or congestion. The excess mucus can get trapped, leading to a build-up of moisture where bacteria can grow and cause infection.

Sometimes, allergies can also contribute to ear infections. If your child experiences recurring ear infections, it's worth considering the possibility of allergies. Foods like sugar, citrus fruits, dairy products (milk, cheese, ice cream), and wheat are common culprits. Removing these potential triggers from your child's diet may help improve their overall health and reduce the frequency of ear infections.

It's important to take ear infections seriously because if left untreated or improperly treated, they can potentially affect your child's hearing. Keep an eye out for early signs like congestion, runny nose, fever, excessive rubbing or pulling of the ear, and irritability. If your child wakes up crying at night and tugging at their ears, it's a clear indication that an infection has taken hold and requires immediate attention.

Many pediatricians prescribe antibiotics for ear infections, which can be effective in acute situations. However, it's important to remember that antibiotics don't address the underlying cause of the problem and can disrupt your child's immune system, making them more susceptible to future illnesses. Overuse of antibiotics is also a concern in our healthcare system and environment.

During an ear infection, ensure that your child gets plenty of rest and avoids going out into cold air too soon. It's a common mistake to think they've fully recovered and send them out to play prematurely. Consider keeping your child at home for a few days until they've fully recovered, even though it may be inconvenient in our busy lives. Taking the time to care for your child during the early stages of illness can help reduce the overall duration of their discomfort.

Avoid giving your child foods that can worsen congestion and aggravate the condition, such as sugary foods, dairy products (especially milk and cheese), wheat products, orange juice, and processed foods. Instead, focus on probiotic cultures like acidophilus, which can be beneficial in supporting their immune system. You can also try a delicious tea made with freshly grated ginger, freshly squeezed lemon, and a touch of honey or maple syrup. It's a refreshing blend that can help decongest. In traditional Chinese medicine, a connection is drawn between the health of the kidneys and the ears. Drinking sufficient fluids like water and cranberry juice can support kidney health. You can also try placing warm packs over the lower back, the area of the kidneys, to provide some relief.

If your herbal home treatments don't show improvement within a day or two, or if the pain and infection worsen, or if you notice pus or blood draining from the ear, it's important to seek medical help immediately. While this may sound alarming, it's important to remember that most ear infections can be effectively treated at home. Ruptured eardrums are rare when infections are promptly addressed, and they usually heal over time without any long-term hearing loss.

Remember, always use common sense and trust your instincts when it comes to your child's health. With proper care, most ear infections can be managed effectively, and your little one will be back to their playful and happy selves in no time.

Supportive Herbs:
- Bayberry
- Black Elder
- Calendula Flower
- Echinacea
- Garlic
- Ginger
- Gingko Biloba
- Ginseng
- Goldenrod Leaf and Flower
- Goldenseal
- Licorice
- Pau D'Arco
- Pine
- Rose
- Slippery Elm
- Valerian
- White Willow
- Wild Indigo
- Witch Hazel
- Marsh Mallow
- Sage Leaf
- Thyme Leaf
- Uva-Ursi Leaf
- Yerba Mansa

Garlic Oil

A quick remedy, with readily available ingredients, common in every household. Beware, using oil as a treatment is only suitable when the ear infection is caused by congestion in the ear canals. If the infection is due to water, using oil can actually worsen the condition. So, it's crucial to determine whether the ear infection is caused by congestion or by water in the ear, also known as swimmer's ear. How can you tell the difference? If your child experiences ear pain along with a runny nose, cough, or other cold and flu symptoms, it's likely that the infection is due to congestion. On the other hand, if there are no signs of congestion or cold and flu symptoms, but your child has recently been swimming or gotten water in their ear during a bath or shower, then the infection is most likely caused by water in the ear.

If the infection is caused by water in the ear, it's important not to use oil as a treatment. Instead, you can try using rubbing alcohol, witch hazel extract, apple cider vinegar, or St. John's wort tincture. These solutions help the water to evaporate. For an added boost against the infection, you can add a drop of tea tree or lavender essential oil to the rubbing alcohol, vinegar, witch hazel, or tincture. Simply put a few drops of the mixture in each ear and gently massage it in. Placing a warm pack over the ear can also provide both pain relief and comfort.

- Crushed Garlic
- Olive oil

Simply:
1. Combine the crushed Garlic and olive oil, leave to steep for at least an hour.
2. After an hour, strain the oil.
3. Bottle the oil and use it as needed once or twice per day.

Ginger Oil (External)

If your outer ear, the portion outside of the ear canal, is swelling, you're in luck.

- Grated Ginger
- Olive oil

Easy steps:

1. Combine the grated Ginger and Olive oil, leave to steep for at least an hour.
2. After an hour, strain the oil.
3. Bottle the oil and use it as needed once or twice per day.

Basil Paste

Basil is a medicinal herb with a wide range of uses. Basil is abundant in antioxidants and has antimicrobial qualities as well. All you need is a handful of basil leaves.

1. Carefully crush five fresh Holy Basil Leaves to extract the juice.
2. Apply the Basil juice to the afflicted ear and the area around it. Avoid getting any of the juice in your ear canal.
3. Wipe the mixture carefully within the ear, around the exterior of the ear, and behind the ear.

Fever

A fever is your body's way of responding to an illness by temporarily elevating your body temperature. It serves as an indication that something out of the ordinary is happening inside your body. In adults, a fever can be uncomfortable but is generally not a cause for immediate concern unless it reaches 103 degrees Fahrenheit (39.4 degrees Celsius) or higher. However, in infants and toddlers, even a slight increase in temperature may be a sign of a potentially serious infection. Fevers typically subside within a few days and can be managed with over-the-counter medications. However, there are instances when it might be better to let the fever run its course. Fevers play a vital role in your child's body's ability to combat various infections. If your child's fever reaches 102°F/39°C or higher, or persists for several days, it's important to seek guidance from your holistic healthcare provider or pediatrician without delay. However, in most cases, it's beneficial to recognize a fever as a valuable tool employed by the immune system. By viewing a fever as part of the body's natural defense mechanism, we can better appreciate its role in fighting off infections. It's important to monitor the fever, provide comfort measures, and ensure your child stays hydrated. If needed, consult a healthcare professional for further guidance and support. Remember, your child's immune system is working diligently to protect and heal, and a fever is a part of that important immune response.

Supportive Herbs:

- Angelica
- Boneset
- Cayenne
- Catnip Leaf and Flower
- Elderflower
- Garlic
- Ginger
- Juniper
- Marigold
- Osha Root
- Oxeye Daisy
- Peppermint Leaf
- Sage Leaf
- Skullcap
- Thyme Leaf
- Tulsi Leaf
- Wild Indigo Root
- Wild Lettuce
- Yarrow Leaf and Flower

Quick Fever Tea

- 1 teaspoon Echinacea Root
- 1 teaspoon White Willow Root
- 1 cup of water

Quick steps:

1. In a pan, combine the roots and cover them with water.
2. Bring to a boil, then lower to low heat and cook for 30 minutes, straining afterward.
3. Take half a cup three times a day, up to four times per day.

Use Cayenne

As you feed your fire, stoke it a bit using cayenne pepper. Pepper helps to boost blood circulation, making your fever that much more effective in kicking the bodies it is fighting.

Punch-Packed Fever Tea

- 1 teaspoon dried Barberry Berries
- 1 teaspoon dried Angelica Root
- 1 teaspoon ground dried Ivy Leaves
- 2 tablespoons dried Peppermint Leaves
- 2 tablespoons dried Blue Vervain Leaves
- 1 tablespoon dried Yarrow
- 1 teaspoon dried Catnip Leaves
- 1 cup of hot water

Simply follow these steps:

1. Combine the herbs listed above.
2. In a cup, put one tablespoon of the mixture; pour boiling water over the herbs; soak for 30 minutes; strain.
3. Consume one cup per day.

Flu

The flu, short for influenza, is a contagious respiratory tract infection that affects the nose, throat, and lungs. It is caused by a virus that can easily spread from person to person, especially during the colder months of the year when flu viruses are most prevalent. When you notice the first signs of a cold or flu in your child, it's important to take action to support their immune system. One helpful approach is to give your child frequent doses of echinacea tincture, a natural remedy that can help boost the immune system. For example, a four-year-old child can take 1/8 teaspoon of echinacea tincture every hour until the symptoms improve. To make it more enjoyable, you can mix the echinacea tincture with an equal amount of elderberry syrup, which not only enhances the taste but also provides additional immune-supportive properties.

In addition to echinacea, it's beneficial to increase your child's intake of vitamin C. This essential nutrient plays a vital role in supporting the immune system's response to infections. Including foods rich in vitamin C, such as citrus fruits, strawberries, kiwi, and bell peppers, can help strengthen your child's natural defenses and assist their body in fighting off the flu. Remember, antibiotics are not effective against viral infections like the flu, so it's best to allow the body to combat the infection on its own. By providing your child with immune-boosting remedies and ensuring they receive proper rest, hydration, and nutritious foods, you can support their body's natural ability to fight off the flu and recover more quickly.

If your child's symptoms worsen or persist, it's always a good idea to consult with a healthcare professional for further guidance and support.

Supportive Herbs:
- Agrimony
- Black Currant
- Black Elder
- Blue Vervain
- Boneset
- Chamomile
- Coltsfoot
- Echinacea
- Elecampane
- Fennel Seed
- Ginger
- Gingko Biloba
- Goldenrod
- Goldenseal
- Horehound
- Indian Root
- Licorice
- Mullein
- Osha
- Oxeye Daisy
- Peppermint
- Pine
- Pleurisy Root
- Queen of the Meadow
- Speedwell
- White Cedar Leaf Tips
- Wild Cherry
- Wild Indigo
- Yarrow
- Yerba Mansa
- Yerba Sante
- Marsh Mallow
- Mullein Leaf
- Sage Leaf
- Thyme Leaf

To get the most out of herbs, we need to know the difference between a hot, dry, irritating cough and a wet, cold, and ineffective cough. You'll have a racking, unrelenting cough if your lungs are dry; we utilize moistening herbs to remedy this.

All-Around Oxymel

What do you get when you combine the vinegar's astringent and stimulating properties with the honey's moistening and calming properties: an oxymel, my personal go-to for coughs of all kinds, thanks to the use of lung-specific herbs.
- 1/3 cup dried Pine Needles
- 1/3 cup dried Sage Leaf
- 1/3 cup dried Thyme Leaf
- 1/4 cup Ginger Powder
- 1 quart apple cider vinegar
- Honey (as needed to top off and sweeten to taste)

Follow these steps:
1. Combine the herbs in a quart-size mason jar.
2. Fill the jar with vinegar until it's four-fifths full, then top it off with honey.
3. Cover the jar and set it aside for 4 weeks to macerate; however, you can start using it immediately.
4. Strain the oxymel and store it in a bottle.
5. As needed, take 1 to 3 tablespoons.

All-Around Flu Fighter
- 30 drops of Echinacea Tincture
- 20 drops of wild Indigo Root Tincture
- 2 cups tea made from White Cedar Leaf Tips

Quick and simple:
Mix all of the ingredients together and drink half a cup at a time, hot. You can take it up to three times per day.

Cough Expectorant for Wet Coughs
- 2 teaspoons of dried Boneset Herb
- 2 teaspoons of Licorice Root
- 2 teaspoons of Wild Cherry Bark
- 2 teaspoons of Ginger Root
- 2 cups of boiling water

In a nonmetallic container, combine the above herbs and cover with boiling water; steep.
Cool for 30 minutes before straining. For a dry tickling cough, take one to two teaspoons at a time, up to two cups per day, as needed.

Mild Burns

Warning: For serious burns, seek medical attention immediately. Burns can be a scary experience, especially when it comes to our little ones. Understanding the different types of burns can help us better care for our children's skin and provide the appropriate treatment. First-degree burns, also known as superficial burns, are the mildest type. They affect the outer layer of the skin, causing redness and discomfort. Think of it like a sunburn, where the skin becomes red but doesn't blister. These burns can be treated at home with cool water, aloe vera gel, or soothing creams to relieve the discomfort.

Second-degree burns, also called partial-thickness burns, go deeper into the skin, affecting both the epidermis and the dermis (the lower layer of the skin). With second-degree burns, you'll notice pain, redness, swelling, and the formation of blisters. It's important not to pop the blisters, as they act as a natural barrier against infection. Cool water, gentle cleaning, and applying a sterile dressing can help promote healing and prevent infection.

Third-degree burns are more severe and penetrate through the dermis, affecting deeper structures. The skin may appear burnt, bleached, or blackened, and the area might be numb because the nerve endings are damaged. Third-degree burns require immediate medical attention. While waiting for professional help, cover the burn with a clean, non-stick bandage or cloth and keep the child calm and comfortable. The most severe type of burn is the fourth-degree burn. These burns can extend beyond the skin, damaging muscles and even bones. Nerve endings are injured or destroyed, so the charred area may not have any sensation or pain. Fourth-degree burns require emergency medical care, and it's crucial to seek immediate help.

Remember, the best way to prevent burns is through prevention. Keep hot objects out of reach, install safety gates around stoves and fireplaces, and teach your children about fire safety. If a burn does occur, providing quick and appropriate care can make a significant difference in the healing process and help minimize scarring.

Always consult with a healthcare professional for proper assessment and treatment of burns, especially for more severe cases.

Supportive Herbs:
- Calendula Flower
- Coneflower
- Echinacea
- Goldenrod
- Hyssop
- Linden Leaf and Flower
- Marsh Mallow
- Peppermint Leaf
- Plantain Leaf
- Rose Petals
- Prunella Vulgaris and Flower
- Sunflower
- Wild Indigo Root
-

Burn Liniment

Use a net or cheesecloth filled with this remedy to help soothe burns.
- 1 tablespoon dried Coneflower Flowers
- 1 tablespoon dried Hyssop Blossoms
- 1 tablespoon dried Goldenrod Flowers
- 1 tablespoon dried Sunflower Petals

Simply:
1. Mix the aforementioned components together, then moisten with boiling water and sandwich between two layers of cheesecloth. Let cool before applying to the affected region.
2. Remoisten when it has dried. Use as often as you need.

Honey Salve

Honey is the single most effective treatment for burns: if all you have is honey, you'll be OK. It's even better when you infuse it with these medicinal herbs ahead of time.
- 1/2 cup fresh Calendula Flower
- 1/2 cup fresh Rose Petals
- 1 pint honey

Follow these steps:
1. In a pint-size mason jar, combine the Calendula and Rose petals.
2. Pour the warm honey into the container. Seal the jar and leave it to infuse for a month in a warm location. It can be used sooner if need be, but one month to cure is optimal.
3. When ready to use, gently reheat the closed jar in a double boiler until the honey has a "smearable" consistency.
4. Apply a layer of the infused honey to a burn site after it has cooled and been cleaned, and cover lightly with a gauze bandage. At least twice a day, refresh the application.

Calendula Paste
- 1/4 cup dried Calendula Flowers
- 1/4 cup dried Violet Leaves
- 1/4 cup dried Plantain Leaves
- 2 tablespoons powdered clay
- 10 drops Lavender essential oil
- 6 ounces hot water

Combine the hot water with the remaining ingredients in a food processor or blender until the paste is smooth and pesto-like. To reach the proper consistency, you may need to add more herbs, clay, or water. Use a few times per day, adding fresh paste as needed when it dries and chips.

Skin Rashes

A rash that appears suddenly usually suggests that the child has come into touch with an irritant, such as an irritating plant, a harmful chemical, or an insect bite or sting. A mild natural soap (a home-made calendula soap is a good option) and water should be used to thoroughly clean the area. Then apply what you've learned about fundamental herbal energetics: If the rash is dry, moistening herbs and preparations should be used; if it's damp and oozy, drying agents should be used.

If there appears to be no direct contact with an irritating plant, chemical, or other direct triggers, the rash could be an external manifestation of an inside imbalance. Of course, allergies and overworked internal detoxification systems might contribute to this. It's time to cure the rash, wash it away, and wait it out in this scenario.

Supportive Herbs:
- Burdock
- Calendula Flower
- Comfrey
- Echinacea
- Evening Primrose
- Goldenseal
- Kelp
- Licorice Root
- Marsh Mallow
- Oregon Grape
- Plantain Leaf
- Rose
- Prunella Vulgaris and Flower
- Slippery Elm
- St. John's Wort Leaf and Flower
- Strawberry
- Uva-Ursi Leaf
- White Oak
- Yarrow Leaf and Flower
- Yellow Dock

All-Around Rash Wash

- 1 teaspoon dried Comfrey Root
- 1 teaspoon dried White Oak Bark or Leaves
- 1 teaspoon dried Slippery Elm Bark
- 2 cups water

Follow these steps:
1. Fill a container halfway with water and add the herbs; bring to a boil and cook for 20 to 30 minutes; cool and drain.
2. As needed, use as a topical wash.

Dry Rash Compound

Because of their oil and wax composition, salves are emollient, especially when they are made with a hydrating oil like olive oil as the base. The soothing and anti-inflammatory properties of the herbs improve the emollient effect in this basic composition.

- 3 fluid ounces Calendula-infused oil
- 3 fluid ounces Plantain-infused oil
- 2 fluid ounces Licorice-infused oil
- 1 ounce beeswax, or until the compound is waxy and spreadable

The steps are simple:
1. Make the salve by combining the oils and beeswax until they become incorporated into a spreadable paste.
2. At least twice a day, apply a thin coating to the affected area.

Weepy Rash Compound

A weepy rash is one that produces fluid, be it through pustules, blisters, or leaking lymph. In this case, it is important to convince the fluid to dry up for the body to begin the healing process or to accelerate it.

- 1 cup dried Calendula Flower
- 1 cup dried Rose Petals
- 1 cup dried Prunella Vulgaris Flowers and Leaves
- 1/2 cup dried St. John's Wort Leaf and Flowers
- 1/2 cup dried Uva-Ursi Leaf
- 1/2 cup dried Yarrow Flower and Leaves

Follow these steps:
1. Place 4 to 6 tablespoons of the herb mixture in a heatproof container.
2. Pour just enough boiling water over the herbs to completely submerge them, but not so hot that they float. Allow 5 minutes for the herbs to steep.
3. Gather up the herbs into a cheesecloth and tie off the satchel to use as a cover. Pat the area, re-wetting the area as it dries. Do this three to four times per day.

Tip: If you don't have access to these herbs, simple green or black tea bags will suffice! Simply get them warm and wet, put them to the rash, and let them on for 20 minutes.

Sore Throat

A sore throat is usually a minor issue that goes away on its own with time. Although the reason for a sore throat is not always known, it is most commonly caused by viral illnesses such as the flu or a regular cold. It can also happen as a result of being exposed to irritants like dust or smoke, allergies, or even talking or screaming too loudly. Swelling of the throat can make swallowing difficult and cause a hoarse voice.

Supportive Herbs:
- Balsam Fir
- Bayberry
- Black Elder
- Blue Vervain
- Canadian Fleabane
- Cayenne
- Cinnamon Bark
- Coltsfoot
- Comfrey
- Echinacea

- Ginger
- Goldenrod Leaf and Flower
- Indian Root
- Licorice Root
- Marsh Mallow
- Osha Root
- Sage Leaf
- Prunella Vulgaris and Flower
- Seneca Snakeroot
- Slippery Elm
- Sumac
- Wild Cherry
- Witch Hazel
- Yerba Sante

Fruity Gargle

- 1 tablespoon Elderberry fruit juice
- 1 tablespoon Sumac extract
- 1 teaspoon Echinacea Root Extract

Simply combine all the ingredients above and gargle. Repeat as needed.

A Coat for the Throat

- 1 cup dried Marsh Mallow Root
- 1/2 cup Ginger Powder
- 1/4 cup Cinnamon Bark
- 1/4 cup dried Licorice root

To create the tea mix:
1. Combine all of the herbs in a small bowl. Keep the container sealed. You'll use this base to create your teas in the future; think of it as having ready-to-go tea leaves in your pantry.
2. When ready, In a covered saucepan over high heat, measure 2 to 4 tablespoons of herbs per quart of water. Cover the pot and add the water. Bring to a boil, then reduce to low heat and cook for 1 hour.
3. Cool the tea completely after decoction to increase the relaxing benefits of the mucilaginous herbs in this blend, then cool for another 1 to 2 hours. Before drinking, strain, and reheat.

Sore Throat Steam Bath

Steaming is a universal remedy for any respiratory system problems, including sinus problems, throughout cultures. Pathogens have a hard time surviving in the presence of heated steam and evaporating volatile oils from the herbs, which increases immunological response in the mucosal membranes. If your sore throat is due to a nasal drip, this should help to clear things out posthaste.

- 1 cup dried Pine Needles
- 1/2 cup dried Sage Leaf
- 1/2 cup dried Thyme Leaf
- 1/2 gallon of water
- 5 chopped Garlic Cloves

Follow these steps to run your steam bath:
1. Fill your pot with the required water and place it on a high burner.
2. As steam begins to rise, add the ingredients.
3. Using a towel or similar length of cloth, tent your head around the pot to take in the rising steam.
4. As your nose begins to run, clear and blow your nose as needed. Repeat this process 2-3 times per day as needed.

Teething

Ah, the joys of teething! It's that exciting time when your baby's little pearly whites start making their grand entrance from beneath the gums. We like to call it the "orthodontiasis" phase, fancy word, right? Teething typically begins around 4 to 7 months of age, but hey, every baby is unique, so don't worry if your little one decides to sprout their teeth on their own timeline. It's all part of their individual journey.

Now, let's talk about the not-so-fun part: the irritability and tears that often accompany teething. Imagine sharp new teeth pushing their way through tender gums— ouch! It's no wonder your baby might be feeling a bit grumpy during this time. But don't worry, there are ways to help soothe those teething troubles.
One of the best things you can do is provide gentle relief for your little one's sore gums. A chilled teething ring or a clean, damp washcloth that has been cooled in the refrigerator can work wonders. The coolness helps numb the discomfort and gives them something safe to chew on. Just make sure to keep an eye on them while they're using these teething aids. Another trick is to gently massage your baby's gums with a clean finger. Applying gentle pressure can help alleviate some of the discomfort and provide temporary relief. Just be sure to wash your hands thoroughly before doing so.

There are also teething gels and natural remedies available that you can discuss with your pediatrician or holistic healthcare provider. These products are specifically designed to help ease the discomfort of teething and provide a soothing sensation for your little one. Remember, during this teething journey, patience and extra cuddles go a long way. Your baby may experience some disrupted sleep patterns and fussiness, but with your love and care, they'll get through it. And soon enough, those adorable little teeth will be proudly on display. So, hang in there! Teething may have its challenges, but it's also an exciting milestone in your baby's development. Enjoy the journey, and before you know it, you'll be capturing those precious toothy smiles in all their glory!

Supportive Herbs:
- Chamomile
- Catnip
- Passionflower
- Valerian
- Mullein

Teething Tinctures

- Twenty drops of herbal tincture (take your pick of the herbal allies)
- One tablespoon olive or coconut oil

Follow these steps:
1. Mix one teaspoon of your selected essential oil well with a teaspoon of carrier oil, usually olive or coconut.
2. Once combined, rub the tincture directly onto the pain point.

Teething Ice Cubes

Using the from above, create a tray of ice cubes using a few droplets of tincture per ice cube. When ready, use the ice cube to massage your baby's sore gums to dull the pain of teeth coming in, as well as to help rub some tincture onto the area.

Teething Cloth

The same process as for ice cubes; however, in this operation, you're wetting a washcloth, adding drops of a tincture, then placing the cloth in the refrigerator or freezer. Once your little one begins to bite and suck on the rag, they'll coat their tiny mouths in the helpful oil, plus have their hands moisturized and soothed as well as they manipulate the cloth.

Upset Stomach

What can you do for tummy troubles? We've all experienced that uncomfortable feeling in our bellies at some point in our lives. It's called abdominal pain, and it can really put a damper on our day. The good news is that most stomach discomfort is nothing to worry about, and your trusty pediatrician can quickly diagnose and treat the issue. Plus, there are plenty of things you can do at home to ease the occasional upset stomach. Now, let's talk about some soothing remedies for your little one's tummy. One trick is to place a warm towel soaked in a calming herbal tea, like chamomile or lavender, on their stomach. Make sure the towel is warm, but not hot, as we don't want any little tummies getting burned. The combination of warm water and the essence of these gentle herbs can work wonders in helping your child relax and relieve those tummy muscles. Another thing you can try is offering small sips of clear fluids to keep your little one hydrated. Opt for gentle options like water, herbal teas, or diluted fruit juices. Avoid fizzy drinks or anything sugary that might upset their stomach even more.

When it comes to food, go for bland and easily digestible choices. Think rice, boiled potatoes, toast, or plain crackers. These gentle foods give their tummies a break and provide some nourishment without adding any extra stress. If your child is experiencing nausea, you can offer them small, frequent meals instead of larger portions. This can help prevent overwhelming their stomach and make it easier for them to keep food down. Remember, it's essential to pay attention to any other symptoms your child may be experiencing, as abdominal pain can sometimes be a sign of a more serious condition. If the pain persists, worsens, or is accompanied by high fever, vomiting, or other concerning symptoms, it's best to consult your pediatrician for a proper evaluation and guidance. In the meantime, offer your little one some extra comfort and TLC. A gentle belly rub or a cozy cuddle session can go a long way in soothing their discomfort and making them feel better.

Supportive Herbs:
- Bayberry
- Catnip Leaf and Flower
- Chamomile Flower
- Chaparral
- Coriander
- Dandelion Root
- Fennel Seed
- Ginger
- Hops
- Kelp
- Licorice Root
- Linden Leaf and Flower
- Marsh Mallow
- Meadowsweet Flower
- Oregon Grape
- Prunella Vulgaris and Flower
- St. John's Wort Leaf and Flower
- Yellow Dock

Stomach-Tamer Tea

- 1 teaspoon dried Catnip Leaves
- 1 teaspoon dried Oxeye Daisy
- 1 cup boiling water

Follow these directions:
1. In a nonmetallic container, combine the herbs and cover with boiling water; soak for 30 minutes; strain.
2. As needed, take a tablespoon at a time.

Heartburn Tea

- 1 teaspoon dried Licorice Root
- 1 teaspoon dried Peppermint Leaves
- 2 cups boiling water

Follow these steps to brew the tea:
1. Combine the above herbs in a nonmetallic container and cover with the boiling water; steep for 15 to 20 minutes; strain.
2. Take as needed, up to one cup a day.

Cold Marsh Mallow Infusion

Taking 2-4 tablespoons of dried Marsh Mallow root, combine the Marsh Mallow with enough cold or room-temperature water to fill a quart-size mason jar. Steep for 4 to 8 hours, covered. Keep refrigerated for 2 to 3 days, depending on the batch.

Activities for Children

In this digital age, kids seem to be glued to their screens, spending more time indoors than ever before. It's a fact that the average American child spends a mere 4 to 7 minutes per day outside, while clocking in over 7 hours in front of various devices. Remember, the great outdoors is not just a place for bugs and dirt—it's an essential playground for our little ones!

Now, picture this: your child stepping outside, taking a deep breath of fresh air, and feeling the warm sun on their face. It's not just a refreshing escape from the four walls of their room; it's a necessary adventure for their overall well-being. Numerous studies have shown that children who embrace outdoor play are not only happier but also more attentive and less stressed than their indoor-bound counterparts.

You see, nature holds endless possibilities for our youngsters. It's a wild playground where they can freely explore, imagine, and create without the boundaries of structured activities. Whether they're climbing trees, building forts, or simply running wild, the great outdoors gives them the chance to develop their independence, boost their confidence, and unleash their creativity.

And let's not forget about the valuable life lessons waiting to be learned in the great wide open. Take caring for a plant, for instance. When kids are responsible for watering and nurturing it, they quickly discover the importance of tending to living things. It's a hands-on experience that teaches them about responsibility, empathy, and the delicate balance of the natural world.

When kids are outside, they are in constant motion. Whether they're chasing butterflies, playing tag, or riding their bikes, they are in an active mode that surpasses any sedentary indoor activity. Not only does this keep their bodies fit and healthy, but it also improves their focus and attention span—a real game-changer, especially for those little ones who may have a touch of the wiggles.

But perhaps one of the most magical aspects of outdoor play is its ability to wash away tension and worries. The freedom and wide-open spaces can do wonders for a child's stress levels. It's like a natural therapy session where they can let their worries fade away amidst the trees, grass, and fresh air.

So, let's encourage our children to step away from the screens and embrace the great outdoors. Let them revel in the wonders of nature, explore their imaginations, and soak up all the benefits that come with being outside. After all, childhood is a time for adventure, and what better place to embark on that adventure than in the beauty of the world around us?

Let's open the doors and let their young spirits roam free!

1. Identify Backyard Plants
Can your little explorers identify the fascinating flora right in your own backyard? Challenge their botany skills by seeing if they can spot and name five different types of plants. Are they able to distinguish between three unique flower types? Encourage them to take note of the vibrant colors of leaves and petals, the distinct shapes of branches and stems, and the varying heights or lengths of these plant wonders.

But let's take it up a notch! Introduce the concept of shapes into their nature exploration. Cut out shapes from colorful paper and challenge your children to find natural objects that match those shapes. Can they find something in the shape of a circle, a triangle, or perhaps even an unexpected shape? It's a playful way to combine art and nature, engaging their creativity and observation skills.

For an added twist, let's mix in some color exploration! Gather bright and colorful household items like old paint swatches, cereal box parts, bathroom towels, or even running shoes. Ask the kids to venture out and hunt for natural items in those same vibrant hues. However, it's essential to emphasize that while we can admire and appreciate the beauty of nature, we must leave it undisturbed in its natural environment.

So, get ready for a nature scavenger hunt in your own backyard, where your little ones can unleash their curiosity, sharpen their observation skills, and discover the wonders of the natural world right at their fingertips. It's a journey that combines learning, creativity, and the joy of exploring the magic that surrounds us every day!

2. Foraged Art
Start by crafting your very own picture frames using cardboard. Don't have any cardboard on hand? No worries! Repurpose a cereal box or tape together a few pieces of newspaper to form a frame. Remember to explain to the kids that they should only gather items found on the ground and avoid anything that is still growing.

Challenge your little artists to collect items in a specific color sequence. First, they can gather green goodies, then move on to yellow treasures, and finally, search for items in vibrant red hues. Engage them in a discussion about why certain colors may be more abundant than others. This is a perfect opportunity to explore the concept of seasons. What colors do you think they would find if they did this activity in winter? How about during autumn?

Once they have their collection of nature's hues, it's time to unleash their imagination! Encourage your children to arrange and combine their gathered items into a captivating nature scene, a mesmerizing collage, or a stunning mosaic within their handmade frames. The possibilities are endless, and their creativity will truly shine!

As they bring their artistic visions to life, they'll not only have a delightful time but also learn to appreciate the beauty of nature in a new way. This activity nurtures their observation skills, sparks their imagination, and encourages them to find inspiration in the world around them.

3. What Makes an Ecosystem?

Find a white or light-colored sheet, or even some towels or an old t-shirt, and head outside. Choose a tree and carefully place the sheet on the ground beneath its branches. Now, let the exploration begin!

Give the tree branches a gentle shake and observe what emerges. Do you see any tiny seeds falling onto the sheet? Are there colorful leaves scattered around? Can you spot specks of pollen floating in the air? Keep a close eye out for any fascinating bugs or insects that make their way onto the sheet.

Take a moment to ponder why certain locations may have more bugs than others. What factors could contribute to this difference? Is it the type of tree, the availability of food, or the surrounding environment? This discussion can open up a world of understanding about the intricate balance and interdependence within ecosystems.

Now, let's imagine performing this activity in the fall. What do you think would fall upon the sheet during this season? Perhaps an array of vibrant autumn leaves, acorns, or even migrating butterflies. This is a perfect opportunity to delve into the topic of seasons and explore how ecosystems change and adapt throughout the year.

As you observe and discuss the elements that appear on the sheet, you're unraveling the fascinating components of an ecosystem. From the smallest seeds to the buzzing insects, every living thing plays a vital role in maintaining the delicate balance of nature.

4. Explore Small Ecosystems

It's time to embark on a microhike and explore the fascinating world of small ecosystems. Are you ready to shrink down and dive into the wonders that exist right beneath your feet?

To begin, gather a hula hoop or a piece of twine and create a circular habitat in your yard. This will be your micro-ecosystem, a special space where nature comes to life. Gather your family members and position yourselves around the circle, ready to embark on this exciting exploration.

Now, let's shift our perspective and imagine ourselves as tiny creatures, like ants, navigating this miniature world. Encourage the kids to use their imagination and shrink down to the size of ants. As you explore, pay close attention to what you see, hear, smell, touch, and even taste. Yes, that's right - let's engage all five senses!

Start by investigating what lies beneath rocks, logs, and leaves. Lift them carefully, and observe the hidden treasures that await. Keep an eye out for tiny insects, fascinating critters, and intricate patterns of life. Discuss the importance of these creatures in the ecosystem and how they contribute to the balance of nature.

As you move through the micro-ecosystem, encourage the kids to search for little objects and discover the beauty in the details. Remind them to be gentle and respectful of the environment, leaving everything as they found it.

To make it more fun, try tossing a bean bag or a frisbee to choose a specific spot in the yard. This will lead the

exploration to a new area, unveiling a fresh realm of nature to discover. Follow the object's landing point and let your curiosity guide you.

Throughout the microhike, engage in lively discussions about the interconnectedness of living organisms, the importance of biodiversity, and the delicate balance within ecosystems. Encourage your children to ask questions, make observations, and share their findings.

Happy exploring!

5. Be Outdoor Painters

Calling all budding artists! It's time to unleash your creativity and become outdoor painters in your very own backyard. Get ready to paint scenes that capture the beauty and memories of this special place.

First, let the children choose a scene in the backyard that inspires them. It could be the towering trees, the playful squirrels, the fluffy clouds, or any other captivating feature. Provide them with watercolors or any other type of paint and scrap paper to bring their vision to life.

Now, here comes the exciting challenge! Encourage the children to close their eyes while they paint. This will unleash their imagination and add a touch of mystery to their artwork. What vivid memories do they have of the area? How do they envision it with their eyes closed?

Once the paintings are complete, have the children hand their masterpieces to someone else in the family. It's time for a fun guessing game! Can the other person guess which section of the backyard was painted based on the colors and brushstrokes? It's a delightful way to celebrate the unique perspectives and interpretations of each artist.

Gather acrylic paint and rocks for another painting adventure. Let the children recreate their masterpieces on the rocks, turning them into lasting works of art. Once the paint is dry, encourage them to display their rock paintings in the yard or garden, where they can admire their artwork whenever they please.

As they paint, encourage the children to reminisce about the fond memories they have of the backyard. It could be the laughter shared with friends, the magical adventures they've had, or the peaceful moments of solitude. Let their imaginations run wild as they infuse their artwork with their personal connection to the space.

6. Create Outdoor Journals

To create your outdoor journals, fold a few sheets of paper in half and punch holes along the fold. Use yarn or staples to bind the pages together, creating a personalized journal just for you. This will be your trusted companion as you explore the outdoors.

Now, let's set the stage for your week-long adventure. Explain to the kids that for the next seven days, they will choose a specific area in the backyard to observe. It could be a patch of grass, a tree, or a corner of the garden. The goal is to note everything you see, hear, and smell in that particular spot.

Before you head outside, let's make some predictions!

Ask questions like:
- What color do you think the sky will be on a sunny day?
- When do you think you'll hear the most birds?
- How do you imagine the air will smell when it rains?

Now it's time to put your observations to the test. Go outside at the same time every day and document what you discover in your journal. Pay attention to changes in weather, colors, animals, or anything else that catches your eye. Take note of what remains the same and what surprises you throughout the week.

As the days pass, you'll start to see the magic of nature unfolding. Perhaps flowers will bloom where there were none before, or you'll notice new sounds as the seasons change. Spring is an especially exciting time for this activity, as nature transforms rapidly around us. Adults can join in too and start their own nature journals alongside the kids.

This game is also a fantastic opportunity to understand the distinction between climate and weather. Discuss how climate represents the expected weather patterns in an area, while weather is what we experience day to day. Encourage the kids to draw or write about their observations and imagine how their journal entries would differ if they recorded the same scene in winter.

Building on your previous activities, take storytelling to the next level. Challenge the children to create tales based on their observations. They can write from the perspective of an ant on the ground or a majestic tree towering above it all.

7. Discover Light and Shadow
Begin by asking your little ones if they notice any shadows when they gaze out into a wide, open area with nothing around them. The answer is no, as shadows require both a light source and an object. Shadows are created when light is blocked by something!

Now, let's conduct a fun experiment. Have someone hold a flashlight up in the air while you stand in front of it. Can you see your shadow on the ground? That's the light being blocked by your body, creating a shadow. It's like you're playing a game of hide-and-seek with the light!

Next, let's talk about natural light sources. Can your kids guess the biggest and most powerful natural light source? That's right—it's the sun! Throughout the day, the position of the sun changes, which affects the way light and shadows behave. Encourage your children to step outside at the same time every hour and observe how the light and shadows transform throughout the day.

Here's a fun challenge: Ask your kids to place their favorite toy outside on the ground. Each time they go outside to check on it, observe how the toy's shadow changes. Does it get longer or shorter? Does it shift direction? It's like the toy is playing its own game with the sun, creating a delightful show of shadows!

While you're outside, take a moment to look up at the sky on a sunny day. Do your children notice that the sun is in a different spot in the morning compared to the afternoon? This is because the sun rises in one direction

and sets in another. You can even research the specific sunrise and sunset times for your area to deepen your understanding of the sun's movement.

Remember, it's important to remind the kids never to stare directly at the sun. Explain to them why it's not safe and how it can harm their eyes.

Throughout the day, engage in conversations about light, shadows, and the sun's journey across the sky. Encourage your little scientists to ask questions and share their observations. Together, you'll uncover the magical world of light and shadows, appreciating the beauty and wonder that surrounds us every day!

8. Go Backyard Camping
Get ready for a backyard camping adventure! Set up a tent in your backyard or create a fort indoors for a cozy camping experience. Cook a delicious campfire-style dinner together and enjoy storytelling by the "campfire." Disconnect from screens and immerse yourselves in nature. Snuggle into your sleeping bags or makeshift beds and fall asleep under the stars. Wake up to a refreshing morning and savor a delightful outdoor breakfast. Create lasting memories as you enjoy the magic of camping right in your own backyard. Happy camping!

9. Start a Scavenger Hunt
Get ready for an exciting adventure in the great outdoors with a thrilling scavenger hunt! It's time to gather your family and embark on a quest to discover the hidden treasures of nature. Scavenger hunts are always a hit with the crowd, and this one will be no exception.

To start off, gather everyone together and create a list of items you anticipate finding outside. Let your imagination run wild as you think about the wonders of nature that await you. It could be spotting a beautiful flower, finding a unique rock, or even identifying different types of leaves. Write each item on separate pieces of paper and make sure everyone has their own list to mark off their discoveries.

Equip each family member with pens, markers, or stickers to track their findings. This will not only make the hunt more interactive but also unleash their artistic side as they mark off the items on their lists. The excitement will build as everyone prepares to venture into the great outdoors.

Step outside and let the scavenger hunt begin! Explore your surroundings, whether it's your own backyard, a local park, or a nearby nature trail. Keep your eyes peeled and your senses alert as you search high and low for the items on your list. Each discovery will bring a sense of joy and accomplishment.

Take your time during the hunt and encourage everyone to fully immerse themselves in the experience. Share stories, laughter, and excitement as you uncover each hidden gem. Admire the vibrant colors of a blooming flower, marvel at the intricate details of a fallen leaf, and appreciate the wonders of the natural world surrounding you.

As the hunt progresses, celebrate each finding together. Pause to observe and appreciate the beauty of nature, discussing interesting facts about the items you come across. This scavenger hunt will not only create lasting memories but also foster a deeper connection with the environment and instill a sense of wonder and curiosity about the world we live in.

Here are some ideas for scavenger hunts:
- Something yellow, orange, red, green, and blue?
- Something bigger than a hand?
- Something that isn't a natural product?
- Something that makes noise?
- Two rocks that resemble each other?
- A bug that flies?

- A blade of tall grass?
- Animal footprints that don't belong to pets?

Conclusion

I hope you have enjoyed reading this book as much as I've enjoyed writing it, and I hope it will accompany you in your ongoing journey to the discovery of Native American herbs and their medicinal uses.

If you found this book useful and are feeling generous, please take the time to leave a short review on Amazon so that other may enjoy this guide as well.

I leave you with good wishes and hopefully a better knowledge of the plants around us and their amazing powers. This volume is part of a seven-books series on Native American Herbalism from foraging and gardening native plants to making herbal remedies for adults and children. Check out the other volumes to gain a deeper understanding of the amazing wisdom and knowledge of our forefathers and to improve not only your health, but the health of our land as well.

Made in the USA
Columbia, SC
07 December 2023

79ab5934-d5ec-4d63-8bd7-6bad10a052abR02